# NMR
# IN
# DRUG
# DESIGN

# CRC Series in
# ANALYTICAL
# BIOTECHNOLOGY

*Series Editor*
## William S. Hancock
*Hewlett-Packard, Inc.*

*Advisory Editors*

**Barry Karger**
*Northeastern University*

**Csaba Horvath**
*Yale University*

**Fred Regnier**
*Purdue University*

**Donald B. Wetlaufer**
*University of Delaware*

## *New and Forthcoming Titles*

Deamidation and Isoaspartate Formation in Peptides and Proteins, *Dana Aswad*

New Methods in Peptide Mapping for the Characterization of Proteins, *William Hancock*

NMR in Drug Design in Biotechnology, *David J. Craik*

Capillary Electrophoresis in Analytical Biotechnology, *Pier Giorgio Righetti*

High Performance Ion-Exchange Chromatography of Proteins, *Istvan Mazsaroff*

Oxidation Reactions in Peptides and Proteins, *Eleanor Canova-Davis*

Methods for Assessing Genetic Stability, *Mickey Williams*

Methods for the Analysis of Antisense Oligonucleotides, *Aharon Cohen*

QC Methods in Biotechnology, *Alan Herman*

Impurity Analysis of rDNA Derived Proteins, *Vince Anicetti*

Chromatographic Separations of Peptide and Protein Samples, *Benny Welinder*

# NMR
# IN
# DRUG
# DESIGN

*Edited by*
## David James Craik, Ph.D.
Professor of Biomolecular Structure
*Centre for Drug Design and Development*
*University of Queensland*
*Brisbane*
*Queensland, Australia*

**CRC Press**
**Boca Raton   New York   London   Tokyo**

**Library of Congress Cataloging-in-Publication Data**

Craik, David James.
  NMR in drug design / David James Craik
      p.    cm. -- (Analytical biotechnology)
    Includes bibliographical references and index.
    ISBN 0-8493-7824-9 (alk. paper)
    1. Drugs--Design.    2. Nuclear magnetic resonance spectroscopy.
  I. Title.   II. Series: CRC series in analytical biotechnology.
  RS420.C73 1995
  615'.1901--dc20                                                              95-34213
                                                                                   CIP

© 1996 by CRC Press, Inc.

No claim to original U.S. Government works
International Standard Book Number 0-8493-7824-9
Library of Congress Card Number 95-34213
Printed in the United States of America  1  2  3  4  5  6  7  8  9  0
Printed on acid-free paper

# FOREWORD

NMR spectroscopy is an extremely useful tool in drug research. In addition to its utility for determining the primary structures of bioactive natural products and chemically synthesized compounds, NMR has the potential to aid in the design of new pharmaceutical agents. This has become possible due to rapid advances in several areas of research. Proteins that function as drug targets can now be rapidly cloned, expressed, isotopically labeled, and purified in large quantities for NMR studies. Heteronuclear multi-dimensional NMR methods have been developed to assign and determine the three-dimensional structures of biomacromolecules and molecular complexes in a relatively short period of time (2 months for a protein of ~100 residues). In addition, computational tools have been developed and refined to take advantage of the structural information that can be obtained from the NMR experiments.

The type of structural information that can be obtained from NMR includes: the conformation of protein-bound ligands, the portion of the ligand that interacts with the biomacromolecule, the protonation state of the ligand, and the location and structure of the ligand-binding site. All of this information is potentially useful in the drug design process. However, some challenges and questions still remain. Is the resolution of the NMR-derived structures sufficient to be used in interactive structure-based design cycles — an approach that has proved to be successful when based on high resolution X-ray structures? Are the computational tools that ignore entropic effects and possible conformational changes in the protein and the ligand good enough for structure-based drug design? Which of the NMR-derived structures in the ensemble does one use in the design of new analogs?

As more experience is gained in the utilization of NMR-derived structures in the drug design process, the strengths and limitations of the method will be revealed. It has only recently become possible to obtain suitable quantities of drug receptors and to rapidly determine their three-dimensional structures. Thus, the use of NMR in this regard is still in its infancy, but the future holds great promise for the application of NMR in drug design.

**Stephen W. Fesik**
Abbott Laboratories
Abbott Park, Illinois

# INTRODUCTION

Nuclear Magnetic Resonance spectroscopy is an exquisitely powerful technique for providing the kind of information that is required by researchers involved in the design and development of new drugs. There is a large amount of literature available in the separate fields of NMR spectroscopy and drug design, and there are several specialist journals devoted to each of these fields. However, there is no existing publication which draws the two fields together as is attempted in the following chapters. This book should be useful both for researchers involved in drug design and for NMR spectroscopists interested in biological applications. In particular, it will allow medicinal chemists and pharmacologists working in drug design to appreciate the scope and limitations of NMR spectroscopy and will assist NMR spectroscopists to understand the problems inherent in drug design, thereby stimulating them to design novel experiments to assist in this important area.

The fields of NMR and drug design are both in phases of rapid expansion. In the case of NMR spectroscopy, there is currently great emphasis on the development of new pulse sequences and methodology for extracting an increasingly detailed level of information from the sample under study. This development is particularly intense in applications to the study of macromolecules and their interactions with ligands. Drug design is expanding on several frontiers, not the least of which is an increasing trend toward computational approaches to drug design. One reason for this relates to the increasing power and decreasing cost of computational and graphics hardware, combined with a significant expansion in available software. The high cost of the synthesis of large numbers of drug analogs for testing can be significantly reduced if computational procedures can provide some initial screening. An issue that is addressed in this book is that while computational approaches are extremely useful guides for the synthesis of lead compounds, it is important to have an **experimental** means of confirming that the synthesized compounds bind to their macromolecular targets in the way in which they were designed to bind. This information is an essential prerequisite to further refinement of lead compounds. X-ray crystallography has traditionally been an important tool for providing this information in receptor-based drug design and is characterized by the high degree of accuracy with which the complex between a drug and its target macromolecule may be determined. It has only been over the last few years that NMR spectroscopy has been able to approach the sort of atomic resolution seen in X-ray crystallography, and knowledge in the field is still evolving rapidly.

From the comments above it is clear that methods which determine not just the structure of a drug, or its receptor, but the nature of their interaction, will be important in the drug design process. NMR offers the opportunity to derive this information. It is hoped that the current volume will, by describing advances so far, stimulate further developments in the field.

This book is divided into twelve chapters. The first provides an overview of the fields of drug design and drug discovery, and traces the history of these alternative starting points for the development of new pharmaceutical compounds. This historical overview is used to set the scene for a discussion of the current state-of-the-art in drug development and to indicate where it may next be heading. It is interesting to see that the two approaches to drug development — discovery (based on traditional medicine, chance observations, or random screening), and design (based on theories of selective toxicity, molecular optimization, and knowledge of biomolecular structures) — are converging and that most major pharmaceutical companies are committed to a combination of both approaches. Chapter 1 highlights the areas in which NMR will play an increasingly important role in the future.

Chapter 2 identifies the contributions that NMR has made in the past to the pharmaceutical sciences, with particular reference to drug development, and gives a brief introduction to the capabilities of modern NMR spectroscopy. Over the last decade NMR has undergone an astounding increase in the capabilities of both instrumentation and methodology, and these have dramatically expanded the potential applications in drug design. Ten years ago the use of NMR to determine protein structures was in its embryonic stages, but today it competes with, and complements, X-ray crystallography as a premier technique for structure determination of medium-sized proteins.

One of the aims of this book is to assist drug researchers who may have little knowledge of NMR to appreciate its potential applications in their field. Drug design and development is a multidisciplinary field that involves chemists, biochemists, pharmacologists, and medically oriented researchers. It is unusual for those at one end of this spectrum of expertise to have been fully exposed to techniques at the other end of the spectrum. In planning this book, it was therefore important to include a chapter in which some of the principles of NMR and some of the important measurable NMR parameters could be described at a level suitable for a non-expert. Chapter 3 achieves this aim and provides an extremely thorough account of the parameters and methods of modern NMR spectroscopy that are relevant in drug design. It provides a basis for the understanding of the many applications and examples described in the following chapters. The chapter is equally useful for NMR experts, as many topics are dealt with at a more advanced level. In particular, the role of chemical exchange is clearly fundamental in drug action, as it is central to receptor binding. The third chapter covers this important field with an attention to detail that makes it valuable as a reference chapter for NMR researchers whose focus may be in fields other than drug design, but who deal with chemical exchange processes in their applications.

Chapter 4 describes the state-of-the-art in protein structure determination by NMR. Proteins of increasing size are being studied in increasing numbers as instrumentation improves and as new NMR methods are developed to overcome some of the limitations present in 'traditional' approaches to structure determination (if it is appropriate to use the word traditional for a field that is essentially only a decade old!). The advantages of labelling proteins with $^{13}C$ and/or $^{15}N$ isotopes are described, and a section on the methods for doing this is included. As with Chapter 3, this chapter provides a valuable reference source for both the expert and nonexpert in the field.

With the scene set by the introductory chapters, and the relevant methods described in Chapters 3 and 4, the remaining chapters focus on applications in drug design and development. Chapter 5 concentrates on drugs themselves. While to some extent the 'glamour' applications of NMR over the last few years have been associated with macromolecules, including many drug targets, it is important to remember that NMR has contributed very substantially to our understanding of molecular structure and conformations of small molecules. The average molecular weight of the most commonly used drugs today is still, after all, only approximately 300 Da. Applications involving the identification and characterization of such species will continue to be of paramount importance.

Peptides, or analogues derived from them, have been widely touted as the drugs of the future. In Chapter 6 the methods that are particularly valuable for the study of these fascinating and potent molecules are described. The possibilities for conformational variability in even small peptides are endless, and approaches to limiting this flexibility are described. NMR plays a crucial role in establishing the nature and effectiveness of many of these conformational constraints. The potential to use conformations derived by NMR for the design of potent peptide mimics is outstanding.

It is important to emphasize that NMR plays a very practical role in drug development and is not just an esoteric technique confined to academic questions of molecular structure. It is therefore particularly gratifying to be able to include several chapters from researchers actively working in the pharmaceutical industry. Chapter 7 is one of these and is packed with examples showing how NMR has contributed vital information in drug design programs. As in the previous chapter, the importance of recognizing differences between solution and receptor-bound conformations is emphasized.

Dihydrofolate reductase is a key target for a number of drugs in clinical use and it provides a classic example of the extent of information that can be obtained by NMR. This enzyme is one of the most thoroughly studied by NMR and the author of Chapter 8 has been at the forefront of this work. This chapter illustrates the incredible level of detail about ionization states, functional group interactions, and binding modes that is provided by carefully designed NMR studies. It also illustrates the value of NMR in identifying multiple binding modes, a factor that complicates drug design if applied in a naive sense. The fact that similar ligands can sometimes bind in quite different orientations shows just how important it is to continue to develop methods that define binding modes with very high accuracy.

Chapter 9 is another contribution from an active NMR research group within the pharmaceutical industry and provides an insight into drug binding to the important target protein, calmodulin. This chapter is an up-to-date account of work in-progress on the binding of calmidazolium, a potent inhibitor of calmodulin function. It emphasizes the central importance of ligand-macromolecule interactions in drug design. Once again the value of using isotope labels is illustrated.

It is increasingly being recognized that it is not only the structure and geometry of molecules that determine their binding but also their dynamics. Both drugs and their receptors may undergo conformational changes on binding, and these changes may have an integral effect on the resulting response. In Chapter 10, NMR approaches to the study of molecular flexibility of an important drug target enzyme, HIV-1 protease, are described. Information obtained from such studies significantly extends our understanding of the mechanism of action of this enzyme.

DNA is another important target for drugs and the final two chapters describe NMR approaches that have been applied in studies of ligand binding to this macromolecule. In Chapter 11, the focus is on compounds that intercalate between the base pairs of DNA. This chapter includes a discussion on the role of DNA as a drug target. In Chapter 12, the minor groove of DNA is the site of interest and studies involving a range of drugs and other ligands are described.

Together these twelve chapters provide an up-to-date account of the contribution of NMR to drug design. Used in combination with other methods, including traditional medicinal chemistry, X-ray crystallography, and computational approaches, NMR promises to increase the success rate and reduce the lead time in drug development.

In closing, I would like to sincerely thank all of the authors for their contributions to this book. Their care in the preparation of their chapters was greatly appreciated and made the editorial process far easier than it might otherwise have been. It has been a pleasure to read the various chapters and to correspond with the authors.

Finally, I would like to thank my colleagues John Gehrmann, Justine Hill, Kathy Nielsen, and Martin Scanlon for their invaluable assistance in proofreading the various manuscripts. Special thanks go to John and Justine for their extra help in the production process, their help with diagrams, and for the countless trips to the photocopier. I am also very grateful to Jacqui King for her invaluable assistance with typing, correspondence, and other editorial matters. I also thank my wife, Robyn, for additional editorial assistance and for her patience with me during the production of this book.

**David J. Craik**

# THE EDITOR

**David J. Craik, Ph.D.,** is Professor of Biomolecular Structure at the Centre for Drug Design and Development, University of Queensland, Brisbane, Australia. He received his B.Sc. (Hons) degree from La Trobe University in 1977 and completed a Ph.D. on applications of NMR spectroscopy in organic chemistry at La Trobe in 1980. Following two years of postdoctoral work in the United States at Florida State and Syracuse Universities, he returned to Australia to a Lectureship, and in 1986 a Senior Lectureship, in Pharmaceutical Chemistry at the Victorian College of Pharmacy in Melbourne. In 1988 he was appointed Professor of Medicinal Chemistry and Dean of the School of Pharmaceutical Chemistry at Victorian College of Pharmacy, Monash University, a position he held until moving to the University of Queensland in 1995.

Professor Craik is a Fellow of the Royal Australian Chemical Institute, a member of the American Chemical Society, and is a Professorial Associate at the University of Melbourne, Australia and the University of Kansas in Lawrence, Kansas. He is Associate Editor of the journal, *Current Medicinal Chemistry*.

His major research interests are in applications of NMR to drug design and development. Current research activities focus on the use of NMR to study macromolecule-ligand interactions and on the study of biologically important peptides and proteins. His contribution to medicinal chemistry applications of NMR was recognized in 1993 by the award of the Adrien Albert Lectureship of the Division of Medicinal and Agricultural Chemistry, Royal Australian Chemical Institute. Professor Craik is the author of more than 120 research publications and a dozen reviews and chapters in the fields of NMR and medicinal chemistry.

# CONTRIBUTORS

**Peter R. Andrews, Ph.D.**
*Centre for Drug Design and Development*
*University of Queensland*
*Brisbane, Australia*

**Chong-Hwan Chang, Ph.D.**
*DuPont Merck Pharmaceutical Company*
*DuPont Experimental Station*
*Wilmington, Delaware*

**Robert M. Cooke, Ph.D.**
*Department of Biomolecular Structure*
*Glaxo Wellcome*
*Medicines Research Centre*
*Stevenage, England*

**David J. Craik, Ph.D.**
*Centre for Drug Design and Development*
*University of Queensland*
*Brisbane, Australia*

**Andrew J. Edwards**
*Analytical Sciences Department*
*SmithKline Beecham Pharmaceuticals*
*The Frythe, Welwyn, England*

**James Feeney, Ph.D.**
*Division of Molecular Structure*
*National Institute for Medical*
*  Research*
*The Ridgeway, Mill Hill,*
*London, England*

**J. T. Gerig, Ph.D.**
*Department of Chemistry*
*University of California*
*Santa Barbara, California*

**C. Nicholas Hodge, Ph.D.**
*DuPont Merck Pharmaceutical Company*
*DuPont Experimental Station*
*Wilmington, Delaware*

**Jerzy W. Jaroszewski, Ph.D.**
*Department of Medicinal Chemistry*
*Royal Danish School of Pharmacy*
*Copenhagen, Denmark*

**Horst Kessler, Ph.D.**
*Institute of Organic Chemistry and*
*  Biochemistry*
*Technical University Munich*
*Garshing, Germany*

**Glenn F. King, Ph.D.**
*Department of Biochemistry*
*University of Sydney*
*Sydney, NSW, Australia*

**Robert Konat, M.Sc.**
*Institute of Organic Chemistry and*
*  Biochemistry*
*Technical University Munich*
*Garshing, Germany*

**Joel Mackay, Ph.D.**
*Department of Biochemistry*
*University of Sydney*
*Sydney, NSW, Australia*

**Linda K. Nicholson, Ph.D.**
*Section of Biochemistry, Molecular and*
*  Cell Biology*
*Cornell University*
*Ithaca, New York*

**Spiro Pavlopoulos**

*Department of Medicinal Chemistry*
*Victorian College of Pharmacy*
*Monash University*
*Parkville, Victoria, Australia*

**David G. Reid, Ph.D.**

*Analytical Sciences Department*
*SmithKline Beecham Pharmaceuticals*
*The Frythe, Welwyn, England*

**Mark S. Searle, Ph.D.**

*Department of Chemistry*
*University of Nottingham*
*Nottingham, England*

**Wolfgang Schmitt, M.Sc.**

*Institute of Organic Chemistry and*
  *Biochemistry*
*Technical University Munich*
*Garshing, Germany*

**Patricia J. Sweeney, Ph.D.**

*Cantab Pharmaceutical Research Ltd.*
*Cambridge, England*

**Geoffrey Wickham, Ph.D.**

*Department of Chemistry*
*University of Wollongong*
*Wollongong, NSW, Australia*

# CONTENTS

Chapter 1
Drug Design and Discovery: Where Next? ...................................................... 1
Peter R. Andrews

Chapter 2
The Role of NMR in Drug Design and Development ................................... 15
David J. Craik

Chapter 3
Studies of Drug–Receptor Interactions by NMR: Theory
and Applications ............................................................................................ 31
J.T. Gerig

Chapter 4
Protein Structure Determination Using NMR Spectroscopy ...................... 101
Glenn F. King and Joel P. Mackay

Chapter 5
Conformational Analysis of Drug Molecules ............................................. 201
Jerzy W. Jaroszewski

Chapter 6
Conformational Analysis of Peptides: Application to Drug Design ............ 215
Horst Kessler, Robert K. Konat, and Wolfgang Schmitt

Chapter 7
Protein–Ligand Interactions: Examples in Drug Design ............................. 245
Robert M. Cooke

Chapter 8
NMR Studies of Ligand Binding to Dihydrofolate Reductase
and Their Application in Drug Design ........................................................ 275
J. Feeney

Chapter 9
Studies of Drug-Calmodulin Binding Using Isotopically
Labelled Protein ........................................................................ 315
**David G. Reid, Andrew J. Edwards, and Patricia J. Sweeney**

Chapter 10
Flexibility and Function in the HIV-1 Protease ........................................... 337
**Linda K. Nicholson, Chong-Hwan Chang, and C. Nicholas Hodge**

Chapter 11
DNA as a Target for Drug Action: Complexes of Intercalating
Antibiotics ............................................................................. 377
**Mark S. Searle**

Chapter 12
Drug Binding to the Minor Groove of DNA ............................................. 423
**David J. Craik, Spiro Pavlopoulos, and Geoffrey Wickham**

Index ..................................................................................... 465

*To Robyn, Andrew, Peter, and Jennifer*

# CHAPTER 1

# DRUG DESIGN AND DISCOVERY: WHERE NEXT?

*Peter R. Andrews*

## CONTENTS

I  Introduction ............................................................................. 2

II  Historical Overview ................................................................ 2
   A  Discovery: Traditional Medicine ...................................... 2
   B  Design: Selective Toxicity ................................................ 3
   C  Discovery: Clinical Observations ..................................... 4
   D  Design: Molecular Optimisation ...................................... 5
   E  Discovery: Molecular Pharmacology ................................ 6
   F  Design: Biomolecular Structure ....................................... 8
   G  Discovery: Biochemical Screening ................................... 8
   H  Design: Chemical Libraries .............................................. 10

III  Where Next? ......................................................................... 11
   A  Discovery or Design? ....................................................... 11
   B  Large or Small? ................................................................. 11
   C  Macromolecules or Mimetics? .......................................... 12
   D  Skeletons or Surfaces? ...................................................... 12

References ................................................................................... 13

0-8493-7824-9/96/$0.00+$.50

# I    INTRODUCTION

New drug development is based on two complementary strategies.

One involves the design and synthesis of new compounds which block or mimic targets identified through basic research in biology and medicine. This strategy, which applies modern computer graphic technology to the detailed three-dimensional structures of biomolecular targets, is commonly referred to as "rational drug design", and has been adopted enthusiastically by most international pharmaceutical companies since its first appearance in university laboratories in the mid-1970s.

The other involves the screening of naturally occurring compounds (such as those in plants and microorganisms) for pharmaceutical activity, and subsequent optimisation of that activity by way of structural modification. Today, about 25% of all prescription drugs consumed in the Western world contain active ingredients extracted from natural sources,[1] and the screening approach has been rejuvenated by the introduction of robotics and similar techniques to allow very rapid assessment of large numbers of compounds in a wide variety of disease or "target-directed" screens.

The purpose of this chapter is twofold. The first part provides an historical overview of the development of these two alternative strategies, drug design and discovery, over the course of the 20th century. The second part uses this historical perspective as the starting point for a discussion of where the discipline of drug design is now, and where we may be heading next. The increasingly important role that will be played by NMR spectroscopy in the future of drug design will be evident from the rest of this book.

# II   HISTORICAL OVERVIEW

The historical development of the two alternative strategies, drug discovery and drug design, over the course of the 20th century is summarised in Table 1. In practice, the divisions between the two strategies are rapidly disappearing, as will be evident from the following discussion.

## A    DISCOVERY: TRADITIONAL MEDICINE

Over one hundred compounds in the Western world's pharmacopoeia were originally derived from plants, and it has been estimated[1] that about three quarters of these were discovered through ethnobotany — the pursuit of leads from the traditional medicine of indigenous cultures.

Many of these compounds are still used in the ways discovered by our ancestors: digitalis, from the leaves of the purple foxglove, as a cardiotonic;

**TABLE 1**

A Century of Drug Design and Discovery

| Chronology | Discovery | Design |
|---|---|---|
| 1900 | Traditional medicine | |
| | | Selective toxicity |
| | Clinical observation | |
| | | Molecular optimisation |
| | Molecular pharmacology | |
| | | Biomolecular structure |
| | Biochemical Screening | |
| | | Chemical libraries |
| 2000 | ? | |

atropine, from the leaves and roots of the deadly nightshade (*Atropa belladonna*), for dilation of the pupil in ophthalmology; quinine, from cinchona bark, for the treatment of malaria. Others have new or adapted uses: reserpine, found in the root of the Indian plant *Rauwolfia serpentina* and used historically in India for the treatment of anxiety, was introduced into Western medicine in the 1950s as an antihypertensive that not only lowers blood pressure but also acts as a tranquilizer; morphine, used by the early Egyptians to induce sleep, is now used primarily to relieve pain; cocaine, used by the South American Indians to allay the onset of hunger and fatigue, is now used mainly as a local anaesthetic.[2]

Clearly, the method used to discover these drugs — primary screening in man — is no longer available to the modern pharmaceutical industry, but industrial interest in the development of compounds based on ethno-botanical leads, which ebbed in the 1950s, is once again becoming high.[1]

## B   Design: Selective Toxicity

Although the phrase *drug design* is itself relatively recent, the basic principles can be traced back to the concept of chemotherapy, pioneered by Paul Ehrlich at the turn of the century.[3]

Ehrlich's concept of chemotherapy, *the use of drugs to injure an invading organism without injury to the host*,[4] was based on his studies of the selective distribution of dyestuffs in the tissues of living animals and in microorganisms. In particular, the observation that bacteria could be stained selectively with certain dyes led him to the "design" hypothesis that toxic derivatives of dyestuffs that bind selectively to bacterial cells might prove useful as selective antibacterials.* It was this design hypothesis that

---

* Dyes continue to be important lead compounds in drug development, and NMR studies now provide a structural explanation for their binding, illustrated, for example, in Chapter 12 in studies of the binding of the dye Hoechst 33258 to DNA.

ultimately led to the development of our first major class of antibacterials, the sulfonamides.

Of particular interest to Ehrlich's followers were the azo dyes, of which many thousands were subsequently synthesised and tested, culminating in the successful demonstration of the *in vivo* antibacterial activity of the sulfonamide Prontosil (**1**) by the German physician Domagk, who used it to cure his young daughter of an almost certainly lethal case of septicaemia.

Can we claim this as the first successful example of drug design? Unfortunately, we cannot. As it turned out, Prontosil proved totally inactive against bacteria *in vitro*, and it was subsequently shown that the dramatic clinical activity demonstrated by Domagk was due to rapid metabolic conversion of Prontosil to sulfanilamide (**2**), which no longer contains the chromophoric azo group. Indeed, as we now know, sulfanilamide relies for its activity entirely on its close structural resemblance to *p*-aminobenzoic acid (**3**), which is essential for the biosynthesis of tetrahydrofolate in bacteria, but not in humans.

Thus, while the postulated role of the dye moiety in Ehrlich's design hypothesis proved to be irrelevant to the ultimate antibacterial activity, his concept of selective toxicity was entirely vindicated, and has formed the basis for most subsequent developments in chemotherapy.

## C   DISCOVERY: CLINICAL OBSERVATIONS

By the middle of the 20th century, the emphasis of drug discovery had shifted away from the subjective and qualitative observations of traditional medicine toward more quantitative clinical observations, with capitalisation on the side effects of existing therapies proving to be one of the most prolific sources of new drugs. The enormous clinical success of the antibacterial sulfonamides, in particular, led to a sequence of drugs for other indications, almost all of which were based on apparently unrelated clinical observations. For example:

- Trials in typhoid fever and other infectious diseases showed that the sulfonamide IPTD (4) also lowered blood sugar. Optimisation of this activity led to the discovery of the mechanistically unrelated tolbutamide (5), which acts by stimulating insulin secretion from the pancreas.
- The antibacterial activity of some sulfonamides was seen to be accompanied by an increase in urine volume. Optimisation of this activity led to antidiuretics and hypotensives such as acetazolamide (6), which inhibits carbonic anhydrase by virtue of the structural similarity between the sulfonamide group (7) and the bicarbonate ion (8).

Today, the requirements of regulatory authorities for new trials before allowing the use of drugs in new indications has reduced the frequency of this route to drug discovery, but examples are still relatively common. The use of low-dose aspirin to reduce platelet aggregation in patients at risk from cardiac disease is a recent example.

## D    DESIGN: MOLECULAR OPTIMISATION

The discovery of Prontosil in 1935 led to the subsequent synthesis and testing of tens of thousands of related sulfonamides, and similarly heavy-handed principles were applied to other promising leads. Although nowadays denigrated as "molecular roulette", such studies were of enormous benefit in establishing the existence of clear-cut qualitative relationships between chemical structure and biological activity.

In the case of the sulfonamides, for example, the following generalisations emerged:[5]

- The presence of the $p$-aminobenzenesulfonyl radical ($H_2N-C_6H_4-SO_2-$) is essential for activity.
- Substitution of the amino group is acceptable, but only if the substituent is readily removed *in vivo*.
- Monosubstitution of the sulfonamido nitrogen results in significant variations in activity.

Generalisations of this type proved of immediate value in guiding the modification of drugs to produce compounds with more desirable pharmaceutical properties. Varying the substituent on the sulfonamido nitrogen, for example, allowed the creation of sulfonamides which are absorbed from the gastrointestinal tract rapidly (for treating urinary tract infections) or poorly (for gastrointestinal infections), and with half-lives ranging from 2.5 h (for acute infections) to 150 h (for chronic infections or prophylaxis).

The extension of these qualitative observations into the first quantitative studies of structure–activity relationships began to emerge in the 1940s. One of the earliest of these was the observation of Bell and Roblin[6] that the antibacterial activity of the sulfonamides was related to the pKa of the sulfonamido group by a bell-shaped curve in which the maximum activity occurred in the pKa range 6.0–7.4. This suggested that optimal activity occurs when the sulfonamides are approximately 50% ionised, reflecting the fact that while the ionised form is required for the ultimate biological activity (to mimic the ionisation state of $p$-aminobenzoic acid [3]), the un-ionised form is required to penetrate the bacterial cell.

Subsequent development of these concepts by Hansch and his colleagues[7] led to the discipline of quantitative structure–activity relationships (QSAR), in which partition coefficients, electronic parameters, and the steric properties of substituent groups are used directly to provide quantitative predictions of biological activity.

## E  Discovery: Molecular Pharmacology

The appearance of the discipline of molecular pharmacology in the 1960s provided both new assays and new targets for medicinal chemists. Of particular importance were the structures and activities of endogenous molecules, since these provided a natural starting point in the development of more selective pharmaceuticals based on the human as the source of new leads. A good example of this approach is provided by the molecular optimisation of histamine to produce cimetidine.

The development by James Black of bioassays for the histamine-induced release of acid in the gut opened the way for the search for specific $H_2$ antagonists as potential anti-ulcer drugs. In the early stages of the search, a range of ring- and side-chain-substituted derivatives of histamine (9) were investigated, but none of these showed anything other than agonist activity. Subsequent modification of the polarity and length of the histamine side chain led to burimamide (10), the first pure competitive $H_2$ antagonist, and ultimately to cimetidine (11).

The structural changes made in the optimisation of burimamide to cimetidine were primarily aimed at producing analogues with the imidazole ring in the same tautomeric form as histamine, in which the electron-withdrawing nature of the side chain results in greater stability of the 1,4-tautomer, whereas in burimamide the 1,5-tautomer is favoured by the electron-releasing character of the longer hydrocarbon chain. This challenge was met[8] by introducing an electron-withdrawing group (S) into the burimamide side chain and an electron-releasing group (Me) adjacent to the preferred nitrogen.

It is instructive to note that, despite the success of this strategy, the presence of the imidazole ring, regardless of its tautomeric form, ultimately proved unnecessary for $H_2$ antagonist activity, as illustrated by the subsequent development of equally powerful $H_2$ antagonists, such as ranitidine (12), based on appending cimetidine-like side chains to quite different ring systems.

## F    Design: Biomolecular Structure

The direct design of ligands to match their macromolecular targets became possible with the ability to determine the crystal structures of proteins and nucleic acids. An early example of this approach was the development of antihypertensive angiotensin-converting enzyme (ACE) inhibitors based on the structure of a closely related enzyme, carboxypeptidase A.

The structures of complexes between carboxypeptidase A and various substrate analogues revealed that catalytic removal of the C-terminal amino acid is mediated by interactions between (1) the carbonyl group of the labile peptide bond and a zinc atom in the active site of the enzyme; (2) the amino acid sidechain and a hydrophobic pocket in the active site; and (3) the negatively charged carboxyl terminal and a positive charge in the enzyme.

Since ACE removes the C-terminal dipeptide from its substrates by a mechanism similar to that of carboxypeptidase A, Ondetti and co-workers[9] proposed a hypothetical active site mode for ACE which incorporated the same three structural features plus a second hydrophobic pocket (for the sidechain of the penultimate amino acid) and a hydrogen-bonding group to interact with the adjacent carbonyl group (Figure 1a). Based on this model, they further proposed that a substrate analogue of the terminal dipeptide in which the labile peptide bond NH was replaced with a methylene group (Figure 1b) should inhibit the enzyme. This proved to be the case, and subsequent optimisation of the two side chains (Figure 1c) and introduction of a more powerful zinc-chelating moiety (Figure 1d) led to the potent antihypertensive drug Captopril (**13**).

Many related ACE inhibitors have since been developed and marketed, but conformational analysis[10] on a range of the structures confirms that the key binding groups of the active site of the enzyme are fully consistent with the original design hypothesis.[9]

A more recent, and strikingly simple example of receptor-based drug design is the development of influenza sialidase inhibitors[11] based on the structure of the enzyme complexed with the nonselective sialidase inhibitor 2-deoxy-2,3-didehydro-D-N-acetyl-neuraminic acid (**14**). This crystal structure revealed the presence of a pocket lined with negatively charged carboxyl groups immediately adjacent to the 4-hydroxyl substituent, and subsequent replacement of this group with a guanidino moiety (**15**) led to a selective reduction in $K_i$ of approximately four orders of magnitude.

## G    Discovery: Biochemical Screening

While the development of Captopril and related angiotensin-converting enzyme inhibitors as antihypertensive drugs during the 1980s was

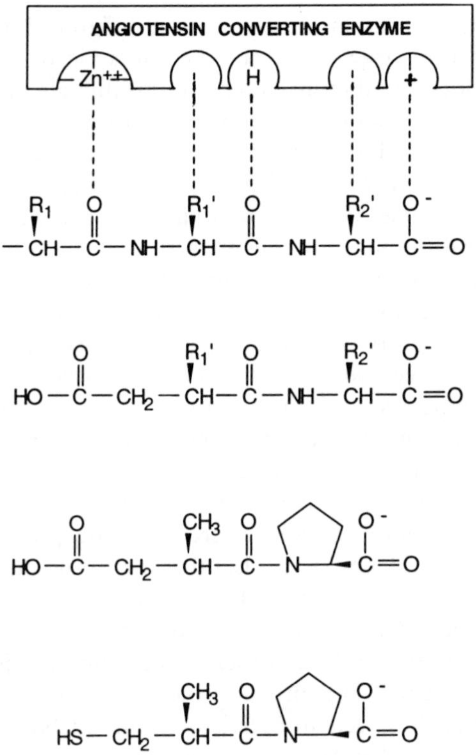


(a)

(b)

(c)

(d)

**FIGURE 1**
Development of the antihypertensive angiotensin-converting enzyme inhibitor Captopril (**13**). Successive stages in development are shown in (a) – (d).

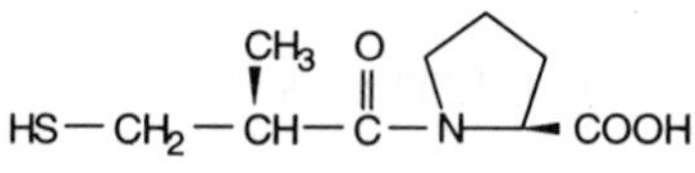

**13**

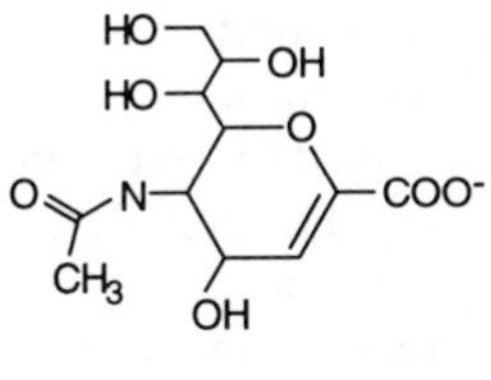

**14**

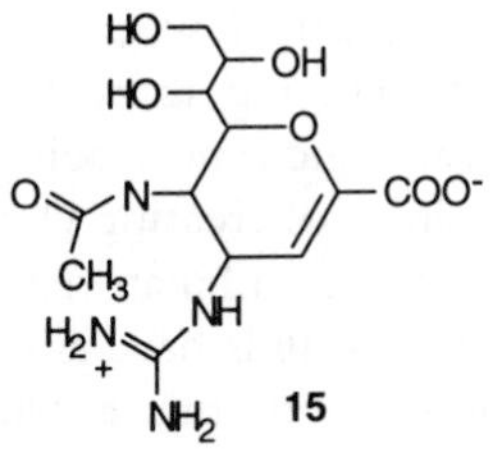

**15**

primarily based on the application of rational drug design techniques to a structural model of the target enzyme, the initial lead came from antihypertensive peptides found in snake venom. It is thus also an example of the so-called ecochemical approach to drug discovery, which relies on observations of the interactions between plants, insects, and animals, rather than the traditional medicine of indigenous cultures.

The best-known example of ecochemical drug discovery is undoubtedly the search for novel antibiotics in soil microorganisms, which has been practised by the pharmaceutical industry since the 1950s. Most of the antibiotic classes in clinical use today are direct outcomes of this process, which is based on the observation that bacteria competing with other bacteria for limited resources will inevitably produce novel antibacterials.

Today, many companies continue to run major programs seeking novel antibiotics by screening fermentation broths from microorganisms, but dramatic reductions in the cost of target-directed screening programs have vastly increased the scope of their activities. This is particularly true for new classes of therapeutic activity, where screening programs have proved remarkably successful, despite the fact that there is no rational basis upon which the discovery of drugs other than antibiotics could reasonably be anticipated in the secondary metabolites produced by microorganisms. The blood-cholesterol-lowering drug lovastatin, for example, is just one of several enzyme inhibitors with potential in various unrelated therapeutic areas discovered in fungal extracts in Merck's screening laboratories.

It is intriguing to note that Merck, early leaders in the development of drug design technology, have also become increasingly involved in biodiversity prospecting, including an agreement with Costa Rica that involves the provision of extracts of plants and insects from Costa Rican rain forests for pharmaceutical screening.

## H   DESIGN: CHEMICAL LIBRARIES

The logic that has led the pharmaceutical industry to increasingly random screening — "You've no way of telling where it is, nor can you tell where it isn't" — is applicable to more than natural products. Many companies are now screening their chemical collections for targets that were not dreamed of when the original compounds were synthesised. Others are purchasing access to chemical collections.

The same logic is now being further extended by researchers moving into the business of creating chemical diversity. For peptides, oligonucleotides, and other combinatorially straightforward polymers, libraries of 1–10 billion compounds have already been created, and current research is aimed at developing libraries with a much broader coverage of structural diversity.

By incorporating structural features suggested by other design strategies into new chemical libraries, we now have the opportunity to complete the merger of drug design and drug discovery, producing larger numbers of compounds with greater probability of activity in new therapeutic targets.

# III  WHERE NEXT?

## A  DISCOVERY OR DESIGN?

As will be evident from the preceding discussion, the distinction between the strategies of drug discovery and drug design is now on the point of disappearing. Novel leads isolated from natural products become the starting points for the design of synthetic compounds with greater potency and better selectivity. Newly identified peptides and proteins from biomedical research laboratories become the starting points for the design of agonists and antagonists with greater stability and better bioavailability. The discovery of distinct enzymes performing the same activity in host and parasite becomes the starting point for the design of selectively toxic inhibitors.

In each case, the key step in the transition from discovery to design is the structural and conformational characterisation of the target molecule. In each case, a key discipline in the determination of the three-dimensional structure of the target molecule is NMR.

## B  LARGE OR SMALL?

It will also be evident that the scales on which the design and discovery strategies can be implemented have both expanded dramatically. Where the cost of individual assays previously precluded study of more than a few compounds or extracts at a time, improved screening technology now allows tens of thousands of compounds to be processed in search of a novel lead. And where the paucity of structural data on macromolecular targets previously restricted designers to a handful of relatively abundant molecules, detailed three-dimensional structures are now available for hundreds of macromolecular targets.

At the same time, the sizes of the systems amenable to routine study, previously at two extremes, have dramatically converged. On the discovery side, we have reduced the complexity of our assay systems from a subjective, whole-animal level (i.e., human) to totally objective (often robotic) screens of individual macromolecular targets. On the design side, we have moved from the atomic level, represented by the azo group in some of Ehrlich's early dyes, to the point where detailed design studies can be routinely undertaken on the three-dimensional structures of the same macromolecular targets.

This shift in scale from small molecule to macromolecule has been paralleled by, and in part has resulted from, a corresponding shift in the size of molecules accessible using NMR. Some of the advances in instrumentation and NMR methodology that have been responsible for this shift are described in Chapters 2–4, and resulting applications are given in following chapters.

## C  MACROMOLECULES OR MIMETICS?

Some of the most exciting of the new drug molecules now emerging from the world's biomedical research laboratories are bioactive peptides, and many of these structures are currently in various phases of clinical trial. Despite these potential successes, however, peptides are far from ideal drugs. In effect, the body treats all peptides as food, breaking them down in both gut and bloodstream to their constituent amino acids. The result is an increasing recognition that the greatest potential for new drugs lies with peptidomimetics — nonpeptidic molecules that mimic the structures of peptides and proteins. In particular, strategies are being developed for the synthesis of conformationally constrained cyclic templates for the synthesis of more versatile peptidomimetic libraries.

In this case, the key prerequisite for the design process is the conformation of the peptide as it binds to its target receptor. To date, the most significant source of information on the conformations of bioactive peptides and their cyclic analogues is NMR, as described in Chapter 6.

## D  SKELETONS OR SURFACES?

The increasing role of peptidomimetics in current thinking on drug design begs intriguing molecular-recognition questions. Is the structure of the peptide as a whole (i.e., backbone and side chains) necessary for bioactivity? If not, is it necessary for the backbone of the peptide to be retained in order to present a surface the primary purpose of which is to mimic the functionality of the side chains?

The cimetidine/ranitidine story (**11** vs. **12**) bears witness to the dangers of thinking too narrowly on these issues. In some cases, such as the inhibition of proteolytic enzymes with substrate analogues, the maintenance of the hydrogen-bonding structure between the enzyme and the amide moieties in the backbone of the substrate/inhibitor is clearly important. In others, such as the design of surface patch analogues of peptide hormones, the development of rigid scaffolds to mimic either continuous or discontinuous arrays of amino-acid side chains is of primary importance.

In both cases, the fundamental requirement is to know which groups are actually involved in interacting with the enzyme or receptor. Once again, the key discipline in eliciting this information is now NMR.

# REFERENCES

1. Joyce, C.; *New Scientist, Prospectors for Tropical Medicines,* 32-36, October 19, 1991.
2. Foye, W.O.; Medicinals of plant origin: historical aspects, in *Principles of Medicinal Chemistry,* 3rd ed.; W.O. Foye, Ed.; Lea & Febiger: Philadelphia, 1989; pp. 623-627.
3. Rost, W.J.; Chemotherapy: an introduction, in *Principles of Medicinal Chemistry,* 3rd ed.; W.O. Foye, Ed.; Lea & Febiger: Philadelphia, 1989; pp. 629-635.
4. Albert, A.; *Selective Toxicity,* 5th ed.; Chapman & Hall: London, 1973; pp. 130-172.
5. Anand, N.; Metabolite antagonism, in *Principles of Medicinal Chemistry,* 3rd ed.; W.O. Foye, Ed.; Lea & Febiger: Philadelphia, 1989; pp. 637-659.
6. Bell, P.H.; Roblin, R.O.; *J. Am. Chem. Soc.,* 1942, 64, 2905-2917.
7. Kubinyi, H.; *Hansch Analysis and Related Approaches,* VCH Publishers: New York, 1993.
8. Ganellin, C.R.; *Farmaceutisch Tijdschrift voor Belgie,* 1978, No. 1.
9. Petrillo, E.W.; Ondetti, M.A.; *Med. Res. Rev.,* 1982, 2, 1-41.
10. Andrews, P.R.; Carson, J.M.; Caselli, A.; Spark, M.J.; Woods, R.; *J. Med. Chem.,* 1985, 28, 393-399.
11. von Itzstein, M.; Wu, W.-Y.; Kok, G.B.; Pegg, M.S.; Dyason, J.C.; Jin, B.; Phan, T.V.; Smythe, M.L.; White, H.F.; Oliver, S.W.; Colman, P.M.; Varghese, J.N.; Ryan, D.M.; Woods, J.M.; Bethell, R.C.; Hotham, V.J.; Cameron, J.M.; Penn, C.R.; *Nature,* 1993, 363, 418-423.

CHAPTER 2

# THE ROLE OF NMR IN DRUG DESIGN AND DEVELOPMENT

*David J. Craik*

## CONTENTS

I  Introduction ................................................................................. 15

II  History of NMR Applications in Drug Research ........................... 16
   A  Overview of Past Applications ................................................. 16
   B  Recent Developments ............................................................. 17

III  NMR in Drug Development ........................................................ 20

IV  NMR in Drug Design ................................................................. 24

References ...................................................................................... 28

## I    INTRODUCTION

The first chapter provided a historical overview of the field of drug design and discovery, and pointed out a trend to the convergence of two alternative approaches to the first stage of new drug development, that is, design vs. discovery. It also indicated the increasing role that structural techniques such as NMR will play in the future development of new drugs. The remainder of this book is concerned with describing how NMR can

0-8493-7824-9/96/$0.00+$.50

be used in this role. At the end of this chapter some of the questions of relevance to drug design that can be addressed by NMR spectroscopy are identified. This sets the scene for elucidation of the answers to these questions in the following chapters. It is first appropriate, though, to briefly outline historical developments in the application of NMR to the study of drugs and their effects. This is done in Section II, which traces the use of NMR in drug-related applications, ranging from analytical measurements, to drug design, to metabolic studies. In Section III, the way in which these various applications fit into a drug development program is described. The discussion for the remainder of the chapter, and indeed the book, then focuses on the design phase of drug development.

## II  HISTORY OF NMR APPLICATIONS IN DRUG RESEARCH

NMR spectroscopy has long been an important tool in the pharmaceutical sciences. Its initial role, which began soon after NMR spectrometers became commercially available, was to identify and characterize chemically synthesized drugs, or biologically active molecules derived from a variety of natural sources, which formed the basis of pharmaceutical products. The methods used in such studies are described in a multitude of textbooks on organic applications of NMR spectroscopy.[1-3] Today, along with mass spectrometry, NMR remains a premier method for the structural characterization of pharmaceutical compounds.

Over the last decade or so this role as an analytical tool has been supplemented by a more fundamental application — providing information to be used in the design of new drugs. This new role has arisen in part because of the tremendous advances in NMR instrumentation and methods that have occurred over recent years, and in part because of important advances in biochemistry and molecular biology that have led to the ability to isolate and purify large quantities of biological macromolecules that have potential pharmaceutical applications.

### A  OVERVIEW OF PAST APPLICATIONS

Applications to drug design had their origins in the 1960s and 1970s, with the use of NMR to determine structures and conformations of biologically important organic molecules,[4] typically with molecular weights of up to 1000 Da. These studies were done initially on 60- to 100-MHz spectrometers, where the conformational information was derived from chemical shifts, coupling constants, and nuclear Overhauser enhancement (NOE) measurements.[5,6] These studies proved extremely valuable for

defining solution conformations, but the limitation that such conformations might not necessarily reflect the biologically active form at the
receptor site had to be kept in mind. Nevertheless, in the case of relatively
rigid molecules, the solution conformation is a valuable starting point in
drug design applications.

The increasing availability of higher-field (200–500 MHz) spectrometers in the late 1970s and early 1980s dramatically increased the complexity of molecules that could be examined by NMR. In addition to the ability
to study more complex organic molecules, it became possible to examine
biological macromolecules in significant detail. Although at this time,
high-resolution three-dimensional (3D) structures of macromolecules could
not be determined by NMR, a variety of NMR-based approaches could be
used to derive selective and qualitative information about structure in small
biopolymers. Studies of the interaction of drugs with enzymes, proteins,
nucleic acids, and membranes became possible, thus greatly enhancing the
physiological relevance of NMR applications in drug research.[7-9]

In parallel with these high-resolution developments, the availability of
wide-bore magnets made it possible to examine intact organs and even
whole animals using surface coil technology. The ability to directly observe
NMR signals in living systems[10] opened up a new range of potential
pharmaceutical applications of NMR,[11] including studies of drug metabolism and studies of the effects of drugs on biochemical energetics.[12] These
studies showed that NMR has potential applications across the whole
spectrum of the drug development process, from design to *in vivo* testing.
The wide range of applications of NMR spectroscopy in drug research up
to approximately 1987 is admirably illustrated in a book arising from an
Alfred Benzon Symposium on the topic held in 1987.[13]

## B    RECENT DEVELOPMENTS

The number of applications of NMR in the pharmaceutical sciences
has increased substantially, and they have become more sophisticated since
the mid-1980s due, on the one hand, to further improvements in instrumentation, and on the other, to new NMR methods that have been
developed since then. In particular, the development of methodology for
assigning and determining the structures of peptides and proteins by 2D
NMR[14] has made possible a variety of new applications in the field of drug
design. As will be seen in the following chapters, these arise because of the
importance of biologically active peptides as potential targets in analogue-
based drug design, and of proteins in receptor-based drug design. Initially,
the new methodology provided the capability to determine the complete
3D structures of small proteins (<10 kDa) based on the determination of
a large number of interproton distance constraints derived from 2D NOE
measurements. With the more recent development of 3D and 4D NMR

methods and high-field spectrometers, the molecular weight limit has been extended to more than 30 kDa.[15-17] In addition, methods have been developed that allow the nature of protein-ligand complexes to be characterized in detail.[18-20] Several recent reviews have described the application of these methods in drug design.[21-24]

In general, many of the methodological advances in NMR over recent years have been based on the development of a vast array of pulse sequences for extraction of different types of information from the sample, as well as a range of different nuclei that can be utilized. By making use of $^1$H, $^{13}$C and $^{15}$N nuclei in uniformly labelled proteins, several approaches can be applied to improve the utility of information contained in NMR spectra. These include the use of the large chemical shift range of the heteronuclei to disperse peaks in multidimensional spectra to thus reduce overlap, the use of heteronuclear coupling constants to provide dihedral angle constraints to assist in structure refinement, and the use of the heteronuclei to selectively edit spectra. Using appropriate pulse sequences, it is possible to create subspectra in which only protons attached to a $^{13}$C or $^{15}$N nucleus are selectively either included or excluded, thus considerably simplifying spectra. Such isotope editing techniques have found widespread application over the last few years in the study of drug–protein complexes.[21-25] Examples are given in several chapters of this book, with the most extensive discussion of the methodology for the study of protein–ligand complexes being in Chapter 7.

Many pulse sequences developed over recent years have benefited from the incorporation of pulsed field gradient technology.[26,27] The use of gradients for the selection of coherence pathways (which determine the nature of multidimensional NMR experiments) and for the suppression of the unwanted signal from solvent water are methodological developments that have resulted in significant improvements in the quality of NMR spectra of biomolecules. The details of this technology are discussed further in Chapter 4.

The instrumental advances that have accompanied these exciting new developments in methodology include further increases in magnetic field strength, improved accuracy and flexibility of the radiofrequency (rf) electronics, the development of pulsed field gradient hardware, and improvements in probe technology. These are discussed briefly below, but it is first useful to define the essential features of NMR instrumentation for drug design applications today.

The basic requirement in a spectrometer to be used in drug design research is for there to be sufficient sensitivity and resolution to detect signals from drugs and/or their receptors when these are dissolved in solution at millimolar or lower concentrations in aqueous media. In particular, the detection of NOEs in various multidimensional NMR experiments is of paramount importance. The minimum instrument frequency suitable for such studies is 500 MHz, and most major pharmaceutical companies have, over recent years, utilised one or more 500- or 600-MHz spectrometers in their drug development programs. While some studies can be done on lower field instruments, the number of NOEs detected on these instruments is usually substantially smaller than for high-field systems, making them less suitable for applications involving 3D structure determination.

Systems of 750 MHz have been commercially available for the last year or two, and they offer significantly increased sensitivity and dispersion over lower-field systems. The importance of such instruments in drug design is demonstrated by the fact that pharmaceutical companies have been amongst the first organisations to purchase them. Their increased sensitivity and dispersion lead to higher-quality data sets, and ultimately, to higher-quality 3D structures. Alternatively, the increased sensitivity can be used to obtain data of a quality similar to that obtained on, say, 600-MHz instruments, but in a shorter time. This is important in cases where the macromolecule under study may degrade over the course of the multidimensional NMR experiments. Another advantage of the greater sensitivity of 750-MHz instruments is that more dilute solutions may be examined. This is important for proteins that tend to aggregate, an occurrence not uncommon at millimolar concentrations. In many cases, dilution from 1 to 0.5 m$M$ can lead to a substantial reduction in the degree of aggregation and hence can reduce spectral linewidths.

Another instrumental advance that has helped in the study of more dilute solutions has been the development of high-resolution probes capable of utilizing larger-volume sample tubes. Dissolution of the same amount of protein in a larger volume results in a more dilute solution, but as the number of spins in the receiver coil is the same, there should be minimal difference in sensitivity. However, in cases where aggregation is a problem, its reduction due to dilution, and consequent improved linewidths, leads to a net improvement in spectral quality. A difficulty with this approach in the past has been the generally poorer homogeneity of both $B_0$ and $B_1$ fields over the larger sample volume, but improvements in probes, shims, and rf systems mean that similar homogeneity can be achieved in 8- or 10-mm tubes to that in 5-mm tubes.

At the other end of the scale there have also been significant developments in microvolume probes over the last few years. These are useful where the amount of sample available is limited, for example, where only small amounts of a natural product lead compound can be extracted, or where submilligram quantities of a protein are available. The latter situation is becoming less common with the increasing availability of recombinant proteins, where production of tens of milligrams of purified protein is often feasible. Nevertheless, in the early stages of protein studies by NMR, a number of preliminary experiments to establish the optimal conditions of temperature, pH, and other solution conditions are performed, and in some cases these lead to destruction of the sample. If preliminary tests can be done on small sample quantities in a microprobe, then the remainder of the sample is preserved for the extended data-acquisition experiments. Another situation where only limited supplies of protein may be available is when specific isotope labelling is used. This may be achieved using molecular biology (where all residues of a particular amino acid type are labelled) or solid-phase peptide synthesis for smaller proteins (where a specific amino acid may be labelled). In either case, moderately expensive labelled amino acid precursors are required, and the amounts of available sample may be limited. The microprobes currently in use require 40–100 µl of solution, compared with 450–600 µl in conventional 5-mm tubes. Thus the reduction in the amount of sample required is more than fivefold. The decrease in sensitivity associated with the smaller amount of sample is offset by the higher sensitivity per unit volume of these probes.

In summary, over the last decade, the size of molecules that can be studied by NMR has steadily increased while the amount of sample required has decreased.

---

## III   NMR IN DRUG DEVELOPMENT

It is apparent from the above discussion that NMR instruments are now sufficiently powerful and versatile to examine samples ranging in complexity from solutions of drug molecules, to their receptor proteins, to intact organs and animals. To illustrate how these capabilities may contribute to a drug design and development program, it is useful to provide a simplified description of such a program, as illustrated in Figure 1.

Figure 1 shows that the drug development process starts with a *design* or *discovery* phase. Discovery refers to the process of identifying a lead

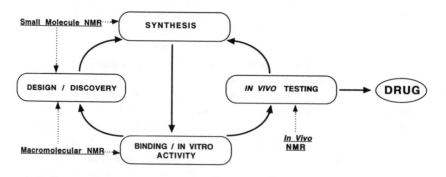

**FIGURE 1**
Schematic illustration of the drug development process, showing the contribution of NMR.

compound from a random screening program or from chance observation. As indicated in Chapter 1, a large proportion of existing drugs were indeed initially discovered in these ways. Design implies a more directed and rational approach to the production of a lead compound. There are several possible design strategies, but two of the most common may be categorised as either "analogue-based" design, where knowledge of the structure or conformation of a known drug or bioactive molecule is used to design either antagonists or more potent analogues, or "receptor-based" design, where knowledge of the structure of a macromolecular drug target is used to design compounds to interact with that target.

In the case of either design or discovery, once an initial drug candidate is identified the next step is chemical synthesis, followed by biological testing. This testing usually takes the form of a simple *in vitro* assay (i.e., receptor binding or enzyme inhibition). At this point, depending on the results of the initial assay, the design hypothesis may need to be modified and there could be several cycles of the left-hand loop in Figure 1, with each cycle producing a compound of higher affinity/activity. The resultant lead compound is then submitted for more extensive *in vivo* testing. At this stage problems with bioavailability, various physicochemical properties, or acute toxicity may become apparent, and it may be necessary to ameliorate these by chemical modification of the lead compound. Further chemical input may be required to protect the active compound from enzymatic breakdown and metabolism *in vivo*, and so there are likely to be several cycles of the right-hand loop of Figure 1 before a drug candidate emerges.

This is a simplified description, but the main purpose of introducing it here is that it allows the NMR approaches that are possible at each stage to be described. Three classes of NMR experiments can be identified — small-molecule NMR (studies of molecules of less than a few kilodaltons in molecular weight), macromolecular NMR (studies of molecules or complexes of tens of kilodaltons molecular weight) and *in vivo* NMR (whole-organ or whole-animal studies). The points at which these contribute to the drug development process are indicated in Figure 1.

Small-molecule NMR contributes both at the synthetic stage, as an analytical tool for the verification of structure, and at the drug design stage, that is, by providing conformational information it is a valuable tool in analogue-based drug design. Macromolecular NMR clearly has the potential to assist in the design stage (of receptor-based drug design) by providing the structures of key protein targets, and it is also extremely valuable at the *in vitro* testing stage. In particular, one of the strengths of NMR is its application to the study of ligand–protein interactions. Once it has been confirmed that a drug candidate binds to a receptor macromolecule (usually done by non-NMR methods), it is important to establish the *mode* of binding so that further development of lead compounds is based on correct information about the intermolecular interactions. Finally, *in vivo* NMR is valuable for investigating the effects of drugs on target organs. This is an area that will not be addressed specifically in this book, apart from one example below, which illustrates the type of applications possible.

The example chosen is the use of $^{31}P$ NMR to study the effects on cardiac metabolism of drugs designed to protect the heart during periods of ischaemia (reduced blood flow). With a simple adaptation of standard Langendorff perfusion apparatus, it is possible to perfuse a rat heart inside the magnet bore of an NMR spectrometer and obtain signals from abundant phosphorus-containing species in the beating heart. These include the high-energy phosphate species adenosine triphosphate (ATP), phosphocreatine (PCr) and inorganic phosphate ($P_i$). With a few minutes of data acquisition it is possible to obtain spectra (Figure 2) in which the relative abundance of ATP, PCr, and $P_i$ may be readily measured. These provide an important measure of the bioenergetic status of the heart. In addition, by measuring the chemical shift of the inorganic phosphate peak, the intracellular pH (another important marker of cardiac viability) can be determined.

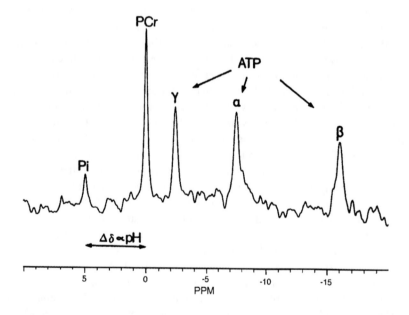

**FIGURE 2**

$^{31}P$ NMR spectrum of an isolated perfused rat heart. Peaks due to $P_i$, PCr, and the three phosphate atoms ($\gamma$, $\alpha$, $\beta$) of ATP are indicated. (From Craik, D.J., and Kneen, M.M., *Chem. Aust.*, 56, 30–32, 1989. With permission.)

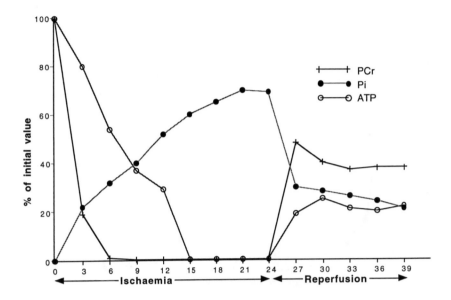

**FIGURE 3**
Response of the phosphorus-containing metabolites in the heart to a period of ischaemia
followed by reperfusion. (Adapted from Craik, D.J., and Kneen, M.M., *Chem. Aust.*, 56,
30–32, 1989.)

By monitoring the spectrum as a function of time following an
ischaemic insult to the perfused heart, the levels of these various metabolites can be followed (together with pH). The profile for a 24-min period
of ischaemia (induced by turning off the flow of perfusate to the heart)
followed by reperfusion is given in Figure 3.[11] Here it is seen that within
3 to 6 min of global ischaemia the PCr levels have dropped to zero, but
the ATP levels decline at a slower rate. Concomitant with these decreases
is a rise in $P_i$, as well as a drop in pH (not shown).

The modulating effects of drugs on the rate of decline of the high-
energy phosphorous metabolites can be readily determined by comparing
the above profiles for control hearts with hearts that have received pretreat-
ment with the drug of interest. Figure 4, for example, shows the reduced
rate of decline of PCr levels in hearts pretreated with anipamil. By comparing different drugs and treatment protocols, improved cardioprotective
drugs or dose profiles can be developed.

This example provides a simple illustration of the fact that NMR can
play a role at the final stages of drug development. The remainder of this
book focuses on applications of NMR to drug design (i.e., those fitting
into the small-molecule NMR and macromolecular NMR categories described above).

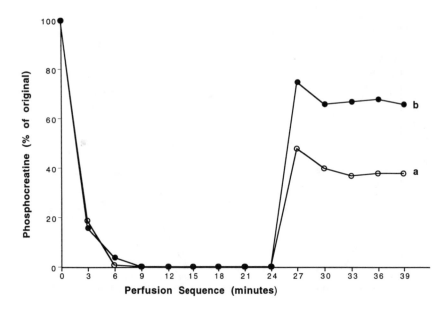

**FIGURE 4**

Recovery in the levels of PCr in isolated perfused hearts following 24 min of ischaemia for (a) untreated rats and (b) rats pretreated with anipamil (3 mg/kg) for three days prior to the experiment. (Adapted from Craik, D.J., and Kneen, M.M., *Chem. Aust.*, 56, 30–32, 1989.)

---

# IV  NMR IN DRUG DESIGN

It is clear in an intuitive sense that knowledge of the nature of bioactive molecules and their macromolecular target sites should be useful in designing new compounds to interact at those sites and potentially act as therapeutic agents. However, it is useful to specifically identify the questions about such interactions that may be relevant in the design process: What is the structure of the bioactive lead compound? What is its bound conformation and what charge state does it bind in? Is there more than one bound conformation, and if so, what are the dynamics at the receptor site? Which parts of the compound interact with the receptor, and which parts (if any) are solvent exposed? Where is the binding site on the receptor, and what functional group interactions are involved in ligand recognition and binding? What effect does ligand binding have on the conformation and flexibility of the target macromolecule?

Some of the answers will have a major impact on drug design (e.g., the discovery of a strong interaction between a positive charge on a bioactive lead compound and a negative charge on a receptor would dictate that newly designed ligands should have an appropriately located positive charge), and others might lead to more subtle design strategies. For example, a knowledge of solvent-exposed parts of a bound drug might encourage modifications to this presumably "redundant" region to improve bioavailability, if necessary, or to improve the economics of synthesis.

Some of the questions can be answered by studies of the bioactive ligands or drugs themselves, but most require examination of the target macromolecule and its complex with the ligand. These are technically demanding problems, and it is for this reason that only relatively recently has NMR spectroscopy been able to make significant contributions to the field of drug design.

In the following chapters the ways in which NMR can provide answers to the questions posed above are described. Chapters 3 and 4 give overviews of the appropriate NMR theory. In particular, Chapter 3 describes a range of relevant NMR parameters and techniques, and provides the background for an understanding of how these are applicable in the study of drug–receptor interactions. The chapter includes some introductory discussion on drug design, making it useful as a stand-alone article for those seeking an introduction to the topic in a single chapter. Its central aim, though, is to provide a foundation for the applications described in Chapters 5–12. Chapter 4 provides a comprehensive description of the state of the art in protein structure determination by NMR, including a discussion on isotope labelling methods and the practical considerations associated with structure determination. Again, the aim is to provide a basis for understanding the applications described in Chapters 5–12.

NMR is of course not the only method that can provide answers to the questions posed above. The traditional medicinal chemistry approach involving a cyclic process of synthesis and assay (Figure 1) provides a direct answer to the question of which parts of a ligand are important for binding and activity, but does not necessarily explain *why* these parts are important. For this it is necessary to enlist one or more of the structure-based methods, including X-ray crystallography, computer graphics/modelling,[28,29] or NMR spectroscopy. Each of these methods promises to significantly contribute to the drug design field over the new few years, but each has some limitations. Since the focus of this book is on NMR-based approaches, it is useful to comment briefly on the advantages and disadvantages of NMR relative to other structure-based methods.

By comparison with X-ray crystallography, NMR has the advantages of providing information in the solution state, not being limited to molecules that can be crystallized, and providing information on the dynamics of drug–receptor interactions. To be fair, it is important not to overemphasize the significance of the first of these advantages, as it is clear that the crystal environment in many protein structures solved by X-ray methods is highly solvated, and therefore probably not too dissimilar from the solution state. Nevertheless, the importance of studies in solution is clear from many of the following chapters, including examples of drugs exhibiting multiple conformers in solution, but not in the crystal (Chapter 4), and enzymes showing multiple drug-binding modes in solution (Chapter 8). The second advantage of NMR over X-ray methods is best illustrated by the studies of peptides described in Chapter 6. Peptides are widely regarded as the next generation of target molecules in drug design applications, but they are notoriously difficult to crystallize. NMR studies of the conformations of native peptides and constrained analogs are currently providing much valuable information that is simply not obtainable using X-ray methods. The third advantage is emphasized in Chapter 10, where the elegance of NMR for defining in detail the flexibility, with implications for function, of the key target enzyme in anti-AIDS drug design, HIV-1 protease, is demonstrated.

The quality of structural information obtainable by NMR methods is comparable to that obtained by X-ray approaches.[30] The major disadvantage of NMR is of course, the size limitation (<35 kDa) on proteins that can be studied. Chapter 4 discusses this limitation and describes approaches that are being used to push the limit higher. Several other chapters illustrate the fact that if only selected information is required (i.e., the conformation of a bound ligand, rather than a complete structure of a protein complex), then much larger protein–ligand complexes can already be examined using NMR techniques such as transferred NOEs.

NMR offers some considerable advantages over computer-based design. While computational and graphics approaches are tremendously useful in providing design leads and in helping to understand or visualise binding modes or enzyme mechanisms, they are not yet sufficiently reliable to replace hard experimental data on biomolecular structures. In any design protocol in which a particular binding mode is proposed, and compounds are synthesized and tested, then even if binding and activity are evident, it is important to experimentally verify that the compounds bind in the way predicted. If this is not done, and it happens that some other binding mode is actually present, then any further development of the lead compound based on the original hypothesis will be misguided.

The potential for quite similar ligands to bind in quite different orientations at a given site has been particularly well documented for substrate and inhibitor binding to the enzyme dihydrofolate reductase. Related to such observations is the fact that even a single ligand may exhibit multiple binding modes. The unique contributions that NMR has made in determining multiple binding modes of ligands for this enzyme are described in Chapter 8. Computer graphics approaches may well be useful in rationalising such findings, but experimental methods are still essential for their discovery.

An even more basic illustration of the importance of experimentally confirming the mode of action of computer-designed compounds relates to structure integrity in solution. It is clearly important to establish that the structure of the designed compound is stable under the physiological conditions at which it will act. An example relating to the design of potential antibacterials serves to illustrate the point.[31] In this study an extensive range of computational procedures was used to design compounds that, as putative transition-state analogues, would be inhibitors of the enzyme alanine racemase, which is essential for the production of the bacterial cell wall. A series of oxazine compounds with the structures shown below (1) was then synthesized and indeed found to have mild antibacterial activity.

However, simple NMR studies showed that in aqueous media the compounds rapidly break down to give the open-chain derivatives (2), together with formaldehye, itself a mild antibacterial. Thus, the activity of the compounds had little to do with the original design hypothesis. Indeed the possibility that they were transition state analogues could not be tested, as they essentially acted as prodrugs for delivery of formaldehyde before they got to the target enzyme!

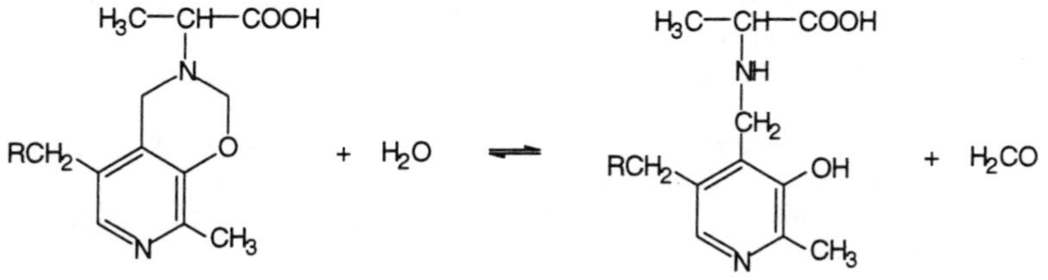

1                                    2

As already noted, this lesson is one that is evident in more subtle ways when drug–receptor interactions are studied. Once a binding mode has been predicted from computer graphics techniques, it needs to be experimentally verified. Likewise, once a conformation is experimentally verified under one set of conditions, it needs to be confirmed under physiologically relevant conditions. This applies in extrapolations of solution conformations to the receptor-bound state, which can in some cases be quite different. For example, NMR studies of the immunosuppressant drug cyclosporin A bound to its target protein cyclophilin[32,33] showed that the bound conformation of this cyclic undecapeptide is completely rearranged compared to the free conformation. Likewise, NMR studies of an FK-506 analogue, ascomycin, bound to FK-506 binding protein do not correlate with the ascomycin structure derived in solution.[34] This may be, in part, due to the nonaqueous environment in which the structures of the free drugs were determined, but the potential of the bound conformation of a molecule to deviate from its free form is clearly evident. These examples are discussed more fully in Chapters 6 and 7.

In summary, this chapter has given a brief overview of past applications of NMR in the pharmaceutical sciences, has traced the developments in NMR instrumentation and methods that now make it such a powerful technique, and has identified some of the important questions in drug design that may potentially be addressed by NMR. Some of the advantages of NMR relative to other structure-based approaches have been described. The combination of medicinal chemistry with NMR, X-ray, and computer graphics approaches promises to be extremely valuable in drug design, but for the remainder of this book the focus is on NMR approaches.

# REFERENCES

1. Jackman, L.M.; Sternhell, S. *Applications of Nuclear Magnetic Resonance Spectroscopy in Organic Chemistry*; Pergamon Press, Oxford, 1969.
2. Becker, E.D. *High Resolution NMR*; Academic Press, New York, 1969.
3. Gunther, H. *NMR Spectroscopy*; John Wiley & Sons, New York, 1980.
4. Casy, A.F. *PMR Spectroscopy in Medicinal and Biological Chemistry*; Academic Press, London, 1971.
5. Noggle, J.H.; Schirmer, R.E. *The Nuclear Overhauser Effect*; Academic Press, New York, 1971.
6. Neuhaus, D.; Williamson, M.P. *The Nuclear Overhauser Effect in Structural and Conformational Analysis*; VCH Publishers, New York, 1989.
7. Dwek, R.A. *Nuclear Magnetic Resonance in Biochemistry*; Clarendon Press, Oxford, 1973.
8. Jardetzky, O.; Roberts, G.C.K. *NMR in Molecular Biology*; Academic Press, New York, 1981.
9. Govil, G.; Hosur, R.V. *Conformation of Biological Molecules: New Results from NMR*; Springer-Verlag, Berlin, 1982.
10. Gadian, D.G. *Nuclear Magnetic Resonance and Its Application to Living Systems*; Clarendon Press, Oxford, 1982.
11. Craik, D.J.; Kneen, M.M. *Chem. Aust.*, 1989, 56, 30-32.
12. Nunnally, R.L.; Bottomley, P.A. *Science*, 1981, 211, 177-180.
13. Jaroszewski, J.W.; Schaumburg, K.; Kofod, H.; Eds. *NMR Spectroscopy in Drug Research*; Munksgaard, Copenhagen, 1988.
14. Wüthrich, K. *NMR of Proteins and Nucleic Acids*; John Wiley & Sons, New York, 1986.
15. Clore, G.M.; Gronenborn, A.M. *Science,* 1991, 252, 1390-1399.
16. Gronenborn, A.M.; Clore, G.M. *Proteins: Structure, Function, and Genetics*, 1994, 19, 273-278.
17. Bax, A.; Grzesiek, S. *Acc. Chem. Res.*, 1993, 26, 131-138.
18. Handschumacher, R.E.; Armitage, I.M., Eds.; *NMR Methods for Elucidating Macromolecule–Ligand Interactions: An Approach to Drug Design*; Pergamon Press, Oxford, 1989.
19. Feeney, J.; Birdsall, B. NMR studies of protein–ligand interactions, in *NMR of Macromolecules: A Practical Approach*; Roberts, G.C.K., Ed.; Oxford University Press, 1993, chap. 7.
20. Craik, D.J.; Higgins, K.A. *Annu. Rep. NMR Spectrosc., Vol.*, 22; 1990, pp 61-138.
21. Fesik, S.W.; Zuiderweg, E.R.P.; Olejniczak, E.T.; Gampe, R.T. *Biochem. Pharmacol.*, 1990, 40, 161-167.
22. Fesik, S.W. *J. Med. Chem.*, 1991, 34, 2937-2945.

23. Fesik, S.W. *J. Biomolec. NMR*, 1993, 3, 261-269.
24. Otting, G. *Curr. Opin. Struct. Biol.*, 1993, 3, 760-766.
25. Otting, G.; Wüthrich, K. *Q. Rev. Biophys.*, 1990, 23, 39-96.
26. Hurd, R.E. *J. Magn. Reson.*, 1990, 87, 422-428.
27. Bax, A.; Pochapsky, S. *J. Magn. Reson.*, 1992, 99, 638-643.
28. Perun, T.J.; Propst, C.L., Eds.; *Computer-Aided Drug Design: Methods and Applications*; Marcel Dekker, New York, 1989.
29. Verlinde, C.L.M.J.; Hol, W.G.J. *Structure*, 1994, 2, 577-587.
30. Clore, G.M.; Gronenborn, A.M. *Protein Sci.*, 1994, 3, 372-390.
31. Leung, D.K.; Andrews, P.R.; Craik, D.J.; Iskander, M.I.; Winkler, D.A. *Aust. J. Chem.*, 1985, 38, 297-306.
32. Weber, C.; Wider, G.; von Freyberg, B.; Traber, R.; Braun, W.; Widmer, H.; Wüthrich, K. *Biochemistry,* 1991, 30, 6563-6574.
33. Fesik, S.W.; Gampe, R.T.; Eaton, H.L.; Gemmecker, G.; Olejniczak, E.T.; Neri, P.; Holzman, T.F.; Egan, D.A.; Edalji, R.; Simmer, R.; Helfrich, R.; Hochlowski, J.; Jackson, M. *Biochemistry,* 1991, 30, 6574-6583.
34. Petros, A.M.; Gemmecker, G.; Neri, P.; Olejniczak, E.T.; Nettesheim, D.; Xu, R.X.; Gubbins, E.G.; Smith, H.; Fesik, S.W. *J. Med. Chem.,* 1992, 35, 2467.

# CHAPTER 3

# STUDIES OF DRUG–RECEPTOR INTERACTIONS BY NMR: THEORY AND APPLICATIONS

*J. T. Gerig*

## CONTENTS

I Introduction ................................................................. 32

II Consequences of Drug–Receptor Interactions ................................. 33

III Finding New Drugs ........................................................ 34

IV Structure-Based Drug Development ......................................... 35

V Structures of Drug–Receptor Complexes ..................................... 37

VI What NMR Can Tell About Drug–Receptor Complexes ............... 39

VII NMR Parameters and the Information They Provide .................... 40
    A Chemical Shielding ...................................................... 41
    B Scalar Coupling ......................................................... 43
    C Spin–Lattice ($T_1$) Relaxation ........................................ 45
    D Transverse ($T_2$) Relaxation .......................................... 46
    E Nuclear Overhauser Effects ............................................ 48

VIII Processes Leading to Relaxation ........................................... 49

0-8493-7824-9/96/$0.00+$.50

**IX**  Chemical-Exchange Effects ........................................................ 55
   A   Lineshapes ................................................................................ 55
   B   Spin–Lattice Relaxation ............................................................. 64
   C   Scalar Coupling ......................................................................... 66
   D   Nuclear Overhauser Effects ....................................................... 66

 **X**  Determination of Dissociation Rates for Drug–Receptor
       Complexes ................................................................................. 66
   A   Saturation Transfer .................................................................... 67
   B   Inversion Transfer ..................................................................... 70
   C   Two-Dimensional Exchange Spectroscopy ...................................71
   D   Lineshape Methods ................................................................... 75
   E   Spin Echo Methods .................................................................... 76
   F   $T_1$ in the Rotating Frame $T_1\rho$ ...................................... 77

**XI**  Nuclear Overhauser Effects ........................................................ 77
   A   Steady-State NOE ....................................................................... 81
   B   NOE Buildup .............................................................................. 82
   C   Transient NOE ........................................................................... 83
   D   Two-Dimensional NOE ............................................................... 83
   E   Rotating-Frame NOEs ................................................................ 85
   F   Transferred NOEs ...................................................................... 86

**XII**  Some Examples .......................................................................... 88
   A   Actinomycin D Conformation ..................................................... 88
   B   Sulindac and Sulindac Sulfide with Albumin .............................89
   C   Hirudin-Derived Peptides Bound to Thrombin ........................91
   D   Calicheamicin with Duplex DNA ................................................ 92
   E   Immunosuppressant–Immunophilin Complexes ........................93

**XIII**  Summary ................................................................................. 96

Acknowledgments ................................................................................ 96

**References** ...................................................................................... 96

---

# I   INTRODUCTION

In the preceding chapters it was noted that most drugs exert their effect because they interact with a specific "site" in the biological makeup of the target organism. This site of interaction is termed a receptor for the drug, and the drug is a ligand for the receptor. A receptor is typically a protein molecule but could be a nucleic acid.[1,2] Protein receptors are often located on or within cell membranes, but intracellular or extracellular proteins of the organism could also be loci of interactions with drug molecules.

The chemical and physical interactions between a drug and its receptor are, of course, the same as those potentially present between any two molecules. Coulombic (electrostatic) attraction or repulsion is possible if the drug and the receptor-binding site contain anionic or cationic groups. Hydrogen bonding between the drug and the receptor may take place if appropriate proton donors and acceptors are present. Ion–dipole, dipole–dipole, and van der Waals interactions within the receptor-binding site could lower the free energy of the complex relative to the separated, hydrated drug and the receptor. Clearly, the energetics of all these interactions are critically dependent on the properties of the solvent and the three-dimensional structures of the receptor site, the drug, and the drug–receptor complex. It is not surprising that minor amino-acid changes in a receptor protein can significantly alter the pharmacological profile of a receptor.[3]

## II  CONSEQUENCES OF DRUG–RECEPTOR INTERACTIONS

Binding of a molecule to a receptor can have several consequences. Most commonly, such binding prevents binding of another molecule to the same receptor site. Drugs that are enzyme inhibitors generally act by interacting with the active site of an enzyme, making approach of the substrate to the catalytic machinery of the active site impossible. A goal in the development of drugs that are enzyme inhibitors is high selectivity for binding to a single member of a group of similar enzymes within the target organism, or selective binding to an enzyme of an invading foreign organism, while not interacting with similar enzymes of the host. Before resistance to the drug developed, sulfanilamide was an effective compound for combating streptococcal infections because, as we saw in Chapter 1, it selectively inhibits an enzyme crucial to folic acid biosynthesis in the invading microorganism. The streptococcal enzyme is the receptor site for the drug, and the drug action involves binding to the receptor in a manner that is competitive with binding of its substrate.

Other consequences of a drug binding to a receptor can be more subtle than simple blockage of access of other molecules to the receptor site. It should not be assumed that the formation of a complex between a ligand (drug) and a receptor takes place without structural changes in both partners. Certainly, proteins and nucleic acids are not rigid molecules, and they may well adopt new three-dimensional structures in the course of interacting with a ligand or after a complex is formed with the ligand.

The importance of molecular flexibility in receptors is illustrated in Chapter 10. The three-dimensional structure of the ligand at the receptor site may not be the dominant conformation in solution. Examples of situations where the solution and bound conformations are different are given in Chapters 6 and 7. Formation of a ligand–receptor complex may alter the rate at which some conformational change of the receptor structure or the ligand takes place. Binding of a ligand may provoke the release or capture of protons by the receptor, thus altering the acidity in the vicinity where the receptor–ligand interactions took place. Similarly, another molecule previously bound to the receptor may be released when binding of the ligand occurs. Lastly, the presence of the bound ligand may alter the rate at which the receptor protein or nucleic acid is metabolized or chemically altered by reactions that take place in the target organism.

## III   FINDING NEW DRUGS

The development of modern structural chemistry and biochemistry over the past century or so has provided increasingly detailed information about the chemical nature of living organisms. Much has been learned, for example, about the molecular basis for adhesion of cells to each other, how the immune system functions, and how chemical signalling between cells can produce changes in cell shape or stimulate DNA synthesis. Each new insight about the way organisms "work" provides additional guidance for the construction of chemical compounds that may produce a desirable pharmacological effect.

Chapter 1 described some examples of the unearthing of new drugs largely through serendipity. There are many other examples; one of the best known is the discovery of penicillin by Fleming, which basically took place through a botched experiment that proved difficult to reproduce.[4,5] Observations made during clinical trials of compounds thought to be potential drugs for one condition may reveal a side effect that is more significant or lucrative. Rogaine (Minoxodil), currently widely advertised as a solution to male pattern baldness, was originally developed and approved for use in the treatment of hypertension.[6,7]

A systematic search for new drugs can be made by screening compounds through biological assays. This process is limited by the budget available, is not guaranteed to produce a favourable result, and may miss potential drugs because the assay chosen was not appropriate. Random screening has led to the discovery of several antibiotics and other important drugs but is clearly inefficient. For example, according to one estimate, between 1983 and 1988 more than 200,000 compounds were evaluated in industrial screening programs as possible inhibitors of binding to the interleukin-1 and interleukin-2 receptors found in the human immune system, but not a single significant discovery was reported.[8]

A compound found to produce a desirable biological effect is like the first clue in a mystery story and becomes a lead compound. Simply determining that a material exerts an effect in a screening experiment, however, does not automatically lead to development of a drug. Transport of the compound to the site of action in the target organism, the toxicity of the material and its metabolites, the specificity of the interaction of the compound with the target receptor in a complex environment where a multitude of other receptors is present, the nature and severity of side effects, and the economics of synthesizing, investigating, and marketing the compound are all considerations along the path of developing a promising lead compound into a useful drug.

---

# IV  STRUCTURE-BASED DRUG DEVELOPMENT

New knowledge can suggest new approaches to drug discovery and development. This is particularly the case if a specific macromolecule can be identified as the receptor or target for a possible drug. The situation is even better if there is knowledge about the three-dimensional nature of the putative binding site for the drug.

The development of new knowledge about protein structure has been explosive. The revolution started in the 1950s with the pioneering efforts of Perutz and Kendrew in finding the three-dimensional structures of haemoglobin and myoglobin by means of X-ray diffraction from protein crystals. X-ray and NMR methods are currently providing the three-dimensional structures of individual proteins, and complexes of proteins with ligands, at the rate of several hundred per year.[9] In 1994, the Protein Data Bank maintained at Brookhaven National Laboratories contained in excess of 2300 structures of proteins and nucleic acids.

Consideration of the types of proteins for which structures are available shows that the structures of many soluble enzymes have been solved but relatively few structures are available for membrane proteins. The number of studies of tertiary structures of oligo-deoxyribonucleotides (as models for DNA) and of RNAs by X-ray diffraction or NMR is smaller than the number of protein structures. While there is much evidence that the tertiary structures of a protein observed in protein crystals by diffraction methods are similar to the average structure of the proteins in solutions observed by NMR, the consensus at present seems to be that the structures of nucleic acids observed in crystals may be imperfect guides to the average structures of these molecules in solution.

Structure-based drug development is the use of atomic-level three-dimensional structural information about a demonstrated or putative macromolecular receptor to guide the design of a drug. A brief introduction to the topic was given in the Chapter 2, and Navia and Peattie[10] have recently provided an excellent survey of the current practice of structure-based drug development. The scheme in Figure 1, guided by a corresponding figure in their article, shows critical steps in the process. After a lead compound is identified, by either serendipity, screening, or imputation

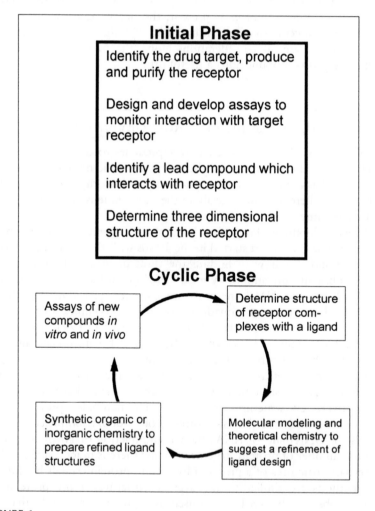

**FIGURE 1**

A representation of structure-based drug design. An initial exploratory phase is followed by cycles of structure determination by X-ray crystallography, NMR or other methods, molecular modelling, synthetic chemistry, and biological evaluation.

based on related systems, and after the structure of its receptor is determined or inferred, a cyclic process can begin in which computer modelling, synthesis of new compounds, and biological testing can be used in some combination to improve binding to the receptor while addressing the concerns mentioned above relating to toxicity, bioavailability, and metabolic stability. It should be noted that the knowledge base and technologies necessary for application of the approach to drug development indicated in Figure 1 have become readily available only in the last 10 years, the recent availability of relatively inexpensive computer hardware and software for molecular modelling being a major factor in the progress made.[11] There are now a number of examples where the structure-based approach has led to improvement in drug performance,[12] and a number of compounds that have had their genesis in the application of structure-based drug development are in clinical trial. These include trials of a topical inhibitor of carbonic anhydrase for control of glaucoma, several inhibitors of HIV-1 protease, and as noted in Chapter 1, inhibitors of influenza sialidase.[13]

---

# V  STRUCTURES OF DRUG–RECEPTOR COMPLEXES

A primary requirement for structure-based drug development is knowledge about the three-dimensional nature of the drug receptor site. An experimental structure determination is preferred, but if the primary sequence of the receptor is known and the structure for a material that has a reasonably similar sequence is available, it may be possible to infer what the tertiary structure of the receptor of interest might be.

There are several steps in defining the three-dimensional structure of a receptor by diffraction methods. The single most important and time-consuming step is adequate purification of the receptor molecule and its subsequent crystallization. Data on the diffraction of X-rays or, less commonly, of neutrons by the crystals are obtained and some procedure is developed for solving the crystallographic phase problem.[9] At this point, a representation of the electron density distribution in the crystal is at hand and an initial guess at the structure, guided by the primary sequence of the biopolymer under study, is made. Refinement procedures then try to optimize the fit between the observed electron density data and the electron density expected for the three-dimensional structure that has been proposed. When the fit is sufficiently good, the structural problem is regarded as being solved. It should be noted that X-ray diffraction studies with proteins and other biomolecules do not locate the positions of hydrogen atoms. These positions have to be inferred from the arrangement of the heavier atoms in the structure. Neutron diffraction is capable of locating hydrogens in these structures to high accuracy, but the ability to do neutron diffraction experiments is severely limited by the scarcity of monochromatic neutron sources.

While it is difficult to generalize, the time scale for obtaining suitable crystals may range from months to years, or even longer. Sufficient data from stable, well-diffracting crystals may be collected in a matter of days, while solution of the phasing problem may require weeks to months. Depending on the complexity of the structure and the availability of reasonable precedents, the final structure may be available months to years after the phase problem is solved. Biomolecule crystallographers are becoming ever more adept at production of useful crystals, and this, coupled with the impact of modern computing and molecular modelling capabilities, is largely responsible for the rapid growth in the number of three-dimensional structures made available by diffraction methods.

A recent structure determination of the enzyme β-galactosidase (*Escherichia coli*) at a resolution of 3.5 Å illustrates the state of the art.[14] The protein was found to be a tetramer of subunits, each subunit consisting of a 1023-amino-acid polypeptide of $M_r$ = 465,412 Da. This is the longest polypeptide chain for which a structure at atomic resolution has so far been obtained.

NMR methodologies for the determination of three-dimensional structures rely on an entirely different set of physical principles. A recent volume provides much practical advice on the determination of NMR spectra of proteins, nucleic acids, and polysaccharides, including discussions of NMR methods for study of ligand complexes with these biopolymers.[15] Techniques for interpreting NMR spectral data, and the reliability of the structures proposed from this evidence, have been extensively discussed.[16-20] For systems of even modest complexity, multidimensional experiments, often involving the use of materials that have been isotopically enriched in carbon-13, nitrogen-15, or deuterium, are necessary to obtain resolved and interpretable spectra, as is outlined in Chapter 4.

As will be discussed below and elsewhere in this book, various observations made by NMR can provide information about internuclear distances, dihedral angles, or the relative orientations of groups of nuclei. Each piece of information acts as a constraint on what the relative positions of some small set of atoms of the molecule under investigation can be. Even though they are relatively short range in their implications, if there are enough constraints of this nature, the three-dimensional structure of the molecule can be defined. In the majority of cases studied, the sample of interest is a protein, and half a dozen or more of these short-range constraints may be obtained for each amino acid in the sequence. An "NMR structure" actually consists of a family of 20 or more, usually very similar conformations that are found by computational methods and molecular modelling to satisfy the various experimental restraints.

NMR methods of structure determination use noncrystalline samples, typically aqueous solutions. The solution conditions (pH, temperature, nature and concentration of buffers or added salts, concentration of the macromolecule) can be varied.* There is thus a contrast to diffraction methods, which employ solid, crystalline samples that are often teased from solutions that have unusual compositions, including the presence of high concentrations of organic solvents or salts. NMR methods are unique in being able to detect the presence of significant amounts of two or more conformations[21-23] and to obtain quantitative information on dynamic processes, including the rates of conformational interconversion, rates of exchange of labile protons, particularly amide NH protons, and rates of segmental backbone and side-chain motions.

The resolution of a structure obtained by X-ray diffraction depends on the quality and stability of the crystals examined, while the resolution of an NMR structure depends on the number and distribution within the molecule of the constraints that led to the definition of the structure. In biopolymers, a resolution of 2 Å or better is needed to trace the backbone chain, detect secondary structural elements, and define side-chain orientations.[25] It should be borne in mind that the two methodologies are based on different physical phenomena and employ samples in different physical states. Thus, the structural "answers" obtained by the X-ray and NMR methods, assuming that both were competently applied, are neither right nor wrong, but are simply two views of the same system.

## VI  WHAT NMR CAN TELL ABOUT DRUG–RECEPTOR COMPLEXES

Like many other spectroscopic methods, NMR can be used in titration experiments to demonstrate the stoichiometry of a ligand–receptor interaction and to provide a value for the equilibrium constant that characterizes formation of the ligand–receptor complex. NMR methods can be used to determine the rate of dissociation of complexes, and are particularly useful when the rates are in the range of $10^{-1}$ to $10^4$ events per second. Detailed examples of these applications are given in Chapter 12 for drug–DNA binding.

The basic suite of experiments used to define the three-dimensional structure of a receptor can also be applied to determination of the structure

---

* It might be noted that the protein concentrations used in such experiments (in the millimolar range) are very high relative to typical concentrations at the locale where the protein plays its biological role in an organism.

(conformation) of a bound ligand,[27] but the details of how these experiments are executed and interpreted depend critically on the rate at which the ligand–receptor complex dissociates. Obtaining the structure of a bound ligand will be considered in more detail later in this chapter, and examples are described in Chapters 6–12.

Beyond three-dimensional structural data, NMR experiments can potentially demonstrate the presence of multiple conformations of the ligand, the receptor, or the complex formed, as well as provide an estimate of the rate of interconversion of these conformations. Thus, the knowledge base for discovery of new pharmaceutical agents by structure-based drug design can be considerably expanded by NMR experiments since these experiments not only can provide three-dimensional structural information, but also can indicate structural flexibility (Chapter 10).

Understanding of the features that control the rate of ligand–macromolecule complex formation and of how such rates respond to changes in the chemical nature of a ligand is presently at a rudimentary level, and such considerations are rarely factored into a drug design procedure. Taking into account the dynamic aspects of molecular flexibility and of complex formation may provide a useful added dimension in structure-based drug design efforts.

---

# VII NMR PARAMETERS AND THE INFORMATION THEY PROVIDE

NMR spectroscopic methods are useful to the structural chemist and biochemist because, even in the simplest experiments, these methods make available a high density of chemically relevant information. Depending on the spectral resolution, information about chemical shielding and nuclear spin relaxation for each NMR-active atom in the molecule is potentially available. Virtually all constituents of biological systems include protons in their structure, and NMR signals from these nuclei are readily detectable. Unfortunately, the chemical-shift range for these hydrogens when considered in units of Hertz is relatively small compared to signal line widths, and resolution of unique proton signals from a complex system is problematic, even at the relatively high magnetic field strengths presently available (corresponding to proton NMR at 750 MHz). The chemical-shift ranges for carbon-13 and nitrogen-15 nuclei are roughly 25 times larger than the proton chemical-shift range, and because relaxation of these nuclei is relatively less efficient, the spectral lines for carbon-13 and nitrogen-15 signals from a biopolymer can be better resolved than the proton NMR signals from the same molecule. But carbon-13 and nitrogen-15 nuclei are present at 1.1 and 0.37% natural abundance, respectively, and this presents a signal-to-noise ratio problem. (The amounts of these species present can be enriched to essentially 100% by appropriate synthetic efforts, with a concomitant increase in signal strength.) There are isotopes of many other elements of biological importance that can give rise to NMR signals, including phosphorus, sodium, magnesium, calcium, and transition metal ions. Elements that are not naturally present in a biological system but are, nonetheless, NMR detectable can be part of a ligand or introduced into a receptor structure by synthesis; these nuclei include fluorine (100% natural abundance), deuterium ($^2$H), or tritium ($^3$H).

The parameters that characterize an NMR spectral result for a single conformation or chemical species include chemical shifts, spin-coupling constants, and spin relaxation rates. All these parameters are structure dependent, and in practice, many depend on the solution conditions mentioned earlier. Moreover, superimposed on observations that report chemical shielding effects, scalar coupling interactions, or nuclear spin relaxation are the effects of reactions that interchange the local environments of the spins under observation and, thus, potentially change or average shielding, scalar coupling, or spin relaxation.

It is also important to note that the chemical shift and spin coupling parameters in principle depend on how a particular molecule is aligned in the magnetic field. In liquid samples of most solutes, the molecules change their orientations rapidly with the result that the shift or coupling constant observed represents the average overall possible positions of the molecule in the magnetic field. The tumbling of molecules in solution averages atomic positions and thus has the effect of simplifying the NMR spectrum observed at the cost of removing some information about molecular positions from the spectrum.[*]

It is not appropriate to discuss in detail here the physical bases for nuclear shielding effects, relaxation, or scalar coupling, and the reader is referred to the excellent texts that are available. However, some comments on each of these classes of NMR parameters that are relevant in the context of biomolecular structure follow.

## A  CHEMICAL SHIELDING

The exact radiofrequency at which a nucleus undergoes the NMR phenomenon depends primarily on the properties of the nucleus and secondarily on its chemical environment. The chemical environment is defined largely by the nature of the electronic structure in the vicinity of

---

[*] There are systems where complete averaging of molecular position may not take place on a time scale rapid enough to average all orientations during the course of an NMR observation. Examples would be intact cells or cell membranes, viruses, and systems that exhibit liquid crystal behaviour.

the nucleus, that is, the number of electrons and type(s) of chemical bonds that link the observed nucleus to a molecule. However, electrons in more distant parts of the molecule, in solvent, or in other solute molecules that may be present also have an effect. Thus the conditions for resonance depend on the details of molecular structure and on factors such as the nature of the solvent, solute concentration(s), temperature, and pressure.

This dependence of the resonance frequency on conditions for a particular nucleus in a molecule and on the chemical nature and environment of the molecule is quantified by the chemical shift. Chemical-shift effects are characterized by a shielding parameter, usually symbolized by $\sigma$. The shielding parameter is dimensionless, and since it is of an order of magnitude $1 \times 10^{-6}$, it is stated in terms of parts per million (ppm). Differences in shielding parameter are the reasons for the range of proton signals observed, for example, in the proton NMR spectrum of a protein or nucleic acid.

The values for shielding parameters in the absence of tertiary structure for each of the nuclei present in the amino-acid or nucleoside subunits of a protein or nucleic acid have long been established.[28] As tertiary structures of proteins or nucleic acids form, water is excluded from between subunits, and many close contacts between subunits develop. The new local interactions are highly structure specific, and the result is that the shielding parameter for, say, a valine methyl group in one part of the protein becomes different from the shielding parameter for the same kind of methyl group located in another part of the protein. In the case of valine methyls, the differences in proton shielding parameters due to tertiary structure may be as large as ±2 ppm.

Aromatic ring current effects and the electronic anisotropies associated with the peptide group and other covalent structures in a protein appear to be the major sources of tertiary structure-specific proton shielding changes in proteins.[29,30] The same factors are important in the proton NMR spectra of nucleic acids although, because of their covalent nature and the kinds of conformations adopted, ring current effects from the heterocyclic bases are more strongly felt by the protons in the hydrogen bonds between base pairs.[31-34]

The carbon, nitrogen, and phosphorus nuclei in molecules are surrounded by more electrons than hydrogen. The shielding parameters for these nuclei are thus larger than those of hydrogen, and are much more sensitive to the details of tertiary structure. The range of values for the shielding parameters of the peptide (NH) protons in proteins is about 5 ppm, while the range of $^{15}N$ shielding parameters for the corresponding $^{15}NH$ positions is about 50 ppm.

The high sensitivity of the shielding parameter to the details of tertiary structure means that, at least in principle, each proton, carbon or nitrogen, within a protein or nucleic acid should give rise to a distinct, characteristic

NMR signal. For small proteins and oligonucleotides, this is often the case, and one thereby has a large number of "observation ports" through which to obtain information about structure and dynamics. As molecular size increases, however, two considerations conspire to make it more difficult to take advantage experimentally of the wealth of chemical-shift information present in an NMR spectrum. Increasing molecular size means that there must be more subunits (amino acids or nucleotides) present, and therefore there will be more signals in a spectrum. Further, as molecules become larger, they move more slowly in solution with the result, mentioned before, that transverse NMR relaxation becomes more efficient. More rapid relaxation means that NMR lines become broader. For both reasons, resolving signals from specific nuclei of a biopolymer becomes more difficult as molecular weight increases.

For studies of tertiary structure by NMR, one must be able to resolve and assign all or most of the proton signals from the molecule of interest, yet it is proton-shielding parameters that have the smallest range. A variety of experiments have been designed that allow the greater range of shielding parameters for carbon-13 and nitrogen-15 to be utilized in accomplishing this task, and with currently available magnetic fields it is usually possible to assign most of the proton signals from a monomeric protein of about 22 kDa[23] or a nucleic acid fragment of about 15 bp.

Binding of molecules to a protein or nucleic acid receptor often produces a change in shielding parameters for the spins of the molecule as a result of the change in environment. Ligands free in solution experience interactions with the electrons and nuclei of solvent molecules that are interrupted and changed on a time scale defined by the strengths of these interactions, the strengths of interactions between solvent molecules, and solution variables such as temperature. When the ligands enter a receptor-binding site, a variety of new interactions with the atoms of the receptor site is developed; these interactions are modulated on a different time scale, which depends on the rate of dissociation of the complex and the motions of the complex. While it cannot be guaranteed that a change in chemical shielding parameter will accompany binding of a ligand to a receptor, this is usually the case, particularly when the shielding parameters of nuclei other than hydrogen are considered. In the absence of detectable changes in shielding parameter, binding may still be detectable through NMR experiments that measure nuclear spin relaxation times, since these are sensitive to the time scales of molecular motions and interactions.

## B   SCALAR COUPLING

Scalar coupling produces fine structure in an NMR spectrum and arises because the NMR behaviour of a given spin can be influenced by the presence of other nuclear spins. The effect is quantitated by means of a scalar coupling constant $J$, which has units of Hertz. The primary mechanism for scalar or $J$ coupling involves transmission of information about nuclear spin orientations through electron spins. The effect is therefore an intramolecular one and is critically dependent on the details of the stereoelectronic structure of molecules. The magnitude of the coupling constant $J$, depends on the number of chemical bonds that intervene between the spin being observed and that which is coupling to it, as well as the number of electrons surrounding each of the coupling partners. The magnitudes of scalar coupling constants for nuclei directly bonded to each other (a one-bond coupling) are large and typically become negligible for nuclei that are separated by more than four bonds. Scalar coupling between carbon-13 or nitrogen-15 and a proton in $^{13}CH$ or $^{15}NH$ groups is typically 125–160 and 80–90 Hz, respectively, while the magnitude of $J$ for coupling between two protons in a methylene ($CH_2$) group, a two-bond coupling, is 10–16 Hz.

Of particular significance for studies of three-dimensional structures by NMR is the variation of three-bond coupling constants with the dihedral angle between them. For example, in the CH–CH fragment, the coupling constant between the two protons varies from about 10, to about 2, to about 12 Hz when the dihedral angle between the C–H bonds is changed from 0 to 90 or 180°, respectively. Importantly, this variation is qualitatively observed for other types of nuclei connected by three bonds, and three-bond carbon–proton, carbon–carbon, and nitrogen–proton coupling constants can also convey dihedral angle information.

Determination of three-bond coupling constants can be a powerful means of defining the conformation of a ligand in the bound and unbound state.[35] Unfortunately, as molecular size increases, it becomes increasingly difficult to resolve the fine structure created by three-bond coupling, so that this parameter cannot be obtained simply by inspection of a one-dimensional (1D) NMR spectrum. More elaborate experiments, including $J$-resolved two-dimensional experiments,[36] consideration of the shapes of cross-peaks in two-dimensional coherence transfer experiments,[38] or analysis of three-dimensional heteronuclear results[39,40] may make this information available.

The effects of scalar coupling — the fine structure that such coupling produces in an NMR spectrum — can be removed from a spectrum by a process known as decoupling. The technical details of how decoupling is accomplished vary with the nature of the spin being observed and the spin(s) being decoupled. While a spectrum obtained with decoupling will lack information about scalar coupling constants, information about shielding parameters is retained. Such loss of information can, in fact, often be desirable; for example, carbon-13 spectra of biopolymers are hopelessly complicated by the effects of one-bond $J$ coupling between carbon and hydrogen because the corresponding coupling constants are so large that fine structure from different carbons of the molecule is strongly interdigitated. When the proton–carbon coupling is removed by decoupling, the carbon spectrum is reduced to a series of singlets, each positioned according to the shielding parameter of a specific carbon nucleus of the molecule. It does not remove the coupling, which is fundamentally dependent on the electronic structure of the molecule being examined.

## C   SPIN–LATTICE ($T_1$) RELAXATION

The discussion which follows will consider only the behaviour of spin 1/2 nuclei such as $^1H$, $^3H$, $^{13}C$, $^{15}N$, $^{19}F$, and $^{31}P$. We focus initially on a small collection of such nuclei, say, all the protons in a small molecule. When placed in a magnetic field, each spin in this collection must take up one of the two allowed orientations for spin 1/2 particles in this situation. Each orientation has associated with it an energy of interaction with the field and, given a system of $n$ spin 1/2 nuclei, there will thus be created $2^n$ possible energy states for the system. An NMR sample consists of a very large number of such molecules or systems. After the sample comes to equilibrium in the magnetic field, the Boltzmann distribution law will apply and the number of molecules found in each of the possible energy states will depend on (1) the number of molecules present, (2) the energy differences between the states, (3) the sample temperature, and (4) the value of the magnetic field. When the sample is at equilibrium, there is only one set of populations that satisfies the Boltzmann law.

Outside the magnet of an NMR instrument, a sample is at equilibrium in the earth's magnetic field. Just after being placed in the much stronger magnetic field of a spectrometer, the sample is not at equilibrium, since the magnetic field that the nuclei experience is now different. Moreover, application of energy to the sample in the form of rf pulses during the course of an experiment may alter the numbers of molecules in some or all of the allowed molecular states. In nature, the spontaneous direction of change is, of course, toward equilibrium and, regardless of how the sample in the spectrometer attained a nonequilibrium condition, when left alone the numbers of molecules in each state will change until the correct numbers, as defined by Boltzmann's law, are present. To get the correct state populations, molecules may have to convert from one allowed energy state to another by either losing or gaining energy. The sink for the energy that must be transferred in these processes has its source in the surroundings of the sample; this is typically called the lattice.

The processes that transfer energy back and forth between the lattice and the spin systems of a sample, so that the correct populations for equilibrium are present, are known collectively as spin–lattice relaxation. Experimentally it is usually observed that spin–lattice relaxation follows a first-order rate law; the rate constant for the process is usually symbolized as $R_1$ (referred to as the spin–lattice relaxation rate) and has units of $s^{-1}$.

It is also common to describe the rate constant for spin–lattice relaxation in terms of the reciprocal of $R_1$ ($1/R_1 = T_1$), which has units of seconds and is referred to as the spin–lattice relaxation time $T_1$. Because spin–lattice relaxation can depend on a number of structure-specific interactions and on the details of molecular motions, the $T_1$ associated with each spin in a biopolymer may be different. A more detailed consideration shows that each line in a multiplet (fine structure) that arises from scalar coupling may have a different $T_1$ value.[41]

Compared to other spectroscopic experiments such as fluorescence or infrared, the time scale for spin–lattice relaxation in NMR is slow. For many protein and nucleic acid systems, spin–lattice relaxation times fall in the range 0.1–10 s. A rule of thumb is that a time equal to about $5 \times T_1$ is needed for a spin to come to equilibrium, so that the time scale for complete spin–lattice relaxation in a protein or nucleic acid is seconds to, perhaps, minutes.

A standard 1D NMR spectrum, obtained with a sample that was at thermal equilibrium before the experiment that produced the spectrum began, contains no information about $T_1$ relaxation, and more complex experiments are needed to obtain values for spin–lattice relaxation times.

## D   Transverse ($T_2$) Relaxation

As discussed above, spin–lattice relaxation is basically an enthalpic process: energy flows into and out of spin systems of the sample until the collection of molecules comes to thermal equilibrium, as defined by the Boltzmann populations. That equilibrium is a dynamic one; molecules are continually interconverting between allowed states, even after the correct numbers of molecules in each state have been achieved. The Boltzmann distribution law only tells us what the average populations of these states will be at equilibrium.

Some rf pulses can also exert an entropic effect on the sample in that they can create a situation in which the spin systems of molecules in the sample are more organized than is the case when the sample is at equilibrium. These pulses can cause all or some of the spins to move in a coherent fashion as they precess around the direction of the magnetic field in which the sample resides. Such coherence or organization of spin motions is temporary, since at equilibrium the sample is in a state of maximum disorder (entropy). After an rf pulse is turned off, any coherence it created starts to dissipate spontaneously as the system comes back to equilibrium.

The loss of coherence in the motion(s) of spins is a kind of relaxation, but it is not like spin–lattice relaxation. Loss of coherence is loss of order within a collection of spins, and is a process that need not obligatorily involve the transfer of energy into or out of individual spin systems. Loss of spin coherence is called spin–spin relaxation or transverse relaxation. Experimentally it is observed that loss of coherence is also a first-order process and, by analogy to the practice used for spin–lattice relaxation, spin–spin relaxation is described by a spin–spin relaxation rate $R_2$, or a spin–spin relaxation time $T_2 = 1/R_2$.

If there are no other means for loss of spin coherence, the width at half-maximum height, $w_{1/2}$, observed for a signal in an NMR spectrum, is given by

$$w_{1/2} = \frac{R_2}{\pi} \tag{1}$$

Unfortunately, loss of spin coherence in a sample can also take place because the magnetic field in which the experiment is done is not perfect. It is not technically possible to create an experimental situation where the magnetic field experienced by the sample is exactly the same in all parts of the sample. Such inhomogeneity produces an experimental effect that is the same as spin–spin relaxation. The width at half-maximum height $w_{1/2}$ observed for a signal in an NMR spectrum is thus given by Equation (2), where the term $\Delta w$ represents the effects field of inhomogeneities.

$$w_{1/2} = \frac{R_2}{\pi} + \Delta w = \frac{1}{\pi T_2} + \Delta w \tag{2}$$

Field inhomogeneity effects can also be expressed in terms of an effective spin–spin relaxation time, $T_2^*$, which is understood to express both the effects of true transverse relaxation $T_2$ and the loss of coherence due to field inhomogeneities $1/T_2^* = 1/T_2 + \pi \Delta w$).

For small molecules, it is generally found that the field inhomogeneity term of Equation (2) is competitive with or larger than the term involving $T_2$. Depending on the value of the magnetic field and the size of the molecule under examination, the field inhomogeneity term can be negligible relative to the $T_2$ term in experiments with proteins and nucleic acids.

Chemical reactions of the species holding the spin under observation can also provide another means by which spin coherence is lost. Thus, processes that convert a species into one with a different structure, conformation, or environment can also lead to broadening of the observed signal. The effects of such chemical reactions or exchange processes are considered in more detail below.

The exchanges of energy that result in $T_1$ relaxation can be accompanied by loss of coherence, so that spin–lattice relaxation may be accompanied by $T_2$ relaxation. Since loss of coherence can also take place by several means, experimentally observed spin–spin relaxation with biological macromolecules is more rapid than spin–lattice relaxation.

## E   NUCLEAR OVERHAUSER EFFECTS

An NMR experiment must at some point produce magnetic effects that are detectable instrumentally. Usually, one or more pulses of rf energy applied to the sample are used to accomplish this. The intensities with which a given signal appears in a spectrum depend on the populations of molecules in the allowed nuclear spin energy states immediately before the analyzing rf pulse is applied. In the simplest instance, these populations are the Boltzmann populations, characteristic of the system at thermal equilibrium. Under these conditions, the signals observed are proportional to the number of spins present, and the relative intensities of signals from various chemically different groups of spins of a molecule are proportional to the relative numbers of spins of each type.

In a variety of circumstances, including an experimental design more complex than the application of a single rf pulse to the sample, the numbers of molecules in some or all of the permitted nuclear energy states may be different from those that are characteristic of thermal equilibrium. In this event, the intensity of a signal observed in the spectrum will be changed. The change in a signal's intensity as the result of perturbation applied to spins other than those associated with that signal is called a nuclear Overhauser effect, or NOE. There are several ways of expressing the NOE quantitatively. We shall use the equation $f_I\{S\} = I_p/I_0 - 1$ for this purpose. In this equation the symbol $f_I\{S\}$ indicates the NOE (or fractional intensity change) on the signal from spin $I$ when there is a perturbation of population levels associated with spin $S$; $I_0$ is the normal intensity of the signal for spin $I$ observed from a sample at thermal equilibrium, while $I_p$ is the intensity of the same signal when there has been a perturbation of the $S$ spins in the sample.

It is also possible to create Overhauser effects through interactions between various coherences formed as the result of the application of rf pulses to the sample.[42] These experiments, called rotating frame NOEs or ROEs, exhibit a different dependence on molecular motion than the NOEs described above. The NOE and ROE experimental results are thus complementary.

It should be apparent that the nuclear Overhauser effect is strongly related to spin–lattice relaxation and, in the case of the ROE, to transverse relaxation as well. Since relaxation processes will resist the effects of a perturbation applied to the sample, which is aimed at altering the thermal populations of the various spin states, the formation and disappearance of the NOE will be time dependent. The formation of the ROE is also time dependent and must compete with the decay of spin coherence by transverse relaxation.

The utility of the NOE is that the bulk of the interactions that lead to $T_1$ and $T_2$ relaxation are dependent on the distance between interacting spins. Thus studies of NOEs and ROEs can provide internuclear distance information about a ligand, a receptor or nucleic acid, or a ligand–receptor complex.

---

# VIII  PROCESSES LEADING TO RELAXATION

Values for $T_1$ and $T_2$ relaxation times depend on two factors: the strength of time-varying magnetic fields and the details of how these fields change with time relative to the spin under observation. Effective spin–lattice and spin–spin relaxation of individual spins and spin systems in a sample require that there be present, near or within the spin systems, fluctuating magnetic fields that vary their orientations with frequencies similar to the frequencies associated with NMR transitions. Relaxation of a carbon-13 nucleus in a $^{13}C-H$ fragment in a magnetic field of 11.75 $T$, for example, will be most efficient when there are magnetic fields near the carbon nucleus that change their orientations relative to the carbon-13 spin at about 125 million and 500 million times per second (125 and 500 MHz, respectively).*

Most NMR studies of ligand–receptor interactions involve observations of spin 1/2 nuclei. An important relaxation mechanism is the magnetic dipole–magnetic dipole interaction that takes place between pairs of such spins. The local magnetic field experienced by any particular spin in a sample will be defined not only by the laboratory field in which the sample is placed, but also by microscopic fields due to nearby spins. Thus, the field experienced by the carbon-13 nucleus in the $^{13}C-H$ fragment mentioned will be the sum of the laboratory field, the field due to the attached $^1H$, and any fields due to nearby nuclear spins. Because molecules jiggle about in solutions, local fields from the proton and the nearby spins will change with time, and if the motions of the molecules are on the right time scale, their local dipolar fields will contribute to the relaxation of the carbon-13 spin.

A model of molecular motion in solution is needed to produce a mathematical treatment of the dipole–dipole relaxation interactions. The simplest view is that (1) the spin of interest and all spins that have interactions producing relaxation are present within one molecule (i.e., all dipole–dipole interactions are intramolecular); (2) the molecule can be represented by a sphere; (3) all spins rigidly retain their relative orientations within the sphere; and (4) the motion of the sphere can be described by the classical Debye–Stokes–Einstein theory for the behaviour of viscous

---

* A more detailed analysis shows that fields with frequencies of variation at 375 MHz (500 − 125) and 625 MHz (500 + 125) also contribute to relaxation. The point at present is to establish the time scale for motions that lead to relaxation.

fluids. The conclusion of a theory based on this set of assumptions is that a molecule of volume $V$ in a fluid of viscosity $\eta$ at temperature $T$ will reorient because of collisions with solvent molecules such that any given orientation of the sphere, on average, will persist for a time $\tau_c$ before it jumps to a new orientation. The parameter $\tau_c$ is called the correlation time. The connection between these variables is given by the equation

$$\tau_c = \frac{V\eta}{kT} = \frac{4\pi r^3 \eta}{3kT} \tag{3}$$

where $k$ is Boltzmann's constant and $r$ is the radius of the sphere that has volume $V$.

The equation is consistent with the expectation that a large molecule will maintain a particular orientation in solution longer than a small molecule. The predicted increase in correlation time as the viscosity of the sample increases is observed experimentally, as is a decrease in correlation time when a sample is warmed. Estimates for $\tau_c$ are available from dielectric relaxation, fluorescence, NMR, and ESR experiments[43] and typically agree with the order of magnitude predicted by Equation (3). As a rough rule of thumb, the correlation time for molecules in typical solvents near room temperature is about $10^{-12} \times M_w$, where $M_w$ is the molecular mass expressed in Da.

The model used to arrive at Equation (3) is clearly nonsensical, since few molecules are spherical and most have several conformations available because of rotation around chemical bonds. This model is, however, a reasonable first approximation for the dynamics of globular proteins. For molecules entrained in a membrane or for nucleic acids of dimensions more than about 10 bp, the molecules are not shaped like a sphere or do not move like a sphere, and the model described is much less appropriate for them. In these cases, the mathematical descriptions of the molecular motions that lead to relaxation are more complex and will be described in terms of additional parameters.

In the case of just two spins, $I$ and $S$, where spin $I$ is observed and spin $S$ leads to relaxation of spin $I$, spin–lattice relaxation and transverse relaxation rates are given by Equations (4) and (5). The symbols $\omega_I$ and $\omega_S$ are the resonance frequencies for the $I$ and $S$ spins, $\gamma_I$ and $\gamma_S$ are the gyromagnetic ratios for these spins, $r_{IS}$ is the distance between them, and $\hbar$ is Planck's constant divided by $2\pi$. It should be noted that $\omega_I$ and $\omega_S$ depend on the laboratory magnetic field used to do an experiment. The expressions for $1/T_1$ and $1/T_2$

$$\frac{1}{T_1} = \frac{1}{10} \frac{\gamma_I^2 \gamma_S^2 \hbar^2}{r_{IS}^6} \tau_c \left[ \frac{3}{1+\omega_I^2 \tau_c^2} + \frac{1}{1+\left(\omega_I - \omega_S\right)^2 \tau_c^2} + \frac{6}{1+\left(\omega_I + \omega_S\right)^2 \tau_c^2} \right] \tag{4}$$

$$\frac{1}{T_2} = \frac{1}{20} \frac{\gamma_I^2 \gamma_S^2 \hbar^2}{r_{IS}^6}$$

$$\tau_c \left[ \frac{1}{1+\left(\omega_I - \omega_S\right)^2 \tau_c^2} + \frac{3}{1+\omega_I^2 \tau_c^2} + \frac{6}{1+\omega_S^2 \tau_c^2} + \frac{6}{1+\left(\omega_I + \omega_S\right)^2 \tau_c^2} + 4 \right] \quad (5)$$

show that spin–lattice and transverse relaxation are independent of magnetic field when the molecules under study are small and, therefore, have small rotational correlation times $\tau_c$. For macromolecular drug receptors, the correlation times are such that spin–lattice and transverse relaxation are dependent on the magnetic field chosen for an experiment.

Equations (4) and (5) are derived under the assumption that $I$ and $S$ have different gyromagnetic ratios. When this is not the case, or when the signals for $I$ and $S$ are not resolved, the equations describing relaxation are somewhat different.[44] In formulating the equations, it has also been assumed that there is no spin coupling between $I$ and $S$; the presence of spin coupling appreciably complicates the equations and may have a nonnegligible effect on relaxation.[45,46]

There is often more than one dipolar interaction producing relaxation of observed spin $I$. In the first approximation, the contributions of each interaction present, calculated according to the above equations, can be merely summed together to get the total effect on spin $I$. A more rigorous treatment requires consideration of the dipolar interactions between *all* spins of the spin system that includes the observed spin, and the degree to which the motions of these spins are correlated with one another.[47-49]

Equations (4) and (5) provide the important information that the dipole–dipole contributions to $T_1$ and $T_2$ relaxation depend strongly on internuclear distances. As shown in Figure 2, the $1/r^6$ distance dependence in these equations causes the effects of a relaxation interaction to decrease very rapidly as internuclear distances increase. The drop-off is so steep that dipole–dipole interactions for effective relaxation of a spin are basically provided only by the nearest neighbours, those spins 2–4 Å away. Provided that knowledge of $\tau_c$ is available, experiments to evaluate dipole–dipole relaxation contributions thus have the potential to provide information about the distances between pairs of spins in a three-dimensional structure.

A useful case of dipole–dipole spin relaxation arises when the interacting spin $S$ is not a nuclear but an electron spin. The magnetic dipole associated with an unpaired electron spin is 658 times larger than the magnetic dipole of the proton. The result is that dipole–dipole interaction with an unpaired electron is a potent mechanism for nuclear spin relaxation, the impact of the electron spin being dependent on the distance

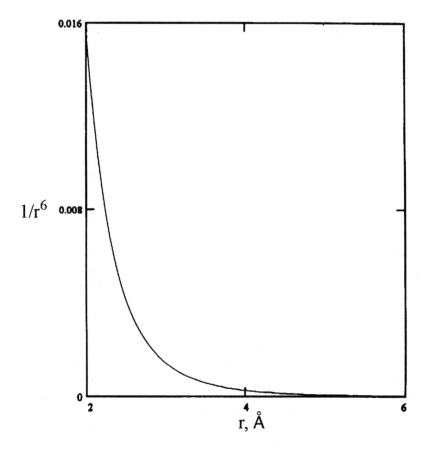

**FIGURE 2**
A plot of $1/r^6$ vs. $r$. For calibration purposes, it may be noted that carbon–hydrogen bonds are 1.1 Å long and the distance of closest approach of two covalently bound hydrogen atoms is about 2.4 Å.

between the observed nuclear spin and the electron. Unpaired electron spins may be present in a particular system in the form of paramagnetic metal ions, nitroxide "spin labels", or other paramagnetic species.*

The especially potent ability of unpaired electron spins to relax nuclear spins has been used in experiments designed to explore protein surfaces[50] and to determine the parts of protein-bound ligands that are exposed to solvent.[51] The cartoon in Figure 3 indicates the physical basis for these

---

* The most common source of unpaired electrons in NMR samples is dissolved (paramagnetic) oxygen and trace transition metal ions. Care should be taken to exclude these species when reliable data for nuclear spin-nuclear spin diplor interactions are desired.

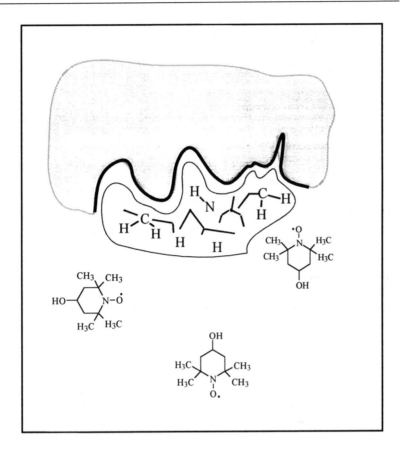

**FIGURE 3**
Identification of solvent-exposed nuclear spins in a drug–receptor complex by means of paramagnetic species present in the solution. In this cartoon the paramagnetic species is the stable nitroxide radical 4-hydroxy-2,2,6,6-tetramethylpiperidinyl-1-oxy.

experiments. A receptor site, indicated by the darker shaded area, interacts with a ligand molecule (lighter area), which is composed of a group of nuclear spins held together by a network of chemical bonds. The spins involved will certainly be protons but may also be carbon-13 or nitrogen-15, or other spin 1/2 nuclei. The unpaired electron of the stable nitroxide shown (4-hydroxy-2,2,6,6-tetramethylpiperidinyl-1-oxy) in the solution can approach those spins on the exterior surface of the ligand but, presuming that the ligand–receptor complex is long lived enough, not those on the interior surface. The unpaired electron spin of the nitroxide moiety will selectively increase the spin–lattice and transverse relaxation rates of those nuclei to which it can come close, thus identifying the portions of the ligand molecule exposed to the solution.

A second mechanism for spin–lattice and spin–spin relaxation that is becoming increasingly important in NMR studies of ligands and their receptors is relaxation due to the anisotropy of chemical shielding. The magnetic field experienced by a spin in a molecule depends on the electronic structure of the molecule and the ease with which the electrons of the molecule move when placed in a magnetic field. Movement of the electrons is more facile in some orientations than in others. Thus, the chemical-shielding parameter $\sigma$ is anisotropic, and the value observed for a particular spin in a specific molecule depends on how the molecule is situated in the magnetic field.

Because molecular motions in fluids are fast, solute molecules rapidly take up all possible orientations. While the experimentally observed shielding parameter is thus an averaged value, in the process of that averaging, the spin being observed experiences a magnetic field that varies randomly with time. Depending on the details of molecular motion and the magnitude of the anisotropy of the shielding, these variations of the field are sufficient to produce relaxation. Equations (6) and (7) show the contribution of chemical shift anisotropy (CSA) to spin–lattice relaxation under certain conditions. It should be noted that these relaxation effects depend on the anisotropy of the shielding, characterized by the parameters $\sigma_\parallel$ and $\sigma_\perp$, and also on $B_0^2$, the square of the spectrometer magnetic field. The anisotropy of the shielding parameter $(\sigma_\parallel - \sigma_\perp)$ will roughly depend on the number of electrons that surround the nucleus under consideration. Thus, the shielding anisotropy of $^1$H is relatively small, at most about 5 ppm, while the anisotropies of heavier elements such as $^{13}$C and $^{15}$N are as large as 300 ppm.[52] It is the $B_0^2$ factor that explains why considerations of the CSA contribution to relaxation cannot be neglected in many contemporary studies. Proton NMR experiments at 1000 MHz ($B_0 = 23\,T$) will soon be feasible, and at this frequency CSA effects will be about nine times larger than those experienced when the experiment is done at 300 MHz. Moreover, detailed consideration of the dipole–dipole and CSA relaxation mechanisms shows that interactions between them can produce observed $T_1$ and $T_2$ effects, even when the CSA mechanism alone is negligibly small.[53-55]

$$\frac{1}{T_1} = \frac{2}{15}\left(\sigma_\parallel - \sigma_\perp\right)^2 \gamma^2 B_0^2 \tau_c \; \frac{1}{\left(1 + \omega^2 \tau_c^2\right)} \tag{6}$$

$$\frac{1}{T_2} = \frac{1}{15}\left(\sigma_\parallel - \sigma_\perp\right)^2 \gamma^2 B_0^2 \tau_c \left(\frac{2}{3} + \frac{1}{2}\frac{1}{\left(1 + \omega^2 \tau_c^2\right)}\right) \tag{7}$$

# IX CHEMICAL-EXCHANGE EFFECTS

The equilibrium dissociation constant for the interaction of a ligand with a receptor is the result of the difference in the free energy of the system when the ligand and receptor are separated and the free energy when the complex between the two has formed. However, the interaction of a ligand with a binding site also depends on time. It is possible that several conformations of the free ligand are present, and it is only one of these that is able to bind to the receptor. There may be only one of several conformations of the receptor that is able to bind the ligand well. There may be several possible structures for the ligand–receptor complex, and these may be interconvertible. The act of entering the binding site is clearly a time-dependent process. There are many examples where binding is a slow event because the ligand (and the receptor) explore many structures and interactions before the one of lowest energy is found. The dissociation constant does not provide information about the rate at which complexes are formed, nor the rate of conformational or structural changes before, during, or after formation of the complex. However, the rates of these various processes can be critical to what is observed during an NMR study of the ligand–receptor interaction. The dependence of observable NMR phenomena on time-dependent processes in the sample must at least be considered in making interpretations of NMR data, and may be the source of information about the rates of these processes.

It is difficult to discuss succinctly the influence of chemical exchange processes on NMR experiments. In many cases, an adequate understanding of these influences in a particular experiment may require detailed computer modelling. In most of the discussion that follows, in order to provide some qualitative understanding of the nature of such effects, chemical or structural changes will be assumed to interconvert two different configurations of a molecule in the sample. This situation would correspond, for example, to a ligand interconverting between a state in which it is free in solution and one in which it interacts with the binding site of a receptor. For actuality's sake, it will be supposed that the spin under observation in a particular experiment is attached to the ligand. However, binding of ligand to a receptor could potentially be followed by observation of signals from nuclei attached to the receptor, and the considerations discussed would be the same for either kind of experiment.

## A  LINESHAPES

Assume that a spin of the ligand gives rise to a signal in an NMR spectrum at a position $\delta_F$ in the absence of receptor. Scalar coupling to the spin will be assumed to be absent, so $\delta_F$ depends only on the shielding parameter $\sigma_F$ for the nucleus under observation. When the ligand becomes complexed to a protein or other macromolecule, the spin will experience a change of local environment and, thus, will likely experience a change in shielding parameter. Therefore, the signal for the bound ligand should appear at a different position in the spectrum $\delta_B$. When the binding process is slow, that is, when the rate of exchange of the ligand between the receptor-bound and free states is slow, then two signals are observed, one at $\delta_F$ and one at $\delta_B$. The relative intensities of these signals depend on the fraction of molecules that, at equilibrium, is in the bound state $X_B$ and the fraction that remains free of the receptor $X_F$. However, the appearance of the spectrum when exchange between free and bound states is not slow depends heavily on the rate of exchange.

Theoretical descriptions of the effects of exchange on NMR spectra are readily available and are the basis for computer programs that can provide simulations of NMR lineshapes or other NMR phenomena.[56] Figure 4 shows computed spectra for the equilibrium

$$B \underset{k_{FB}}{\overset{k_{BF}}{\rightleftharpoons}} F \tag{8}$$

when the amounts of the two interconvertible species $F$ and $B$ present in the sample are equal and the linewidths of both species are the same. When the rate of conversion of $F$ to $B$ is slow ($k_{FB}$ is small), the spectrum consists of the expected two lines of equal intensity, with widths corresponding to the widths of the $F$ and $B$ signals in the absence of exchange. When the interconversion process is faster, the signals for $F$ and $B$ are broadened, and when the exchange rate is fast enough, the signal positions are shifted toward each other. At a certain rate, the resonances for $F$ and $B$ have broadened and shifted to such an extent that they merge to a single line. Even faster exchange leads to sharpening of the single (averaged) line until, at very fast exchange of $F$ and $B$, the signal appears at the average position $\delta_{OBS}$.

$$\delta_{OBS} = X_B\delta_B + X_F\delta_F \tag{9}$$

When equal amounts of free and bound ligand molecules are present and the line-widths of both the free and bound forms are the same, algebraic expressions relating characteristics of the spectrum (peak separation, linewidth) to the rate constant $k_{FB}$ for conversion of the free-ligand molecules to receptor bound can be written (Reference 15, Chapter 6). For the equal-concentrations case, there will be a rate of interchange where the separate lines for free and bound species are no longer discernible. This

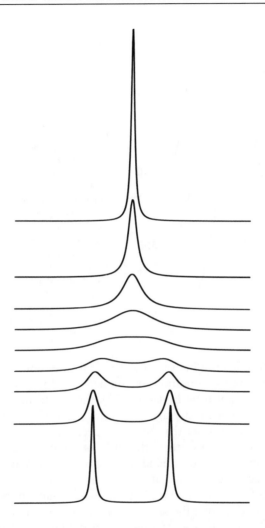

**FIGURE 4**
Computed NMR spectra for sample of two species undergoing interchange during the course of the NMR experiment. For this example, the amounts of the two species are equal and their linewidths at half-maximum peak height $w_{1/2}$, are the same (5 Hz). Each plot is 300 Hz wide and the chemical shift difference between the two signals is 100 Hz. The left signal is arbitrarily assigned to the free ligand molecule $F$; from top to bottom, the rate constants for change of free ligand to bound ligand $k_{FB}$ are 10,000, 2000, 667, 333, 222, 133, 67, 33 and 0.33 s$^{-1}$, respectively.

is the so-called coalescence rate and is given by Equation (10). Here, $\Delta$ is the

$$k_{FB} = \frac{\pi\Delta}{\sqrt{2}}$$

(10)

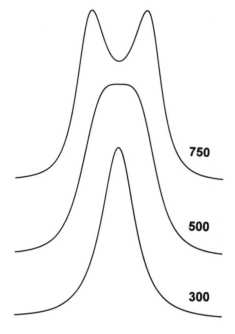

**FIGURE 5**
Magnetic-field dependence of a sample of two exchanging species present at equal concentrations. The signals for each are separated by 0.5 ppm and their linewidth in the absence of exchange was 3 Hz. In all cases the rate constant for conversion of one species to the other was 555 s$^{-1}$. Each plot is 1 ppm wide. It was assumed that the sample was observed at 750, 500, and 300 MHz, respectively. Magnetic-field dependence for the transverse relaxation times of the two species was neglected for these calculations. The vertical scale is arbitrary for the plots.

chemical shift difference between the signals for free and bound ligand *in units of Hertz*. For the conditions mentioned, if the rate constant is larger than the number given by Equation (10), the spectrum will consist of a single line centred at the averaged chemical shifts of the free and bound ligand, and if $k_{BF}$ is smaller than this, the spectrum will show two signals, though not necessarily exactly at the shifts of the free and bound ligand.

It is important to bear in mind that the parameter $\Delta$ in Equation (10) depends on the magnetic field at which a spectrum is obtained. Figure 5 shows spectra for a system consisting of equal amounts of both exchange partners with both having the same linewidth $w_{1/2}$. The rate of exchange is identical in all three spectra. At a high magnetic field, corresponding to a 750-MHz spectrometer in the example, the spectrum exhibits two peaks; at the lowest field (300 MHz), the spectrum is a single line, and at the intermediate field (500 MHz), the system is exactly at the coalescence rate. One often hears the expression "the NMR time scale" in discussions of rate effects in an NMR spectrum. The calculated spectra in Figure 5 show that this phrase has little meaning unless the shift difference in Hertz is specified.

When the ligand is bound to a receptor, it will likely tumble more slowly than when it is in free solution. Transverse $T_2$ relaxation will be more efficient in the complex, and the linewidth of the signal for the bound ligand will probably be substantially broader than that for the free ligand. Figure 6 shows computed NMR lineshapes for a situation identical to that used for the generation of Figure 4, except that the line for the bound species $B$ is five times broader than the line for the free species.

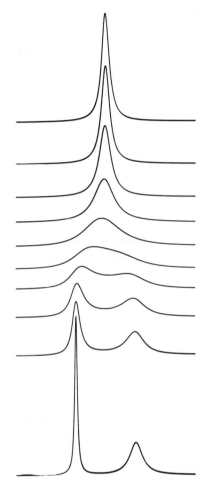

**FIGURE 6**
Computed NMR spectra for a sample of two species undergoing interchange during the course of the NMR experiment. The amounts of the two species are equal, but the left signal, assigned to the free ligand, has a width of 5 Hz, while the signal for the bound ligand has a width of 25 Hz. Each plot is 300 Hz wide and the chemical shift difference between the two signals is 100 Hz. The rate constants for change of free to bound ligand $k_{FB}$ are the same as those used in the simulations given in Figure 4 and, top to bottom, are 1,000,000, 10,000, 2000, 667, 333, 222, 133, 67, 33, and 0.33 s$^{-1}$, respectively. The vertical scale was the same for all plots.

Again, at a slow rate of interchange, separate signals for the free and bound species are expected, and as the exchange rate increases, these signals merge and eventually evolve into a single resonance. At fast exchange, the position of the average resonance is given by Equation (9); the signal width observed is the weighted average of the widths for the free, $w_{1/2}(F)$, and bound, $w_{1/2}(B)$, species in the absence of any exchange:

$$w_{1/2}(OBS) = X_F w_{1/2}(F) + X_B w_{1/2}(B) \tag{11}$$

Inhomogeneity of the magnetic field has been neglected in Equation (11) but will add to the observed linewidth, as indicated in Equation (2).

As a result of the differences in widths of lines merged by the exchange process, the spectra near the coalescence point are decidedly asymmetric.

This asymmetry could easily be masked by baseline noise in a real experiment, or by maladjustment of the phasing parameters when processing experimental results. It is essential when dealing with spectra with broad lines to ensure that sufficient baseline is plotted so that the nature of the experimental lineshape can be judged, especially when exchange may be influencing lineshape.

The appearance of the spectrum for a system between the slow and fast exchange limits depends, in perhaps unexpected ways, on the amounts of free and bound ligand present. Figure 7 shows spectra for a system in which 10% of the ligand present is bound to the receptor. For these calculations, the linewidths of both the free and the bound ligand are the same, so the spectra can be compared to those in Figure 4. Note that, even at relatively slow rates of exchange, there is appreciable broadening of the signal for the bound ligand, while the signal for the free species, although also broadened at these exchange rates, is not broadened as much. At certain rates the signal for the bound species is so broad that it would not be likely to be detectable in the presence of the noise in a real spectrum. At these intermediate exchange rates, it would be quite reasonable to conclude that the spectrum, and the sample, consist of only a single species. It is only at fairly rapid exchange rates that the single observable signal shifts to the averaged position, as given by Equation (9), and narrows to the average linewidths, Equation (10). Possible misinterpretation of NMR spectra for systems that have unequal populations present and are in the intermediate-exchange regime has been discussed in more detail.[57,58]

There are algebraic expressions that give the line position and width of the spectrum of a system of two species undergoing exchange when the amount of one species is in large concentration excess, that is, for the present discussion, when $X_F \gg X_B$.[59] Comparison of the predictions of these equations with those of the exact theory indicate that they should be valid for ligand–receptor studies when $X_B$ is less than 0.2.[60] According to these results, the position of the observed resonance is shifted by the exchange process from the position of the resonance corresponding to the major species in the absence of exchange by the amount $s$ (in Hertz).

$$s = \frac{X_B k_{BF}^2 \Delta}{\left(\dfrac{1}{T_{2B}} + k_{BF}\right)^2 + \Delta^2} \tag{12}$$

In this equation, $k_{BF}$ is the rate constant for conversion of the bound form of the ligand to the free form, $T_{2B}$ is the transverse relaxation time for the spin observed in the bound ligand, and $\Delta$ has the same significance as earlier. For the shift in line position $s$ to be directly proportional to the

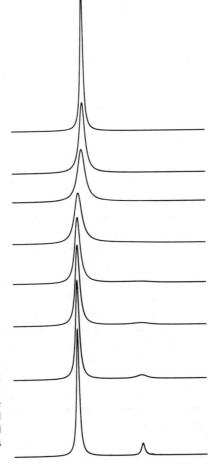

**FIGURE 7**

Computed NMR spectra for a sample of two species undergoing interchange during the course of the NMR experiment. For this example, the amounts of the two species are not equal although their linewidths at half-maximum peak height $w_{1/2}$, are the same (5 Hz). Each plot is 300 Hz wide, and the chemical shift difference between the two signals is 100 Hz. The left signal is assigned to the free ligand molecule $F$, which is present in ninefold excess over the amount of bound ligand, represented by the signal to the right. From top to bottom, the rate constants for change of free to bound ligand $k_{FB}$ are $1 \times 10^6$, 200, 100, 33, 17, 10, 5, and 0.33 s$^{-1}$, respectively. The vertical scale was the same for all plots.

amount of bound ligand present $X_B$, as is indicated by Equation (10), it is necessary that $k_{BF}$ be much greater than $\Delta$ and $1/T_{2B}$.

When $X_F \gg X_B$, the linewidth of the signal observed in the spectrum is given by

$$w_{1/2}\left(OBS\right) = \frac{1}{\pi T_2\left(OBS\right)} = \frac{1}{\pi T_{2F}} + \frac{X_B k_{BF}}{\pi X_F}\left[\frac{\dfrac{1}{T_{2B}}\left(\dfrac{1}{T_{2B}} + k_{BF}\right) + \Delta^2}{\left(\dfrac{1}{T_{2B}} + k_{BF}\right)^2 + \Delta^2}\right] \quad (13)$$

where $w_{1/2}(OBS)$ is the observed peak linewidth at half-maximum height. This equation shows that it is only when $k_{BF} \gg \Delta^2$ and $k_{BF} \gg 1/T_{2B}$ that the linewidth observed in the spectrum will be at the fast exchange limit given by Equation (11). As indicated by the calculated spectra in Figure 6 and Equations (12) and (13), the conditions for averaging of line positions in the case of a two-site exchange process are different from those that must obtain for averaging of the linewidths. The observed line will appear at the position that is the weighted average of the positions of the component species at a slower rate of exchange than that required to produce the average of the linewidths.

When a single, broadened line is observed in an NMR spectrum of a ligand–receptor system, it can be challenging to determine whether the line corresponds to a single species that (1) is influenced by a long rotational correlation time, (2) is experiencing some efficient pathway for transverse relaxation possibly involving the presence of a paramagnetic species near it, or (3) is involved in an exchange process in which one of the exchanging species is "silent" in the spectrum because of the rate of exchange or the relative amount that is present. Careful sample preparation can exclude factors such as paramagnetic species. Increasing the sample temperature would be expected to increase the rate of exchange processes and thereby narrow lines that are broadened by exchange. However, increasing sample temperature also has the effect of decreasing solution viscosity and decreasing the correlation time, as indicated in Equation (2), so interpretation of the observation of a narrowed line with increased temperature can be ambiguous. Another way to diagnose the influence of exchange on the appearance of a spectrum is to compare spectra taken at two or more magnetic field strengths; an increase in magnetic field should shift the spectrum toward the appearance of the slow-exchange limit spectrum. However, as shown in Equations (5) and (7), the dipole–dipole and CSA relaxation effects that define the intrinsic linewidths of NMR signals depend on magnetic field strength at the correlation times typical of drug receptors. Any changes in the exchange contributions to the experimental lineshape when the magnetic field is changed could be obscured by concomitant changes in intrinsic $T_2$ relaxation times.

Equations (9) and (11) give the expected averaged line position and linewidth for a two-site exchange under conditions of fast exchange. What is observed when the rate of interconversion is neither in the slow-exchange limit nor in the fast-exchange (averaged) limit depends on the difference between $\delta_B$ and $\delta_F$ (expressed in Hertz), the fraction of each species present ($X_B$, $X_F$), the transverse relaxation times of the free and bound spins, and the rate of interconversion. London[58] has provided expressions that may be useful in the analysis of certain situations in the intermediate-exchange region, but probably the easiest way to be certain of correctly predicting what is to be expected from a given combination of these variables is computer simulation.

When more than two species are involved in an exchange process, the observed NMR lineshape can become quite misleading. Computed spectra for a hypothetical example are shown in Figure 8. In this case, the exchange process is represented by the equilibria

$$F \underset{k_{B1F}}{\overset{k_{FB1}}{\rightleftarrows}} B1 \underset{k_{B21}}{\overset{k_{B12}}{\rightleftarrows}} B2 \tag{14}$$

This would correspond, for example, to the binding of free ligand $F$ with a receptor to give an initial complex $B1$, which then rearranges in some way to give the final complex $B2$.[*] As presented, it is not possible for $F$ to bind directly to give the complex $B2$, that is, $k_{FB2}$ is very small. It has been assumed for these calculations that the amounts of $F$ and $B2$ are equal, while 10% of the ligand is in the intermediate state $B_1$. The linewidths of all three species are the same, and the rates of conversion of $F$ to $B1$, characterized by the rate constant $k_{FB1}$, is equal to the rate of conversion of $B2$ to $B1$ ($k_{FB1} = k_{B21}$). When the rates of interconversion of $B1$ to $B2$ and of binding of $F$ to $B1$ are slow, the spectrum shows the expected three lines with intensities proportionate to the amounts indicated. At faster rates of interconversion, all signals show broadening due to the exchange process, but the signal corresponding to the intermediate broadens more than do the more intense lines, as would be anticipated from the behaviour illustrated in Figure 6. At some rate of exchange, the signal for the intermediate disappears from the spectrum, particularly if the baseline noise level is high enough, and the lines that remain suggest the spectrum of a *two-species* system at or near the slow-exchange regime. At more rapid rates of interchange, the two remaining lines broaden, coalesce, and then sharpen to give lineshapes similar to those for the standard two-site exchange situation illustrated in Figure 4. However, the rate constants that might be adduced by analysis of these spectra are not the rate constants that characterize the conversion of $F$ to $B2$, which remains slow for all the spectra shown in Figure 8, but are approximately the rate constants that correspond to the interconversion of $F$ to $B1$ and $B1$ to $B2$! The spectra, and their interpretation, would be even more mysterious if the linewidths for the three species were different and the rates of interconversion of $F$ to $B1$ and $B1$ to $B2$ were not identical. While this example is rather artificial, it serves to emphasize the points that complex exchange processes can give

---

[*] The model discussed could also correspond to a situation in which a minor conformation of the ligand is the one that binds to the receptor. The interconversion of $F$ to $B1$ in Equation (14) would then correspond to conversion of the dominant form of the ligand to the minor form, while the step taking $B1$ to $B2$ would correspond to interaction of the minor conformation with the receptor.

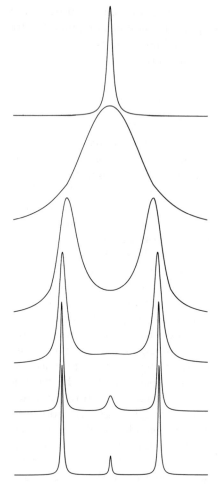

**FIGURE 8**
Computed NMR spectra for a sample of three species undergoing interchange during the course of the NMR experiment according to the equilibria given in Equation (14). For this example, the amounts of free $F$ and $B2$ species were equal, with the intermediate $B1$ species present to the extent of 10% of the mixture. The linewidths for all species were the same (5 Hz). The chemical shift difference between $F$ and $B1$ signals was 100 Hz, while the shift difference between $F$ and $B2$ was 200 Hz; each spectrum was 400 Hz wide. From top to bottom, the rate constants $k_{FB1}$, for conversion of $F$ to $B1$, and $k_{B21}$, for conversion of $B2$ to $B1$, were 12,700, 1000, 220, 44, 5.6, and $4 \times 10^{-7}$, respectively. The vertical scales for the plots were arbitrary.

apparently simple spectra and that rate constants evaluated from such spectra can be incorrect. It is the author's opinion that it is wise to have at least two independent determinations of a rate constant obtained from NMR data to guard against erroneous conclusions that could arise from the incorrect interpretation of exchange effects.

## B   SPIN–LATTICE RELAXATION

The spin–lattice relaxation time $T_1$, is usually determined by an experiment in which an initial rf pulse is used to perturb the populations of the various energy levels of the spin system away from those that exist at thermal equilibrium. After a defined amount of time (the mixing time) during which the system begins to return to equilibrium, a second rf pulse is applied to produce a spectrum from which can be determined signal intensities and, thus, population levels that existed at the end of the mixing time. The experiment is repeated several times using a range of mixing times, and analysis of the intensities of the lines of the spectrum is carried out to provide an experimental $T_1$ relaxation time. If this experiment is done in a selective way, that is, if only one particular spin is affected by the pulses, the value for $T_1$ obtained by the experiment, to a good approximation, is that given by the sum of all the effects that produce relaxation of the spin. The contribution of each dipole-dipole interaction to the relaxation can be computed by means of Equation (4), while Equation (6) gives the CSA contribution.

When the spin observed in a $T_1$ experiment is involved in a chemical exchange process, the value of $T_1$ obtained will be a mixture of the $T_1$ values characteristic of each of the species interconverted by the exchange reactions, and it may also become intermingled with the rate of the exchange process itself.

If we consider the case of a two-site exchange in which a ligand or receptor is found, either free in solution or bound together in a ligand–receptor complex, the $T_1$ measured for a signal from either the ligand or the receptor must represent a composite of the relaxation behaviour of both the free and complexed species. For rapid exchange between sites, the spin–lattice relaxation time is averaged according to

$$\frac{1}{T_1}\left(OBS\right)=\frac{X_F}{T_{1F}}+\frac{X_B}{T_{1B}} \tag{15}$$

That is, at a fast rate of interchange, the observed $1/T_1$ is simply a weighted average of the $1/T_1$ values of the two species involved in the exchange. It is found that the condition for fast exchange averaging of spin–lattice relaxation rates is a rather loose one, namely $(k_{FB} + k_{BF}) \gg (1/T_{1A} + 1/T_{1B})$.[60] Since $R_1 (= 1/T_1)$ for receptor-bound spins is probably in the range $1-10$ s$^{-1}$, this condition is usually much easier to meet than are the requirements for bringing the signal position or linewidth of the observed spins to the fast-exchange average limit, as discussed previously. Thus, $1/T_1$ may be found to be in the fully averaged limit indicated by Equation (15), even though the appearance of the observed spectrum may be near the slow-exchange limit with respect to signal positions and linewidths.

For most complex situations, including those where the fast-exchange conditions are not met or where the experiment performed is not the selective one described, it may be necessary to employ computer simulations to obtain a meaningful interpretation of spin–lattice relaxation data.

## C   SCALAR COUPLING

The ligand (or receptor) spin involved in an exchange process may appear in the NMR spectrum as a multiplet because of spin coupling to other spins. When the dissociation of the ligand–receptor complex is slow, separate multiplets for the free and bound states will be present, provided that the linewidth for each species, defined by its respective $T_2^*$ value, is less than the separation of the multiplet components. With rapid dissociation, a single averaged multiplet will be present representing both forms. The observed spin-coupling constant in the multiplet under fast exchange conditions will be the average of the coupling constants for the ligand in the free and bound states:

$$J(OBS) = X_F J_F + X_B J_B \qquad (16)$$

The appearance of the observed ligand spin when the lines for the bound ligand are broad enough that the multiplet structure of this species cannot be resolved, or when the rate of dissociation of the ligand–receptor complex is such that neither slow nor fast exchange conditions are present, will depend on a number of variables, including $k_{BF}$, $\Delta$, and the transverse relaxation times $T_2$ for the free and bound ligand molecules. Computer simulation is the only reliable way to obtain information about spin-coupling constants under these conditions. However, it may be preferable to eliminate complications from $J$ coupling by spin decoupling or some other means, or simply to ignore the effects of spin coupling when the coupling constants are expected to be small.

It might be noted that spin coupling to nitrogen-14 nuclei (the form of nitrogen normally present in biological systems) and deuterium ($^2H$) is usually not observed when these spins are in large molecules or when they are attached to ligands that become bound to large molecules. An additional mechanism for spin–lattice relaxation arising from the quadrupolar nature of nitrogen-14 and deuterium results in very efficient spin–lattice relaxation for $^{14}N$ and $^2H$, and has the effect of decoupling these nuclei.[61]

## D   NUCLEAR OVERHAUSER EFFECTS

Exchange processes greatly influence the outcome of nuclear Overhauser effect (NOE) experiments; these effects are considered in more detail later in the chapter.

---

# X   DETERMINATION OF DISSOCIATION RATES FOR DRUG–RECEPTOR COMPLEXES

The rate of dissociation of a drug–receptor complex is a critical variable in determining what can be learned about the complex by NMR experiments. A variety of methods is available for estimating ligand binding or dissociation rates. Some are based on absorption or fluorescence spectroscopy and thus require the presence of a chromophoric group within the ligand or receptor that is responsive to the binding process. NMR methods for determining these rates can be especially effective. In this case, the chromophore is a distinct and assignable NMR signal from the free ligand or receptor or the ligand–receptor complex. Provided there is a change in one or more of the NMR parameters (chemical shift, coupling constant, $T_1$, $T_2$, NOE) that are characteristic of this signal, an experiment can often be devised that will define $k_{BF}$, the rate constant for dissociation of the complex. NMR methods are most likely to be productive when the $k_{BF}$ is in the range $10^0$ to $10^5$ s$^{-1}$. As indicated above, when the exchange process is slow, the spectral parameters observed experimentally are simply those characteristic of the individual species present in the slow exchange. When the interchange process is very fast, the NMR spectrum is described by parameters that are weighted averages of those that are characteristic of the interchanging species, and it makes no difference to the (averaged) values observed how fast the exchange process may be.

For the equilibrium shown in Equation (8), the rate constant for dissociation of the complex represented by $B$ is given by

$$k_{BF} = k_{FB}K_D \qquad (17)$$

where $K_D$ is the dissociation constant of the complex. The dissociation constants for effective drugs are typically in the range $10^{-9}$ to $10^{-6}$ $M$, and if we assume that the association of the receptor and ligand to form the complex is near the diffusion limit ($k_{FB} \approx 10^{10}$ $M^{-1}$ s$^{-1}$, Reference 43, page 547), $k_{BF}$ can be expected to be in the range 10 to $10^4$ s$^{-1}$. While there are many examples of drug binding that is slower, sometimes much slower, than the diffusive encounter rate, it is a reasonable hope that an NMR technique will provide information about the dissociation rate of a drug–receptor complex.

The discussion below will briefly indicate some of the common experiments that have been applied to the determination of ligand dissociation rates from ligand–macromolecule complexes. In each case, the discussion will assume that a two-site exchange process is being observed, with one site corresponding to the free ligand (or the free receptor) and the other to the ligand–receptor complex. Thus, the signal(s) observed will be characterized by two sets of NMR parameters, one for the free and one for the bound states.

## A   SATURATION TRANSFER

Saturation is the result of a process by which a population difference between nuclear spin energy levels is reduced to zero. Experimentally, this state can be achieved by supplying rf energy in large enough quantities that transitions between the nuclear spin states take place so rapidly that the natural processes that try to keep the population levels at their Boltzmann values ($T_1$ relaxation) are overwhelmed. If the populations of two nuclear spin levels connected by a transition are equal, then the intensity of that transition, which depends on the population difference, will be reduced to zero. The transition is then said to have become saturated. The experimental conditions needed to achieve saturation can conflict with requirements for selectivity, and it may not be possible to achieve complete saturation of a specific signal, but only a reduction in its intensity. In this case, the signal is regarded as partially saturated.

Now consider a situation in which there are two species present in a sample, $F$ and $B$, and an exchange process that interconverts them. The rate of the exchange must be slow enough that separate $F$ and $B$ signals are observed. Selective saturation of one of the signals, say $F$, will reduce its intensity in the spectrum. However, because of conversion of the spins corresponding to this signal to spins of the second type $B$, the intensity of the $B$ signal will also decrease. The intensity observed for the $B$ signal depends on the rate of the interconversion process *and* on the rate of spin–lattice relaxation for the $B$ spins. Algebraic analysis of this experiment is straightforward.[62] Let $F_0$ and $B_0$ correspond to the intensities of the respective signals when the system is at equilibrium, while $F_t$ and $B_t$ represent these signal intensities at some time $t$ after the saturation of the $F$ signal has begun. The change in the $B$ signal intensity with time is given by

$$\frac{dB_t}{dt} = k_{FB}\left(F_t - F_0\right) - \left(R_{1B} + k_{BF}\right)\left(B_t - B_0\right) \qquad (18)$$

where $R_{1B}$ is the spin–lattice relaxation rate for the spins represented by signal $B$, $k_{FB}$ is the first-order or pseudo-first-order rate constant for conversion of $F$ spins to $B$ spins, and $k_{BF}$ is the first-order or pseudo-first-order rate constant for conversion of $B$ spins to $F$ spins. The rate constants in Equation (18) could be evaluated by following the change in intensity of the $B$ signal with time after saturation of the $F$ spin begins. If saturation of the $F$ signal continues long enough that a steady state is reached ($dB_t/dt = 0$), some algebraic manipulation shows that

$$k_{BF} = \frac{R_{1B}\left(1 - \dfrac{B_e}{B_0}\right)}{\dfrac{B_e}{B_0} - \dfrac{F_e}{F_0}} \qquad (19)$$

where $F_e$ and $B_e$ are the intensities, respectively, for the $F$ and $B$ signals when the steady state is achieved, and $F_0$ and $B_0$ are the intensities of these signals at equilibrium in the absence of any perturbation. This result is even simpler if it can be arranged experimentally that the saturation of the signal for $F$ is complete, that is, $F_e = 0$.

If the spin–lattice relaxation time $(1/T_{1B} = R_{1B})$ for the $B$ spins is known, the rate constant for conversion of $B$ spins to $F$ spins can be evaluated from the relative intensities of the $B$ signal in the presence and absence of saturation of the $F$ signal. It should be noted that obtaining the spin–lattice relaxation time for $B$ may not be trivial, since there may be an exchange contribution to the apparent relaxation time measured by an experiment intended to measure $T_1$ (Section IX.B).

Equation (19) shows that the range of values for the rate constant $k_{BF}$ that can be measured experimentally by this method is basically determined by the value of the spin–lattice relaxation rate $R_{1B}$. If it is assumed that a 2% reduction in the $B$ signal could be reliably detected and that the signal for the $F$ species is completely saturated, then the product $T_{1B}k_{BF}$ cannot be smaller than 0.02. If the experiment is able to detect the $B$ signal when it has been reduced 98% by saturation transfer, the product $T_{1B}k_{BA}$ cannot be larger than 49. Given typical values for $T_1$ in ligand–receptor systems, these considerations indicate that saturation transfer experiments should be useful for the determination of rate constants in the range $10^{-1}$ to $10^2$ s$^{-1}$.

It might be noted that saturation transfer can be an undesirable feature of some proton NMR studies of ligand–receptor systems. Observation of peptide NH resonances in proteins and of NH protons hydrogen-bonded between base pairs in nucleic acids is often an essential feature of structural studies in these systems. These hydrogens are labile (exchangeable) with respect to the protons of water. Therefore, experiments must be carried out using $H_2O$ rather than $D_2O$ as the solvent, since the NH groups would be converted to ND groups in $D_2O$ and the corresponding signals would disappear from the $^1H$ NMR spectrum. The molar concentration of water protons in solvent water is approximately 110 $M$, vastly greater than the concentration of solute protons in a typical NMR sample. Because of dynamic range limitations inherent in the detection systems of NMR spectrometers, it is necessary to reduce the water signal in some other way.[63] A convenient way to reduce the water signal is simply to saturate it, but when this is done, transfer of saturation to NH protons may take place and may lead to full or partial disappearance of these signals as well. Sample pH and temperature can possibly be adjusted so that the rate of exchange between water protons and NH protons is slow enough that such saturation transfer can be neglected, but when this is not feasible, some other means of minimising the water signal in the proton NMR spectrum must be implemented.[63]

### B    INVERSION TRANSFER

A variation of the saturation transfer experiment — inversion transfer — may be useful, particularly in cases where it is not practical to determine $T_1$ relaxation times in the absence of the exchange process. In the inversion transfer experiment, a series of rf pulses is used to establish initial conditions in which the signal for, say, the $F$ spins is inverted. For inversion of a particular transition the spin population characteristic of the high-energy state involved in the transition is transferred to the low-energy spin state, and vice versa. Since the population of the low-energy state is then less than the population of the high-energy state, net emission of energy is observed; that is, the signal for the transition, if observed immediately, appears upside down in the usual display. Inverted spin populations cannot be a permanent condition for the sample, since the Boltzmann distribution law is being violated and, over time, the populations of the spin energy levels return to those characteristic of thermal equilibrium by means of spin–lattice relaxation processes.

When interchange of species $F$ and $B$ takes place, inverted $F$-spin magnetization is changed to $B$-spin magnetization. This will have the effect of temporarily reducing the intensity of the $B$ signal. In following the $F$ and $B$ signal intensities as a function of time after application of the pulses that inverted the $F$ signal, a recovery of the $F$ signal to its normal position will be observed. The signal for $B$ is initially at its equilibrium value; it decreases temporarily and then recovers back to its equilibrium intensity as the effect of the $F$ signal inversion is propagated through the system. Analysis of the intensity–time curves for the $F$ and $B$ signals using a mathematical formulation that starts with equations similar to Equation (18) can provide values for $k_{BF}$ and $T_{1B}$.[64] The range of rate constants that can be adduced by inversion transfer experiments is roughly the same as that for the saturation transfer method.

A potentially significant experimental consideration when executing either saturation transfer or inversion transfer experiments is the extent to which one is able to achieve selective saturation or selective inversion of one resonance in the spectrum. This is especially a problem in the case of saturation transfer, since application of rf energy to specific spins of a sample can involve some "spillover" of the radiation to neighbouring spins. The selectivity with which saturation can be obtained depends on $T_1$ and $T_2$ for the observed and saturated spins, the separation of their respective signals in Hertz, and the intensity of the applied field.[65]

Saturation transfer and inversion transfer experiments have been used to examine the conformation of the seven-membered ring in Valium, (next page). The two methylene protons in this ring are not equivalent, and their NMR signals are sufficiently separated to allow selective saturation or inversion of one of them to be accomplished; a variety of experiments shows that the ring flexes about fives times per second.[66]

Valium

## C   Two-Dimensional Exchange Spectroscopy

Two-dimensional (2D) NMR methods for mapping exchange processes and determining their rates are basically elaborations of the inversion
transfer experiment.[62] Two-dimensional experiments have the advantages
that (1) selectivity of the inversion part of the experiment is not a consideration, as the selectivity of inversion is essentially limited only by the
linewidth $T_2^*$ of signals of the spectrum; and (2) the signals in the NMR
spectrum that are connected by an exchange process are clearly identified.
This latter feature can be especially useful when there is an exchange
between signals of unequal intensity to the extent that it is difficult to
detect the weaker of these against the noise level of the standard one-
dimensional spectrum. This point is discussed in more detail below and in
Chapter 6, in relation to studies of peptides that exist in multiple conformations in solution.

Space does not permit a lengthy exposition of 2D exchange experiments, and the original literature should be consulted for further details
and discussions of methods to extract quantitative information from them
(Reference 41, Chapter 9). A compact summary of the experiments, is
given by Homans.[67] However, consideration of Equations (18) and (20)
may indicate the basic principles. The signals for the $F$ and $B$ spins involved
in a two-site exchange process appear at characteristic frequencies in the
NMR spectrum, $\delta_F$ and $\delta_B$, when exchange is slow enough. The intensity
of the signal for the $B$ spins as a function of

$$\frac{dB_t}{dt} = k_{FB}\left(F_t - F_0\right) - \left(R_{1B} + k_{BF}\right)\left(B_t - B_0\right) \tag{18}$$

$$\frac{dF_t}{dt} = k_{BF}\left(B_t - B_0\right) - \left(R_{1F} + k_{FB}\right)\left(F_t - F_0\right) \tag{20}$$

time is described by Equation (18), given earlier, but repeated here for
convenience, while Equation (20) describes the behaviour of the intensity
of the signal corresponding to the $F$ spins. Any solution of these equations
to give $B_t$ and $F_t$ at some specific time $t$ will have to include knowledge of

the signal intensities when the system is at equilibrium $B_0$ and $F_0$, as well as the starting (initial) values $B_i$ and $F_i$.

In the two-dimensional exchange experiment, a series of rf pulses is applied to the sample before detection of the signals that make up the spectrum. The timing of the application of these pulses is such that it is convenient to break the progress of the experiment into three distinct phases. The last phase of the experiment consists of simply detecting the signals corresponding to the $F$ and $B$ spins. During the middle phase of the experiment, which is usually referred to as the mixing time, transfers of signal intensity from the signal for $B$ to the signal for $F$, and vice versa, take place according to Equations (18) and (20). In the first period of the experiment, the pulses applied have the effect of making the initial values $F_i$ and $B_i$ for the mixing time dependent on the frequencies $\delta_F$ and $\delta_B$, respectively. Therefore, the signal intensity detected for, say, species $B$ will depend on frequency $\delta_B$ and, if there has been exchange during the mixing period, also on frequency $\delta_F$.

Presentation of the results of the 2D exchange experiment is usually by means of a contour map in which signal intensity is represented by contour lines as a function of two frequency variables. This kind of display for the $F \rightleftarrows B$ interconversion appears schematically in Figure 9. Frequencies along the axis labelled $f_2$ are those that would appear in a standard one-dimensional spectrum of this system. The exchange information provided by the experiment is obtained by considering a trace along the second frequency axis $f_1$. Reading vertically at $\delta_F$, for example, one finds a feature at a frequency $\delta_F$. Its intensity depends on the $T_1$ relaxation time for the $F$ spins, the rate of exchange, and the duration of the mixing time. A second feature at $\delta_B$ arises only if there is significant $F \rightleftarrows B$ exchange; this corresponds to nascent $F$-signal intensity, which was characterized by the frequency $\delta_B$ at the start of the mixing period.

Those features of the map shown in Figure 9 that lie at the coordinates $f_1 = f_2 = \delta_F$ and $f_1 = f_2 = \delta_B$ are called the diagonal peaks of the spectrum and would be present with or without exchange, since $T_1$ cannot be zero; there is always spin–lattice relaxation. The other, off-diagonal features in this 2D spectrum are cross-peaks; these can appear only if there is appreciable interconversion of spins from the $F$ environment to the $B$ environment, and from $B$ to $F$, over the course of the mixing time.

The neurohypophyseal hormones, oxytocin and arginine-vasopressin, are nonapeptides that contain a proline residue in their sequence. There is

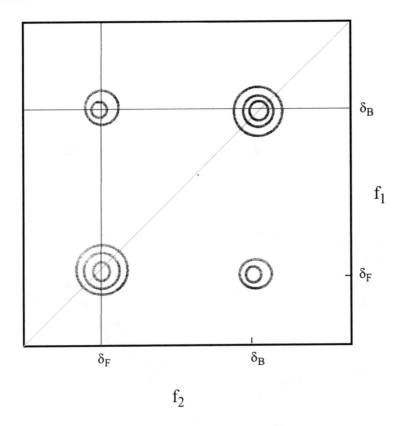

**FIGURE 9**
Schematic representation of the contour map that is the result of a two-dimensional experiment for detecting exchange. Quantitative analysis of the relative intensities of the features shown can lead to an estimate of the rate at which an exchange process takes place.

the possibility that appreciable amounts of two conformational isomers of these peptides will be present due to the presence of *cis* and *trans* isomers at the proline peptide bond, as indicated.

Figure 10 shows the NH regions of a 1D $^1$H NMR spectrum of arginine-vasopressin and the result of a 2D exchange experiment. At first glance, only one set of NH resonances for the hormone is apparent in the spectrum. The appearance of cross-peaks in the 2D exchange spectrum clearly establishes weak signals involved in an exchange process with the major signals present. The strong NH signals correspond to a conformation of the peptide in which the proline residue is in the *trans* conformation, with the minor signals arising from the *cis* conformation. The rate constant for the *trans* to *cis* conversion was determined to be 0.03–0.05 s$^{-1}$, depending on the solvent.[68]

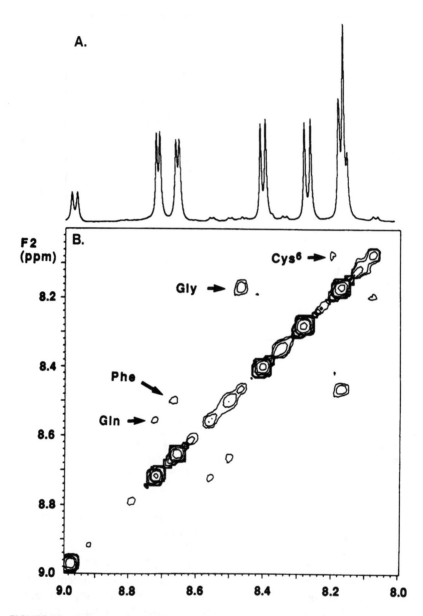

**FIGURE 10**

(A) One-dimensional proton NMR spectrum of the hormone arginine vasopressin dissolved in methanol at 37°C. Only the amide NH region of the spectrum is shown, with the amide NH doublets from a number of residues in the nonapeptide identified. (B) Two-dimensional proton NMR experiment, which includes the effects of exchange with the same sample used for spectrum A. The off-diagonal features of the spectrum arise because exchange between the dominant conformation and a minor conformation of the peptide takes place. (Adapted from Larive, C.K. and Rubenstein, D.L., *J. Am. Chem. Soc.*, 115, 2833–2836, 1993.)

A comparison of 1D and 2D methods for determination of exchange rates in the slow-exchange regime has been given.[69]

## D  LINESHAPE METHODS

Saturation transfer, inversion transfer, and 2D methods for measuring the rates characteristic of a ligand–receptor interaction require that signals corresponding to the free and bound forms of the ligand or receptor be sufficiently close to the slow-exchange limit that separate signals for each of these forms are observable. When the exchange process is more rapid, there may be appreciable line broadening, merging of signals, or when one species is present in small amounts, disappearance of signals. Computer simulations of NMR lineshapes as a function of the relevant NMR variables are readily accomplished, at least for relatively simple systems, and comparison of such simulations with experimental results may make it possible to estimate the dissociation behaviour of a ligand–receptor complex.[70]

An important limitation of lineshape methods applied to drug–receptor interactions is the necessity of knowing the chemical-shift difference between the free and bound states of the nucleus being observed. A change in sample temperature or pH could be used to take the system into the slow-exchange region to enable measurement of this difference, but it may not be possible to find conditions under which the exchange process can be slowed sufficiently to make the necessary observations that are compatible with the biochemical system under study.

The complex formed between dihydrofolate reductase and the difluorinated analogue of methotrexate (shown below) has been examined by fluorine NMR spectroscopy by Clore et al.[71] Some of their results are shown in Figure 11. The two fluorine nuclei in the drug analogue are rendered nonequivalent because of the inherent asymmetry of the binding site on the protein and the slow rate of rotation of the difluorinated aromatic ring in the complex. The complex is stable over the temperature range 0–35°, and within this range, the fluorine spectrum exhibits two-site exchange behaviour, as shown previously in Figure 4. Analysis of the spectra at each temperature was accomplished by computing theoretical lineshapes (shown) and comparing them to the experimental results. Thus, it was determined that the difluoroaromatic ring rotates within the drug–protein complex about 7300 times per second at room temperature.

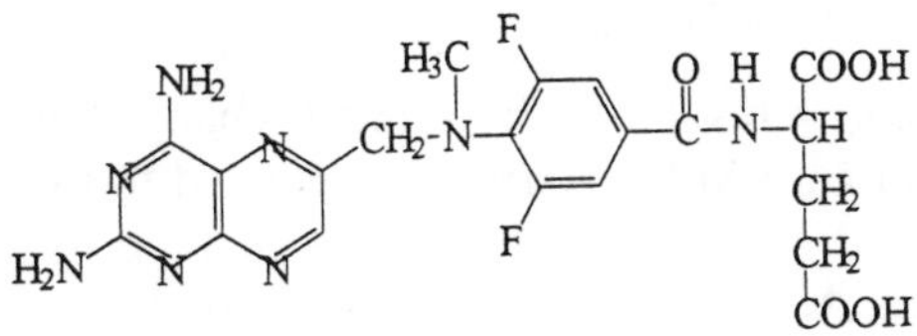

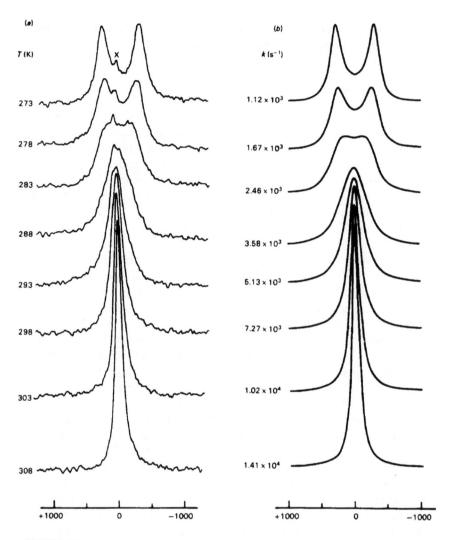

**FIGURE 11**

Observed (a) and calculated (b) 188.0 MHz fluorine NMR spectra of 3′,5′-di-fluoromethotrexate bound to dihydrofolate reductase (*Lactobacillus casei*). For the spectra shown, all the ligand present was bound to the enzyme. (Adapted from Clore, G.M., et al., *Biochem, J.,* 217, 659, 1984.)

## E   SPIN ECHO METHODS

When exchange rates approach the fast-exchange limit, their effects on the appearance of an NMR spectrum are reduced to mere broadening of the averaged signal observed. These effects may be so slight, relative to experimental error, that it may not be possible to obtain accurate information about exchange rates by consideration of the line-shape. This apparent limit on exchange rate determinations by NMR techniques can be extended a little by the use of spin echo experiments. A spin echo is a pattern of signals that can appear during or after the application of two or more rf pulses to a sample. The echo pattern may be collected and transformed to a one-dimensional spectrum that has many features of a standard spectrum, but will usually have distorted peak shapes and intensities, depending on the details of the experiment. Spin echoes decay in amplitude with time because of transverse (spin–spin) relaxation, as well as spin–lattice relaxation. Chemical-exchange processes provide a means of line broadening; thus an increase in the measured $T_2^*$ relaxation time, following the decay of the intensity of spin echo signals, is a means of extracting exchange rate information.

The most common spin echo experiment involves a series of pulses designed to remove the effects of magnetic field inhomogeneity from $T_2^*$, leaving a residual relaxation effect that is due to the intrinsic relaxation interactions and any exchange processes present. As has been noted, the field inhomogeneity term can be the major contributor to $T_2^*$, so these other effects become much more apparent in its absence. Spin echo observations have been used to determine ligand–protein exchange rates,[60,72] although the technique has not been popular, possibly because of the considerable requirements it places on the quality of an NMR spectrometer.[73,74] Jen[75] has given an analysis of the experiment with more than two exchanging sites.

### F  $T_1$ IN THE ROTATING FRAME $T_1\rho$

Under equilibrium conditions, the magnetization associated with a group of equivalent spins in an NMR sample is aligned along the direction of the laboratory magnetic file $B_0$. "Spin locking" is a procedure that involves holding the magnetism associated with a group of spins in a plane that is at right angles to the direction of $B_0$. The spins undergo relaxation under these conditions by spin–lattice and spin–spin relaxation processes. This relaxation can be characterized by a relaxation time $T_1\rho$ which is a combination of $T_1$ and $T_2^*$.[76] When an exchange process is present, $T_1\rho$ can also include terms dependent on the rate of that process, particularly when the rates are near the fast exchange limit.[77] A recent study of conformational isomerization in cyclohexane illustrates how the rotating frame relaxation technique can be used to extend the range of rates that can be measured by NMR.[78]

# XI  NUCLEAR OVERHAUSER EFFECTS

NMR spectra arise because of the absorption or emission of energy by nuclear spins. It was indicated above that a definite number of energy states is present for a given configuration of spins, and that molecules containing these spins must be in one of these allowed states. Absorption or emission of energy corresponds to molecules changing between allowed states by the absorption or emission of photons of the appropriate frequency. The larger the population difference between these states, the stronger will be the signal.[*]

There are many ways to temporarily alter the population of molecules in a given state, including application of an rf pulse to the sample that is selective for only one spin or one subgroup of the states, or by continuously irradiating the sample with rf energy. During and after any such perturbation of the sample, spin–lattice relaxation processes act to bring the sample back to thermal equilibrium. If the perturbation is applied continuously, the sample comes to a steady state in which the effects of the perturbation and relaxation balance one another in some way.

All the allowed nuclear spin states for a molecular system are connected by spin–lattice relaxation pathways, and a possible result of an experiment that selectively alters the populations of particular states away from their values at thermal equilibrium is alteration of the populations of states *not* directly affected by the selective perturbation. The intensities of the signals that arise because of transition between these latter states will thus be changed. A change in intensity of an NMR signal assignable to one nucleus of a spin system as the result of selective perturbation of the populations of states associated with signals assigned to another spin of the system has been defined above as the nuclear Overhauser effect, or NOE. NOEs can be positive (enhancement of signal strength as a result of the selective perturbation) or negative, and may be such that a signal disappears completely as a result of a perturbation that has been applied. The volume by Neuhaus and Williamson[47] provides an excellent discussion of contemporary NOE experiments.

To gain some insight into the nature of several NOE experiments, and thereby indicate the utility of these experiments in structural studies of ligand–receptor complexes, we consider the behaviour of two spins, $I$ and $S$, in a network of spins (Figure 12). We will assume that the chemical shielding parameters of these spins are sufficiently different that well-separated signals for each spin are present in the spectrum. Spin coupling between spins will be neglected, although in many cases, if the integrated

---

[*] The energy difference between allowed spin states increases when the magnetic field used for the NMR experiment increases. According to the Boltzmann distribution law, the larger the energy difference between two states, the larger the difference in the number of molecules in each state. Signal intensity increases when the laboratory magnetic field used for an NMR experiment is increased because the population difference between states increases. This is an inducement to use the highest possible magnetic field when doing an NMR experiment. However, consideration of other factors, particularly the dependence of relaxation on magnetic field, may indicate that somewhat lower magnetic fields will be better for a particular system.

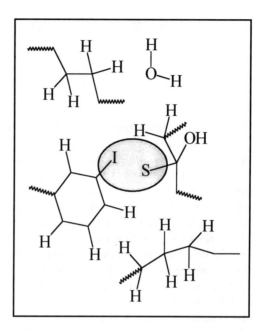

**FIGURE 12**

Hypothetical network of spins in a biological macromolecule. The various spins shown may be within bonding distance of each other; many spins not directly bonded will likely be within van der Waals contact of each other.

intensity over the multiplet associated with a spin or a group of equivalent spins is considered, the equations and other concepts given below will be good approximations, even if spin coupling is present. However, rigorous treatments of NOEs in coupled spin systems are available.[54,79]

The network of spins indicated in Figure 12 could be the collection of protons attached to the amino acid residues of a protein, a collection of protons within a given volume of the protein, or a group of spins that includes several different types of nuclei, say, carbon-13, nitrogen-15, and protons, which would be present in a protein that had been specifically enriched with the carbon and nitrogen isotopes. Proteins are nearly perfectly packed,[80] and many of the hydrogen atoms of the amino acid residues present in them are nearly within the van der Waals contact (2 Å) of each other. Certainly, in a protein or nucleic acid where tertiary structure is well developed, there will be many networks of spins in close proximity to each other.

Spin–lattice (and spin–spin) relaxation of spins within the network depicted will depend on a variety of internuclear interactions, particularly those between hydrogen nuclei. Spin $I$ will experience a number of magnetic dipole–dipole interactions that contribute to its relaxation, including the interaction with spin $S$. Spin $S$ also has a number of partners for relaxation. Both spin $I$ and spin $S$ may relax by processes that do not involve interactions with other spins, such as that due to the anisotropy of the chemical shielding parameter. If we arbitrarily choose to observe spin $I$ in the spectrum, and focus only on the contribution of spin $S$ to the relaxation of spin $I$, in the simplest treatment (the Solomon equations;

Reference 47, page 25 *et seq.*), the behaviour of the signal intensity for spin $I$ is given by

$$\frac{dI_t}{dt} = -\rho_I \left( I_t - I_0 \right) - \sigma_{IS} \left( S_t - S_0 \right) \tag{21}$$

where $I_t$ is the signal intensity of $I$ at time $t$, $I_0$ is the intensity for this signal observed when the network is at thermodynamic equilibrium, and $S_t$ and $S_0$ are the corresponding quantities for spin $S$.[*] Without further discussion, it will simply be stated that $\rho_I$ depends on *all* the relaxation interactions and mechanisms that produce thermal equilibration of the populations of spin states that give rise to the $I$ signal(s), including the interaction with spin $S$. Experimentally, it is the case that $\rho_I$ is equal to $R_1 = 1/T_1$, the spin–lattice relaxation rate for spin $I$. In virtually all practical applications of the NOE, the parameter $\sigma_{IS}$ depends *only* on the specific dipole–dipole inter-action between spin $I$ and spin $S$. In this case, the magnitude and the sign of $\sigma_{IS}$ depend on the nature of spins $I$ and $S$, their separation (as $1/r_{IS}^6$), and the correlation time, $\tau_c$ for the network, as shown in Equation (22). An evaluation of $\sigma_{IS}$ is the goal of an NOE experiment because of the distance information it contains. It should be noted, in considering Equa-tion (22), that if the correlation time $\tau_c$ is large enough, the value of $\sigma_{IS}$ is dependent on the laboratory magnetic field used to do the experiment, since the resonance frequencies $\omega_1$ and $\omega_S$ change with field. Also, because of the negative sign in Equation (22) it is possible to encounter conditions under which $\sigma_{IS}$ will be zero, even if the internuclear distance is small.

$$\sigma_{IS} = \frac{\frac{1}{10} \gamma_I^2 \gamma_S^2 \hbar^2 \left[ \dfrac{6\tau_c}{1 + \left( \omega_I + \omega_S \right)^2 \tau_c^2} - \dfrac{\tau_c}{1 + \left( \omega_I - \omega_S \right)^2 \tau_c^2} \right]}{r_{IS}^6} \tag{22}$$

---

[*] The utilization and discussion of the Solomon equations given here is rather imprecise. 1D NMR spectra are produced by the application of rf pulses to the sample of interest in such a way that magnetization associated with the spin that was originally oriented along the same axis as the direction of the laboratory magnetic field $B_0$ is turned so that it has a component in the plane that is at right angles to the laboratory field. An NMR spectrom-eter can only directly detect magnetization components in this plane. Thus, the amplitudes of signals detected by an instrument are directly proportional to the amplitude of the magnetization components that were aligned along the direction of $B_0$ immediately before the observation pulse was applied. The "signal intensitites" used in the version of the Solomon equations discussed in the text actually refer to the components of spin magne-tization along the direction of the laboratory field, since it is these that will ultimately be represented in the spectrum.

## A STEADY-STATE NOE

A steady-state NOE on spin $I$ is created when spin $S$ is saturated for a long enough time that the entire spin system reaches a steady state, that is, when the populations of molecules in the various allowed nuclear spin energy states are no longer changed by the saturation of spin $S$. If a steady state is present, then $dI_t/dt = 0$ and $S_t = 0$ (because spin $S$ is saturated), and Equation (22) can be rearranged to

$$\frac{I_{OBS} - I_0}{I_0} = f_I\{S\} = \frac{\sigma_{IS} S_0}{\rho_I I_0} \tag{23}$$

where $I_{OBS}$ is the intensity of the signal for spins of type $I$ when the steady state is achieved. If $I$ and $S$ are the same kind of spin, say, both are protons, and there are equal numbers of $I$ and $S$ spins in the molecule, then the NOE depends only on $\sigma_{IS}/\rho_I$ spins. Recall that $\rho_I$ is the result of all interactions that lead to $T_1$ relaxation of spin $I$. In the unlikely event that spin $I$ relaxes only because of its interaction with spin $S$, it can be shown by manipulating Equation (4) and Equation (22) that $\rho_I = 2\sigma_{IS}$ when the molecule containing the $[I,S]$ spin pair has a short correlation time, and that $\rho_I = -\sigma_{IS}$ when the molecule is large and, thus, has a long correlation time. For these idealized conditions, the NOE for small molecules would be $f_I\{S\} = 1/2$, corresponding to a 50% enhancement of the $I$ signal intensity. For large molecules, $f_I\{S\} = -1$, which means that $I_{OBS} = 0$, that is, the $I$ signal would disappear from the spectrum. In real molecules, $\rho_I$ is larger than the values calculated for the ideal cases discussed, with the result that the NOE is less than a 50% enhancement for small molecules and the $I$ signal does not completely disappear in large molecules.

For situations where $I$ and $S$ are not the same kind of nuclei, but are present in equal numbers, the ratio $S_0/I_0$ can be replaced by $\gamma_S/\gamma_I$, the ratio of the gyromagnetic ratios of the two nuclear spins. As indicated by Neuhaus and Williamson,[47] for some spin pairs the ratios will be of opposite sign.* Moreover, the NOE observed in the limit of slow motion will be a complicated function of the resonance frequencies of both $I$ and $S$. Lastly, the presence of additional relaxation contributions to $\rho_I$, other than the relaxation resulting from the interaction of $I$ with $S$, will produce a reduction of the magnitude of NOE.

---

* It should be kept in mind when working with Equations (4) and (22) that when a gyromagnetic ratio is negative, the corresponding resonance frequency $\omega$ is also negative.

## B   NOE Buildup

Another useful NOE experiment is one in which the saturation of spin $S$ starts at time $t = 0$ and the change in the intensity of the $I$ signal is followed as a function of time after saturation has started. We will assume that the saturation of $S$ is done in such a way that $S$ is saturated instantly, so that $St = 0$ at the start and for the course of the experiment. Under these conditions, Equation (22) becomes

$$\frac{dIt}{dt} = -\rho_I \left( It - I_0 \right) + \sigma_{IS} S_0 \qquad (24)$$

Integration of this equation gives

$$\frac{It - I_0}{I_0} = \left( f_I \{ S \} \right) t = \frac{\sigma_{IS} S_0}{\rho_I I_0} \left[ 1 - \exp\left( -\rho_I t \right) \right] \qquad (25)$$

This equation has the correct behaviour at $t = 0$, where the $f_I\{S\}$ NOE is 0, and at long times, where the steady-state NOE is the same as that given by Equation (23). Equation (25) shows that the time scale for generation of the NOE after the start of saturation is defined by $\rho_1 = R_1 = 1/T_1$ for spin $I$. It takes about $5T_1$ for the NOE due to perturbation of spin $S$ to become fully developed, and at least that long for the system to return to thermal equilibrium.[81]

A potentially more useful NOE buildup experiment is one in which the spin network, initially at thermal equilibrium, is saturated at spin $S$ starting at time = 0. Initially, $I_t = I_0$, and if the saturation of $S$ can be assumed to be instantaneous, the *initial rate* of change of the observed $I$ signal intensity is given by

$$\left. \frac{dI_t}{dt} \right|_{\text{initial}} = \sigma_{IS} S_0 = \left. \frac{I_0 d\left[ \left( I_t - I_0 \right) / I_0 \right]}{dt} \right|_{\text{initial}} \qquad (26)$$

This initial rate approximation for any spin–pair interaction is valid regardless of the complexity of the spin network that makes up the molecule. Since $\sigma_{IS}$ is dependent on $1/\tau_{IS}^6$, a study of relative initial rates can provide a measure of the relative distances between the various spins in the network. Unfortunately, in experiments with real molecules, it may be difficult to measure reliably the rather small initial changes in signal intensity, so that reliable estimates of relative distances may not be possible in practice.

## C   Transient NOE

Another kind of NOE experiment can be appreciated by referring to Equation (22). Suppose that the spin network starts at equilibrium and is perturbed from equilibrium by application of a pulse or series of rf pulses that have the effect of selectively inverting the populations of energy states associated with the $S$ spin. (This kind of perturbation was mentioned earlier in the context of determining spin–lattice relaxation times.) If selective inversion of the $S$ spin is achieved at the start of the experiment, $S_t = -S_0$. With these initial conditions, the initial rate of change of the $I$ spin intensity is

$$\left.\frac{dI_t}{dt}\right|_{\text{initial}} = 2\sigma_{IS}S_0 = \left.\frac{I_0 d\left[\left(I_t - I_0\right)/I_0\right]}{dt}\right|_{\text{initial}} \tag{27}$$

Presuming that a selective inversion can be achieved, this is a better experiment than the initial rate study of NOE buildup indicated above, since the initial rate of change of $I_t$ is twice as large.

Note that after the initial change of $I$ signal intensity produced by the inversion (perturbation) of spin $S$, the system must eventually return to equilibrium. The expected behaviour for the $I$ signal intensity over time in this experiment is shown schematically in Figure 13, where curves corresponding to spin networks characterizable by a short $\tau_c$ (small molecules) and a long $\tau_c$ (macromolecules) are shown. It is seen that $f_I\{S\}$ is time dependent and an NOE is detectable only transiently before equilibrium is reestablished. The initial slope of a plot of $I$ signal intensity against time depends on $\sigma_{IS}$, but the recovery phase of the experiment and the time at which the maximum NOE is observed depends on the details of spin–lattice relaxation.

## D   Two-Dimensional NOE

In analogy to the two-dimensional exchange experiment discussed earlier, an experiment (NOESY) can be devised in which $I_t$ and $S_t$ can be made to have initial values that depend on their respective chemical shift positions in the one-dimensional spectrum of the system $\delta_I$ and $\delta_S$. At the end of a mixing time $t_{mix}$ in which the initial rate approximation is valid, the intensity of signal for spin $I$ (observed at $\delta_I$) can be written

$$I_{t_{mix}} = \left[-\rho_I\left[f\left(\delta_I\right)-I_0\right]-\sigma_{IS}\left[f\left(\delta_S\right)-S_0\right]\right]t_{mix} \tag{28}$$

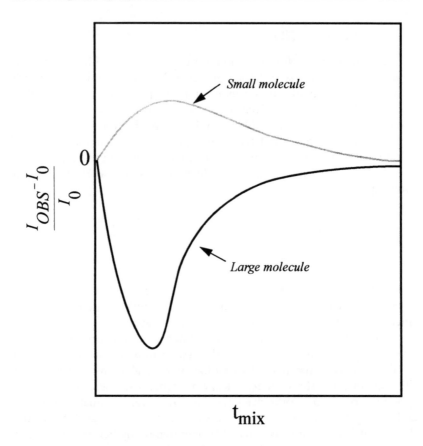

$$\frac{I_{OBS}-I_0}{I_0}$$

**FIGURE 13**
Schematic representation of the outcome of transient NOE experiments for large and small molecules. The experiment consists of perturbation of one spin or group of spins by a 180° pulse, followed by a mixing time $t_{mix}$, after which the spectrum of the observed spin is collected.

where the expression in Equation (21) has been integrated over the short time $t_{mix}$, and $f(\delta_I)$ and $f(\delta_S)$ represent the initial values for $I_t$ and $S_t$ which have become dependent on their respective chemical shifts. A similar expression describes the dependence of the $S$ spin intensity, detected at frequency $\delta_S$, on the initial conditions. The results of this kind of experiment are displayed as a 2D contour map very similar to that described in Figure 8. However, the intensities of the diagonal features now depend on $\rho_I$ and $\rho_S$, while the intensity of the off-diagonal cross-peaks depend on $\sigma_{IS}$. In the exchange experiment the appearance of a cross-peak at the coordinates $(\delta_I, \delta_S)$ or $(\delta_S, \delta_I)$ indicated that spins of type $S$ change by some kinetic process into spins of type $I$, and vice versa. A cross-peak at $(\delta_I, \delta_S)$ or $(\delta_S, \delta_I)$ appears in a 2D NOE spectrum because $\sigma_{IS}$ is not zero, that is, because spins $I$ and $S$ are physically proximate to each other in the molecule being examined. The intensity of this cross-peak can be an indication of the $I$–$S$ distance. Generally, because of the $1/r_{IS}^6$ factor found in the expression for $\sigma_{IS}$, cross-peaks are not observed if $r_{IS}$ is greater than about 4.5 Å. However, since there are conditions under which $\sigma_{IS}$ is zero even when the $I$–$S$ internuclear distance is short, the *absence* of a cross-peak in a 2D NOE cannot be interpreted to mean that a particular internuclear distance is longer than 4.5 Å.

The sequences of rf pulses used to carry out 2D NOESY and 2D exchange experiments are similar, and it is possible for cross-peaks to appear from both effects in the 2D spectrum produced by either experiment.

## E    ROTATING-FRAME NOEs

The NOEs described in Sections XI.A–D involve only $T_1$ relaxation. A derivation similar to that used to produce Equation (22) can be done to describe NOEs under the spin-locked condition where both $T_1$ and $T_2$ relaxation processes can operate.[82] It is found that development of these rotating-frame NOEs involves a factor similar to $\sigma_{IS}$.

Rotating-frame NOEs can be generated in one-dimensional experiments that are analogues to the steady state and NOE buildup experiments indicated in Sections XI.A–D.[82] Two-dimensional rotating-frame NOE experiments are often called ROESY experiments and produce results that are presented in the same format as NOESY experiments.

The ROESY experiment has several advantages over the NOESY experiment for detecting the proximity of two spins. Although the magnitude of the $\sigma_{IS}$-like factor in the equations describing the rotating-frame NOE is somewhat dependent on the strength of the laboratory magnetic field used for the experiment and the correlation time for the spin system under study, this factor is always positive. Thus, a cross-peak will not go missing, as can be the case in the NOESY experiment when the correlation time or magnetic field conspires to make $\sigma_{IS}$ zero. Moreover, analysis shows that the cross-peaks arising from Overhauser effects and from chemical exchange in ROESY spectra have the opposite sign,[42] making it possible to identify unambiguously the spectral features that are due to exchange effects and those due to the relaxation interactions of adjacent spins. Unfortunately, there are also situations when the ROESY experiment can produce cross-peaks between nuclei merely because they are spin coupled to each other. Moreover, the effects of spin coupling can become intertwined with Overhauser effects, so that a spin that is quite distant from the one under observation may still exhibit a cross-peak to the observed peak. Such artifacts can usually be sorted out by running variants of the ROESY experiment and by alteration of the instrumental conditions used for the experiment.[83]

## F  Transferred NOEs

The discussions so far have assumed that the system under study can be described in terms of a single network of spins. The study of a ligand–receptor complex, however, must potentially consider the behaviour of at least two networks of spins that are undergoing exchange with each other. To particularize, suppose that the $[I, S]$ spin pair of Figure 12 is part of the network of spins associated with the ligand. When the ligand–receptor complex forms, the network containing $I$ and $S$ will most likely be different from the network characteristic of the free ligand, both in terms of the three-dimensional arrangement of the spin in the network, and because the correlation time(s) that characterize motion(s) of the ligand in solution will change when the ligand is part of the complex. Thus, the strength of the various dipole–dipole interactions, including the $I$–$S$ interaction, could be different in the bound state. Even if there are no changes in the geometrical properties of the ligand upon binding to the receptor, the change in correlation time will produce a change in NOEs from those found for the free ligand. What is observed from an NOE experiment with a system where free ligand and complexed ligand are interchanging with each other depends on the rate of exchange between the two environments. If fast exchange conditions prevail, the characteristics of the signal for the observed spin $I$ will be the population-weighted average of those for $I$ in the free and bound states. Spin $S$ will also be present in the spectrum with averaged properties. The NOE on the (averaged) signal for $I$ when the (averaged) signal for spin $S$ is perturbed will thus depend on the NOEs characteristic of the free and bound molecules. Should the system be at the slow exchange limit with separate signals present in the spectrum for free and bound $S$, the NOE experiment can be carried out on each species independently, with results that will be the same as those that would be obtained if each could be studied in separate samples.

It may be recalled that the nuclear Overhauser effect is intimately connected to spin–lattice relaxation, and that the conditions for fast exchange averaging of $T_1$ relaxation times are quite modest. The upshot is that a spectrum can exhibit separate signals for a spin in two environments, yet exhibit the Overhauser effects characteristic of the averaged system. Interpretation of the NOE experiments when a ligand–receptor system is in neither the fast nor the slow exchange limit as regards relaxation is more difficult and clearly depends on having information about the rate of the exchange process that connects the two spin networks. The importance of having this information was one reason for mentioning earlier the variety of NMR experiments available for obtaining rates of dissociation of ligand–receptor complexes.

NOE experiments on systems where exchange is taking place are referred to as transferred NOE experiments. It is often the case that the NOE peculiar to one state of the system, usually the ligand–receptor complex, is transferred by exchange to signals of another state of the system, usually the signals of the free ligand. A number of authors have provided mathematical analyses of the transferred NOE experiment.[84-88] We can get some notion of these treatments and how NOEs are transferred. Assume that the spin pair $I$ and $S$ is found in two separate networks of spins corresponding to, say, the free $F$ and bound $B$ ligand. The fraction of molecules in each state is given by $X_F$ and $X_B$, respectively, and when starting from thermal equilibrium, the signal intensities for spin $I$ in the free and bound states are $I_0^F$ and $I_0^B$, respectively, with similar terms for the intensities of the free and bound $S$ spins. Again, we assume that spin $S$ is the one that will be perturbed during the course of the experiment, while spin $I$ is the one observed. As before, there are potentially many interactions leading to relaxation of both spins.

Considering first the free ligand, Equation (21) is extended to

$$\frac{dI_t^F}{dt} = -\rho_I^F \left( I_t^F + I_0^F \right) - \sigma_{IS}^F \left( S_t^F - S_0^F \right) - k_{FB} \left( I_t^F - I_0^F \right) + k_{BF} \left( I_t^B - I_0^B \right) \tag{29}$$

and for the bound ligand

$$\frac{dI_t^B}{dt} = -\rho_I^B \left( I_t^B - I_0^B \right) - \sigma_{IS}^B \left( S_t^B - S_0^B \right) + k_{FB} \left( I_t^F - I_0^F \right) - k_{BF} \left( I_t^B - I_0^B \right) \tag{30}$$

where $I_t^F$ and $I_t^B$ are the intensities of the signals associated with the free and bound signals, respectively, of spin $I$, and the superscripts $F$ and $B$ on the various components indicate quantities for the free and bound states. The additional terms appearing in Equations (29) and (30) relative to Equation (21) arise because the exchange process converts molecules that are represented by the signal for $I^F$ to molecules represented by $I^B$. The first-order or pseudo-first-order rate constants for the process that converts free ligand to bound ligand and the reverse reaction are $k_{FB}$ and $k_{BF}$, respectively. If it is assumed that the exchange process is fast enough to average spin–lattice relaxation of the $I$ spins in both environments ($k_{FB} > R_t^F$, $k_{BF} > R_t^B$) and the experiment is one in which both $S^F$ and $S^B$ are saturated ($S_t^B = S_t^F = 0$) until a steady state is reached, the NOE for both the free and bound $I$ spins is given by

$$f_I^F \{ S \} = f_I^B \{ S \} = \frac{X_F \sigma_{IS}^F + X_B \sigma_{IS}^B}{\rho_I^{AVE}} \tag{31}$$

where $\rho_I^{AVE}$ is the fast-exchange averaged spin–lattice relaxation rate, $\rho_I^{AVE} = X_F \rho_I^F + X_B \rho_I^B = R_I^{AVE} = X_F R_I^F + X_B R_I^B$ (Reference 47, page 149 *et seq.*). It is important to note that the NOEs in this situation are not simply the average of the NOEs that would be characteristic of the free and bound states of the systems but, rather, are obtained by averaging of the $\sigma_{IS}$ and $\rho_I$ terms separately.

The utility of the transferred NOE arises because it is often the case that $\sigma_{IS}^B$ for the bound ligand is significantly larger in magnitude than the corresponding term for the free ligand. Thus, even though the fraction of the ligand bound $X_B$ may be relatively small, the NOE observed is largely the one characteristic of the bound state. It is therefore possible to obtain information about intranuclear distances within the drug–receptor complex by observing signals that largely correspond to those of the free drug.

Although the discussion here has been couched in terms of spins $I$ and $S$ being present in the ligand, this is not a necessary feature of the discussion, and the $I–S$ interaction under study could involve one spin being located on the ligand while the other is part of the receptor. In this case, the $\sigma_{IS}$ term for the free ligand would be negligible because the separation of the $I$ and $S$ spins in the free state would be large.

# XII SOME EXAMPLES

## A ACTINOMYCIN D CONFORMATION

Actinomycin D is a powerful antibiotic isolated from streptomyces strains. The orange-red material has the covalent structure indicated below and consists of two pentapeptide lactone rings linked to an aminophenoxazone chromophore. Actinomycin D is used in clinical treatment of some cancers; the drug apparently acts by binding to DNA such that the chromophore intercalates between base pairs, with the peptide side chains lying in the minor groove.

Molecules of this size are ideal candidates for structural studies by proton NMR spectroscopy, since standard 1D and 2D homonuclear experiments are usually sufficient to afford complete assignment of the spectrum. The conformation of actinomycin D in solution has been determined by proton NMR methods.[89] The proton signals from the amino-acid residues in each pentapeptide lactone ring were assigned by COSY-type experiments and confirmed by correlating proton chemical shifts to those of the corresponding carbon atoms. About 40 NOEs were observed between various proton pairs in each pentapeptide lactone ring. The presence of an NOE exerts a constraint on the conformation of the molecule, since whatever conformation is present must position the pair of nuclei exhibiting the NOE proximate to each other. For the referenced study, and as is standard practice, the structural constraints implied by the observed NOEs were used in the data analysis in terms of a range of permissible distances. Computer methods, including distance geometry and restrained molecular dynamics, produced a conformation of the drug in solution that is similar to the structure found in the solid state by X-ray crystallography. Proton NMR methods have also been used to examine an actinomycin D–DNA oligomer complex.[90] Chapter 11 contains a detailed description of binding studies to DNA of a number of other antibiotics.

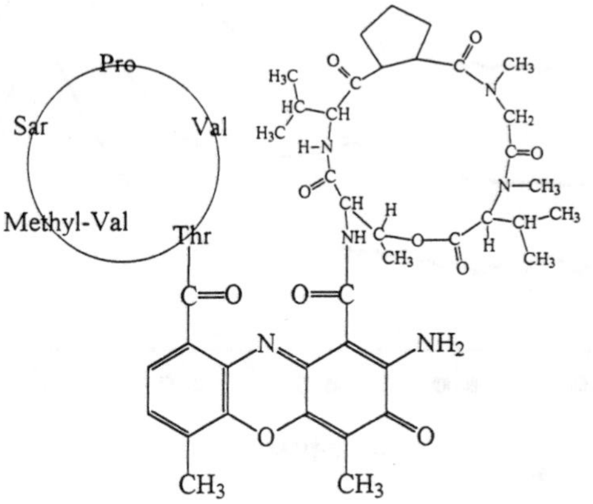

Actinomycin D

There are two identical cyclic pentapeptides attached to the aminophenoxazone chromophore in Actinomycin D. One of these is shown explicitly in the structure above.

## B SULINDAC AND SULINDAC SULFIDE WITH ALBUMIN

Human serum albumin (HSA) is a plasma protein of 69 kDa mass that is a receptor for a large number of drugs, fatty acids, and endogenous ligands. Several of these species may be bound simultaneously. Sulindac has been developed as an anti-inflammatory. The fluorine nucleus, which is part of its structure, provides a convenient means of examining the interaction of this drug and its metabolite, sulindac sulfide, with HSA.[91]

The fluorine-19 NMR spectrum of sulindac in the presence of HSA (Figure 14A) shows a broad, asymmetric signal at low sulindac to HSA

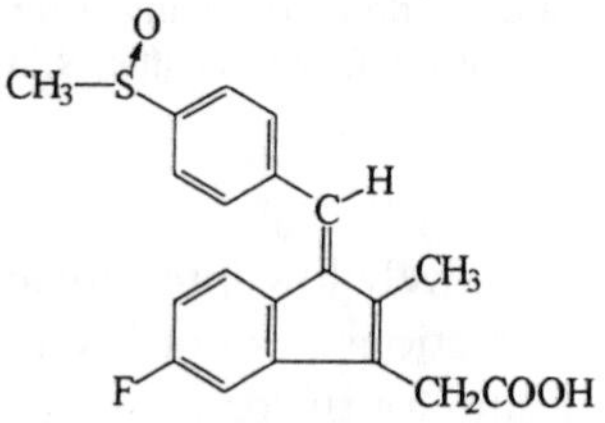

Sulindac 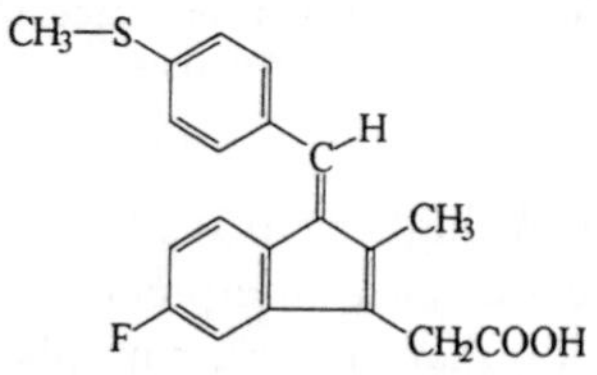                          Sulindac sulfide

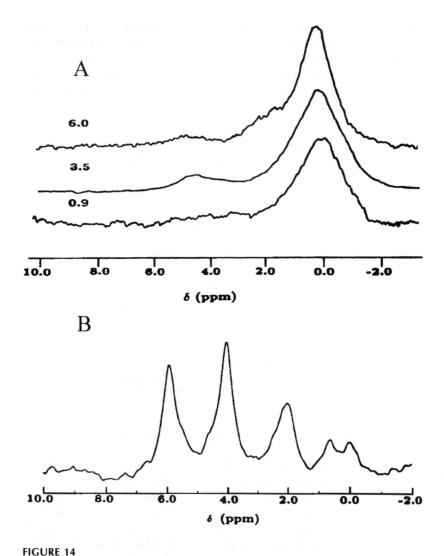

**FIGURE 14**
Fluorine-19 NMR spectra obtained with samples of sulindac (A) and the metabolite sulindac sulfide (B) in the presence of human serum albumin. Spectra were obtained at 338 MHz under conditions where the instrumental contribution to the signal line-widths was about 2 Hz. In series A, the ratio of the concentration of drug to protein concentration is indicated at the left of each trace. (Adapted from Jenkins, B.G. and Lauffer, R. B., *Mol. Pharm.*, 37, 111–118, 1990.)

ratios. At higher ratios additional peaks of relatively low intensity appear. While a detailed interpretation of these observations has not been made, it is clear that there are a number of binding sites for the drug on HSA and that the rate of dissociation of complexes formed at these sites is slow enough that slow-exchange conditions apply. The active metabolite, sulindac sulfide, shows a higher affinity for HSA; fluorine spectra (Figure 14B) suggest the formation of at least five complexes. It has been indicated that other ligands can selectively displace sulindac sulfide from these binding sites.[91] While the fluorine spectra in this case do not provide three-dimensional structural information, they do indicate that a panoply of receptor sites for a single drug molecule is present. Fluorine NMR provides a means of exploring the kinetics of drug binding, as well as competition and cooperation in the interaction of other ligands with these sites.

## C   HIRUDIN-DERIVED PEPTIDES BOUND TO THROMBIN

Thrombin is a central enzyme in blood coagulation and is involved in the conversion of circulating fibrinogen to the fibrin clot. The enzyme interacts with several components of the coagulation cascade and stimulates platelet aggregation. Hirudin is a small protein of 65 amino acids and is a very potent anticoagulant. Proteolytic removal of the C-terminal residues leads to an appreciable loss of activity, and it has been suggested that peptides derived from this region of hirudin may interact with a site on thrombin that is involved in its interaction with fibrinogen. These peptides are thus lead compounds for the development of antithrombotic agents. Proton NMR has been used to examine the interaction of the tetradecapeptide HR1 ($Asn_{52}$–$Asp_{53}$–$Gly_{54}$–$Asp_{55}$–$Phe_{56}$–$Glu_{57}$–$Glu_{58}$–$Ile_{59}$–$Pro_{60}$–$Glu_{61}$–$Glu_{62}$–$Tyr_{63}$–$Leu_{64}$–$Gln_{65}$) with thrombin.[92] This material corresponds to the 14 residues at the C-terminal of hirudin.

Figure 15A shows the NH and aromatic proton region of the spectrum of HR1. The various signals in the spectrum were assigned by 2D coherence transfer methods (COSY, TOCSY). Some of the signals are significantly broadened when thrombin is present in the sample (Figure 15B), particularly the NH proton signals for the residues from $Glu_{58}$ to $Gln_{65}$. Many side-chain resonances are also broadened by the presence of thrombin. The broadening effects observed are clear evidence that the peptide binds to the enzyme and that the rate of dissociation of the complex is at least sufficiently fast to provide some exchange broadening of signals from the peptide. Determination of proton–proton NOEs for HR1 alone showed only the expected NOEs between adjacent residues of the peptide, consistent with the peptide having a random conformation in solution. Transferred NOEs are characteristic of the bound peptide. Using the available NOE data as constraints, it was concluded that residues 55–65 of thrombin-bound HR1 take up a definite conformation in the complex, with amino acids from $Glu_{61}$ to $Leu_{64}$ involved in a helical structure.

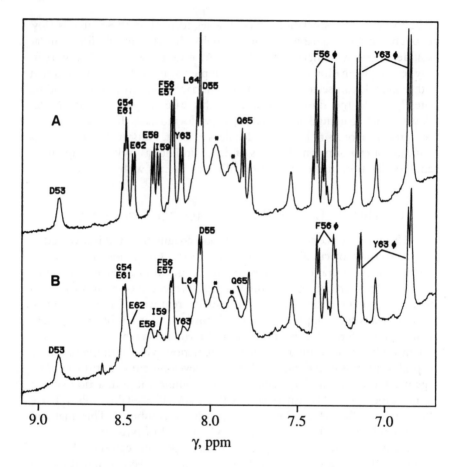

**FIGURE 15**

(A) The NH and aromatic proton region of the $^1$H NMR spectrum (500 MHz) of the peptide HR1 in water at 25°C at a concentration of 8 m$M$. (B) The same spectral region of HR1 when 0.36 m$M$ bovine thrombin is present. The labels shown correspond to residues in the peptide; the symbol $\phi$ indicates the aromatic ring protons of Phe 56 and Tyr 63. The asterisks mark an impurity in the samples. Because of the approximately 20-fold difference in concentration, the $^1$H NMR signals of thrombin appear as a broad distortion in the baseline of the spectra. (Adapted from data in Ni, F. et al., *Biochemistry,* 29, 4479–4489, 1990. With permission.)

## D    CALICHEAMICIN WITH DUPLEX DNA

Compounds containing the enediyne functionality have emerged as an important class of antitumour antibiotics. Their mechanism of action appears to involve site-specific cleavage of DNA and, ultimately, cell death. Such compounds include the calicheamicins, experamicins, neocarzinostatins, kedarcidins, and their derivatives.

Calicheamicin $\theta_1^I$, shown below, binds to the minor groove of DNA duplexes and, once bound, exhibits high sequence selectivity in DNA cleavage. A detailed study of the structures of complexes formed by this compound with the duplex $d$(GCATCCTAGC)·$d$(GCTAGGATGC) by proton NMR methods has been carried out.[93] More than 200 NOEs observed between DNA protons, between drug protons, and between protons of the drug and the DNA provided distance constraints that were used to develop a model of the complex.

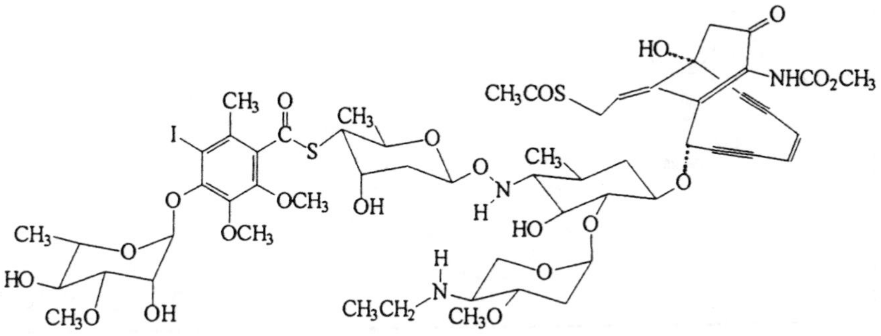

Calicheamicin $\theta_1^I$

A portion of proton NMR spectra of the complex obtained at various temperatures is shown in Figure 16. Upon lowering the sample temperature below 27°C, several of the drug and DNA signals split into two distinct signals, present with an intensity ratio of about 3:1. These must arise because two energetically similar conformations of the complex are present. Analysis of the lineshapes indicates that the lifetimes for the major and minor forms of the structure are <19 and <6 ms at the temperature (47°C) where coalescence of the signals is observed. The authors proposed that the conformations of the DNA–calicheamicin complex detected in these experiments differ because of movement of the aglycone portion of the drug in the minor groove. Studies of a range of other minor groove-binding drugs are described in Chapter 12.

## E  IMMUNOSUPPRESSANT–IMMUNOPHILIN COMPLEXES

Peptide prolyl *cis–trans* isomerases, enzymes that catalyse the interconversion of *cis* and *trans* isomers at proline peptide bonds (*cf.* Section X.C) appear to be targets of immunosuppressive drugs such as

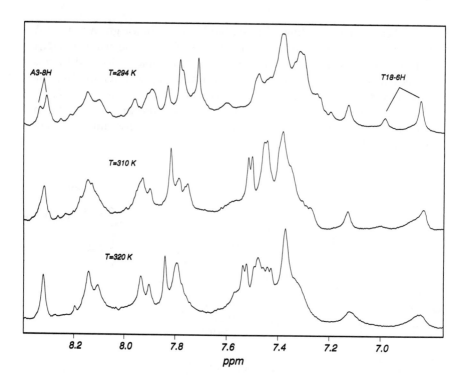

**FIGURE 16**

Aromatic region of the proton NMR spectrum at 500 MHz of a calicheamicin $\theta_I{}^I$–DNA complex; signals for protons 8H of base A3 and 6H of base T18 are indicated at different temperatures. The pairs of peaks observed for each proton at low temperature first coalesce, then merge to averaged lines above 310 K. (Spectra modified from Paloma, L.G., et al., *J. Am. Chem. Soc.*, 116, 3697–3708, 1994.)

cyclosporin A. The effects of these drugs probably also involve interaction with proteins important for T-cell activation. Both the ligands and the receptor proteins, particularly cyclophilin and FK506-binding protein, are sufficiently small that NMR methods provide a powerful means of deducing the structure of free and bound ligand and the free and bound receptor. NMR studies of various drug-receptor complexes of this nature have been nicely summarized by Fesik and Neri.[94] The work of their group and others provides a long list of examples of state-of-the-art applications of NMR in providing information of potential value in the development of drugs.

The FK506-binding protein has a mass of 11.8 kDa (107 amino acids) and, thus, is of a size where standard 1D and 2D proton NMR experiments may become difficult because of resonance overlap. The protein has been expressed in *Escherichia coli* and is preparable in forms in which all nitrogen positions are enriched in nitrogen-15 by use of [15]N-enriched ammonium chloride in the culture medium or enriched in carbon-13 by including labelled acetate. These methods are described in more detail in Chapter 4. Methods are also available for producing drugs such as ascomycin, shown below, in carbon-13 enriched forms.

A nitrogen-15 in a peptide bond will spin-couple directly to the adjacent peptide NH proton, less strongly to carbon-bound protons two

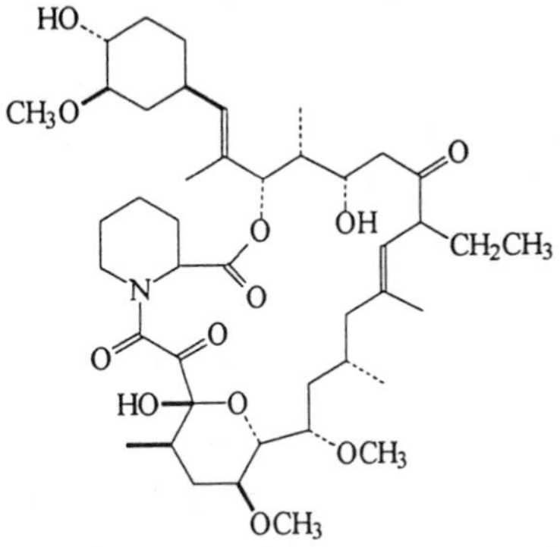

Ascomycin

and three bonds away, and to adjacent carbon-13 nuclei. Carbon-13 spins in such structures are also coupled to protons one, two, and three bonds away. It is this dense network of spins interconnected by coupling constants that is the basis for the effectiveness of the various multidimensional heteronuclear NMR experiments that are essential to providing data upon which tertiary structures of proteins and protein–ligand complexes can be based when such structures become larger than about 10 kDa. In the case of the FK506-binding protein–ascomycin complex, constraints on the structure produced by NMR included 1724 proton–proton nuclear Overhauser effects and more than 100 values of dihedral angles derived from vicinal coupling constants.[95] Further details on the structures of related complexes are given in Chapter 7.

The presence of the carbon and nitrogen isotope labels (and the corresponding coupling constants) in such systems also makes possible experiments in which the signals for the protons attached to the carbon or nitrogen spins may be selectively included or excluded from proton NMR spectra. Depending on which partner bears the carbon-13 and nitrogen-15 nuclei, [1]H NMR spectra of drug–receptor complexes could be obtained in which signals from only the drug or only the receptor portion of the structure appear in the spectrum.[96,97]

## XIII SUMMARY

The remainder of this book demonstrates the scope of contemporary applications of NMR spectroscopy to many aspects of drug design and evaluation. The unique abilities of NMR methods to provide information about the structures and conformations of ligand molecules, receptors, and ligand–receptor complexes, as well as the dynamic aspects of these species, can only expand as technological advances make possible experiments at magnetic fields corresponding to proton NMR observations at 1000 MHz or beyond. The use of *in vivo* NMR in the evaluation of drug performance and in elucidation of the basic mechanisms of drug action, still rather limited in its scope, offers a potentially important extra dimension for drug development efforts.

## ACKNOWLEDGMENTS

This chapter was prepared with the partial support of the National Institutes of Health (Grant GM25975). I am indebted to the researchers mentioned, who made drawings and other materials available, and to members of my laboratory and my wife, who provided helpful comments and editorial assistance.

# REFERENCES

1. Hurley, L.H.; *J. Med. Chem.* 1989, 32, 2027-2033.
2. Propst, C.L.; Perun, T.J. Eds.; *Nucleic Acid Targeted Drug Design*; Marcel Dekker: New York, 1989.
3. Oksenburg, D.; Marsters, S.A.; O'Dowd, B.F.; Jin, H.; Hovlik, S.; Peroutka, S.J.; Ashkenazi, A.; *Nature* 1992, 360, 161-163.
4. Hare, R.; *The Birth of Penicillin*; Allen & Unwin: London, 1970.
5. Wainwright, M.; *Miracle Cure. The Story of Penicillin and the Golden Age of Antibiotics*; Blackwell Scientific: Oxford, 1990.
6. Campese, V.M.; *Drugs* 1981, 22, 257-278.
7. Meisheri, K.D.; Johnson, G.A.; Puddington, L.; *Biochem. Pharmacol.* 1993, 45, 271-279.
8. Devlin, J.P.; *Today's Chemist at Work*, September 1993.
9. Perutz, M.F.; *Protein Structure. New Approaches to Disease and Therapy*; Freeman: New York, 1992.
10. Navia, M.A.; Peattie, D.A.; *Immunology Today* 1993, 14, 296-302 (and in *TiPS* 1993, 14, 189-195).
11. Bowen, J.P.; Charifson, P.S.; Fox, P.C.; Kontoyianni, M.; Miller, A.B.; Schnur, D.; Stewart, E.; Van Dyke, C.; *J. Clin. Pharmacol.* 1993, 33, 1149-1164.
12. Whittle, P.J.; Blundell, T.L.; *Annu. Rev. Biophys. Biomol. Struct.* 1994, 23, 349-375.

13. von Itzstein, M.; Wu, W.-Y.; Kok, G.B.; Pegg, M.S.; Dyason, J.C.; Jin, B.; Phan, T.V.; Smythe, M.L.; White, H.F.; Oliver, S.W.; Colman, P.M.; Varghese, J.N.; Ryan, D.M.; Woods, J.M.; Bethell, R.C.; Hotham, V.J.; Cameron, J.M.; Penn, C.R.; *Nature* 1993, 363, 418-423.

14. Jacobson, R.H.; Zhang, X.-J.; DuBose, R.F.; Matthews, B.W.; *Nature* 1994, 369, 761-763.

15. Roberts, G.C.K., Ed.; *NMR of Macromolecules*; IRL: Oxford, 1993.

16. Wüthrich, K.; *Biochem. Pharmacol.* 1990, 40, 55-62.

17. Clore, G.M.; Gronenborn, A.M. *Science* 1991, 252, 1390-1399.

18. Kaptein, R.; Boelens, R.; Scheek, R.M.; van Gunsteren, W.F.; *Biochemistry* 1988, 27, 5389-5395.

19. Bax, A.; Grzesiek, S.; *Acc. Chem. Res.* 1993, 26, 131-138.

20. Clore, G.M., Gronenborn, A.M., Eds.; *NMR of Proteins*; CRC Press: Boca Raton, FL. 1993.

21. Hinck, A.P.; Eberhardt, E.S.; Markeley, J.L. *Biochemistry* 1993, 32, 11810-11818.

22. Kim, Y.; Prestegard, J.H.; *J. Am. Chem. Soc.* 1990, 112, 3707-3709.

23. Birdsall, B.; Tendler, S.J.B.; Arnold, J.R.P.; Feeney, J.; Griffin, R.J.; Carr, M.D.; Thomas, J.A.; Roberts G.C.K.; Stevens, M.F.G.; *Biochemistry* 1990, 29, 9660-9677.

24. Wagner, G.; *J. Biomol. NMR* 1993, 3, 378-385.

25. Lesk, A.M.; *Protein Architecture*; IRL Press: Oxford, 1991; p. 15.

26. Billeter, M.; *Quart. Rev. Biophys.* 1992, 25, 325-377.

27. Fesik, S.W.; *J. Biomol. NMR* 1993, 3, 261-269.

28. Wüthrich, K.; *NMR of Proteins and Nucleic Acids*; Wiley-Interscience: New York, 1986.

29. Perkins, S.J.; *Biol. Magn. Reson.* 1982, 4, 193-336.

30. Williamson, M.P.; Asakura, T.; *J. Magn. Reson. B* 1993, 101, 63-71.

31. Reid, B.R.; *Methods Enzymol.* 1979, 59, 21-57.

32. Bolton, P.H.; Kearns, D.R.; *Biol. Magn. Reson.* 1978, 1, 91-138.

33. Wemmer, D.E.; *Biol. Magn. Reson.* 1992, 10, 195-264.

34. Varani, G.; Tinoco, I.; *Quart. Rev. Biophys.* 1991, 24, 479-532.

35. Xu, R.X.; Olejniczak, E.T.; Fesik, S.W.; *FEBS Lett.* 1992, 305, 137-143.

36. Sanders, J.K.M.; Hunter, B.K.; *Modern NMR Spectroscopy;* Oxford University Press: Oxford, 1987; p. 114 et seq.

37. Szyperski, T.; Guntert, P.; Otting, G.; Wüthrich, K.; *J. Magn. Reson.* 1992, 99, 552-560.

38. Byrd, R.A.; Dawson, W.H.; Ellis, P.D.; Dunlap, R.H.; *J. Am. Chem.Soc.* 1978, 100, 7478-7486.

39. Billeter, M.; Neri, D.; Otting, G.; Qian, Y.Q.; Wüthrich, K.; *J. Biomol. NMR* 1992, 2, 257-274.

40. Kay, L.E.; Bax, A.; *J. Magn. Reson.* 1990, 86, 110-126.

41. Ernst, R.R.; Bodenhausen, G.; Wokaun, A.; *Principles of Nuclear Magnetic Resonance in One- and Two-Dimensions;* Clarendon Press: Oxford, 1987; p. 49.

42. Brown, L.R.; Farmer, B.T., II; *Methods Enzymol.* 1989, 176, 199-216.

43. Marshall, A.G.; *Biophysical Chemistry*; John Wiley & Sons: New York, 1978; p. 709 et seq.

44. Goldman, M.; *Quantum Description of High-Resolution NMR in Liquids*; Clarendon Press: Oxford, 1988; chap 9.

45. Noggle, J.H.; Schirmer, R.E.; *The Nuclear Overhauser Effect*; Academic Press: New York, 1971; app. I.

46. Harbison, G.S. *J. Am. Chem. Soc.* 1993, 115, 3026-3027.

47. Neuhaus, D.; Williamson, M.P.; *The Nuclear Overhauser Effect in Structural and Conformational Analysis*; VCH Publishers: New York, 1989; Chapter 4.
48. Borgias, B.A.; James, T.L. *Methods Enzymol.* 1989, 176, 169-184.
49. Bull, T.E.; *J. Magn. Reson.* 1987, 72, 397-413.
50. Petros, A.M.; Mueller, L.; Kopple, K.D.; *Biochemistry* 1990, 29, 10041-10048.
51. Fesik, S.W.; Gemmecker, G.; Olejniczak, E.T.; Petros, A.M.; *J. Am. Chem. Soc.* 1991, 113, 7080-7081.
52. Duncan, T.M.; *A Compilation of Chemical Shift Anisotropies*; Farragut: Chicago, 1990.
53. Dalvit, C.; *J. Magn. Reson.* 1991, 95, 410-416.
54. Keeler, J.; Sanchez-Ferrando, F.; *J. Magn. Reson.* 1987, 75, 96-109.
55. Daragan, V.A.; Mayo, K.H.; *Chem. Phys. Lett.* 1993, 206, 393-400.
56. Sandstrom, J.; *Dynamic NMR Spectroscopy*; Academic Press: London, 1982.
57. Feeney, J.; Batchelor, J.G.; Albrand, J.P.; Roberts, G.C.K.; *J. Magn. Reson.* 1979, 33, 519-529.
58. London, R.E.; *J. Magn. Reson. A* 1993, 104, 190-196.
59. Swift, T.J.; Connick, R.E.; *J. Chem. Phys.* 1962, 37, 307-320.
60. Gerig, J.T.; Stock, A.D.; *Org. Magn. Reson.* 1975, 7, 249-255.
61. Bovey, F.A.; Jelinski, L.; Mirau, P.A.; *NMR Spectroscopy*, 2nd ed.; Academic Press: San Diego, 1988; p. 265.
62. Led, J.J.; Gesmar, H.; Abildgaard, F.; *Methods Enzymol.* 1989, 176, 311-329.
63. Gueron, M.; Plateau, P.; Decorps, M.; *Prog. NMR Spectrosc.* 1991, 23, 135-209.
64. Perrin, C.L.; Engler, R.E.; *J. Magn. Reson.* 1990, 90, 363-369.
65. Gerig, J.T.; *J. Am. Chem. Soc.* 1977, 99, 1721-1725.
66. Campbell, I.D.; Dobson, C.M.; Ratcliffe, R.G.; Williams, R.J.P.; *J. Magn. Reson.* 1978, 29, 397-417.
67. Homans, S.W.; *A Dictionary of Concepts in NMR*; Clarendon Press: Oxford, 1989; p. 113.
68. Larive, C.K.; Rabenstein, D.L.; *J. Am. Chem. Soc.* 1993, 115, 2833-2836.
69. Boyd, J.; Brindle, K.M.; Campbell, I.D.; Radda, G.K.; *J. Magn. Reson.* 1984, 60, 149-155.
70. Nageswara-Rao, B.D.; *Methods Enzymol.* 1989, 176, 279-311.
71. Clore, G.M.; Gronenborn, A.M.; Birdsall, B.; Feeney, J.; Roberts, G.C.K.; *Biochem. J.* 1984, 217, 659-666.
72. London, R.E.; personal communication.
73. Hughes, D.G.; Lindblom, G.J.; *J. Magn. Reson.* 1977, 26, 469-479.
74. Hughes, D.G.; *J. Magn. Reson.* 1977, 26, 481-489.
75. Jen, J.; *J. Magn. Reson.* 1978, 30, 111-128.
76. Bull, T.E.; *Prog. NMR Spectrosc.* 1992, 24, 377-410.
77. Deverell, C.; Morgan, R.E.; Strange, J.H.; *Mol. Phys.* 1970, 18, 553-559.
78. Campbell, D.M.; Mackowiak, M.; Jonas, J.; *J. Chem. Phys.* 1992, 96, 2717-2723.
79. Dalvit, C.; Bodenhausen, G.; *Adv. Magn. Reson.* 1990, 14, 1-33.
80. Richards, F.M.; Lim, W.A.; *Q. Rev. Biophys.* 1994, 26, 423-498.
81. Opella, S.J.; Nelson, D.J.; Jardetzky, O.; *J. Chem. Phys.* 1976, 64, 2533-2535.
82. Bothner-By, A.; Stephens, R.L.; Lee, J.; Warren, C.D.; Jeanloz, R.W.; *J. Am. Chem. Soc.* 1984, 106, 811-813.
83. Hwang, T-L.; Shaka, A.J.; *J. Am. Chem. Soc.* 1992, 114, 3157-3159.
84. Clore, G.M.; Gronenborn, A.M.; *J. Magn. Reson.* 1983, 53, 423-442.
85. Anderson, N.H.; Eaton, H.L.; Nguyen, K.T.; *Magn. Reson. Chem.* 1987, 25, 1025-1034.
86. Campbell, A.P.; Sykes, B.D.; *J. Magn. Reson.* 1991, 93, 77-92.

87. Campbell, A.P.; Sykes, B.D.; *Ann. Rev. Biophys. Biomol. Struct.* 1993, 22, 99-122.
88. London, R.E.; Perlman, M.E.; Davis, D.G.; *J. Magn. Reson.* 1992, 97, 79-98.
89. Yu, C.; Tseng, Y.-Y.; *Eur. J. Biochem.* 1992, 209, 181-187.
90. Liu, X.; Chen, H.; Patel,; D.J. *J. Biomol. NMR* 1991, 1, 323-347.
91. Jenkins, B.G.; Lauffer, R.B.; *Mol. Pharm.* 1990, 37, 111-118.
92. Ni, F.; Konishi, Y.; Sheraga, H.A.; *Biochemistry* 1990, 29, 4479-4489.
93. Paloma, L.G.; Smith, J.A.; Chazin, W.J.; Nicolaou, K.C.; *J. Am. Chem. Soc.* 1994, 116, 3697-3708.
94. Fesik, S.W.; Neri, P.; Multidimensional NMR studies of immunosuppressant/immunophilin complexes, in *NMR of Proteins*, Clore, G.M.; Gronenborn, A.M.; Eds.; CRC Press: Boca Raton, FL, 1993; Chap. 4.
95. Meadows, R.P.; Nettesheim, D.G.; Xu, R.X.; Olejniczak, E.T.; Petros, A.M.; Holzman, T.F.; Severin, J.; Gubbins, E.; Smith, H.; Fesik, S.W.; *Biochemistry* 1993, 32, 754-765.
96. Petros, A.M.; Kawai, M.; Luly, J.R.; Fesik, S.W.; *FEBS Lett.* 1992, 308, 309-314.
97. Petros, A.M.; Gemmecker, G.; Neri, P.; Olejniczak, E.T.; Nettesheim, D.; Xu, R.X.; Gubbins, E.G.; Smith, H.; Fesik, S.W.; *J. Med. Chem.* 1992, 35, 2467-2473.

# CHAPTER 4

# PROTEIN STRUCTURE DETERMINATION USING NMR SPECTROSCOPY

*Glenn F. King and Joel P. Mackay*

## CONTENTS

I  Introduction ................................................................................... 103

II  Overexpression of Recombinant Proteins ..................................... 104
  A  Overview ................................................................................ 104
  B  Generating DNA for Cloning ................................................. 105
  C  Choice of Host Expression System ........................................ 106
  D  Choice of Cloning Vector and Purification Strategy ............. 109
  E  Isotopic Labelling of Proteins for NMR Studies ................... 112
    1  Overview .......................................................................... 112
    2  Uniform $^{13}C/^{15}N$ Labelling .......................................... 112
    3  Random Fractional Deuteration ...................................... 113
    4  Selective Labelling .......................................................... 115

III  Sample Preparation ....................................................................... 116
  A  Heterogeneity of the NMR Sample ........................................ 116
  B  Paramagnetic and Microbial Contamination ......................... 118
  C  Sample pH .............................................................................. 118
  D  Sample Temperature ............................................................... 120

0-8493-7824-9/96/$0.00+$.50
© 1996 by CRC Press, Inc.

**IV**  Acquisition of Structural Data.................................................. 121
   A  Overview ...................................................................... 121
   B  Homonuclear Resonance-Assignment Strategies .................... 122
      1  Overview .................................................................. 122
      2  Suitability of a Protein for Homonuclear
         Assignment Techniques ........................................... 125
      3  Spin System Identification ..................................... 127
      4  Sequence-Specific Resonance Assignment ................ 129
      5  Three-Dimensional Homonuclear NMR .................... 130
   C  Heteronuclear Resonance Assignment Strategies .................. 132
      1  Overview .................................................................. 132
      2  Heteronuclear-Edited Homonuclear Experiments ........... 135
      3  Triple-Resonance Experiments ................................. 140
      4  Summary of Resonance-Assignment Strategies ............. 148
   D  Recent Advances.............................................................. 153
      1  Pulsed Field Gradients ........................................... 153
      2  Heteronuclear Cross-Polarisation ............................ 157
      3  Other Areas ............................................................ 158
   E  Extraction of Structural Constraints ................................ 161
      1  Overview .................................................................. 161
      2  NOEs ...................................................................... 161
      3  Scalar Coupling Constants....................................... 165
      4  Amide-Proton Exchange .......................................... 169
      5  Chemical Shifts as Structural Parameters .................... 170

**V**  Calculation of Tertiary Structures from NMR Data .................... 170
   A  Overview ...................................................................... 170
   B  Distance Geometry.......................................................... 171
      1  Overview .................................................................. 171
      2  Metric-Matrix DG Algorithms ................................. 171
      3  Torsion-Space DG Algorithms ................................. 174
      4  (Dis)advantages of Torsion-Angle vs. Metric-Matrix
         DG Algorithms ........................................................ 175
   C  Energy Minimisation and Restrained Molecular
      Dynamics ...................................................................... 176
   D  Dynamical Simulated Annealing....................................... 178
   E  Use of Time-Averaged NMR Constraints ............................ 180
   F  Direct Refinement Against NOE Intensities .......................... 182
   G  Optimal Filtering............................................................ 185
   H  Assessing the Quality of the Calculated Structure(s).............. 187

**VI**  Conclusions and Future Prospects ..................................... 189

Acknowledgments ...................................................................... 191

**References** ............................................................................. 191

# I   INTRODUCTION

As noted in earlier chapters, currently available drugs have arisen either from serendipitous discovery or from systematic screening of large numbers of natural or synthetic compounds. While the latter approach is often successful, it can be very expensive. It is not guaranteed to produce a lead compound, and even if it does, considerable effort may be required to transform the lead compound into a drug with desirable properties such as low toxicity, high bioavailability, and economical means of manufacture.

Our increased understanding of the molecular basis of numerous disease processes has paved the way for a more direct method of drug design, which promises to supplant or supplement these speculative traditional approaches. In the process of structure-based drug design described in Chapters 1 to 3, one starts with the three-dimensional structure of the target molecule, generally a protein, and attempts to *rationally* design a drug molecule that will interact *specifically* with the target. Several drugs designed in this manner are currently in clinical trial, including inhibitors of HIV protease, thymidylate synthase, thrombin, and influenza neuraminidase.[1,2]

The rate-limiting step in the application of this rational approach to drug design is the determination of the tertiary structure of the target protein. Currently, there are only two methods that can be used to elucidate the structures of proteins at close to atomic resolution, namely, X-ray crystallography and NMR spectroscopy. While the first crystallographic images of proteins were produced by Perutz and Kendrews in the early 1960s,[3,4] the first complete determination of a protein structure using NMR spectroscopy was not achieved until 1985.[5] However, despite their relative infancy, NMR-based structure-determination techniques have already led to the deposition of coordinates for more than 100 protein structures in the Brookhaven protein databank.[6]

A particularly attractive feature of NMR-based methods for structure determination is that, once the hard work of assigning resonances and calculating the structure has been completed, substantially less groundwork is required to do further NMR studies to probe other aspects of protein function such as molecular dynamics, ligand binding, and reaction kinetics. This is in contrast to X-ray crystallographic studies, which generally provide only structural data and which frequently have the growth of suitable crystals as the rate limiting step. The latter process defies generalisation, even between closely related compounds (such as a protein and the same protein bound to a ligand).

Thus, NMR spectroscopy promises to make an important contribution to the field of structure-based drug design. The aim of this chapter is to review the state of the art with respect to this rapidly evolving field. We shall survey methods for overproduction and isotopic labelling of the target proteins, salient aspects of sample preparation, homonuclear and heteronuclear strategies for NMR resonance assignment, the types of structural data that can be elucidated using NMR techniques, and strategies for calculating three-dimensional protein structures from NMR data. Finally, we shall offer some speculations on the future prospects for this exciting and rapidly advancing field of research.

## II  OVEREXPRESSION OF RECOMBINANT PROTEINS

### A  OVERVIEW

Protein structure determination using NMR spectroscopy requires reasonably large amounts of protein. Typically, the minimum requirement is a 400- to 500-µl solution of ~1 m$M$ protein, which corresponds to 0.6–7.5 mg of protein for the currently feasible molecular weight range of 3–30 kDa. While the NMR technique itself is essentially noninvasive, thus enabling samples to be recovered at the end of the NMR study for biochemical testing and for other biophysical experiments, in practice there is often deterioration of the sample during the many days or even months[7] that the sample needs to spend in the spectrometer probehead. In combination with the fact that some protein is often irretrievably degraded in initial experiments designed to establish the optimal parameters for spectral acquisition, this means that several times the minimum quantity mentioned above will generally be required. Thus, tens of milligrams of protein will likely be needed for NMR structural studies of a 30-kDa protein.

Proteins smaller than 10 kDa, for which isotopic labelling is not essential (although it may be desirable), can be purified from a native source if it is sufficiently abundant (a minimum of ~0.6–2 mg will be required). An economically viable alternative for proteins less than about 50 residues, or structurally autonomous modules of larger proteins,[8,9] is automated solid-phase peptide synthesis.[10] Proteins larger than ~10 kDa need to be uniformly enriched with nonradioactive $^{15}$N and $^{13}$C isotopes (so-called heteronuclei); in these cases, recombinant DNA technology represents the only economically feasible means of producing the requisite quantities of isotopically labelled protein. Not only do recombinant DNA techniques facilitate isotopic labelling, thus extending the complement of NMR experiments that can be performed on the protein, but they also enable easy introduction of point mutations to test structure-function hypotheses.[11]

The overproduction of a protein using recombinant DNA techniques essentially involves four stages: generation of the DNA sequence that encodes the target protein, ligation of the foreign DNA into a cloning vector, introduction of the vector into a host cell (this step must include some means of selecting correctly transformed cells), and overexpression and purification of the protein from the background of host proteins.[12] The ligation and transformation steps are reasonably standard and are covered in detail in a number of practical manuals.[13,14] The major variables of concern to the molecular biologist, which we discuss in the following sections, are the methods available for generating the DNA sequence, and the choice of host and cloning vector, to which the purification strategy is often inextricably linked.

## B   GENERATING DNA FOR CLONING

It is beyond the scope of this chapter to provide more than a brief outline of the methods available for generating the desired DNA sequence. By far the most favoured host for overexpression of heterologous proteins is the Gram-negative bacterium *Escherichia coli*. Since prokaryotes lack a mechanism for removing introns, these regions must be removed when cloning eukaryotic genes for expression in bacteria. Thus, the cloning process most often begins with a cDNA library, which is derived from the mRNA and therefore lacks intron sequences. Traditional methods for cloning genes from cDNA libraries are outlined in detail in most genetic engineering texts and practical manuals[12-14] and therefore will not be covered here.

More recently, the polymerase chain reaction (PCR)[15] has been developed to allow facile amplification of desired gene sequences from cDNA.[13,14,16] The PCR protocol involves repetitive cycles of template denaturation, primer annealing, and extension of the annealed primers, according to the template cDNA sequence, by DNA polymerase. Because the initial phase of template denaturation is performed at high temperature, extension is generally achieved using *Taq* polymerase, a thermostable DNA polymerase isolated from the thermophilic eubacterial microorganism *Thermus aquaticus*, which was first isolated from a hot spring in Yellowstone National Park.[16] Unfortunately, *Taq* polymerase lacks the 3'–5' exonuclease proofreading activity found in *E. coli* DNA polymerase I, which is most commonly used in conventional cloning procedures. While this leads to a somewhat reduced copying fidelity, the error rate is still estimated to be negligible at $\sim 2 \times 10^{-4}$ nucleotides per cycle.[16] The PCR fidelity problem might be ameliorated or completely obviated by the discovery of thermostable DNA polymerases that have proofreading activity.[17] Thus, if a cDNA library is available, PCR amplification is probably the simplest method for obtaining the desired DNA sequence.

The aforementioned strategies generate DNA fragments that are exact replicas of the parental cDNA. A potential problem with this approach is that the DNA may contain codons which are rarely used by the host organism, which might cause low translation efficiencies,[18,19] misincorporation of amino acids,[20] and deletion of amino acids due to translational hopping.[21] Thus, an alternative strategy for small proteins or protein modules is to generate the DNA fragment using synthetic oligonucleotides constructed using only codons that are known to be efficiently translated in the host organism. The synthetic gene approach also allows for inclusion of engineered restriction enzyme sites in order to facilitate site-directed mutagenesis, introduction and/or removal of exon homologues,[22] and addition of flanking protein modules.

Synthetic genes are constructed by annealing and subsequently ligating a number of overlapping oligonucleotides.[22,23] The terminal 3′ oligonucleotide is designed to encode translation–termination codons, and restriction enzyme sites can also be included in the terminal oligonucleotides in order to facilitate directional cloning into the chosen expression vector. This approach has been used to generate the leucine zipper module of the human c-Jun oncoprotein (a 92-residue dimer) for NMR structural studies.[23] The recent construction of a synthetic gene for human tropoelastin, which codes for a protein of 732 residues,[22] indicates that this technique could be used to generate a synthetic gene for any protein in the size range suitable for NMR structural studies (i.e., less than 35 kDa).

## C   CHOICE OF HOST EXPRESSION SYSTEM

There are numerous hosts available for heterologous protein expression, the best studied being *E. coli*, the Gram-positive bacterium *Bacillus subtilis*, yeast, and various mammalian cells; interested readers should refer to an excellent recent review of these systems.[24] More recently, a baculovirus/insect cell system has been developed.[25] The choice of which host to use depends on the properties of the protein being expressed and whether posttranslational modification of the protein is required.

By far the most popular host for heterologous protein expression is *E. coli*. There are several advantages of this system: (1) our knowledge of *E. coli* genetics is superior to that for any other organism, and a wide range of cloning vectors is available; (2) many more proteins have been overexpressed in this host than any other, thus providing an extensive database to guide overexpression of new proteins; (3) heterologous proteins can either be expressed intracellularly or, by use of an appropriate signal sequence, secreted into the periplasmic space (secretion into the extracellular medium is more difficult);[26] (4) a particular advantage for NMR studies is that *E. coli* can grow to very high cell densities, even in minimal medium, thus limiting the amount of expensive medium required for isotopic labelling (see Section II.E below); (5) our extensive knowledge of *E. coli* metabolic pathways facilitates specific, as opposed to uniform, labelling of proteins (see Section II.E below). However, there are several potential disadvantages with this host: (1) while heterologous proteins can be overexpressed intracellularly in very high fractional abundance (30–50% of total cell protein is not uncommon), they are often found in insoluble inclusion bodies from which the protein has to be recovered and renatured, a process that can be fraught with difficulties;[26,27] (2) while secretion into the periplasm generally increases protein stability by enabling formation of disulphide bonds and by limiting exposure to intracellular proteases, yields of secreted protein are often quite low, since periplasmic proteins typically represent only ~4% of total cell protein;[26] (3) *E. coli* does not perform eukaryotic posttranslational modifications such as glycosylation; (4) unless the protein is expressed as a fusion construct (see Section II.D) or it contains a cleavable N-terminal signal sequence that directs the protein into the periplasm, a methionine residue will be appended to the N-terminus of the protein (since the translation-initiation codon in *E. coli* codes for methionine).

*Bacillus subtilis* and yeast (*Saccharomyces cerevisiae*) have the advantage of enabling the overexpressed protein to be secreted into the culture medium. While yields are generally lower than those for proteins overexpressed in the cytoplasm, the lower concentration of protein in the culture medium enhances the prospects of obtaining correctly folded and soluble protein, especially since disulphide bonds can be formed.[24] Secretion into the culture medium also facilitates purification since the background of contaminating proteins is very low. Thus, these systems may be particularly suited to proteins that are difficult to refold from a denatured form or those that are refractory to purification. Secretion systems also yield proteins with authentic N-termini as the signal peptide is removed during export. It might be expected that yeast has the additional advantage of allowing intron splicing from eukaryotic genes, thus obviating the necessity to clone from cDNA. However, *S. cerevisiae* does not excise introns correctly from genes cloned from higher eukaryotes, apparently because these introns do not contain yeast-specific splicing signals.[12]

Some eukaryotic proteins undergo posttranslational modifications such as hydroxylation of proline, N-terminal acetylation, N- and O-linked glycosylation, and phosphorylation of Ser, Thr, or Tyr residues. These modifications cannot be achieved using prokaryotic expression systems. Thus, the NMR spectroscopist has to decide whether any of these posttranslational modifications are absolutely essential for structural studies. For example, unless glycosylation is critical to the function of the protein or it significantly aids protein stability and/or solubility, it is often best avoided as it can unnecessarily complicate NMR spectral analysis and it can significantly increase the molecular weight of the protein.

Only proteins destined for the secretory pathway of eukaryotic cells are glycosylated. Thus, recombinant mammalian proteins are glycosylated in yeast secretion systems. However, the outer core of sugars at each attachment site will typically be simple high-mannose type compared to the more complex and highly branched outer core of higher eukaryotes.[12] Thus, a mammalian expression system will be necessary if authentic glycosylation is important, although even then it is possible that the type of glycosylation will be cell and species specific. However, mammalian expression systems are most commonly used for transient expression of DNA introduced to the cell by microinjection, electroporation, transfection with transient expression vectors, or various chemical-mediated processes.[24] The DNA is expressed over a period of several days to several weeks before being lost from the cells.[24] Stable overexpression of heterologous proteins in mammalian cells is more difficult and generally requires the DNA to be introduced by either: (1) contransformation of the target gene with a selectable marker (e.g., a gene encoding antibiotic resistance), thus enabling selection of cells that have integrated the foreign DNA into their genome;[13] or (2) infection of the cells with a virus containing the DNA of interest;[13,24] in this approach, the virus usurps the protein-synthesis machinery of the host cell and directs synthesis of the heterologous protein. It remains to be seen whether mammalian expression systems can be developed sufficiently to enable routine provision of adequate amounts of isotopically labelled protein for NMR studies.

A viral infection strategy is also employed in the baculovirus/insect expression system.[25] Cultured *Spodoptera frugiperda* insect cells are co-transfected with wild-type DNA from *Autographa californica* multiple nuclear polyhedrosis virus (AcMNPV) and a transfer vector in which the gene of interest is linked to the strong polyhedrin gene promoter sequence. Homologous recombination, which occurs *in vivo* at a frequency of 1–5%,[13] results in overexpression of the heterologous protein. Cells containing the required viral recombinants can be readily selected from cells infected with only wild-type baculovirus DNA as the latter form occlusion bodies due to the production of large amounts of polyhedrin protein. The polyhedrin gene is lost in the successful recombinants and, since the desired heterologous protein is overproduced instead of the polyhedrin protein, occlusion bodies are not formed. It is claimed that this system is capable of producing up to 500 mg of heterologous protein per litre of cultured cells.[25] This high level of overexpression may make this system suitable for producing isotopically labelled proteins for NMR structural studies in cases where posttranslational modifications such as glycosylation and phosphorylation are essential.

Table 1 attempts to summarize the major properties of the various expression systems from the perspective of pursuing NMR structural studies. While the vast majority of recombinant proteins used for NMR studies have been produced using *E. coli* expression systems, several have been produced using yeast secretion systems,[28,29] one has been constructed using a mammalian cell line by Abbott Laboratories,[30] and one has been produced by growing *Bacillus* strain PB92 on either [15]N-labelled yeast or

**TABLE 1**

Properties of Host Systems for Heterologous Protein Expression

| Property | E. coli | B. subtilis | Yeast | Baculovirus | Mammalian |
|---|---|---|---|---|---|
| Ease of vector construction and transformation | +++ | ++[a] | + | + | + |
| High levels of protein expression | +++ | ++ | ++ | +++ | ++ |
| Likelihood of soluble, correctly folded protein | + | ++ | ++ | ++ | ++ |
| Secretion to culture medium possible? | + | ++ | ++ | + | + |
| Correct N-terminus? | No | +[b] | + | ++ | ++ |
| Extent of posttranslational modification | None | None | + | ++ | +++ |
| Ease of isotopic labelling for NMR[c] | +++ | ++ | ++ | Difficult | Difficult |

[a] Homology between the plasmid vector and B. subtilis chromosomal DNA can cause plasmid instability because of the high frequency of homologous recombination in this bacterium.

[b] This assumes that the signal peptide is excised during secretion to the culture medium.

[c] This reflects the ability of the host cells to grow to high cell density in a well-defined minimal medium, conditions that are conducive to economical isotopic labelling (see Section II.E).

a $^{13}$C/$^{15}$N-labelled carbohydrate/amino acid medium.[51] Partially labelled antibodies have been produced using a mouse hybridoma cell line.[31] We are unaware of any heteronuclear NMR studies thus far in which the target protein has been produced using a baculovirus expression system.

## D    CHOICE OF CLONING VECTOR AND PURIFICATION STRATEGY

It is not our intention to summarise the bewildering array of cloning vectors that are available for overexpression of heterologous proteins in the various host systems outlined above; extensive practical and theoretical accounts of cloning vectors can be obtained from numerous sources.[13,14,24,32] Rather, we hope to convey some points of special interest to the NMR spectroscopist, with special reference to E. coli, which is presently the preferred host for protein overexpression.

As the ultimate goal for NMR structural studies is to produce large amounts of isotopically labelled protein, it is desirable for the protein to be highly overexpressed (so that isotopic labelling is economical) and for purification to be reasonably facile (to avoid loss of expensive labelled protein). The first requirement can usually be met by using plasmid vectors with high-copy number and with the target gene linked to a strong inducible promoter. Facile purification can often be achieved by strategically arranging for the protein to be purified using some form of affinity chromatography; this frequently enables single-step purification of the heterologous protein from the background of host-cell proteins. In many cases, however, the protein will not have any natural ligands, or affinity chromatography media with covalently attached ligand may not be available. In these cases, it may be worth considering overexpression of the heterologous protein as a fusion with a carrier protein for which affinity purification media are available.

Numerous vectors have now been constructed that facilitate this approach. In the pGEX family of vectors, the heterologous protein is expressed intracellularly as a fusion with the C-terminus of glutathione S transferase (GST, ~26 kDa)[13,33] from the parasitic helminth *Schistosoma japonicum*. The fusion protein is purified using glutathione (GSH) affinity chromatography, since GSH is a natural substrate of GST. In most pGEX vectors, the heterologous protein is released from GST by either Factor Xa or thrombin cleavage at a specifically engineered recognition site. An important consideration when choosing a pGEX vector for cloning is that Factor Xa gives flush cleavage, whereas thrombin cleavage leaves a vestigial Gly-Ser appended at the N-terminus of the protein. Several protein modules have been overexpressed for NMR studies as GST fusions, including domain I of the T lymphocyte CD2 antigen[34] and the Jun leucine zipper domain;[23] Figure 1 shows efficient one-step purification of the latter fusion protein using GSH-agarose affinity chromatography.

The MAL-c2 and MAL-p2 vectors enable overexpression of the heterologous protein as a fusion with the C-terminus of *E. coli* maltose binding protein (MBP, 40 kDa).[13,35] In the MAL-c2 vectors, the signal sequence is deleted from the MBP gene (*malE*), which results in cytoplasmic expression of the fusion protein in 20–40% fractional abundance.[13] This signal sequence is retained in the MAL-p2 vectors, thus enabling secretion of the fusion protein into the periplasm; as outlined in Section II.C, this leads to significantly decreased yields of protein (5–10% fractional abundance)[13] but increases the likelihood of obtaining soluble, correctly folded protein. Soluble fusion protein can be readily purified using amylose affinity chromatography. The heterologous protein is detached from MBP using Factor Xa cleavage at the engineered recognition site. This can be done on the amylose column or following elution of the fusion protein with maltose. Several proteins have been produced for NMR studies using the MBP-fusion approach.[36,37]

Numerous other fusion methods are currently available (see Reference 38 for a review), and more are likely to become accessible in the near future. An increasingly popular method involves linking the heterologous protein to an N-terminal polyhistidine tag, thus allowing purification of the fusion protein using either $Zn^{2+}$, $Cu^{2+}$, or $Ni^{2+}$ chelation chromatography.[39] An important consideration when choosing a fusion vector to

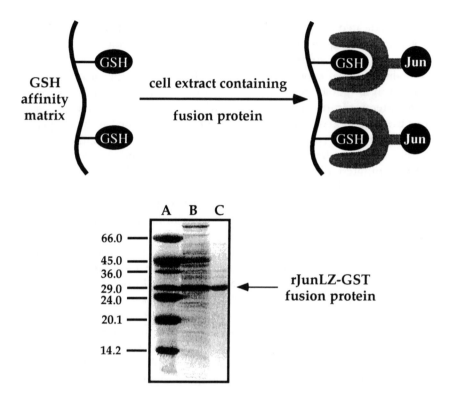

**FIGURE 1**

Purification of the recombinant JunLZ-GST fusion protein using affinity chromatography. The leucine zipper domain of the Jun oncoprotein (JunLZ) was overexpressed in *E. coli* as a fusion with glutathione *S*-transferase (GST), enabling ready purification of the overexpressed fusion protein using glutathione (GSH)-agarose affinity chromatography.[23] This is illustrated schematically in the upper half of the diagram, where the JunLZ module is depicted as a black sphere and the GST fusion protein as a grey U-shaped object. The lanes of the SDS-PAGE gel at the bottom of the figure correspond to (A) standard proteins (molecular masses in kilodaltons at the left of the gel); (B) total soluble-protein fraction resulting from induction of cells; (C) a small fraction of the GSH-agarose beads after the soluble cell fraction has been added (lane B) and unbound components have been washed off. The running position of the rJunLZ-GSH fusion protein is marked on the right of the gel.

produce isotopically labelled proteins for NMR studies is that a considerable portion of the expensive $^{13}$C and $^{15}$N label will be lost in the unwanted carrier protein (although the carrier protein and host-cell proteins can be hydrolysed to give labelled amino acids that can be added to the growth medium in future labelling experiments). Thus, labelling is more economical using smaller carrier proteins. For this reason, fusions with β-galactosidase (116 kDa),[13,24] which have been used extensively in other applications, are less suitable for NMR studies.

As indicated above, purification is generally easier when the heterologous protein is expressed in a soluble form (whether fusion or nonfusion). There are several strategies that can be employed to enhance protein solubility if initial experiments indicate that most of the protein is expressed in insoluble inclusion bodies. *Escherichia coli* can synthesise proteins at temperatures ranging from 10 to 43°C,[13] and it has been observed that the likelihood of obtaining soluble protein is increased as the temperature is decreased[40] (presumably due to more reliable folding of the protein as the rate of translation from the mRNA is reduced, thereby reducing the chances of intermolecular association). Small changes in temperature can lead to spectacular changes in solubility; for example, the majority of Jun leucine zipper-GST fusion protein is expressed in insoluble inclusion bodies when cells are grown at 37°C, but the fusion protein is completely soluble when cells are grown at 32°C.[23] Protein solubility can often be enhanced by reducing the concentration of isopropyl β-D-galactopyranoside (IPTG) when using vectors with IPTG-inducible promoters, and this approach can be used in combination with lower temperatures. Overexpression of active subtilisin in an *E. coli* vector system employing an IPTG-inducible *lac* promoter was increased 16-fold when the induction conditions were altered from 2 m$M$ IPTG/37°C to 0.005 mM IPTG/23°C.[41] A last resort for increasing protein solubility is to reclone the gene for the heterologous protein into a low-copy-number plasmid,[13] although this may make it difficult to obtain enough protein for NMR studies.

## E    Isotopic Labelling of Proteins for NMR Studies

### 1    Overview

In the past five to six years, isotopic labelling of proteins, in combination with triple-resonance assignment strategies that take advantage of large heteronuclear $J$ couplings (see Section IV.C), has revolutionised the field of protein structure determination using NMR spectroscopy. This revolution has extended the size limit for NMR structural studies of proteins from ~10 kDa to perhaps as high as 35 kDa. No laboratory seriously engaged in using NMR to determine the structure of large proteins can do without its own isotopic labelling facilities or at least access to such facilities through collaborators.

### 2    Uniform $^{13}C/^{15}N$ Labelling

Most resonance-assignment strategies for large proteins (*vide infra*) require the protein to be uniformly labelled with stable $^{15}N$ and $^{13}C$ isotopes. There are two basic strategies by which this can be achieved with *E. coli*, the host organism most commonly used for biosynthetic labelling. The cheapest approach is feasible only if sufficient quantities of heterologous protein are obtained for NMR studies when the cells are grown in minimal medium (such as M9).[14] In this case, economical labelling can be readily achieved by growing cells in a modified minimal medium containing either $^{15}NH_4Cl$ or $(^{15}NH_4)_2SO_4$ as the sole nitrogen source and a uniformly $^{13}C$-labelled metabolic precursor such as glucose, succinate, acetate, or glycerol as the sole carbon source; vitamins and antibiotic supplements are added as required.[23,42,43] In favourable circumstances, this approach can provide sufficient $^{15}N/^{13}C$-labelled protein for NMR studies for as little as $500 US.

Some expression systems, however, provide sufficient protein only if the host cells are grown in rich medium. In this case, a fully labelled, rich growth medium is required. Hydrolysates of algae grown on $K^{15}NO_3$ and $^{13}CO_2$ as the sole nitrogen and carbon sources, respectively, are most commonly used for this purpose.[44] These are commercially available, but are very expensive (up to $5000 US for enough double-labelled algal hydrolysate to constitute 1 l of culture medium). It might be possible, however, to produce the labelled algal hydrolysate in house using a low-cost algal culture system as described recently.[45] Even if the target protein can be successfully labelled in minimal medium, the rich-medium approach may be more economical if much larger amounts of the heterologous protein are produced in the more complex algal medium. Algal hydrolysates are also suitable for growing yeast.

Production of labelled protein using mammalian cells is a much more difficult exercise. These cells are generally more sensitive to toxic substances than bacteria, and they require a culture medium that is supplemented with serum, amino acids, vitamins, and cofactors.[30] However, a method was recently devised for uniform $^{13}C/^{15}N$ labelling of proteins overexpressed in mammalian cells.[30] The cells were grown in a complex medium that contained a commercial, double-labelled algal hydrolysate, fetal bovine serum from which unlabelled amino acids had been removed by dialysis, and supplementary amounts of $^{15}N/^{13}C$-labelled cysteine and glutamine. The double-labelled cysteine and glutamine were not readily accessible at the time of the original study, but they are now commercially available. It was estimated by the authors that this rich medium costs ~$4000 US per litre,[30] although this would be marginally higher if commercial sources of labelled cysteine and glutamine were used.

## 3  Random Fractional Deuteration

The primary factor limiting NMR structural studies to proteins less than ~35 kDa is the rapid increase in transverse relaxation rates (and hence linewidths) as the size of the protein increases above 10 kDa (see Sections IV.B.2 and IV.C.3 for more detailed discussions of this point). Since $^1H$–$^1H$ dipolar interactions constitute the primary determinant of $^1H$ relaxation rates, then any method of limiting these interactions will decrease linewidths and increase the efficiency of coherence transfer through scalar couplings.

The $^1H$–$^1H$ dipolar interactions can be significantly diminished by random fractional deuteration of the protein. In this approach, which promises to become more widely used in NMR studies of larger proteins, all protons in the protein are randomly (stochastically) deuterated to the same fractional amount.[43] While this leads to an automatic decrease in signal intensity due to the smaller concentration of protons at any one site in the protein, it is anticipated that, for large proteins, this will be more than compensated for by decreased proton relaxation rates (and hence narrower resonances), since $^2H$–$^1H$ dipolar interactions are only one sixth as efficient as $^1H$–$^1H$ dipolar interactions.[46] As an example, Figure 2 shows the dramatic reduction in proton linewidths obtained for bacteriophage T4 thioredoxin (~12 kDa) following 75% random fractional deuteration. In NMR spectra that exhibit $^1H$–$^1H$ scalar couplings, there will be an

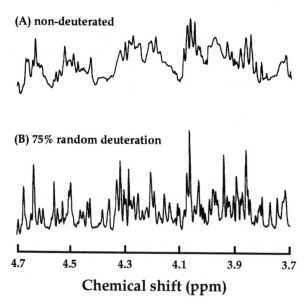

**(A) non-deuterated**

**(B) 75% random deuteration**

| | | | | | |
|---|---|---|---|---|---|
| 4.7 | 4.5 | 4.3 | 4.1 | 3.9 | 3.7 |

**Chemical shift (ppm)**

**FIGURE 2**

The effect of random fractional deuteration on $^1H$ NMR linewidths. A portion of the $^1H$ NMR spectrum is shown for (A) nondeuterated bacteriophage T4 thioredoxin (BT4T), and (B) BT4T that had been stochastically deuterated to a level of 75%. The spectra were collected and processed under similar conditions. Note the much narrower linewidths in the spectrum of the fractionally deuterated sample. (Adapted from LeMaster, D.M., *Methods Enzymol.*, 177, 23–43, 1989. With permission.)

additional gain in signal-to-noise ratio due to the suppression of passive $^1H$–$^1H$ couplings.[43,46] Furthermore, the reduced proton density in fractionally deuterated proteins leads to a decrease in spin-diffusion effects in NOE experiments (see Section IV.E.1 and Chapter 3).[43,46,47]

Random fractional deuteration using *E. coli* is achieved by growing the cells in $^2H_2O$ medium using a deuterated substrate. It may be necessary to gradually adapt the *E. coli* strain to $^2H_2O$ by growing the cells on progressively higher concentrations of heavy water.[43] The culture medium must contain a higher level of $^2H$ than the required value, since there is 5–10% discrimination against the label during biosynthesis.[48] Thus, one might achieve 75% random fractional deuteration by growing cells on a minimal medium in 80% $^2H_2O$ supplemented with sufficient quantities of [80% U-$^2H$] glucose or some other metabolic precursor.

Since transverse relaxation of amide-$^{15}N$ and $^{13}C^\alpha$ nuclei in $^{15}N/^{13}C$-labelled proteins is dominated by dipolar coupling with their directly attached proton, then it might be expected that random fractional deuteration would be most valuable when used in combination with uniform $^{15}N$ and/or $^{13}C$ labelling, thus increasing the efficiency of coherence transfer through heteronuclear couplings in 3D triple-resonance experiments[49] (see Section IV.C.3). This approach appears not to have been attempted thus far, probably because suitable labelled substrates are not available. However, uniformly $^{15}N$-labelled, fractionally deuterated protein could be readily obtained by growing cells in minimal $^2H_2O$ medium with $^{15}NH_4Cl$ or $(^{15}NH_4)_2SO_4$ as the sole nitrogen source and appropriately deuterated glucose as the sole carbon source.

### 4   Selective Labelling

Many early heteronuclear NMR studies of proteins employed amino-acid-selective labelling in order to simplify spectra for the purposes of resonance assignment.[50] Generally, however, spectral ambiguities in $^{15}N/$ $^{13}C$-labelled proteins can be resolved by extending the spectra into a third or fourth frequency dimension (see Section IV.C), and hence this degree of labelling selectivity is most often not required. Amino-acid-selective labelling is most efficiently achieved using mutant strains of *E. coli* that are auxotrophic for the amino acid to be labelled. These cells are grown in a minimal medium to which is added glucose (or some other carbon source), a mixture of unlabelled amino acids (excluding that to be labelled), and a labelled amino acid that matches the auxotrophic requirement.[43] The alternative approach of adding excess labelled amino acid to cells grown in a rich medium gives less-optimal labelling due to isotopic dilution.[42]

# III SAMPLE PREPARATION

## A HETEROGENEITY OF THE NMR SAMPLE

Two major factors affecting the outcome of the NMR analysis are the purity and oligomeric nature of the protein sample. Sample impurities can lead to false peak assignments, particularly in NOESY spectra, and they will exacerbate any spectral overlap problems; a purity of ≥90% is essential, and ≥95% is desirable. A generally more difficult problem to overcome is aggregation of the protein sample at the millimolar concentrations required for NMR analysis. It is absolutely essential that the oligomeric state of the protein sample is known *prior* to beginning the NMR investigation. Dimerisation of a 20-kDa protein will preclude high-resolution structural studies by taking it beyond the currently accessible molecular weight range. Dimerisation of a 14-kDa protein will leave it in the accessible molecular weight range, but special experimental and/or calculational strategies will be required to unravel the intra- and intermolecular NOEs.

There are several methods available for monitoring protein self-associations. An often-used approach is to examine the linewidths of resonances in one-dimensional (1D) NMR spectra of the protein sample as a function of the protein concentration. An increase in linewidths is taken to indicate aggregation of the protein, and the protein concentration is thus reduced below that at which the increase in linewidth is first noticeable. This is an extremely crude approach and must be used with tremendous caution. The protein will not necessarily be monomeric below the point at which linewidth increases occur; the protein may actually dimerise with a low dissociation constant, and the observed increase in linewidth with increasing concentration would correspond to aggregation of dimers. Furthermore, it is doubtful whether one would notice significant increases in resonance linewidths if ~20% of a supposedly monomeric sample were actually dimeric. However, the dimer might contribute significant cross-peaks in the NOESY spectra from strong dipolar couplings, thus leading to incorrect attribution of intermolecular NOEs to intramolecular NOEs and subsequent calculation of an incorrect structure, or at least one with many unexplained NOE conflicts.

There are several more robust methods for determining the molecular weight and heterogeneity of protein samples. By far the best are sedimentation-equilibrium experiments performed using an analytical ultracentrifuge.[51] Since this method is based firmly on thermodynamic principles, it can be used to measure the molecular weights of protein solutions, at chemical equilibrium, with an accuracy of 1–2%.[51] No assumptions need to be made about the shape of the molecule or its degree of hydration. Furthermore, it enables quantitative analysis of protein self-association from fitting of mathematical models of self-association to the sedimentation-equilibrium data.[51,52] A potential problem with the application of sedimentation-equilibrium experiments to NMR samples is that, if absorbance optics are being used to measure the protein concentration or concentration gradient, light absorbance by the highly concentrated protein sample may exceed the linear range of the optical detector; however, in this case one could either reduce the path length of the optical cell or use Schlieren optics for detection.[51]

Measurements of protein molecular weight and heterogeneity can also be obtained using dynamic, or quasielastic, light scattering (QELS). [53,54] This technique enables the translational diffusion coefficient $D$ of a protein to be measured from an analysis of the temporal fluctuations in scattered light intensities when the protein solution is illuminated by a beam of monochromatic (laser) light.[54] The hydrodynamic radius of the protein $r_h$ can then be estimated from $D$ using the Stokes–Einstein relationship;[55] however, this conversion assumes a hard-sphere model for the protein. The protein molecular weight is then estimated (with an accuracy as low as $\pm 20\%$) using a relationship between molecular weight and $r_h$ that has been empirically derived from an analysis of globular proteins. This method can also be used for quantitative analysis of bimodal distributions of protein species (e.g., a mixture of monomer and dimer),[54] but not for higher-order distributions. Protein molecular weights estimated using QELS are considerably less accurate than those obtained from sedimentation-equilibrium experiments, and the latter also provide more quantitative details about protein self-association.

Finally, there are various NMR-based methods for measuring protein molecular weights; while not as accurate as sedimentation-equilibrium analysis, these methods may be particularly convenient in that they can be applied directly to the sample to be used for structure determination and they obviate the need for access to other specialised equipment. The simplest NMR-based approach is to estimate the protein's molecular correlation time (e.g., from the average transverse relaxation time of the amide protons),[56] from which the hydrodynamic radius can be calculated using the Stokes–Einstein relationship given in Equation (1), Section IV.B.2; as indicated above, this can then be used to estimate the protein molecular weight. Alternatively, the translational diffusion coefficient of the protein can be estimated using pulsed-field-gradient spin echo (PFGSE) NMR,[57,58] and this can be used to derive estimates of the protein molecular weight.[59] The latter method is simple and might become increasingly attractive as more and more NMR spectroscopists begin to use PFG techniques for protein structure determination (see Section IV.D.1).

## B  Paramagnetic and Microbial Contamination

Paramagnetic ions such as $Cu^{2+}$, $Mn^{2+}$, $Cr^{3+}$, high-spin $Fe^{3+}$, and low-spin $Co^{2+}$ can cause contact-broadening of the resonances of nearby nuclei. While paramagnetic ions can be used to probe protein structure,[60] these are special NMR applications and these ions must be rigorously excluded from samples to be used in high-resolution structure determinations. This can be achieved by treating samples with a metal-chelating agent such as Chelex, or by adding a small amount (5–50 $\mu M$) of EDTA to the NMR sample.[61]

Microbial contamination is clearly a potential problem as the highly concentrated protein sample represents an excellent growth medium for algae, bacteria, and fungi during the weeks and months over which the NMR experiments are performed. Algal growth can be eliminated by minimising exposure of the sample to light. Azide and fluoride are often used to prevent microbial contamination, but azide is volatile below pH 7 and fluoride cannot be used in the presence of metal ions.[61] Broad-spectrum antibiotics such as chloramphenicol are excellent alternatives; chloramphenicol is chemically inert and is effective against both Gram-positive and -negative bacteria at low concentrations (10–50 $\mu M$).[61]

It should be emphasised that unlabelled additives such as EDTA and chloramphenicol are not problematic in heteronuclear NMR studies as they give no signals in $^{13}C/^{15}N$-isotope-filtered experiments. For example, it is common practice in heteronuclear NMR studies to add large quantities (5–15 m$M$) of dithiothreitol to preserve reduced cysteine residues.[62] High concentrations of nondenaturing detergent (25 m$M$) have also been used to prevent protein aggregation.[56,59] For purely homonuclear studies, it may be necessary to use deuterated additives if their concentrations are sufficiently high that they would otherwise obscure resonances from the protein.

## C  Sample pH

Sample pH is a critical parameter in the NMR experiment for a number of reasons. First, it can dramatically affect the solubility of the sample — at millimolar concentrations, most proteins become insoluble when the pH approaches their isoelectric point (pI), and this caveat should be especially remembered when trying to form protein–peptide complexes since the pI of the individual protein and peptide, as well as the complex, will be important.

Of crucial concern to the NMR experiment is the effect of pH on the rate of exchange of the labile backbone amide protons with solvent protons (most often $H_2O$). The backbone amide protons are often the starting point for obtaining resonance assignments using scalar correlations (see the discussion on TOCSY "skewers" in Section IV.A.3), they provide critical NOE connectivities (especially for $\alpha$-helical regions of the protein), and they often constitute one of the correlated nuclei in heteronuclear triple-resonance experiments. Thus, in most NMR experiments it is desirable to observe as many of the backbone amide-proton resonances as possible.

The exchange of amide protons with solvent water protons is both acid and base catalysed, as evident in the exchange-rate vs. pH profile in Figure 3. The rate of exchange is lowest at ~pH 3 and ~pH 5 for the backbone-amide and side-chain-amide protons (Asn and Gln residues), respectively.[63] Thus, while it might be desirable to work in the pH range 3–5 to maximise the intensity of amide-proton resonances, the protein may be insoluble or may extensively aggregate at these pH values, or it may even have an altered conformation.[64] In these cases, the lowest pH consistent with native conformation, tolerable solubility, and negligible aggregation should be chosen for the NMR study. Even a reduction in the pH from 7 to 6 will lead to a 10-fold reduction in the rate of amide-proton exchange. The amide-proton exchange rate can also be reduced by decreasing the temperature, but this has other consequences as outlined in the next section.

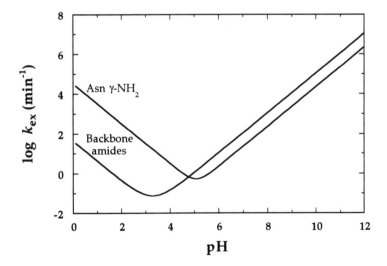

**FIGURE 3**

The pH dependence of the rate of hydrogen–deuterium exchange for backbone and Asn side-chain amide protons. The pseudo-first-order rate constants ($k_{ex}$) at 20°C were calculated using Equations (1) and (3) from Bai *et al.*[63] together with the second-order rate constants given by these authors for acid-, base-, and water-catalysed exchange.

## D   Sample Temperature

While not strictly a sample parameter, the temperature has an important influence on various aspects of the NMR experiment. Increasing the sample temperature will generally increase signal amplitudes (as long as aggregation of the protein is not induced) because the resonances will narrow as a result of the decrease in molecular correlation time $\tau_c$. This in turn increases the efficiency of coherence transfer through scalar couplings. However, for peptides and very small proteins, increasing the temperature could have a deleterious effect on NOE intensities as the maximum possible NOE intensity depends intimately on $\tau_c$, as illustrated in Figure 4.[65] For most proteins, however, variations in temperature will have little bearing on the maximum possible NOE of $-1.0$. The rate of exchange of amide protons with solvent water is reduced at lower temperature, thus making it easier to observe labile amide protons. However, for some experiments, suppression of the water resonance may be better at higher temperatures because of its reduced linewidth.

The overriding factor in decisions regarding temperature are the solubility, state of aggregation, and most importantly, long-term stability of the protein sample. Thus, there has been a general trend toward decreased sample temperatures in NMR studies of proteins as the size of protein being studied has increased. While most early studies of small

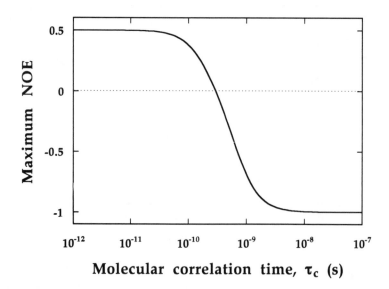

**FIGURE 4**

Dependence of the maximum value of the $^1H$–$^1H$ NOE on molecular correlation time, $\tau_c$. Note that $\tau_c$ is plotted on a log scale. The data are for a field strength of 14.1 Tesla (600 MHz), and it is assumed that $^1H$ relaxation occurs solely by the dipole–dipole mechanism.[65]

proteins were performed above room temperature (30–50°C), many recent studies of larger proteins have been performed at 20–30°C due to sample instability at higher temperatures.[62,66]

# IV ACQUISITION OF STRUCTURAL DATA

## A OVERVIEW

The general strategy for the determination of three-dimensional protein structures using NMR spectroscopy involves several stages: (1) the assignment of NMR resonances ([1]H and, increasingly [15]N and [13]C) to specific atoms or atom groups in the protein; (2) the extraction of experimental constraints from the NMR data that provide information on the relative spatial positions of these atoms in the protein (see Section IV.E); and (3) the use of these constraints as input into a computer program that attempts to derive a family of structures for the protein, each of which "satisfies" the experimental constraints (see Section V).

There are two general approaches through which Stage 1, resonance assignment, may be accomplished, and the choice between them is determined essentially by the molecular mass of the protein. The first approach, pioneered in the laboratory of Kurt Wüthrich,[67] traditionally involves the use of two-dimensional (2D) [1]H–[1]H (homonuclear) NMR experiments (such as COSY, NOESY, and TOCSY; see below). This approach is still widely used today, but is generally limited to proteins of less than ~10 kDa, as explained below. The applicability of a strictly homonuclear assignment strategy was expanded somewhat with the introduction of three-dimensional (3D) methods, but for proteins larger than ~10 kDa, a second approach, entailing the introduction of isotopic labels such as [13]C and [15]N, has proved to be the route of choice. The presence of these labels may be used either to simply edit homonuclear 2D spectra according to the chemical shifts of their attached [15]N/[13]C nuclei, providing a dramatic increase in resolution, or to facilitate the acquisition of so-called triple-resonance NMR experiments. These experiments correlate the chemical shifts of subsets of [1]H, [15]N, and [13]C atoms in a uniformly [15]N/[13]C-labelled protein through scalar connections, providing an alternative method of achieving sequence-specific resonance assignments. These methods have yielded resonance assignments for proteins of up to 31 kDa (interferon-$\gamma$[64]), with the prospect of some further increase in this size limit in the near future.

Homonuclear and heteronuclear strategies for resonance assignment are outlined in turn below. The most recent methodological advances in data-acquisition techniques are then discussed, and finally the generation of experimental constraints from NMR data is considered.

## B Homonuclear Resonance-Assignment Strategies

### 1 Overview

The advent of 2D NMR techniques in the early 1980s was the breakthrough that allowed detailed structural information to be extracted from proteins in solution. If information concerning the interactions between spins is to be extracted from one-dimensional (1D) experiments, pulses must be selectively applied to particular resonances and their effect(s) on other spins gauged from changes to the 1D spectrum. This method is adequate in the absence of significant spectral overlap, but soon becomes impractical even for molecules of modest size. By contrast, extending such measurements into a second dimension alleviates the overlap problem to a significant degree. These 2D experiments[68] consist of discrete elements: a preparation period; an evolution period $t_1$, where spins are "labelled" as they precess in the $xy$ plane according to their chemical shift; a mixing period, during which correlations are made with other spins; and a detection period $t_2$, where a free induction decay (FID) is recorded (see Figure 5A). Note that these elements may be combined to create more complex experiments; this is the basis of higher-dimensional (3D and 4D) NMR as outlined in Section IV.B.5. The FID is signal averaged as usual (as required for both signal-to-noise and phase-cycling considerations),[68] and then the process is repeated a number of times with incremented values of $t_1$. After Fourier transformation of the series of $t_1$-incremented experiments, the amplitude of each signal through the series is found to be modulated according to both its frequency and the frequency of the proton(s) to which it is correlated during the mixing period (see Figure 6). In addition, transverse relaxation, which occurs during the pulse sequence, will result in smaller peak intensities for increasing values of $t_1$, so that cross-sections of the $t_2$-transformed data have the form of exponentially decreasing sinusoids (cf. FIDs). A Fourier transformation of these cross-sections (i.e., with respect to $t_1$) thus yields a planar spectrum with two frequency dimensions ($F_2 \times F_1$; termed the directly and indirectly detected dimensions, respectively) where, in most homonuclear 2D experiments, the 1D spectrum (sometimes simplified) is present as a diagonal, and correlations between spins are represented by off-diagonal elements known as cross-peaks (see Figure 9 in Chapter 3).

Experiments are distinguished by the nature of the correlations that are probed during the mixing period. Scalar couplings between protons up to three bonds apart are revealed using correlated spectroscopy (COSY),[69] or preferably double-quantum-filtered COSY (DQFCOSY),[70] which has superseded basic COSY as the experiment of choice for elucidating these couplings, due to the narrower lineshapes it produces. Nuclear Overhauser effect spectroscopy (NOESY)[71,72] connects protons that are close (< ca. 5 Å) in space (see Section IV.E.1 and Chapter 3 for an explanation of the

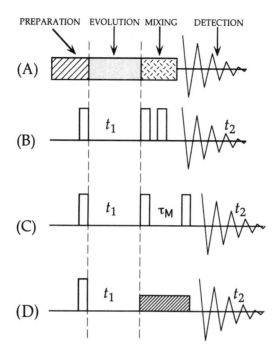

**FIGURE 5**

(A) The elements of a generalised two-dimensional NMR experiment. Basic pulse sequences are given for (B) DQFCOSY, (C) NOESY, and (D) TOCSY experiments, illustrating that the nature of the mixing period determines the types of correlations observed in the experiment. Phase cycling of certain pulses serves to select the desired components of the magnetisation, and to remove instrumental artifacts, but this is omitted here (and in subsequent diagrams) for clarity. Unfilled rectangles represent 90° pulses, and the hatched region in (D) is the isotropic mixing (spin-lock) pulse (see text), which transfers magnetisation between nuclei within a spin system; $\tau_m$ is the mixing time that allows development of the NOE (see text).

nuclear Overhauser effect). The basic pulse sequences for the COSY and NOESY experiments are given in Figures 5B and 5C, respectively, and it can be seen that an important difference between them lies in the nature of the mixing period. In DQFCOSY, this consists of two 90° pulses separated by a brief delay (*ca.* 3 µs), while in NOESY two 90° pulses sandwich an extended mixing time (~50–400 ms) during which the NOEs build up (there are also phase-cycling differences). A further invaluable experiment, total correlation spectroscopy (TOCSY,[73] also called HOHAHA for homonuclear Hartmann–Hahn spectroscopy;[74] Figure 5D), also yields scalar connectivities. In TOCSY spectra, correlations are observed between (potentially) all protons within a spin system (i.e., a group of protons that share mutual coupling partners, such as the $H^N$, $H^\alpha$, and $CH_3^\beta$ protons of an alanine residue) whether or not they are directly coupled to each other. The coupling is developed during the application of a

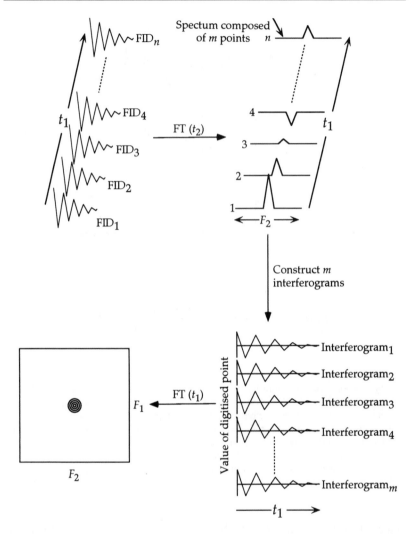

**FIGURE 6**   Processing of a two-dimensional experiment. *n* FIDs are collected, with the value of $t_1$ incremented sequentially throughout the series. Fourier transformation of each FID gives *n* 1D spectra in which the signal intensities are modulated because of the chemical shift precession during $t_1$. Interferograms are then created by taking the corresponding points from each of the *n* spectra; if each FID is composed of *m* points, then *m* interferograms result. These interferograms have the same form as an FID (i.e., exponentially decaying sinusoids), and they can be Fourier transformed to give a second frequency dimension. Thus each signal in the 2D spectrum is characterised by two frequencies, one reported during $t_1$ and the other during $t_2$. If no magnetisation transfer occurs during the mixing period, a signal at $F_2 = F_1$ results. An off-diagonal peak, or so-called cross-peak, arises when magnetisation is transferred from one spin to another (with a different frequency) during the mixing period. The 2D spectrum, which actually comprises two frequency dimensions and one amplitude dimension, is usually displayed as a two-dimensional contour plot, where the number of contour lines in each cross-peak is taken as an indication of its intensity (*cf.* a geographical contour map).

spin-locking pulse (termed the isotropic mixing period), and the extent to which magnetisation is propagated along a spin system depends on the duration of this spin-lock pulse (typically 30–100 ms). These three experiments form the basis of the sequential assignment method proposed originally by Wüthrich[67] for the complete assignment of resonances in polypeptide $^1$H NMR spectra.

In the first stage of this procedure, the individual spin systems of each amino acid are identified from the scalar-coupled 2D experiments, that is, DQFCOSY and TOCSY. Note that all cross-peaks in these experiments correspond to *intraresidue* connectivities, since there are no interresidue pairs of protons within three bonds of each other (Figure 7). Thus, residue types are distinguished, but no information is provided on the positions of the residues within the polypeptide sequence. This information comes from the second stage of the approach, where the characteristic patterns of through-space correlations generated in the NOESY experiment are used to connect sequential pairs of residues and thereby achieve sequence-specific resonance assignment.

## 2 Suitability of a Protein for Homonuclear Assignment Techniques

It has generally been found that homonuclear resonance assignment cannot be applied successfully to proteins larger than around 10 kDa. There are two reasons for this. First, the complexity (number of cross-peaks) in two-dimensional spectra increases in an approximately linear fashion with the number of chemically inequivalent protons in the molecule. Thus, for proteins larger than around 10 kDa, spectral overlap will generally prevent the exhaustive assignment of resonances necessary for structure determination. The second, more fundamental reason arises from the dependence of the transverse relaxation time $T_2$ (and hence, the linewidth $v_{1/2} = 1/(\pi T_2)$ in the absence of field inhomogeneity; see Chapter 3, Section VII), on molecular correlation time $\tau_c$ (see Figure 8).

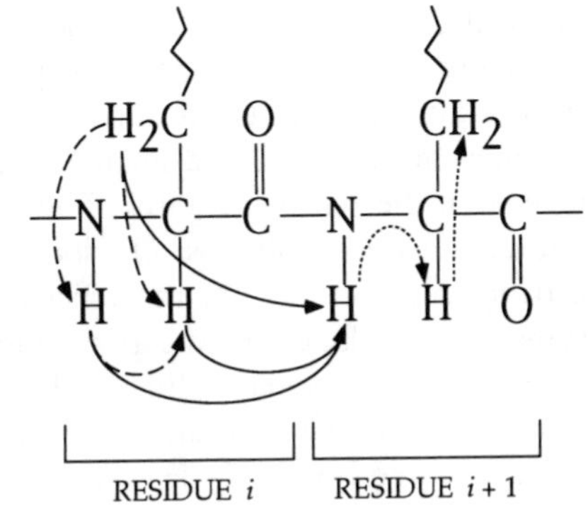

**FIGURE 7**
Intra- and interresidue connectivities used to achieve sequential assignment using the homonuclear strategy developed by Wüthrich.[67] A two-residue segment of a polypeptide is shown. Dotted lines represent scalar $J$ couplings, which are all intraresidue and are used to identify the residue type. Dashed lines indicate intraresidue NOEs, which may assist in this process, and solid arrows show interresidue NOEs, which are used to connect individual spin systems and thereby make sequential assignments.

RESIDUE $i$       RESIDUE $i + 1$

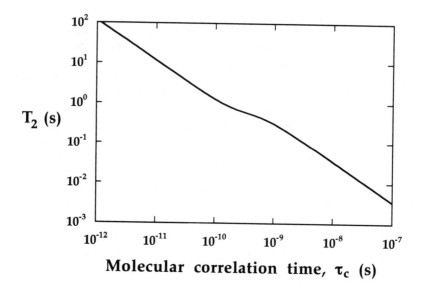

**FIGURE 8**

Logarithmic plot showing the dependence of the ¹H transverse relaxation time, $T_2$ on molecular correlation time $\tau_c$. Transverse magnetisation decays more quickly in larger molecules, a fact that plays a crucial part in determining which NMR experiments are feasible for a particular protein (see text). The curve was computed for two protons separated by 1.8 Å, with resonance frequencies of 600 MHz, using the assumption that relaxation is dominated by dipolar coupling.

Molecular correlation time $\tau_c$ is a measure of how rapidly a molecule tumbles in solution (actually the time taken for a molecule to rotate through 1 rad) and is given for a spherical molecule by the Debye equation:

$$\tau_c = \frac{4\pi\eta r_h^3}{3kT} \tag{1}$$

where $\eta$ is the solvent viscosity, $r_h$ is the hydrodynamic radius of the molecule, $k$ is Boltzmann's constant, and $T$ is the temperature. Note that the derived correlation time is an approximate upper limit. It can be seen from Figure 8 that, as the molecule tumbles more slowly, $T_2$ relaxation becomes more efficient (a small $T_2$ implies efficient relaxation as $T_2$ is the inverse of the relaxation rate). This increase in linewidth with molecular size causes two problems: (1) spectral overlap will clearly be worse for broader signals, and (2) the efficiency of information transfer between spins in the scalar coupled experiments (coherence transfer) becomes very poor when the resonance linewidths start to exceed the magnitude of the spin–spin coupling constants. For example, a 7-Hz coupling (an average value for three-bond ¹H–¹H couplings, $^3J_{HH}$) between protons with 20-Hz linewidths gives a COSY-type transfer efficiency of only *ca.* 2%.[75] Note, however, that the 10-kDa size limit is only a rough guide and that the exact limit depends on the shape of the protein (which influences the tumbling rate) and the chemical shift dispersion; for example, $\alpha$-helical domains generally display less dispersion than $\beta$-sheets, so that the size limit for predominantly helical proteins will be somewhat lower than for other proteins.

In order to ascertain whether or not these homonuclear methods will provide complete resonance assignments, a DQFCOSY spectrum of the protein in $H_2O$ (prepared as outlined in Section III) should be recorded. Note that it will be necessary to attenuate the huge signal arising from the solvent. This is most commonly achieved by selective preirradiation (although see Section IV.D.1), in which case a sequence such as SCUBA[76] should be inserted following the preirradiation to minimise the loss of cross-peaks due to saturation of $H^\alpha$ resonances under/near the $H_2O$ signal. The majority of the cross-peaks in the so-called fingerprint region of this spectrum ($F_2 \approx 10.0–6.0$ ppm, $F_1 \approx 3.0–6.5$ ppm) will be due to correlations between amide protons and the $H^\alpha$ proton of the same residue. The number of $H^N$-$H^\alpha$ cross-peaks should be $\geq$ *ca.* 90% of the number of residues in the protein for homonuclear methods to be adequate. However, cross-peaks may be lost for a number of reasons, including transfer of saturation from the preirradiated $H_2O$ signal to rapidly exchanging $H^N$ protons, saturation of $H^\alpha$ signals lying under the water signal, and the cancellation of antiphase components of the cross-peaks when the linewidths are large compared to the coupling constant. All these problems can be circumvented to some degree (see Chapter 4 in Reference 77), and attempts should be made to do so before casting the homonuclear assignment strategy aside.

### 3   Spin System Identification

Once it has been decided to employ the homonuclear strategy for resonance assignment, good-quality DQFCOSY and TOCSY spectra must be collected in $H_2O$. Preferably TOCSY spectra should be acquired with two to three different mixing times, as the intensity profile for TOCSY cross-peaks is complex.[78] It may also be useful to record either one or both of these experiments in $D_2O$, especially if it is suspected that artifacts resulting from incomplete solvent suppression are obscuring cross-peaks involving $H^\alpha$ protons near the water signal. The two spectra complement each other in information content, with TOCSY skewers providing connectivities between most (or often all) protons in the same spin system, and the DQFCOSY distinguishing between direct and indirect connectivities. These spectra are used to identify the type of spin system associated with each $H^N$–$H^\alpha$ cross-peak, and these spin system types can be matched either to specific amino acids or to groups of amino acids. Note that complete assignment of the longer spin systems in particular (e.g., Met, Lys, Arg) is not crucial for sequential assignment, or frequently even for the generation of NOE constraints. Because these latter residues generally lie on the surface of proteins with their side chains oriented toward the solvent, the distal side-chain protons often do not exhibit structurally useful NOEs.

Figure 9 shows the assignment of several residue types in the synthetic leucine zipper domain of the transcriptional activator protein Jun (sJunLZ), using both TOCSY and DQFCOSY data.[9] Note that the table of random

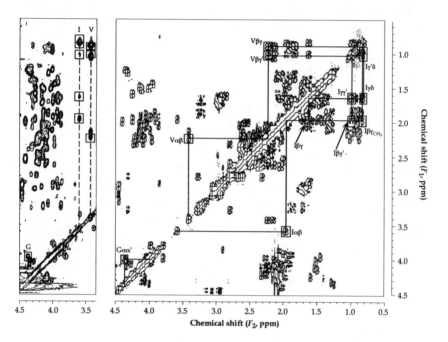

**FIGURE 9**

Identification of spin systems using 2D homonuclear $^1$H NMR experiments. Aliphatic region of a DQFCOSY spectrum of sJunLZ (right side), an 86-residue homodimeric coiled coil domain of the eukaryotic transcription factor Jun. Connectivity patterns are shown for three residue types: Val, Gly, and Ile. Note that the γCH$_3$ and δCH$_3$ resonances of the Ile residue are coincident and that there are two Val residues with coincident H$^\alpha$ signals. Solid black and dashed grey lines represent positive and negative contours, respectively. Section of a 2D TOCSY spectrum (left) of the same protein (spin-lock mixing time = 105 ms). "Skewers" of TOCSY connectivities arising from H$^\alpha$ resonances are shown as dotted lines — the H$^\alpha$ signals are correlated to distant protons in the side-chain spin system. Note that the dispersion of H$^\alpha$ signals is relatively poor for a protein of this size. This lack of dispersion arises because sJunLZ is entirely α-helical, and H$^\alpha$ frequencies are correlated with secondary structure. Note also the complementary nature of the two experiments; the TOCSY provides the power to potentially assign all protons in a residue from a single skewer, but often the extra information it provides can lead to ambiguity and increased spectral overlap. The more selective nature of the DQFCOSY can frequently resolve such problems.

coil chemical shift values for the common amino acids published by Bundi and Wüthrich[79] is invaluable in this assignment process. Some useful information may also be obtained from the fine structure of DQFCOSY cross-peaks.[77]

## 4   Sequence-Specific Resonance Assignment

Once all traceable spin systems have been delineated as described above, they need to be matched to specific residues in the sequence. This is achieved using through-space connectivities derived from a NOESY spectrum — or in the case of smaller polypeptides (those with MW ≈ 1000–3000 Da) a ROESY spectrum[80] — which correlates pairs of protons less than *ca.* 5 Å apart in space, regardless of their relative positions in the primary structure. A series of NOESY spectra in $H_2O$ should be collected, with mixing times ranging from ~50 up to 150–600 ms, depending on the size of the protein; the longer mixing times are suitable for smaller peptides. In general, the shortest mixing times that give good-quality spectra are preferable, since indirect effects are observed at longer values. That is, at longer mixing times magnetisation may effectively be transferred between protons that are > 5 Å apart (see Section IV.E.1).

The sequential assignment procedure relies on the observation of connections between the $H^N$, $H^\alpha$, and $H^\beta$ protons of adjacent residues in the sequence. It has been shown[67] that, irrespective of secondary structure, at least one (generally more) of these pairs of protons will be less than *ca.* 3.5 Å apart, and should consequently give rise to a medium-to-strong intensity NOE. The most useful of these are the $d_{\alpha N}(i, i + 1)$ (i.e., the $H^\alpha$ of a residue $i$ to the $H^N$ of residue $i + 1$), $d_{NN}(i, i + 1)$, and $d_{\beta N}(i, i + 1)$ correlations (see Figure 7).

Before commencing this stage of the procedure, it is useful to record a NOESY spectrum in $D_2O$. In this spectrum, the only signals downfield of ~6 ppm correspond to carbon-bound protons from His, Phe, Trp, and Tyr, so these cross-peaks may be marked as such on the $H_2O$-NOESY to simplify the assignment task. Note that complete exchange of the backbone amide protons for deuterons may take days, weeks, or even months for some protons, depending on sample temperature and pH (high temperature and pH favour exchange). In fact, partial hydrogen–deuterium exchange may be used to simplify (edit) both scalar-coupled and NOESY spectra if spectral overlap proves to be a problem (as is often the case for predominantly α-helical proteins). DQFCOSY/TOCSY and NOESY spectra collected soon after dissolution of the protein in $D_2O$ will exhibit only a subset of the $H^N$ protons, together with their associated connectivities. Similarly, a sample that has been quantitatively exchanged with $D_2O$ may be freeze-dried and reconstituted in $H_2O$, and data collected on this so-called reverse-exchanged sample will contain a complementary subset of correlations.

Thus the presence in the $H_2O$-NOESY of any of the three classes of NOE listed above is used to infer a sequential juxtaposition of the two amino acids concerned. It should be realised, however, that these types of NOEs can (and often will) be observed between residues that are not neighbours in the sequence, so that caution, as always, should be exercised. Consequently, it is more reliable to base a sequential connection on the evidence of more than one of these three types of NOE. Breaks in the sequential assignment will inevitably occur; these can be the result of spectral overlap (e.g., two amide protons with identical chemical shifts will prevent the observation of sequential NOEs) or of the structure itself (e.g., the presence of a proline). Sometimes the $H^\delta$ protons of Pro can be used to continue the assignment sequence [i.e., using $d_{\delta N}(i, i + 1)$ connectivities], although this requires prior complete assignment of the proline spin system, usually a difficult task in the early stages of the procedure. Once short sequences of spin systems (3–4 residues) have been picked out, these can be mapped onto the polypeptide sequence. In some cases, a unique match may be found, but often several possible assignments will exist, and the segment must be extended in either or both directions as described above, until all but one of the possibilities can be excluded. However, for a 200-residue protein containing all 20 types of amino acids, there is a 99% probability that a tetrapeptide segment will be unique.[67] This process is repeated until all possible assignments have been made.

Although homonuclear resonance assignment is almost exclusively carried out using the sequential assignment method, one other approach has found use in some applications. The main-chain-directed (MCD) method[81] is based on the identification of cyclic patterns of NOEs that are characteristic of the different types of secondary structure. Because of this, it is less suitable for the assignment of unstructured or irregularly structured sections of a protein.

## 5    Three-Dimensional Homonuclear NMR

In the late 1980s, a further increase in dimensionality of NMR spectra was proposed and realised — the extension of two-dimensional experiments to a third dimension. A three-dimensional experiment may be considered to be a combination of two 2D experiments (Figure 10A) in which the detection period ($t_2$) of the first experiment is replaced by a second experiment (of which at least the first 90° pulse of the preparation period will be removed). Thus the 3D experiment entails two evolution times ($t_1$ and $t_2$), two mixing periods, and a detection period ($t_3$). The two evolution times are incremented independently, and a 3D Fourier transform, analogous to the 2D transform described above, yields three orthogonal frequency axes in a cubic arrangement (Figure 10B). Two implementations of this technique involve the combination of the 2D NOESY and TOCSY experiments to give the 3D NOESY-HOHAHA[82] (and the

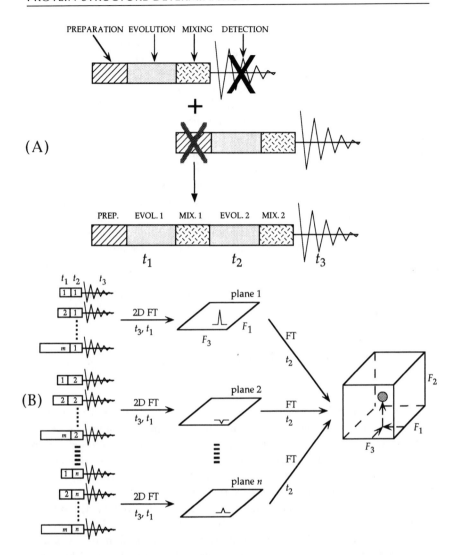

**FIGURE 10**

(A) The construction of a three-dimensional NMR experiment from two 2D experiments. The detection period of the first pulse sequence is deleted together with at least part of the preparation period of the second. Note that the two evolution times become $t_1$ and $t_2$, and the detection period is now $t_3$. (B) Processing of a 3D experiment. In this example, the evolution times $t_1$ and $t_2$ have been incremented $m$ and $n$ times, respectively; the lengths of the boxes indicate the lengths of the associated evolution time. First, a series of $m$ spectra are recorded in which $t_1$ is incremented $m - 1$ times from its starting value, while $t_2$ is held at its initial value. Next, $t_2$ is incremented once, $t_1$ is reset to its initial value, and a second series of $t_1$-incremented spectra is collected. This process is repeated $n$ times, and $m \times n$ spectra are recorded in total. The 3D Fourier transformation (FT) can be thought of as a series of $n$ 2D transforms with respect to $t_3$ and $t_1$, yielding $n$ 2D spectra. The signals in these spectra are modulated in intensity because of the incrementation of $t_2$, and a third FT extracts the frequencies of this modulation, generating a third frequency axis.

closely related HOHAHA-NOESY[83]) experiments, and of two NOESY sequences, giving a NOESY-NOESY.[84] The extension into the third dimension offers a potential increase in resolution since cross-peaks are now characterised by three frequencies. If, for example, both the $H^N$ and $H^\alpha$ signals for two Ala residues were coincident, their scalar correlations would still be distinguishable in a HOHAHA-NOESY if their $H^\beta$ protons (to which they would show NOEs) had distinct chemical shifts. Note that this chemical shift difference needs to be larger than the digital resolution of the spectrum in that dimension; this is less likely than in the corresponding 2D spectra, as the increase in dimensionality requires a decrease in digital resolution because of time and data-storage considerations. Thus, in some cases this approach can partially alleviate the spectral overlap problem, which hampers the use of homonuclear assignment techniques for larger proteins, and can allow some assignment ambiguities to be overcome.[83,85] However, these experiments have not been used widely and have largely been superseded by their heteronuclear counterparts (see below). Consequently, it appears that for proteins that are not amenable to a straightforward 2D homonuclear approach, isotopic labelling is probably the method of choice.

## C   HETERONUCLEAR RESONANCE ASSIGNMENT STRATEGIES

### 1   Overview

As mentioned above, the homonuclear strategy will fail to provide complete and unambiguous assignments for larger proteins, where a slower correlation time with its consequent increase in the efficiency of transverse relaxation translates to broader lines and poor coherence transfer via $^1H$–$^1H$ scalar couplings. The increase in the number of protons also contributes to poorly resolved spectra. Homonuclear 3D NMR techniques, while providing some relief, still rely heavily on these inefficient (for large proteins) $^1H$–$^1H$ scalar couplings for resonance assignment. The gain in resolution from the added dimension is also tempered by both the limited frequency range of $^1H$ and the large increase in the number of cross-peaks generated in such experiments (compared to either of the constituent 2D experiments).

The advent of recombinant DNA technology has allowed the relatively facile production of proteins bearing isotopic labels in a variety of arrangements (see Section II). For example, specific amino acid types may be labelled (*e.g.*, 100% $^{13}C$ labelling of all carbons in all Leu residues) or the whole protein may be labelled uniformly with $^{13}C$ and/or $^{15}N$. In general, either uniform $^{15}N$- or $^{15}N/^{13}C$-labelling is used. The magnetic properties of these nuclei (both with spin quantum number $I = 1/2$) allow them to be utilised in high-resolution NMR, most commonly by exploiting

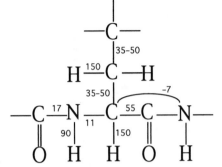

**FIGURE 11**

Segment of a polypeptide chain showing the magnitude of the scalar *J*-couplings exploited in heteronuclear NMR experiments.

their often large, short-range, one- and two-bond scalar couplings to each other and to directly attached protons (Figure 11). These large couplings constitute a major advantage of heteronuclear over homonuclear multidimensional NMR, as magnetisation transfer is very efficient in comparison with the homonuclear case (where $^3J_{HH} \approx 3$–$14$ Hz). Thus, the $^1H$–$^{15}N$ heteronuclear single quantum coherence (HSQC) experiment,[86] which correlates the chemical shifts of $^{15}N$ nuclei (both backbone and side chain in a uniformly labelled protein) to their directly attached proton(s), has very high sensitivity. The pulse sequence (see Figure 12A) involves the initial transfer of $^1H$ magnetisation to $^{15}N$ through the one-bond coupling (using a sequence known as insensitive nuclei enhanced by polarisation transfer—INEPT[87]), an evolution period $t_1$ where the magnetisation is labelled with the $^{15}N$ chemical shift, and transfer back to $^1H$ (with reverse-INEPT) for $^1H$ chemical shift detection during $t_2$. Double Fourier transformation yields a 2D spectrum with no diagonal and a single in-phase cross-peak representing each $H^N$–$N$ correlation.

Figure 12B shows a $^1H$-$^{15}N$ HSQC spectrum of the replication terminator protein from *B. subtilis*, which is a 29-kDa dimer.[62] This type of experiment, together with the related HMQC[88] (heteronuclear multiple quantum coherence spectroscopy), has formed the cornerstone of a wide range of 2D, 3D, and even 4D experiments designed to facilitate the resonance assignment and structure determination of proteins. Note that the HSQC technique is the one of choice for correlation of $^1H$ and $^{15}N$ shifts due to narrower linewidths in the $^{15}N$ dimension.[89,90] Its incorporation into these more complex multidimensional experiments, however, has been more recent than that of the HMQC. Furthermore, because these and most of the other heteronuclear experiments described below observe amide protons, the sample must be in $H_2O$ (rather than $D_2O$). Consequently, a means of suppressing the $H_2O$ resonance is required; preirradiation (as for homonuclear experiments) is commonly used, although application of a spin-lock purge pulse[91] has become the preferred

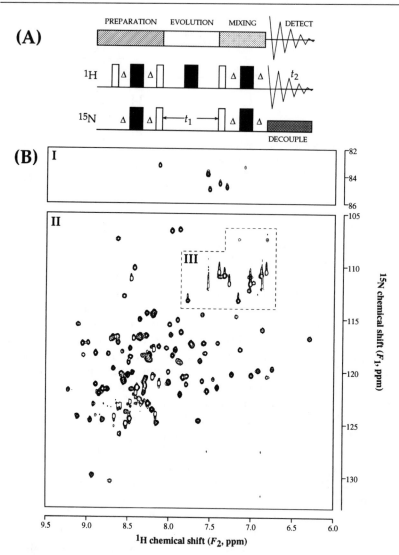

**FIGURE 12**

(A) Pulse sequence for the 2D $^1$H-$^{15}$N HSQC experiment. Unfilled and filled rectangles represent 90 and 180° pulses, respectively. The delays $\Delta$ are tuned to $1/4J_{NH}$ to allow magnetisation transfer between $^1$H and $^{15}$N (and similarly in later diagrams). The hatched box on the $^{15}$N line indicates decoupling of that nucleus during signal acquisition. (B) $^1$H–$^{15}$N HSQC spectrum of uniformly $^{15}$N-labelled replication terminator protein (RTP), a 29-kDa dimer. The spectrum was recorded at 600 MHz using the pulse sequence given in (A), with suppression of the $H_2O$ signal achieved by addition of a 1.5-ms spin-lock pulse[91] at the end of the second $\Delta$ period. The $^1$H–$^{15}$N correlations are seen for backbone amide protons (region II), Asn and Gln side-chain amides (region III), and Arg N$^\varepsilon$ protons (region I). The Asn and Gln side-chain cross-peaks each have a weak partner 0.5–0.6 ppm upfield in the $^{15}$N dimension that results from the deuterium isotope effect produced by the ~10% semideuterated NHD moieties present in the 90% $H_2O$/10% $D_2O$ solution. (Adapted from Kralick, A. V. et al., *Biochemistry*, 32, 10216–10223, 1993.)

method since it was first described (see also Section IV.D.1). A few of these new experiments simply use the heteronucleus to edit a standard homonuclear experiment, while a second, increasingly prevalent class (triple-resonance experiments) achieve resonance assignment by correlating the chemical shifts of $^1$H, $^{13}$C, and $^{15}$N nuclei in a complementary fashion.

## 2    Heteronuclear-Edited Homonuclear Experiments

Concatenation of the HSQC (or HMQC) sequence with a $^1$H–$^1$H NOESY gives rise to the 3D NOESY-HSQC (or 3D NOESY-HMQC) experiment (Figure 13A).[92-94] Here, two of the frequency dimensions represent the amide $^1$H and $^{15}$N chemical shifts, while the third holds the chemical shift of protons with which each amide proton is dipolar coupled. The spectrum is routinely viewed as narrow two-dimensional ($^1$H–$^1$H) strips taken at the $^{15}$N chemical shift of each cross-peak in the $^1$H–$^{15}$N HSQC spectrum (see Figure 14). The increase in resolution compared to a simple NOESY is dramatic, due in part to the lack of a straightforward correlation between $^{15}$N chemical shift and the secondary structure in which a residue is located (in contrast to the case of $H^N$, $H^\alpha$, and $C^\alpha$ chemical shifts; see Section IV.E.4). An analogous combination of TOCSY

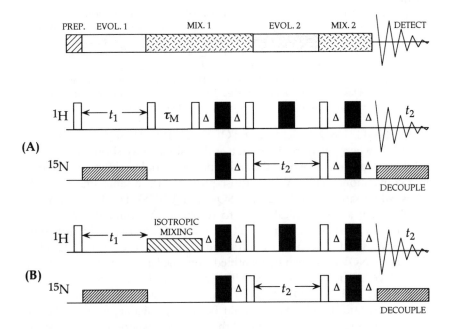

**FIGURE 13**

Pulse sequences for $^1$H–$^{15}$N (A) NOESY-HSQC and (B) TOCSY-HSQC experiments. The sequences consist of the standard 2D homonuclear NOESY or TOCSY experiments, to which an HSQC is appended (minus the first $^1$H 90° pulse of the latter experiment).

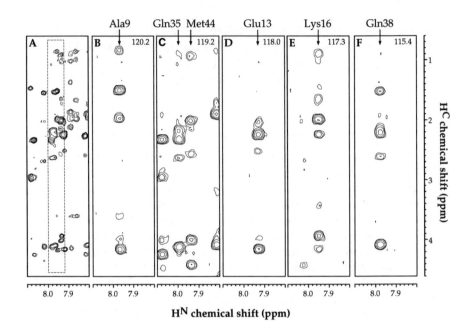

**FIGURE 14**

Comparison of 2D NOESY and 3D $^{15}$N NOESY-HMQC spectra of the recombinant Jun leucine zipper domain.[23] (A) Segment of the amide–aliphatic region of the 2D NOESY. The region enclosed by a dashed box contains cross-peaks from six different amide protons. (B–F) Strips of 2D $^1$H–$^1$H planes taken from the 3D NOESY-HMQC at the chemical shifts of the $^{15}$N nuclei attached to each of the six amide protons referred to in (A). The NOEs to all six amide protons are now clearly resolved. The $^{15}$N chemical shift (in ppm) at which each plane was taken is given at the top of each slice. H$^C$ indicates the aliphatic protons. (Adapted from Junius, F.K. et al., *Biochemistry*, 34, 1995, 6164–6174.)

and HMQC/HSQC yields 3D-TOCSY-HMQC/HSQC (see Figure 13B),[95, 96] where the third dimension as described above shows the chemical shifts of protons to which the amide protons would exhibit correlations in a conventional TOCSY (i.e., those protons in the same spin system). Thus, when satisfactory NOESY-HSQC and TOCSY-HSQC spectra can be obtained, a semiclassical route to resonance assignment can be followed. TOCSY skewers from the TOCSY-HSQC are used to identify spin system types and to account for intraresidue NOEs in the NOESY-HSQC. Sequential NOEs can then be identified from the latter spectrum and used to deduce interresidue connectivities as usual. Information from 2D DQFCOSY and 2D NOESY spectra may aid assignment, as many direct scalar correlations and NOEs should be distinguishable, even for larger proteins. In addition, 2D versions of these two 3D experiments, consisting of $^{15}$N shifts in one dimension $F_1$ and skewers of NOE/TOCSY correlations to the directly attached amide proton in the other $F_2$, have been described (2D-NOESY-HMQC,[89,97] 2D-TOCSY-HMQC).[89,97] These 2D experiments have the advantage of smaller demands on spectrometer time and easier implementation, although their effective resolution compared to the 3D experiments is obviously much poorer.

Analogous experiments can be carried out on $^{13}$C-labelled proteins, such as 3D $^{13}$C-HMQC-NOESY.[98] These experiments suffer a number of drawbacks however:

1. The $^{13}$C transverse relaxation rates (especially C$^\alpha$) can be very large, such that the signal intensities at the end of a multistep pulse sequence are very small.

2. Dipolar coupling of $^{13}$C nuclei to $^1$H increases the relaxation rate of the latter (compared to a $^{12}$C–$^1$H pair), further reducing signal intensity.

3. The $^{13}$C chemical shifts are correlated to secondary structure, as are the $^1$H shifts, thus partially thwarting the gain in resolution potentially available in such heteronuclear-edited experiments.

Despite these drawbacks, the $^{13}$C-edited experiments remain a very powerful way of resolving NOEs that involve carbon-bound protons. A fourth frequency dimension can be introduced in a fashion analogous to the third (i.e., by concatenation of a further 2D sequence), increasing the number of incremented evolution times to three. Such spectra cannot be visualised directly, but instead must be viewed as a number of 3D spectra (or, more usefully, 2D planes of these 3D spectra). Figure 15 illustrates the progression from 2D through to 4D experiments with the concomitant increase in spectral resolution. For instance, the 3D $^{15}$N-NOESY-HMQC should achieve complete (or nearly complete) resolution of amide-proton NOE skewers because of the good dispersion of $^{15}$N chemical shifts. However, a significant problem remains in the identification of the aliphatic-aromatic protons that are giving rise to the NOEs; the overlap in the aliphatic region is much worse than in the amide-proton region. Thus the 4D $^{15}$N/$^{13}$C HMQC-NOESY-HSQC[99] provides further editing of the 3D spectrum by also labelling these NOEs according to the frequency of the carbon to which the carbon-bound protons are attached. Similarly, the $^{13}$C/$^{13}$C-resolved NOESY[100] characterises each NOE (between $^{13}$C-bound protons) by the frequencies of the two protons concerned and of the carbons to which they are directly attached. In favourable circumstances, this can further reduce the chance of overlap, even for proteins of several hundred residues in size. These experiments are very demanding, requiring spectrometer hardware that is capable of irradiating three different nuclei (in the case of the $^{15}$N/$^{13}$C HMQC-NOESY-HSQC) and often-complex processing protocols. At the time of writing, many commercially available data-processing packages are not equipped to handle 4D datasets satisfactorily. Note also that $^{13}$C resonance assignments must be known for an NOE analysis such as this to succeed. These must be obtained from

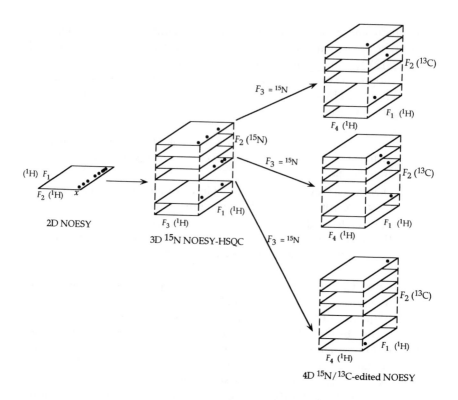

**FIGURE 15**

The advantage of increasing dimensionality in heteronuclear-edited NMR experiments. On the left is a section of a 2D NOESY showing eight NOEs at a single amide proton frequency ($x$ ppm) in $F_2$. The number of amide protons resonating at that frequency cannot be distinguished. A $^{15}$N-edited NOESY-HSQC reveals that there are three amide protons at $x$ ppm. However, the identities of the aliphatic protons giving rise to the NOEs are obscured by the overlap in this region of the spectrum. Separating each plane of the 3D spectrum according to the chemical shift of the $^{13}$C attached to the aliphatic protons gives rise to a 4D $^{15}$N/$^{13}$C-edited NOESY, where each cross-peak is identified by four frequencies, that is, the two protons sharing the NOE and the heteronuclei to which they are attached.

experiments that rely solely on scalar couplings, such as the HCCH-TOCSY and triple-resonance methods, both of which are discussed below.

The 3D (and 4D) HCCH experiments,[101-105] that is, HC(C)H-COSY and HC(C)H-TOCSY (these are the 3D versions, although the parentheses are generally dropped), provide the capability to obtain assignments for side-chain protons and carbons in larger proteins (estimated up to 30 kDa) where TOCSY-HSQC will fail because of the large $^1$H linewidths. In these experiments, proton magnetisation is first transferred to carbon ($^1J_{CH} \approx$ 125–150 Hz) from where it is propagated along the carbon skeleton of the residue via the one-bond $^{13}C$–$^{13}C$ couplings ($^1J_{CC} \approx$ 30–55 Hz) using either HOHAHA- or COSY-type methods. Finally, $^1H$ magnetisation is detected during the acquisition period following transfer of magnetisation from $^{13}C$ to directly attached protons via the large $^1J_{CH}$ coupling. In this way, indirect proton correlations (such as are normally found in TOCSY) are observed using only couplings > *ca.* 30 Hz. Each cross-peak is characterised by the frequencies of two (directly or indirectly coupled) protons and the carbon to which the magnetisation was first transferred. Consequently there is much redundant information in these spectra, since the transfer will proceed in both directions. The HCCH-COSY works in an analogous manner, except that a single-step $^{13}C \rightarrow {}^{13}C$ transfer is used, such that correlations are seen only between directly coupled protons (i.e., protons separated by no more than three bonds).

The HCCH experiments avoid the pitfalls caused by proton linewidths being greater than $^3J_{HH}$ couplings by transferring magnetisation exclusively via large one-bond couplings. These experiments have proven extremely useful in the assignment of both proton and carbon side-chain resonances in medium- to large-sized proteins. They are most profitably used in tandem with triple-resonance experiments, which are used for the assignment of backbone resonances in doubly labelled proteins (see below). Note also that the HCCH experiments are best carried out in $D_2O$, in order to avoid the large water signal that could otherwise obscure a number of the $H^\alpha$ resonances and their associated correlations.

A further implementation of heteronuclear editing of homonuclear spectra can be carried out when specifically labelled samples are available (e.g., $^{15}N$ labelling of all Leu residues). Normal 2D homonuclear pulse sequences to which a so-called difference echo is appended yield $^1H$-$^1H$ spectra where only the residues carrying the labels appear.[106,107] This can be useful for resolving ambiguities that may be present even in the 3D experiments. Some workers have made full assignments by generating many such specifically labelled samples and applying these techniques to each one,[108,109] but this represents a rather time- and labour-intensive approach requiring a very well-behaved expression system, and is consequently not expected to be widely applicable.[109]

The most significant limitation of this resonance-assignment strategy is that some of the experiments still rely on the transfer of magnetisation via small homonuclear couplings ($^3J_{\alpha N}$ is as low as 3 Hz for residues in $\alpha$-helical structure), and hence will fail for larger proteins, as noted earlier. Further, the sequential assignment process requires the use of NOEs, which do not provide unambiguous connections as readily as scalar couplings; assignment consequently involves a pattern-matching process, which is very time consuming. The next section describes a recently developed approach that circumvents these problems to some extent, and promises to allow resonance assignment for proteins up to perhaps 35 kDa in favourable cases.

### 3    Triple-Resonance Experiments

As previously discussed, the large size of one- and two-bond heteronuclear (and homonuclear $J_{CC}$) couplings (Figure 11) results in very efficient magnetisation transfer (using either HSQC or HMQC sequences) relative to homonuclear scalar transfer through either COSY- or TOCSY-type techniques. Therefore, the recent development of an alternative method for the assignment of protein NMR spectra that makes use of these large couplings represents a very significant breakthrough in the field. Although two of these couplings ($^1J_{NC\alpha}$ and $^1J_{NC'}$) are quite small, the experiments have been (and still are being) carefully designed and optimised, so as to minimise the problems presented by these couplings (see below). The concept underlying this class of experiments is that magnetisation is transferred between nuclei via scalar couplings, such that the frequencies of some or all of the atoms involved in the transfer pathway are sampled. Thus a 3D (or 4D) spectrum is obtained that correlates the chemical shifts of three (or four) nuclei as defined by the coherence pathway chosen. In this way, a number of different interresidue correlations can be made, providing unambiguous sequential assignments (*cf.* NOE-based connections). The size of these one-bond $J$ couplings is generally rather insensitive to conformation, allowing the delays in the pulse sequences to be accurately tuned to the coupling constants.

Magnetisation pathways and pulse sequences for two of these experiments are shown in Figure 16. Names are usually designated on the basis of the nuclei involved in the transfer pathway, where nuclei having a chemical shift that is not sampled are given in brackets. Thus the HNCO is an interresidue experiment correlating $H^N(i)$, $N(i)$, and $C'(i-1)$ resonances (where $C'$ signifies the carbonyl carbon). In the pulse sequence name, the term "HN" implies that both the amide proton and its attached nitrogen are frequency labelled; CO refers to the carbonyl carbon, and CA, CB, HA, and HB refer to $C^\alpha$, $C^\beta$, $H^\alpha$, and $H^\beta$, respectively. The order in which the atoms are listed indicates the direction of the magnetisation transfer. In virtually all cases, magnetisation will start on $^1H$ and be passed to a heteronucleus (using either an INEPT or HMQC transfer), so that the sensitivity of the experiment is increased relative to starting with the magnetisation on the heteronucleus.[110] In addition, $^1H$ magnetisation is always detected in the direct dimension, again for sensitivity reasons, meaning that experiments such as the HNCO are termed "out-and-back" experiments. That is, after transfer to $C'$, the reverse pathway is traced, so that the entire experiment is described by $H^N(i) \rightarrow N(i) \rightarrow C'(i-1) \rightarrow N(i) \rightarrow H^N(i)$. The HN(CA)CO,[118] also an out-and-back experiment, selects a symmetrically related intraresidue pathway: $H^N(i) \rightarrow N(i) \rightarrow C^\alpha(i) \rightarrow C'(i) \rightarrow C^\alpha(i) \rightarrow N(i) \rightarrow H^N(i)$, with $C^\alpha$ not frequency labelled. Note that the $C^\alpha$ nuclei (together with $C^\beta$ nuclei in other experiments) are treated separately from the carbonyl carbons in these sequences; to make this possible, pulses that excite, for example, the C′ region of the carbon spectrum but not the aliphatic region must often be generated. This requires either a spectrometer with four separate amplifiers or, if this is not available, the use of off-resonance frequency-selective pulses (for a review of selective pulses, see Reference 111).

A formidable array of these triple-resonance experiments has been developed since the concept was first introduced.[99,112] Consequently a number of strategies are available with which to make assignments, depending on the size, and hence the relaxation properties, of the protein concerned (in particular, $C^\alpha$ and $H^\alpha$ atoms; see below). These experiments in general exist in complementary pairs, with one providing exclusively interresidue connectivities and the other providing both intra- and interresidue connections. This situation arises because $C^\alpha(i)$ is coupled both to $N(i)$ ($^1J_{C\alpha N}$) and to $N(i-1)$ ($^2J_{C\alpha N}$), so that any sequence passing magnetisation between $C^\alpha$ and N will branch off in two directions. Cross-peaks resulting from these two pathways are generally distinguishable in the final spectrum by the lower intensity of the interresidue signals, which arise from the smaller $^2J_{C\alpha N}$ coupling constant. Conversely, the interresidue pathway can be selected exclusively by routing magnetisation (originating from either $N(i)$ or $C^\alpha(i-1)$) through $C'(i-1)$.

The HNCA[112,113] and HN(CO)CA[113,114] experiments form a pair of this type (see Figure 17). The HNCA correlates the $N(i)H(i)$ unit with both $C^\alpha(i)$ and $C^\alpha(i-1)$, while the HN(CO)CA, by virtue of the transfer through $C'(i)$, provides only the interresidue $NH(i) \rightarrow C^\alpha(i-1)$ connection. In theory, these two experiments should suffice to elucidate sequential assignments for all $H^N$, N, and $C^\alpha$ nuclei. However, in practice, overlap and/or missing signals precludes this, and a second linkage between residues, involving an atom other than $C^\alpha$, is required. One possibility is to use $H^\alpha$; the HN(CA)HA[115] and HN(COCA)HA[116] experiments achieve this connection (see Figure 18A–B). Note that a [15]N-TOCSY-HSQC also gives the intraresidue $H^N$–$H^\alpha$ connection, although the homonuclear $^3J_{\alpha N}$ coupling constant will reduce the effectiveness of this experiment for larger proteins (especially those with a high helical content). Another method uses the C′ as the linking atom. The HNCO[113,117] is one of the most sensitive triple-resonance experiments (see below), correlating the $H(i)N(i)$ unit with $C'(i-1)$, while the complementary experiment HN(CA)CO gives the intraresidue $H(i)N(i) \rightarrow C'(i)$ correlation (and often a weaker interresidue cross-peak). Unfortunately, this latter experiment suffers lower sensitivity because of a long residence time on $C^\alpha$, which has a fast transverse-relaxation rate (see below).

Thus, two of these sets of two 3D spectra can provide a pair of interresidue links; the same result can be arrived at by recording two complementary 4D experiments that sample an extra chemical shift each during the magnetisation-transfer pathway. For example, the HNCAHA[119-121] and HN(CO)CAHA[119,121] combine the first four 3D

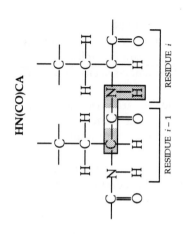

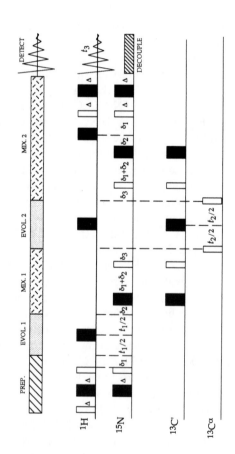

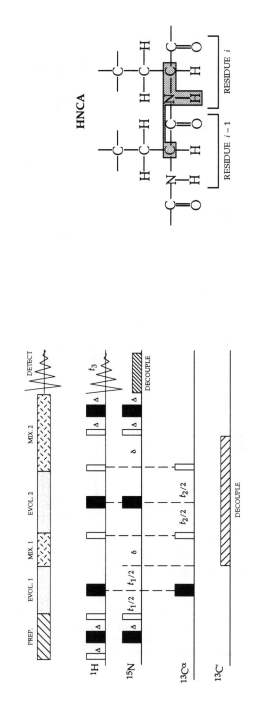

**FIGURE 16**

Basic pulse sequences for the (A) HN(CO)CA and (B) HNCA triple-resonance experiments. The $^{15}N$ and $^{13}C^\alpha$ chemical shifts evolve during $t_1$ and $t_2$ respectively, and the delays $\Delta$ and $\delta$ allow the development of the $^1H-^{15}N$ and $^{15}N-^{13}C/^{13}C^\alpha-^{13}C'$ couplings, respectively. The nuclei involved in the magnetisation transfer pathway(s) in these experiments are boxed. Nuclei shaded grey give rise to frequency axes in the final spectrum, while unshaded nuclei are used in the transfer but are not chemical shift labelled. The thin line in the HNCA pathway indicates that magnetisation is transferred via the two-bond $^2J_{NC\alpha}(i, i-1)$ coupling.

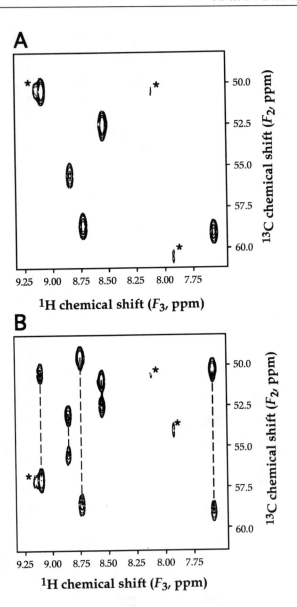

**FIGURE 17**

Sections of 2D $^{13}$C–$^1$H planes taken from triple-resonance (A) HN(CO)CA and (B) HNCA spectra of uniformly $^{15}$N/$^{13}$C-labelled human ubiquitin. These planes were taken at a $^{15}$N chemical shift of 123.7 ppm. In the HN(CO)CA, a single signal is observed per residue, correlating the amide proton and nitrogen of each residue with the C$^\alpha$ of the preceding residue. The HNCA often gives rise to two correlations per residue — from each amide proton-nitrogen pair to the intraresidue and preceding C$^\alpha$ atoms. These pairs are connected by dashed lines in the figure. Correlations marked with an asterisk have their intensity maxima at other nitrogen frequencies. In combination, these two experiments potentially allow the assignment of all HN, N, and C$^\alpha$ atoms of nonprolyl and nonglycyl residues.

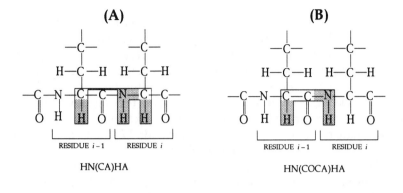

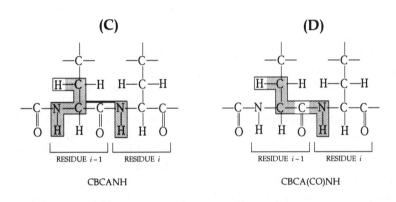

**FIGURE 18**
Correlations observed in the (A) HN(CA)HA, (B) HN(COCA)HA, (C) CBCANH, and (D) CBCA(CO)NH triple-resonance experiments. Note that the insertion of a frequency-labelling period for $C^\alpha$ in experiments (A) and (B) would give rise to the 4D experiments HNCAHA and HN(CO)CAHA, respectively.

triple-resonance experiments described above, resulting in two connections between residues ($H^\alpha$ and $C^\alpha$ chemical shifts) in each experiment. An alternative and powerful method for providing two interresidue links is achieved using only two recent 3D experiments, the CBCANH[122] (or the very similar, but more sensitive HNCACB)[123] and the CBCA(CO)NH.[124,125] These experiments describe the transfer pathways shown in Figure 18C–D, and connect H($i$)N($i$) units of one residue with the $C^\alpha$ and $C^\beta$ atoms of both the same and the preceding residues, in a manner similar to the HNCA/HN(CO)CA pair (i.e., up to four cross-peaks are seen at each combination of N/H$^N$ frequencies). Thus the HNCACB yields the frequencies of up to six nuclei from a single 3D dataset (H$^N$($i$), N($i$), $C^\alpha$($i$), $C^\beta$($i$), $C^\alpha$($i-1$), and $C^\beta$($i-1$)). Interpretation of the spectra is simplified, however, by the opposite signs of $C^\alpha$ and $C^\beta$ correlations. Two further features add to the utility of these experiments. First, the chemical shifts of $C^\alpha$ and $C^\beta$ directly identify the spin systems of several residues (Ala, Thr, Ser, and also Gly from the absence of a $C^\beta$ correlation), providing entry points for sequence-specific assignments. Second, the measured $C^\alpha$ and $C^\beta$ chemical shifts also provide useful overlap with the HCCH-TOCSY and HCCH-COSY experiments, which can be used to assign the side-chain protons. A closely related experiment that correlates $(i - 1)$ side-chain protons rather than carbons with the interresidue $i$ amide unit has also been described, HBHA(CBCACO)NH.[124,125]

Two further experiments, which together provide multiple interresidue connectivities, have been proposed. In the 3D H(CCO)NH-TOCSY[126,127] and H(C)NH-TOCSY,[126,128] magnetisation begins on the side-chain protons of residue $(i - 1)$ and is first transferred to the attached carbon using INEPT. It is then propagated along the side chain via an isotropic (TOCSY-like) mixing sequence. In the former experiment, the magnetisation that arrives at $C^\alpha(i - 1)$ at the end of the mixing period is transferred to $C'(i - 1)$ and then to $N(i)$ and finally $H^N(i)$ for detection. In the latter sequence, direct transfer from $C^\alpha(i - 1)$ to nitrogen, $N(i - 1)$ and $N(i)$, yields, as for HNCA, both intra- and interresidue connectivities (although the latter are rather weak). During these experiments, the chemical shifts of the side-chain protons $H^x(i - 1)$, $N(i)$, and $H^N(i)$ are sampled, as are $N(i - 1)$ and $H^N(i - 1)$ in the H(C)NH-TOCSY. In principle, the information provided by the latter experiment is available in a $^{15}$N-TOCSY-HSQC, although in practice this is not always the case, as the transfer along the side chain is via small homonuclear couplings in the TOCSY-HSQC (*cf.* the large $^1J_{CH}$ and $^1J_{CC}$ couplings in the H(C)NH-TOCSY). Thus the side-chain protons are correlated to the amide unit of both the same and the succeeding residue, providing a useful tool for making sequential assignments. Further, these experiments can be recorded in four dimensions with the side-chain carbons comprising the fourth dimension, that is, HCNH- and HC(CO)NH-TOCSY,[126] in order to provide $^{13}$C chemical shifts and a potential increase in resolution (but see below) if ambiguities still remain. Note also that the H(CCO)NH-TOCSY is very similar in concept to the HBHA(CBCACO)NH described above. The main difference is that transfer from $C^\beta$ to $C^\alpha$ in the latter case is via a COSY-type step. This excludes magnetisation that may have started on $C^\gamma$ from being observed, in contrast to the isotropic mixing sequence used in the two TOCSY-type experiments.

The 3D HCACO[112,129-131] and 3D HCA(CO)N[112,129-131] are also very useful experiments. The HCACO has high sensitivity (because the small $J_{C\alpha N}$ couplings are avoided) and correlates three intraresidue atoms; it is therefore used widely to complement the other triple-resonance experiments. The HCA(CO)N is one of the less sensitive experiments, but its particular benefit lies in its ability to provide correlations to amide nitrogens that are connected to broadened amide protons.[132] Such protons may occur in flexible regions (such as loops and the N- and C-termini) and may fail to provide cross-peaks with sufficient intensity in many of the other triple-resonance experiments that both begin with and detect $H^N$ magnetisation. Because both of these experiments detect $H^\alpha$ in the direct dimension, the spectra must be recorded in $D_2O$, in common with the HCCH experiments. This may give rise to a small isotope shift of the $^{13}C$ resonances (C′ and $C^\alpha$), although such shifts are readily accounted for.[112] The suppression of residual water can also saturate $H^\alpha$ protons that lie directly underneath the water resonance, thus preventing the observation of correlations for these residues.[133]

Finally, a number of more specialised experiments have been proposed, which deal with specific problems in the assignment process. For example, the side chains of the four aromatic residues have traditionally been assigned using NOE connectivities between $H^\beta$ and $H^\delta$ protons. However, Yamazaki et al.[134] describe an experiment that correlates $C^\beta$ with $H^\delta$ and $H^\varepsilon$ with the exclusive use of scalar couplings. Another problem can lie in the detection of Gly residues. Neither of the 4D triple-resonance backbone experiments, HNCAHA and HN(CO)CAHA, generates detectable cross-peaks to Gly $H^\alpha$ atoms.[135,136] This gives rise to breaks in the sequential assignment process, which have been circumvented with the HNHA(Gly) experiment.[135] This experiment correlates Gly $H^\alpha$ protons with both intra- and interresidue NH atom pairs. Alternatively, ambiguities arising from missing Gly correlations may be resolved by recourse to $^{15}N$-TOCSY-HSQC and $^{15}N$-NOESY-HSQC,[136] which may well be recorded as part of the assignment procedure anyway.

Because of the relatively recent development of this branch of NMR, these triple-resonance experiments are undergoing a constant refinement process, whereby the factors limiting two of the key facets of any NMR experiment, sensitivity and resolution, are identified and addressed. In fact, in many cases where more than one reference is given for a single experiment in this section, the later one(s) describe improvements to the original experiments. Because of the complex, multistep nature of these experiments, their main adversary is transverse relaxation $T_2$. First, $T_2$ (and hence linewidth) for a particular nucleus determines how efficient coherence transfer via scalar couplings will be for that nucleus. As described above, when linewidths become larger than the magnitude of the scalar couplings concerned, transfer efficiency declines markedly. The linewidths in a 20-kDa globular protein at 25°C will be $\approx 12$ Hz for $H^N$, $\approx 7$ Hz for N when proton coupled ($\approx 4$ Hz when decoupled), $\approx 15$ Hz for $^{13}C^\alpha$, and $\approx 25$ Hz for $H^\alpha$ (attached to $^{13}C$).[7] These are in general smaller than the couplings used in these experiments, although it is clear that the small $^1J_{C\alpha N}$ coupling will become a primary determinant of which experiments may be carried out with reasonable sensitivity as the protein size increases. A second problem is that the transverse magnetisation associated with a particular nucleus loses phase coherence (and therefore intensity) at a rate characterised by $T_2$ for that nucleus. Thus it is important to minimise the length of time spent on nuclei such as $C^\alpha$, which have comparatively short $T_2$ times (~20 ms for $C^\alpha$). Thus experiments such as 4D HC(CO)NH-TOCSY, which correlate side chain atoms with sequential backbone amides, are significantly more sensitive than the intraresidue HCCNH-TOCSY, as the former avoids the $J_{C\alpha N}$ coupling. For INEPT-type transfer between two nuclei, magnetisation must be resident on each nucleus for around $1/2J$ s. This corresponds to 50 ms spent on $C^\alpha$ for $C^\alpha \rightarrow N$ transfer, but only 9 ms for $C^\alpha \rightarrow C'$ transfer. Clearly the latter pathway allows less transverse relaxation. For similar reasons, the 3D CBCANH, although a powerful experiment in combination with CBCA(CO)NH as outlined above, will decrease rapidly in efficiency for proteins above $ca.$ 20 kDa. This is in contrast to the CBCA(CO)NH, which avoids the $^1J_{C\alpha N}$ coupling, and was applied successfully to the 31.4-kDa interferon-$\gamma$. Similarly, the HNCO is one of the more sensitive of triple-resonance experiments as it avoids the fast-relaxing $C^\alpha$ and $H^\alpha$ altogether. The HN(CO)CA also bypasses $^1J_{C\alpha N}$, and consequently has a sensitivity comparable to the CBCA(CO)NH.[125] It is obviously also important to limit the total length of the pulse sequences so as to minimise $T_2$ relaxation prior to signal sampling. Simple concatenation of magnetisation-transfer and free-precession (frequency-labelling) periods as described above produced the first triple-resonance experiments, but recently it has been shown that these periods may be overlaid such that both free precession and magnetisation transfer occur during the same time interval. This gives rise to so-called constant-time experiments with significantly shortened pulse sequences.[113,131] Further recent methodological advances are discussed in Section IV.D below.

## 4  Summary of Resonance-Assignment Strategies

With such an array of possible approaches to resonance assignment, it must be decided for a particular protein which is the most suitable. Although many smaller proteins may be amenable to a homonuclear approach as described in Section IV.B, there are a number of advantages in using either $^{15}N$- or $^{15}N/^{13}C$-labelled protein. As long as a suitable expression system is available, labelling is relatively straightforward and (at least for $^{15}N$) not excessively expensive (although when the cost of the high-field NMR spectrometer time is taken into account, the price of introducing $^{13}C$ labels becomes more acceptable). For smaller proteins, $^{15}N$ labelling will significantly simplify the resonance-assignment process by making use of $^{15}N$-NOESY-HSQC and $^{15}N$-TOCSY-HSQC, and a number of medium-sized proteins have been assigned using this $^{15}N$-directed strategy.[95,108,137,138] Note, however, that the $^{15}N$-NOESY-HSQC only yields NOEs that involve at least one amide proton, and NOEs between carbon-bound protons will have to be obtained from analysis of

2D NOESY spectra. However, the additional advantages of $^{15}$N labelling, such as the ability to measure amide-proton exchange rates conveniently (see Section IV.E.3 below) and probe backbone dynamics (Chapter 10), combine to make labelling an attractive strategy, even for proteins smaller than 10 kDa.

For proteins smaller than *ca.* 15 kDa (perhaps a little less for α-helical proteins and a little more for predominantly β-sheet proteins), the $^{15}$N-only approach may prove adequate. If not, double labelling with both $^{15}$N and $^{13}$C is necessary, and assignment is most readily achieved using triple-resonance experiments. There are a number of combinations of these experiments that can potentially yield assignments, and for smaller proteins all should give adequate sensitivity. The earlier approaches assigned backbone resonances with combinations of out-and-back experiments such as HNCO, HNCA, and HN(CO)CA, while more recent efforts attempt to integrate both backbone and side-chain assignments in experiments such as the 4D HCC(CO)NH-TOCSY. A feature of the triple-resonance strategy is that nearly all resonance assignments can be made on the basis of scalar couplings. A further advantage is that they provide $^{15}$N and $^{13}$C chemical shifts; the former are used in amide exchange and backbone dynamics studies, while the latter contain information on secondary structure (see below). A decision on which of the armoury of triple-resonance experiments to use will be partly based on the relaxation properties (i.e., size) of the protein. This is essentially due to the rapid transverse relaxation of C$^{\alpha}$ and H$^{\alpha}$; experiments that involve long residence times on these nuclei will often be of limited use for proteins larger than *ca.* 20 kDa, (e.g., CBCANH and HN(CA)CO).

The basic heteronuclear assignment strategy is to create clusters of atoms with known assignments and then to link these clusters (preferably in two or more independent ways), thus generating chains of sequential residues. These chains are then placed within the sequence using spin system information.

For example, in the first study that employed triple-resonance experiments,[112] HNCA, $^{15}$N-TOCSY-HMQC, and HCACO spectra were used to build clusters consisting of H$^N$($i$), N($i$), C$^{\alpha}$($i$), H$^{\alpha}$($i$), and C'($i$) for calmodulin. Then HNCO and HCA(CO)N provide the intercluster connections; HNCA also provided HN($i$) → C$^{\alpha}$($i - 1$) connectivities. This method is still applicable, although HCA(CO)N and $^{15}$N-TOCSY-HMQC will generally be less effective for proteins >20 kDa. Basically the same core of experiments (i.e., HNCO, HNCA, HCACO, and the $^{15}$N-edited TOCSY and NOESY), with the addition of HN(CO)CA, has since been used to obtain backbone assignments for a number of proteins.[139-142] These early experiments remain some of the most sensitive examples, and were used successfully to assign both interferon-γ (a 31.4-kDa symmetrical homodimer)[64] and subtilisin 309 (a 27-kDa monomer).[133] The strategy used in the assignment of interferon-γ involved building atom clusters with HNCO, HN(CO)CA, and HCACO, that is, $H^\alpha(i-1)$, $C^\alpha(i-1)$, $C'(i-1)$, $N(i)$, and $H^N(i)$, and connecting them simultaneously using HNCA, $^{15}$N-TOCSY-HMQC, and $^{15}$N-NOESY-HMQC (Figure 19). Remerowski et al.[133] used the same atom clusters for the assignment of the 269-residue subtilisin 309, but used two extra experiments, HN(COCA)HA and HCA(CO)N, to define the clusters, and an extra one, HN(CA)HA, to connect them. In addition, a CBCA(CO)NH was necessary to resolve ambiguities in the cluster connections.

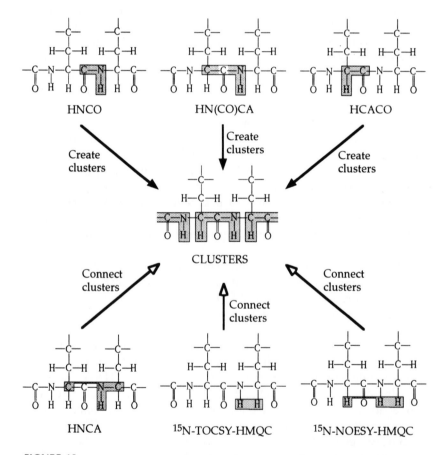

**FIGURE 19**
Summary of the strategy used by Grzesiek et al.[66] in the assignment of interferon-γ. Clusters of correlated nuclei were built up using the HNCO, HN(CO)CA, and HCACO experiments. These clusters were connected in three different ways, as shown in the lower part of the figure, so that sequences of connected clusters were created. Identification of some spin systems then allowed these sequences of clusters to be positioned in the protein sequence.

Two "second-generation" approaches, which have been shown to be very powerful on a small (8.2 kDa) and a medium-sized (20 kDa) protein, respectively, are the 3D H(C)NH-TOCSY/H(CCO)NH-TOCSY[143] and CBCA(CO)NH/CBCANH[122,125,143] combinations. Both of these procedures, however, are predicted to fail for larger proteins. In the first case, both experiments entail significant residence times for magnetisation on $C^\alpha$ (10–50 ms), although the problem is significantly smaller for H(C)NH-TOCSY. In the second case, CBCANH suffers a similar problem as the magnetisation proceeds through the small $^1J_{C\alpha N}$ coupling. However, CBCA(CO)NH, as mentioned previously, is much more sensitive. Because of this sensitivity, combined with the valuable information it provides, this combination has been used widely since it was first described, both with CBCANH[144-146] or with other experiments.[132,145,147,148] H(CCO)NH-TOCSY may prove to have a similar utility.

A number of the recent innovations in the triple-resonance field have focussed on integrating backbone and side-chain assignment strategies. Most of the published assignments of side-chain atoms use 3D HCCH-COSY and HCCH-TOCSY (see, e.g., References 136, 140, 146, 147, 149) although, even for larger proteins, the $^{15}$N-edited TOCSY-HMQC has been shown to provide much useful information.[64,133] These HCCH experiments have a useful overlap with the CBCA(CO)NH, and using the latter for main chain assignments would greatly facilitate the analysis of the former for side-chain connectivities. As noted already, the recent 3D/4D HCNH-TOCSY/HC(CO)NH-TOCSY experiments are potentially very powerful, especially for smaller proteins, as they correlate side-chain atoms (H and/or C) to the backbone NH units.

The 4D scalar experiments (e.g., HNCAHA, HN(CO)CAHA) have not yet become routine, although a few reports of assignments utilising them have been published.[56,136,146,149] It has been noted[126] that a combination of three 4D datasets, the HNCAHA, HN(CO)CAHA, and HC(CO)NH-TOCSY, may be generally sufficient for the complete sequential assignment of larger proteins. Such 4D-centred strategies could well become more popular in the near future, as increased computing power and the widespread adoption of refinements such as the use of pulsed-field gradients (see Section IV.E.1) reduce the long acquisition and processing times generally required for these experiments. Note, however, that 4D datasets do not *necessarily* offer any advantages over their lower-dimensionality counterparts. The 3D and 4D experiments can be considered as mathematical products of the corresponding 2D sequences,[150] such that they do not actually provide any new information per se, but simply resolve overlapping resonances in the 2D or 3D spectrum, respectively. A similar increase in resolution may be achieved in the lower-dimensionality experiment by simply increasing the number of points (*viz.*, the acquisition time) in the indirectly detected dimension. This will be effective until the indirect acquisition time becomes longer than *ca.* $T_2$ for the signals of interest. Beyond that point, the inherent sensitivity of the experiment (per unit time) drops sharply, as the magnitude of the signal collected is lower at longer acquisition times (due to $T_2$ relaxation), so that beyond about $t_1$ $\approx T_2$, the increase in resolution obtained by collecting extra points is insufficient compensation for the decline in sensitivity. Consequently, an increase in dimensionality *is* warranted when suitable resolution cannot be obtained in a lower-dimensional experiment with $t_1 \leq T_2$. It is also not generally desirable to increase dimensionality beyond that which is suffi- cient, as in the same period of time required to record, for example, a 4D HNCAHA, a pair of 3D HN(CA)HA and HNCA experiments with superior digital resolution could be collected that would provide the same information.[7] In summary, an increase from $n$D to $(n + 1)$D is probably beneficial only when the resolution in the $n$D spectra is limited by the natural linewidths of the signals and not by the use of indirect acquisition times much shorter than $T_2$.

Although several discrete triple-resonance strategies have been out- lined here that in theory can yield complete assignments, in practice a whole battery of these experiments are often applied to a protein. For example Anglister *et al.*[56] recorded a total of two 4D, nine 3D, and two 2D spectra to obtain the resonance assignments of calcineurin B. This is generally the result of problems that arise during the assignment that could not be predicted *ab initio*; one example is the chemical-shift coincidence of several atoms in a cluster with those from another cluster. Alternatively, some cross-peaks may be weak or absent in a given spectrum, for one of a number of reasons. For example, amide protons in less-ordered regions may exchange rapidly with solvent protons; this will broaden their NMR signal, reducing the obtainable signal-to-noise ratio for the corresponding cross-peak(s) in multidimensional spectra (this can sometimes be remedied by manipulation of sample conditions; see Section III). Conversely, the carbon atoms of such mobile regions will be much sharper than those of the remainder of the protein (since they are effectively rotating indepen- dently of the bulk of the protein, and therefore exhibit longer $T_2$s). The observation of weaker correlations in the presence of such narrow, intense ones can be exacerbated by artifacts such as $t_1$ noise associated with the stronger cross-peaks.[132] The decision on which triple-resonance experi- ments to use therefore remains to some degree empirical, and often needs to be determined separately for individual cases, and for individual spec- trometers (as some of these experiments require four RF channels). As a starting point, however, the more sensitive of the out-and-back experi- ments, HNCO, HNCA, HN(CO)CA, HCACO, will almost always pro- vide much useable information. If one is confident about the relaxation properties of a protein, one of the second-generation strategies may be attempted straightaway instead.

## D   RECENT ADVANCES

### 1   Pulsed Field Gradients

The use of pulsed-field gradients (PFGs), that is, RF pulses that are (deliberately) inhomogeneous over the volume of the sample, to construct a three-dimensional image of a sample has been routine for a number of years in magnetic resonance imaging applications.[151] Following recent advances in hardware design,[152] they have also been introduced as building blocks in multidimensional solution-state NMR for the selection/suppression of coherences (see Reference 153 and references therein), the generation of which form the basis of all multipulse NMR experiments.[68] The principle governing their use is as follows. The precession frequency of a spin (in rad s$^{-1}$) in the transverse ($xy$) plane after application of an RF pulse is determined by the magnetic field strength at that nucleus:

$$\omega = -\gamma B_{eff} \tag{2}$$

where $\gamma$ is the gyromagnetic ratio and $B_{eff}$ the effective field strength at the nucleus. Furthermore, the phase of the transverse signal after time $t$ is described by a term

$$\exp\left(-ip\gamma B_{eff}t\right) \tag{3}$$

for the evolution of magnetisation with coherence order $p$. Consequently, if a field gradient is applied to the sample during evolution, then equivalent spins in different physical locations within the sample will evolve at different frequencies, and at a given time they will have different phases as indicated by Equation (3) (i.e., the signal will become phase incoherent). Gradients can therefore be used in their simplest form to spoil (dephase) unwanted transverse magnetisation. For instance, at a particular stage of an experiment, the desired component of the magnetisation may be aligned along the $z$ axis, while undesirable components lie in the $xy$ plane, and would otherwise affect the quality of the final spectrum. The application of a field gradient pulse can therefore be used as a so-called $z$ or $zz$ filter.[154-156]

However, the coherence dephasing induced by a gradient pulse can be reversed by the application of a complementary gradient (i.e., one with the same field strength and duration), thus restoring phase coherence. This rephasing may be achieved either by changing the sign of the gradient or by first applying a 180° pulse and then applying the same gradient as was used initially to dephase the magnetisation (Figure 20). In the latter case (but not the former), chemical shifts will also be refocussed. As a result, gradient pulses can be used to select particular coherences, according to either the order or the nuclear identity of the coherence, a task traditionally

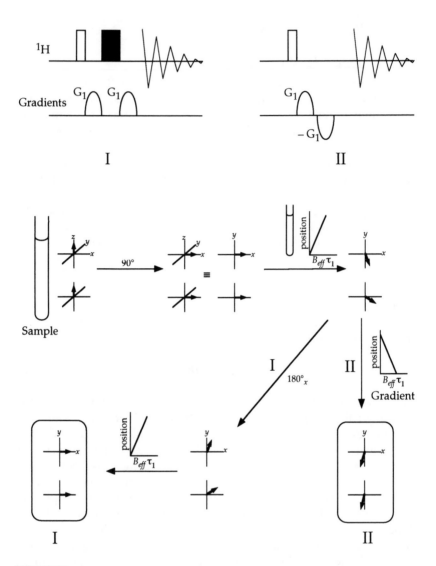

**FIGURE 20**

Defocussing and refocussing of transverse magnetisation using pulsed-field gradients. The behaviour of two identical spins in different physical locations within the sample tube is shown for the two pulse sequences labelled I and II. The first PFG causes the two nuclei to precess at different rates as they experience different effective magnetic fields. In sequence I, a $180°_x$ pulse flips the spins around the $x$ axis. Application of a second, identical PFG causes the upper of the two spins to again precess faster, so that at the end of the gradient pulse, phase coherence is regained *and* chemical shifts are refocussed. In sequence II, the sense of the gradient is reversed (without the 180° pulse), so that the upper spin now precesses slower. After the time $\tau_1$, the spins are again phase coherent, but their chemical shift is not refocussed.

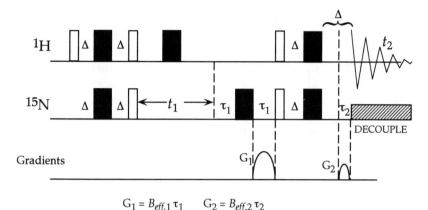

$$G_1 = B_{eff,1}\,\tau_1 \qquad G_2 = B_{eff,2}\,\tau_2$$

**FIGURE 21**

Pulse sequence for a $^1H$–$^{15}N$ HSQC using gradients for coherence selection. During $G_1$ all magnetisation is dephased (at this stage the desired magnetisation is on $^{15}N$). After transfer back to $^1H$, a second gradient described by $G_2 = 0.1\,G_1$ is applied, and only magnetisation that was present on $^{15}N$ during the first gradient $G_1$ will be refocussed and therefore detected during $t_2$.

accomplished by phase-cycling procedures. For example, in a gradient-enhanced $^{15}N$-HSQC experiment[157] using the pulse sequence given in Figure 21, all magnetisation is dephased by the first gradient ($G_1$, applied for a period $\tau_1$) at the end of the $^{15}N$ evolution time $t_1$. Following transfer of magnetisation back to $^1H$ by reverse-INEPT, a second gradient $G_2$ is applied for $\tau_2$ seconds. If this second gradient is generated such that

$$\gamma_H B_{eff,2}\tau_2 = \gamma_N B_{eff,1}\tau_1 \qquad (4)$$

then only the magnetisation that was located on $^{15}N$ during the first gradient period will be refocussed. Since $\gamma_H/\gamma_N \approx 10$, this refocussing can be accomplished by making $10.B_{eff,2}\tau_2 = B_{eff,1}\tau_1$. This can be achieved by reducing either the strength or duration of the second gradient pulse by a factor of 10, while leaving the other variable unchanged (in practice, nonlinearities in available gradient amplifiers may make adjustments of gradient strength problematic). Any magnetisation that was not on $^{15}N$ during $\tau_1$ will be defocussed. Thus coherence selection is achieved in a single scan. This is in contrast to phase-cycling procedures, where successive scans with incrementally altered phases for particular pulses are co-added. The phase incrementation is arranged such that signals arising from desired and undesired magnetisation-transfer pathways have opposite sign; thus, co-addition of FIDs results (ideally) in cancellation of signals arising from the undesired pathways and reinforcement of the desired signal. Unfortunately, this co-addition is often imperfect, so that artifacts such as

$t_1$ noise can result. Further, the cycling of phases for several pulses in a sequence must often be carried out separately, resulting in a minimum number of scans necessary to achieve coherence selection. This minimum can be significantly greater than the number of scans required for adequate signal-to-noise ratio, imposing what can be an inconvenient lower limit on total experimental time, especially for multidimensional experiments. Coherence selection by PFGs avoids both of these problems, although some minimal phase cycling is still carried out for artifact suppression. The elimination of long phase cycles allows a potential increase in resolution in indirectly detected dimension(s) for samples of suitable concentration. An additional feature of PFGs is that, as opposed to actively selecting a particular pathway, they can be used to suppress unwanted magnetisation-transfer pathways at each step of an experiment (e.g., the $z$ filters described above).[158-162] This provides an excellent alternative to the traditional methods for suppression of the $H_2O$ solvent signal. In particular, some of the problems associated with preirradiation are alleviated, such as the saturation of nearby resonances. In some applications, saturation transfer to labile amide protons, which results in intensity reduction, can also be avoided.[163]

Until recently, however, there have been problems associated with the use of PFGs for coherence selection (although these do not apply to coherence rejection strategies). Using the method described, only half of the desired magnetisation (either N- or P type;[164] the meaning of these terms is unimportant for this discussion) is refocussed by the second pulse. The other half is further dephased, so that there is an intrinsic $\sqrt{2}$ loss of sensitivity involved in recording spectra using PFGs for coherence selection. Note that this loss can often be more than compensated for by the reduction in artifacts and the potential increase in $t_1$ resolution associated with the use of gradients for coherence selection.[157] A further problem with PFG coherence selection has been that, because only one component of the magnetisation is detected, signals in the transformed spectra have undesirable phase-twisted lineshapes. This latter problem has recently been overcome by collecting P- or N-type signals on alternate scans and combining them during processing of the spectrum.[165,166] Perhaps even more significantly, a modification of the standard pulse sequences for conventional (i.e., nongradient) heteronuclear 2D experiments has been described[167,168] resulting in an enhancement in sensitivity for such experiments of up to *ca.* $\sqrt{2}$. When these improved sequences are further modified to use PFGs for coherence selection,[169-171] not only is the $\sqrt{2}$ improvement resulting from the new scheme gained, but the original sensitivity loss described earlier for gradients is avoided. Thus, in these very new experiments, all the advantages of PFGs described above (i.e., reduction of artifacts, shorter phase cycles) are retained with no loss in sensitivity compared to equivalent nongradient experiments. Note that one drawback of PFGs is that specialised hardware is required to execute them, but as this hardware becomes more widespread, PFG-assisted NMR experiments will undoubtedly become *de rigeur* for biological NMR spectroscopists.

## 2 Heteronuclear Cross-Polarisation

There are essentially two ways to transfer magnetisation between atoms *via* scalar couplings. The first is to use pulsed free precession, as seen in COSY- and INEPT-type schemes. The second is to use cross-polarisation, as seen for example in the homonuclear TOCSY experiment. In this latter method, an RF field, generally consisting of a train of pulses of intermediate power, is applied to a sample in which transverse magnetisation has been created. A number of these pulse trains (e.g., MLEV,[172] DIPSI,[173] WALTZ,[174] and FLOPSY)[175] have been developed. This spin-locking field ($B_1$, typically 5–10 kHz) consequently becomes the quantising field around which precession occurs. However, because $B_1$ is substantially weaker than the static field ($B_0$, several hundred MHz), the chemical-shift differences between nuclei, which are proportional to the applied field, become insignificant compared to the $J$-coupling terms. In such a situation (termed strong coupling), where the effective fields experienced by two coupled nuclei are identical, an exchange of spin-locked magnetisation takes place. This is the so-called Hartmann–Hahn condition.[176] There are several advantages of this coherence transfer mechanism. First, the cross-peaks arising in a TOCSY are absorption mode, thus avoiding the cancellation of antiphase components that occurs in COSY spectra when linewidths are larger than the coupling constant. Second, relay and multiple-relay peaks appear in the spectrum, potentially yielding cross-peaks which link all spins within a spin system with each other. Third, because transfer between remote spins within a spin system begins at the commencement of the spin-locking period, TOCSY is a more efficient technique for the correlation of such spins (compared to a number of sequential COSY-type steps).

This polarisation transfer method can equally be applied to heteronuclear systems; heteronuclear cross-polarisation (HCP) has long been used in solid-state NMR to observe insensitive spins with long relaxation times, such as $^{13}C$.[177] In this case, spin-locking fields are simultaneously applied to the two nuclear species (e.g., $^1H$ and $^{13}C$). The strengths of these two fields are chosen such that the effective fields experienced by both nuclei are again identical. Thus for the case of $^1H$ and $^{13}C$, where $\gamma(^1H) \approx 4 \times \gamma(^{13}C)$, the Hartmann–Hahn match requires that

$$\gamma_H B_{1,H} = \gamma_C B_{1,C} \tag{5}$$

that is,

$$B_{1,H} = \frac{1}{4} B_{1,C} \tag{6}$$

That is, the $^1$H spin-lock field strength is a quarter that of the $^{13}$C spin-lock. Under these conditions, magnetisation transfer takes place, as for the homonuclear case. Recently this technique was shown to be more effective in solution NMR than the traditionally used INEPT sequence,[178-180] although both should achieve complete magnetisation transfer (and enhancement of $^{13}$C sensitivity by a factor of 4) between two coupled spins in $1/J$ seconds. The superiority of the HCP sequence lies in technical rather than theoretical considerations; for example HCP is less sensitive to RF inhomogeneity.[157] An HCP version of HCCH-TOCSY, the HEHOHEHAHA (for heteronuclear-homonuclear-heteronuclear-Hartmann-Hahn spectroscopy) was shown to be more sensitive than the INEPT-HOHAHA-INEPT equivalent[104] (see Figure 22). Further, HCP between $^{15}$N and $^{13}$C has been investigated, and could well prove beneficial in the $^{13}$C $\rightarrow$ $^{15}$N transfer steps necessary in many of the triple-resonance experiments described above.[181]

## 3 Other Areas

There are a number of other fields of endeavour within NMR that promise (or already are beginning) to make a significant impact on the multinuclear, multidimensional studies of biomolecules that are the subject of this chapter and this book in general. Some of these will be mentioned briefly here.

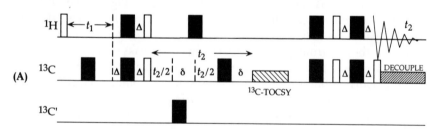

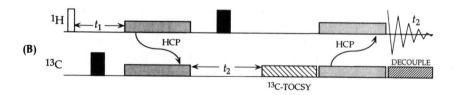

**FIGURE 22**

Pulse sequences for HCCH-TOCSY experiments using either (A) INEPT or (B) heteronuclear cross-polarisation to achieve $^1$H $\rightarrow$ $^{13}$C and $^{13}$C $\rightarrow$ $^1$H transfers. All filled rectangles represent periods of composite pulse decoupling, used either to transfer magnetisation or decouple $^{13}$C during signal acquisition (as labelled).

First, the concept of time-shared $^{13}C$ and $^{15}N$ chemical-shift evolution, first described by Sørensen[182] and Farmer,[183] allows the simultaneous acquisition of $^{13}C$- and $^{15}N$-edited experiments. For example, simultaneous $^1H$–$^{15}N$ and $^1H$–$^{13}C$ versions of the 2D HSQC[184] and 3D NOESY-HQSC[159] experiments have been reported. This arrangement reduces measuring time significantly, allowing more time for increasing digital resolution in the indirectly detected dimension(s). The costs in terms of additional spectral artifacts and reduced signal intensities are very small in comparison.

Nonlinear sampling of data points has been proposed as another way to significantly reduce measuring time for multidimensional experiments.[185-187] It is a requirement of the discrete Fourier transform (FT) that data points be linearly sampled (i.e., evenly spaced in the time domain), but if an alternative algorithm is used to construct the frequency domain from time-domain data, then sampling may be tailored to match the signal. As resolution is essentially determined by the length of the sampling period, alternative, nonlinear sampling schemes that collect fewer points over the same sampling period may be implemented. This is of little advantage in the directly detected dimension of an $n$D experiment ($n \geq 2$), as this sampling time has a relatively small effect on total measuring time. However, in the indirectly detected dimension, where each data point represents a significant investment of time, a reduction in the number of data points required for a given digital resolution will obviously allow for an increase in either sensitivity or resolution per unit time. One factor that has impeded the introduction of nonlinear sampling is the greater computational cost of alternative algorithms, such as maximum entropy (see below), for the reconstruction of the frequency-domain spectrum. With the continual developments in computer performance, however, such approaches to data collection should soon become more widespread.

The maximum-entropy method (MEM) is a general-purpose procedure for data processing[188] that has been considered as an alternative to the Fourier transform in NMR.[189-191] It works essentially in the opposite sense to the conventional FT; whereas the FT calculates a spectrum directly from the data, MEM constructs spectra in the first instance (without knowledge of the real data), reconstructs the hypothetical FIDs that would have given rise to these spectra, and compares these FIDs to the actual experimental FID. After numerous iterations a number of spectra will be found that are consistent with the experimental data; the spectrum containing the least information (i.e., the one with maximum entropy or "least bias") is selected. There are a number of advantages of this approach. For example, baseline noise (some of which is created by the FT) is minimised. In addition, truncation artifacts ("sinc wiggles") arise in Fourier-transformed spectra where the sampling period has been terminated before the signal has completely decayed. This is very common in the indirectly detected dimension(s) of multidimensional spectra as a result of time restrictions.

These artifacts are avoided when data is processed using MEM, which can significantly improve the quality of such spectra, especially at low contour levels where weak signals may be otherwise obscured. Unfortunately, as noted above, this method carries a large penalty in computational time compared to the FT. Further refinement of the MEM procedure, together with the increasing accessibility of powerful computers, may see the MEM method become more commonplace, especially for multidimensional datasets containing truncated data.

Another class of computational methods for improving the quality of multidimensional experiments is centred around the extension of the effective sampling time in indirect dimensions, through postacquisition processing routines. Of these methods, linear prediction (LP) is quite well established.[191-193] This is a technique whereby the data points that have been acquired are used to predict the values of successive data points which have not actually been recorded, given only that the FID is a sum of exponentially decaying sinusoids. This is advantageous up to a certain point (the prediction of around half as many extra points as were actually recorded is common), and the resolution in the predicted dimension is consequently increased significantly. In addition, the artifacts associated with applying an FT to truncated data are reduced correspondingly. Further development of this technique is still in progress,[194,195] although implementations of it are currently available on commercial processing software. Again the application of LP is computationally intensive, but the improvement in resolution is generally well worth the time invested. A related and more recent approach to the same resolution problem is the application of Bayesian probability theory to extrapolate indirectly de-tected data in constant-time experiments.[196] This method employs a proba-bilistic analysis to find the more likely sinusoidal model that accounts for the experimentally recorded data, and uses this model to extend the data in a manner similar to LP.

Increasingly important for the interpretation of a series of multidi-mensional datasets, between which connectivities must be established for up to several hundred residues, is the development of sophisticated software to simplify the process. Resonance assignment for a 200-residue protein is an arduous task, and a number of laboratories are developing software packages that allow the simultaneous display and overlap of planes extracted from several datasets, incorporate assignment databases that are updated for other spectra when an assignment is made on a single spectrum, and so on.[136,197-200] Another aspect of this field is the introduction of algorithms that can automate the assignment process itself. Such programs may start with the processed spectra and initially perform a peak-picking routine. Then, with a list of derived cross-peak frequencies (from several experiments) together with the polypeptide sequence, lists of possible assignments are generated. This represents a very challenging problem; such programs must take account of false peaks (i.e., noise and spectral artifacts), imprecision in frequencies corresponding to the same atoms in different spectra, and the degree of overlap in the data. In this respect, 3D and particularly 4D experiments, where overlap is reduced, are more suitable for such automated procedures. In addition, functions must be developed with suitable criteria to evaluate different possibilities from a list of potential assignments. A number of approaches to this problem have been described and are currently being further refined.[112,201-204]

## E  EXTRACTION OF STRUCTURAL CONSTRAINTS

### 1  Overview

Once the resonance assignment process is completed, the next step in the structure determination process can be tackled; that is the extraction from NMR data of conformation-dependent information. Every such piece of information can then be used as a constraint in an algorithm that, in some way, attempts to generate a three-dimensional structure for the protein (or generally a family of structures) that satisfies the experimental constraints. The most important source of conformational information is homonuclear $^1H-^1H$ NOEs, which are observed between protons less than ca. 5 Å apart in space. Scalar coupling constants (especially $^3J$ couplings) also provide information on torsion angles that can be used as structural constraints. The presence of hydrogen bonds involving backbone amide protons is inferred from slow hydrogen–deuterium exchange rates for these protons, and these are often included in structure calculations. Finally, the chemical shifts of various nuclei have been shown in many cases to be reliable indicators of secondary structure. The information content of each of these classes of data is considered in turn.

### 2  NOEs

When two protons are close in space ($\leq$ ca. 5 Å), they are said to be dipolar coupled (as opposed to scalar coupled, which is a through-bond coupling mechanism). The modulation of this dipolar coupling as a result of molecular tumbling allows relaxation of the protons, and this relaxation may be manifested as a nuclear Overhauser effect (NOE), which can be observed as a cross-peak between the two protons in a two- or higher-dimension NOE experiment (NOESY). For large molecules such as proteins, this relaxation occurs predominantly through coupling of the dipole modulation to a simultaneous mutual spin flipping of the protons, which is essentially a zero-frequency process. As the molecule gets larger, its tumbling (and hence the dipole modulation) occurs at a slower frequency, Equation (1). The prevalence (spectral density) of low-frequency processes[68] therefore increases, and coupling to the zero-frequency proton–proton cross-relaxation process becomes more efficient. As relaxation becomes more efficient, the rate of buildup of an NOE during the mixing period of a NOESY increases. The buildup rate $\rho$ also depends on the strength of the dipolar interaction between the two protons, so that

$$\rho = \frac{1}{r^{-6}} \tau_c \qquad (7)$$

This $r^{-6}$ dependence means that the buildup rate falls off very rapidly with internuclear distance, and NOEs are not generally observed between protons separated by more than *ca.* 5 Å in space (although see below). Consequently, the observation of cross-peaks between protons in the NOESY spectra of a protein provides extremely valuable information concerning its three-dimensional structure. Since several thousand NOEs will be observed for a protein of even modest size, NOEs are the most important information used in structure calculations. But first they need to be assigned to specific proton pairs, quantified, and converted into distance information.

First the assignment of NOEs in the NOESY must be considered. Complete or nearly complete assignment of NOE connectivities can usually be accomplished by visual inspection of a 2D NOESY for a small protein ($\leq$ 5–6 kDa; see Reference 205 and references therein). Many of these NOEs will have been identified as a matter of course if the homonuclear sequential assignment procedure described in Section IV.B was employed. Any ambiguities in NOE assignments may be resolved by an iterative back-calculation procedure,[206,207] whereby structure calculations are first carried out using only unambiguously assigned NOEs. The resulting preliminary structures are used to resolve multiple assignment possibilities for unassigned NOEs by excluding those possibilities that are grossly inconsistent with the calculated structures. The newly assigned NOEs are included in a second round of calculations, and the new, better-defined structures are used to assign NOEs that remained ambiguous after the first iteration. This procedure can be repeated until no further ambiguities are resolved. However, for a larger protein, severe overlap will preclude a simple 2D approach, and resolution enhancement through the incorporation of an extra dimension (or two) into the experiment is required. This can potentially be achieved in a 3D homonuclear experiment (3D NOESY-HOHAHA or NOESY-NOESY, Section IV.B), but far more preferable is editing of the NOESY according to the frequencies of attached heteronuclei, using an isotopically labelled sample. Thus a range of experiments is available, depending on the labelling pattern present in the protein: 3D $^{15}$N-edited NOESY, 3D $^{13}$C-edited NOESY, 4D $^{13}$C, $^{13}$C-edited NOESY, and 4D $^{13}$C, $^{15}$N-edited NOESY (Section IV.C). These experiments, in particular the 4D versions, provide dramatic increases in resolution (see, e.g., Reference 100), despite restricted digital resolution (Section IV.C), because so few cross-peaks appear in each plane. In fact, it has been predicted that 4D spectra with a virtual lack of overlap and adequate sensitivity should be obtainable for proteins of up to 400 residues.[209] Note that a disadvantage of the $^{15}$N-edited experiments is that only NOEs between protons at least one of which is bonded to $^{15}$N can be observed. Thus for a high-resolution structure, $^{13}$C-edited experiments that contain no $^{15}$N magnetisation-transfer step are essential (e.g., 4D $^{13}$C–$^{13}$C NOESY), so that NOEs between pairs of carbon-bound protons can be detected.[136,210]

Once the identity of all or most of the observable NOEs is established, the proximity of each proton pair must be gauged. As noted above, the rate of buildup of an NOE is proportional to the distance between the two protons. However, because all other proton pairs in a molecule give rise to oscillating fields at similar frequencies (as a result of molecular tumbling), these pairs can contribute to the cross-relaxation of a proton. This phenomenon is termed spin diffusion (SD), since it comes about through a stepwise (diffusive) transfer of magnetisation away from a given proton pair *via* other neighbouring protons. The observable results of spin diffusion are (1) a change in the shape of the buildup curve for direct NOEs (see below), and (2) the appearance of cross-peaks between protons that are distant in the molecule. Obviously this latter effect reduces the useful information content of a NOE experiment, and SD should therefore be minimised as far as possible. Since SD is a indirect phenomenon, its buildup has an initial lag phase in comparison to direct NOEs, and the use of short mixing times allows its effects to be discarded to a first approximation. Note that since cross-relaxation is more efficient for larger values of $\tau_c$, SD becomes more of a problem the larger a protein is, necessitating the use of shorter and shorter mixing times.

The buildup of direct NOEs is approximately linear at short mixing times. In this regime (the isolated spin-pair approximation, ISPA)[211] it is assumed that the intensity of the observed cross-peak is directly proportional to $r^{-6}$. The proportionality can be estimated by measuring the intensities $I_{ref}$ of NOEs between protons that are separated by a fixed, conformation-independent distance $d_{ref}$, such as geminal methylene (1.7 Å) or *ortho*-aromatic (2.45 Å) protons. Unknown distances $d_{ij}$ can therefore be calculated as

$$d_{ij} = d_{ref} \left( \frac{I_{ref}}{I_{ij}} \right)^{1/6} \tag{8}$$

where $I_{ij}$ is the intensity of the cross-peak of interest. In this procedure, the intensity of cross-peaks involving a methyl group should first be divided by 3 (or by 9 for NOEs between two methyl groups). Because ISPA is an approximation, care should be taken not to overinterpret the distances derived from Equation (8). These derived distances represent upper limits for the interproton distance, since a number of mechanisms may operate to reduce the observed NOE intensity and lead to the estimation of an artificially longer distance. In addition, the use of a single reference distance can induce systematic errors into the process.[212] Consequently, a better way to derive distances is to use two **different** types of reference distances in combination. This approach has been shown to produce less-biased distance estimates.[212] Error ranges now need to be placed on the derived distances; the most conservative method is to simply assign an upper distance bound of 5–6 Å to all proton pairs that display an NOE, irrespective of their intensity. This can be a useful (and speedy) method for estimating the coarse fold of a protein, but clearly it discards useful information. A more usual approach is to divide the distances into broad categories, for example, 1.8–2.8 Å, 1.8–3.3 Å, and 1.8–5.0 Å, where 1.8 Å is the van der Waals contact distance between two hydrogen atoms (see Reference 213). If stereospecific assignments are unavailable for pairs of methylene protons or Leu and Val methyl group pairs, a so-called pseudoatom is created midway between the pair for the purpose of the structure calculations, and the upper distance bound is relaxed for those NOEs (by *ca.*1 Å for a methylene pair).[214] In addition, 0.5–1.0 Å is normally added to methyl group constraints to account for changes in orientation of the methyl group. It may appear that even this categorisation procedure discards information, but it is certainly better to slightly underinterpret than to overinterpret the data. In any case, it has been established that the most important factor in determining the final quality of an NMR structure is the **number** of distance constraints rather than their **precision**.[67,215]

It is notable that the extraction of distances from NOEs using the above ISPA-based approach involves the implicit assumption that the correlation time for each interproton vector is the same. In fact, regions with greater mobility will have a faster component to their tumbling, resulting in a smaller effective $\tau_c$ and correspondingly different NOE buildup curves. Such effects can be taken into account using recent forms of the complete relaxation matrix approach,[216] as described in Section IV.E. Finally, it is not clear how NOE intensities obtained from different types of experiment (e.g., 2D NOESY and 3D $^{15}$N NOESY-HMQC) should be integrated in the construction of distance constraints, given the additional magnetisation-transfer steps that take place in the heteronuclear experiments. In such situations it is again probably better to err on the side of caution, and define less restrictive sets of bounds.

## 3 Scalar Coupling Constants

It has long been known that the magnitude of scalar coupling constants between atoms depend on the environment in which the coupled atoms reside.[217] In particular, three-bond coupling constants have a characteristic dependence on the dihedral angle $\theta$ between the two coupled atoms. This dependence is described by a Karplus equation[218] of the type

$$J(\theta) = A \cos^2 \theta - B \cos \theta + C \qquad (9)$$

where the constants $A$, $B$, and $C$ have been determined empirically for different types of dihedral angle, such as the $H^N–H^\alpha$ angle in proteins.[219] This function has the form shown in Figure 23, where $\theta = |\phi - 60|$ ($\phi = 0°$ is defined as the conformation where the carbonyl carbon is *trans* to the amide proton). Although there are potentially multiple solutions for $\theta$ at a given value of $^3J$, in practice the dihedral $H^N–H^\alpha$ angles in proteins are concentrated in the range $\phi = -30$ to $-180$,[220] such that unique solutions are possible for all values of $^3J_{HN\alpha}$. Regular secondary structural elements have characteristic values of $^3J_{HN\alpha}$: $\alpha$-helix $\approx$ 3–5 Hz and $\beta$-sheet $\approx$ 8.5–12 Hz. Intermediate values between these two ranges may represent rigid structures with a well-defined angle, but more often indicate averaging of the torsion angle through internal motion (e.g., in loop or terminal regions). Thus, values of $^3J_{HN\alpha}$ are measured for all residues, but only those that lie in the two secondary structural ranges are converted to angles (or ranges of angles, to allow for some flexibility) and used as constraints in structure calculations.

There are numerous methods for measuring coupling constants. The traditional method is to record a DQFCOSY spectrum with extremely high resolution in $F_2$. The coupling constants may then be measured simply from the magnitude of the $F_2$ antiphase splitting in the $H^N–H^\alpha$ cross-peaks.[221] However, this method is compromised in most proteins larger than 5–6 kDa, where linewidths are generally greater than *ca.* 10 Hz.[222] Irrespective of the coupling constant, the minimum separation of the antiphase components in a COSY cross-peak is 0.576 times the linewidth,[212] so that for proteins where the linewidths are 10 Hz, couplings smaller than *ca.*5 Hz will be overestimated. It is often still possible to broadly group the couplings into <5 and >9–13 Hz, but even these estimations become unreliable for proteins larger than *ca.*15 kDa. Alternative methods for measuring $^3J_{HN\alpha}$ that do not rely on the measurement of an antiphase splitting, but instead utilise the large one-bond $^{15}N–^1H$ coupling, have been developed. These experiments facilitate the measurement of $^3J_{HN\alpha}$ values in proteins at least up to 20 kDa. The $J$-modulated

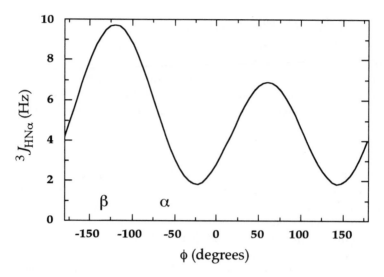

**FIGURE 23**

Plot of the coupling constant $^3J_{HN\alpha}$ as a function of the associated torsion angle $\phi$. The approximate regions of $\phi$ space associated with $\alpha$-helix and $\beta$-sheet are indicated, and it can be seen that these two secondary structural elements give rise to distinct values of $^3J_{HN\alpha}$. The curve was generated using data from Reference 219.

$^1H$–$^{15}N$ HSQC[223,224] consists essentially of a normal HSQC with an extra delay $\tau_2$ appended prior to signal acquisition. During this delay the amide-proton magnetisation, which has been labelled during $t_1$ with the attached $^{15}N$ frequency, evolves according to its coupling to $H^\alpha$. Consequently, the intensity of the observed cross-peaks is modulated according to both $^3J_{HN\alpha}$ and $\tau_2$, according to the equation

$$\bar{V} = A\left[\cos\left(\pi J\tau_1\right)\,\cos\left(\pi J\tau_2\right) - 0.5\,\sin\left(\pi J\tau_1\right)\,\sin\left(\pi J\tau_2\right)\right] \times \exp\left(-\tau_2/T_2'\right)$$

(10)

where $\bar{V}(\tau_2)$ is the cross-peak volume as a function of the delay time $\tau_2$, $A$ is the cross-peak volume at $\tau_2 = 0$, $J$ is the $^3J_{HN\alpha}$ coupling, and $T_2'$ is the apparent $^1H$ transverse relaxation time. A number of spectra with incremented values of $\tau_2$ are recorded, and the change in cross-peak intensity with $\tau_2$ can be fitted to Equation (10) using a nonlinear least-squares algorithm that varies $^3J_{HN\alpha}$, $A$, and $T_2'$ (Figure 24). A modification of the basic pulse sequence for this experiment has also been proposed that is optimised for larger proteins where fast transverse relaxation is especially problematic.[224]

In a second procedure, the $^1H$–$^{15}N$ HMQC-J experiment,[225] $^3J_{HN\alpha}$ is measured as an in-phase splitting of the HMQC-type cross-peaks in the $^{15}N$ dimension $F_1$. However, because the linewidths in this dimension are

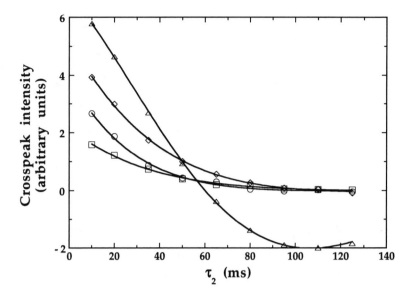

**FIGURE 24**

Determination of $^3J_{HN\alpha}$ coupling constants using the $J$-modulated HSQC method of Billeter et al.[224] The intensity of cross-peaks for several residues in a series of HSQC experiments is plotted against $\tau_2$, a delay inserted at the end of the pulse sequence to generate the $J$-modulation. The data are fitted to Eq. (10) to derive values for the $^3J_{HN\alpha}$ couplings. Residues Ile 8 (○, $^3J_{HN\alpha}$ = 5.0 Hz), Thr 28 (□, $^3J_{HN\alpha}$ = 3.6 Hz), Gln 35 (◇, $^3J_{HN\alpha}$ = 4.5 Hz), and Asn 45 (△, $^3J_{HN\alpha}$ = 8.0 Hz) are shown. (Adapted from Junius, F. K., et al., *Biochemistry*, 34, 1995, 6164–6174.)

significantly narrower than in the homonuclear DQFCOSY, small splittings are resolvable even for large proteins (e.g., an 18-kDa staphylococcal nuclease complex).[225] In addition, the relatively narrow $^{15}N$ frequency range (*ca.* 1.5–2 kHz) allows good digital resolution to be achieved in a realistic time. A further advantage of these heteronuclear methods is that cross-peaks are not lost as a result of being "under" the water signal.

The other dihedral angle that can be readily probed from $^1H$–$^1H$ couplings is $\chi^1$, the angle between $H^\alpha$ and $H^\beta$. This angle is generally found to exist as one of the three possible staggered rotamers, where each atom attached to $C^\beta$ is either in one of the two *gauche* positions relative to $H^\alpha$ or in the *trans* position (Figure 25). Consideration of the appropriate Karplus equation[208] shows that for an amino acid with a β-methine proton (Val, Thr, Ile), the size of the $^3J_{\alpha\beta}$ coupling reveals whether the $H^\beta$ proton is *trans* or *gauche*. For amino acids with a β-methylene group, there are two relevant homonuclear couplings, $H^\alpha$–$H^{\beta2}$ and $H^\alpha$–$H^{\beta3}$. Figure 25 shows their values for the three different staggered rotamers. For the amino acids with a single $H^\beta$ proton, a standard DQFCOSY recorded in $D_2O$ (to eliminate any multiplet structure arising from the $^3J_{HN\alpha}$ coupling

| Structure | | | |
|---|---|---|---|
| Conformation | $g^2g^3$ | $g^2t^3$ | $t^2g^3$ |
| $\chi_1$ | 60° | 180° | −60° |
| $^3J_{\alpha\beta2}$ (Hz) | < 5 | < 5 | > 10 |
| $^3J_{\alpha\beta3}$ (Hz) | < 5 | > 10 | < 5 |
| $d_{\beta2N}(i, i)$ | weak | strong | strong |
| $d_{\beta3N}(i, i)$ | strong | strong | weak |
| $^3J_{\beta2N}$ (Hz) | ~ 5 | ~ 1 | ~ 1 |
| $^3J_{\beta3N}$ (Hz) | ~ 1 | ~ 1 | ~ 5 |

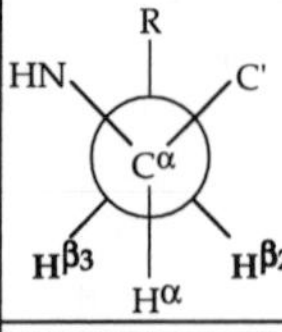

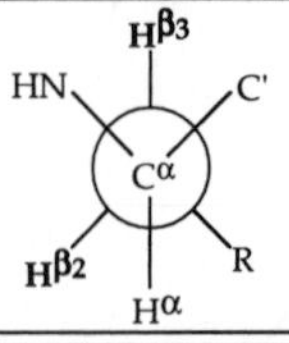

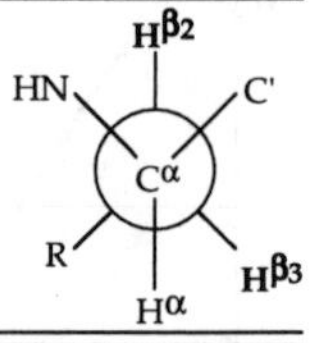

**FIGURE 25**

Newman projections of the three possible staggered conformers about the torsion angle $\chi^1$. The expected values of several coupling constants and NOEs shown can be used to determine which conformer is present, and hence the stereospecific assignments of the $H^{\beta2}$ and $H^{\beta3}$ protons. This information can be used to provide additional constraints for structure calculations.

and to reduce the loss of signals under the solvent peak) may be used to measure $^3J_{\alpha\beta}$. However for amino acids with a β-methylene group, modified COSY experiments such as E.COSY[226] or P.E.COSY[227], which simplify the multiplet structure of the $H^\alpha$–$H^\beta$ cross-peaks, are better suited to the task. These experiments rely on a splitting of the cross-peak of interest by a further large passive coupling; in the case of an $H^\alpha$–$H^{\beta2/3}$ system, the splitting is by the geminal $H^{\beta2}$–$H^{\beta3}$ coupling (*ca.* 14 Hz). As a consequence, couplings can be measured between signals with substantially broader lines than is possible in a simple DQFCOSY, up to perhaps 12–15 kDa.[212] However, spectral overlap, exacerbated by broader lines, still thwarts these experiments in large proteins, and heteronuclear experiments are again an attractive alternative. A modified 3D HCCH-TOCSY experiment, where proton decoupling is not applied during the $^{13}$C chemical-shift evolution time, has been used for this purpose.[233] 2D planes showing $^{13}$C and $^1$H are taken through the indirect proton dimension, and the cross-peaks in the resulting $^1$H–$^{13}$C correlation spectra have an E.COSY format. That is, the cross-peaks consist of two in-phase signals, separated in the $^{13}$C dimension by the passive $^1J_{CH\alpha}$ and in the $^1$H dimension by $^3J_{\alpha\beta}$, which can be measured directly. Alternatively, Clore et al.[228] have shown that the size of the $^3J_{\alpha\beta}$ coupling for each β proton is directly reflected in the intensity of $H^N \rightarrow H^\beta$

correlations in a 3D HOHAHA-HMQC. That is, for the $g^2t^3$ and $t^2g^3$ conformations, only one $H^N \rightarrow H^\beta$ is generally visible (or else one is much stronger), corresponding to the $H^\beta$ with the large $^3J_{\alpha\beta}$ coupling. For $g^2g^3$, both correlations are absent, while disordered side chains sampling some or all of the possible rotamers display two cross-peaks of similar intensity.

Clearly, the two rotamers $g^2t^3$ and $t^2g^3$ cannot be distinguished on the basis of the two $^3J_{\alpha\beta}$ coupling constants unless the identities of the pro-$R$ and pro-$S$ $\beta$-methylene protons are known. Stereospecific assignment of methylene pairs obviates the need for pseudoatom corrections and significantly improves the quality of calculated structures (see, e.g., References 228–230). In this respect, further information is available from a consideration of relative NOE intensities between each of the two $\beta$ protons and the intraresidue $H^N$ and $H^\alpha$ protons (Figure 25). In the $g^2t^3$ conformer, the two $H^\beta$ protons will show similar NOEs to $H^N$, while $t^2g^3$ should yield one NOE ($d_{\beta 3N}$) weaker than the other. The intensities of a number of interresidue NOEs such as $d_{\beta 2N}(i, i + 1)$ and $d_{\beta 3N}(i, i + 1)$ can also assist in the stereospecific assignment process. In addition, three-bond heteronuclear coupling constants can be used to probe torsion angle conformations. For example, a $^1$H-coupled $^{15}$N HSQC-TOCSY[231,232] allows the measurement of the heteronuclear $^3J_{\beta 2N}$ and $^3J_{\beta 3N}$ couplings, which show a conventional Karplus-type dependence on torsion angle (Figure 25).[232] Other experiments that take advantage of the presence of global $^{15}$N and $^{13}$C labelling to measure couplings involving these heteronuclei have also been described,[233-235] but to date they have been little used to provide constraints for structure calculations.

Thus, several different types of data can be used to determine stereospecific assignments. These data can be sorted either manually or by a program such as STEROSEARCH[236] which searches a database comprising torsion angles, associated coupling constants, and interproton distances for a set of data that matches that provided by the user for a given residue. Two databases are used, one comprising a set of crystal structures and the other a set of short hypothetical peptide fragments with systematically varied values of $\phi$, $\psi$, and $\chi^1$ (the presence of which ensures that an unusual conformation is not missed). Note that the two *gauche* conformations of the three $\beta$-methine residues can be discerned in a similar manner.

Finally, note that stereospecific assignments can also be obtained by specific labelling of suitable atoms (see Reference 237 and references therein), although such labelling strategies are generally quite expensive in both time and funds.

## 4 Amide-Proton Exchange

The exchange of amide protons with solvent can be slowed by many orders of magnitude in folded proteins, compared to unstructured peptides.[238,239] This slow exchange is largely due to the existence of hydrogen bonds involving the amide proton, often in regular elements of secondary structure. Measurement of amide-proton exchange rates is usually carried out by monitoring the change in intensity with time of amide cross-peaks in a 2D spectrum following dissolution of the protein in 100% $D_2O$. Several types of 2D spectra can be used for this purpose, including TOSCY, COSY, or best of all, a $^1H$–$^{15}N$ HSQC if $^{15}N$-labelled protein is available. The advantages of the latter method are that the dispersion is generally better and that an HSQC with adequate signal-to-noise ratio can be collected much faster than a comparable homonuclear 2D experiment. The change in peak intensity with time is fitted for each residue to a single exponential function to derive pseudo-first-order rate constants for exchange. The rate constants for the exchange of each residue in an unstructured peptide[11,66,240] are then divided by the observed rate constants for that residue in the protein under investigation, yielding a so-called protection factor for each residue. Large protection factors (>*ca.* $10^3$), when observed for amide protons that exhibit NOEs and coupling constants characteristic of regular secondary structure, can be used to generate constraints for structure calculations. Thus the amide protons concerned are assumed to be part of the hydrogen-bonding pattern characteristic of that type of secondary structure, and distance constraints between the proton and its acceptor carbonyl oxygen, or between the attached nitrogen and the carbonyl oxygen are created.

### 5   *Chemical Shifts as Structural Parameters*

The chemical shift of an atom is exquisitely sensitive to its chemical environment. It has been shown that the chemical shifts of many nuclei, including $H^\alpha$,[241] and the carbon atoms $C^\alpha$,[242] $C^\beta$, and $C'$,[243] are strongly correlated with the type of secondary structure of which they are part. For example, $H^\alpha$ protons involved in an $\alpha$-helix display a marked upfield shift relative to values tabulated for random coil peptides,[67] while the opposite is true for residues that are part of a $\beta$-sheet. These patterns have been interpreted in terms of "chemical-shift indices" for $H^\alpha$, $C^\alpha$, $C^\beta$, and $C'$,[241,243] which allow quite accurate predictions of secondary structure. Such indices could potentially be incorporated into structure calculation strategies, but no examples of this have yet been reported.

# V   CALCULATION OF TERTIARY STRUCTURES FROM NMR DATA

## A   OVERVIEW

An essential step in the application of NMR methods to protein structure determination has been the development of computational approaches that can use the semiquantitative NMR-derived structural constraints to generate tertiary structures. While numerous calculation methods have been suggested, most investigators use either a distance geometry[244] or restrained molecular dynamics approach,[245,246] or a combination of the two. We shall discuss each of these in turn before examining more recent developments, such as relaxation-matrix-based methods for refining structures directly against NOE intensities,[247] an optimal filtering approach for calculating probabilistic descriptions of protein structures from sparse NOE data,[248] and calculation strategies in which the NOE-derived interproton distances are treated as time averages in order to account for motional averaging.[249]

## B  DISTANCE GEOMETRY

### 1  Overview

Distance geometry (DG) is a branch of applied mathematics concerned with building structures from internal distances,[250] and therefore DG algorithms are well suited to constructing three-dimensional protein structures from a subset of experimentally derived intramolecular distance estimates. There are two fundamentally different DG algorithms used for calculating protein structures from NMR data; one operates in distance space (the so-called metric-matrix approach) while the other works in torsion-angle space (see Figure 26). We shall outline each of the two approaches before analysing some of their relative advantages and disadvantages.

### 2  Metric-Matrix DG Algorithms

The first DG program developed for NMR structure calculations (DISGEO)[244] incorporated a metric-matrix-based algorithm; numerous programs incorporating similar approaches are now available for general use (e.g., DG-II, DSPACE, DGEOM). The metric-matrix-based approach involves five distinct stages: generation of a matrix of distance bounds, bounds smoothing, generation of trial distances, embedding, and optimisation.[213,251] In the first step, a matrix is constructed that contains upper and lower bounds for every pair of atoms in the protein; a symmetric matrix of this kind contains $(N^2 - 1)/2$ distances for a protein with $N$ atoms. The lower bounds are initially the sum of the van der Waals radii of the two atoms, while either the upper bounds are derived from the NOE data (as outlined in Section IV.E.1) or, if no experimental information on these distances is available, they are initially set to an arbitrarily large distance, which must be larger than the longest dimension of the protein. Standard covalent bond lengths and angles,[252] predetermined by the primary structure of the protein, are also used as input constraints.

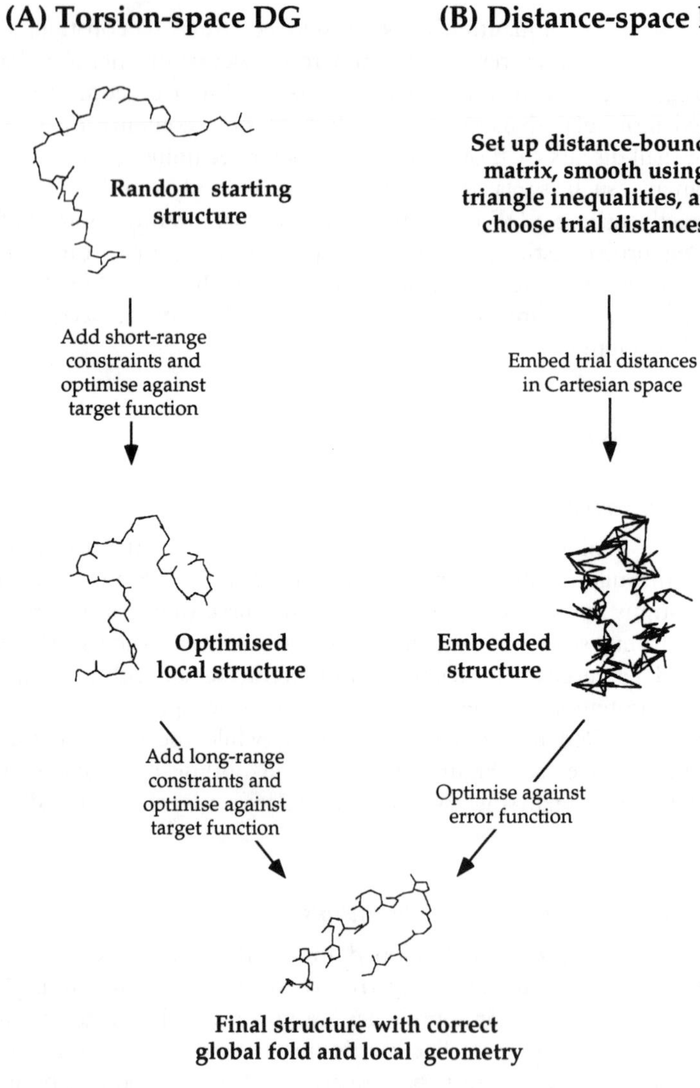

## (A) Torsion-space DG          (B) Distance-space DG

**Random starting
structure**

**Set up distance-bounds
matrix, smooth using
triangle inequalities, and
choose trial distances**

Add short-range
constraints and
optimise against
target function

Embed trial distances
in Cartesian space

**Optimised
local structure**

**Embedded
structure**

Add long-range
constraints and
optimise against
target function

Optimise against
error function

**Final structure with correct
global fold and local geometry**

**FIGURE 26**

Comparison of distance geometry calculations performed in (A) torsion space and (B) distance space. Torsion space algorithms begin with random but stereochemically correct structures, which are gradually folded by first adding short-range distance constraints in order to optimise the local geometry, and then introducing sequentially more distant constraints in order to establish the global fold of the polypeptide. In distance-space methods, a distance-bounds matrix is first constructed from the experimentally derived distance constraints, then this is smoothed using triangle inequality relationships. Trial distances are chosen within the final distance bounds, then these distances are "embedded" into Cartesian coordinate space. The local geometry and global fold of the protein are then simultaneously optimised by minimising an error function.

The region of conformational space available to the protein is then reduced by a procedure known as bounds smoothing. The simplest smoothing approach uses the triangle inequality relationship to increase the lower bounds and decrease the upper bounds until they are geometrically self-consistent.[213,251] Consider three atoms $i$, $j$, and $k$ with corresponding experimentally derived or arbitrarily defined upper distances $u_{ij}$, $u_{ik}$, and $u_{jk}$. The furthest that $j$ can be from atom $i$ corresponds to $i$, $j$, and $k$ being collinear with $k$ lying between atoms $i$ and $j$. Thus

$$u_{ij} \leq u_{ik} + u_{kj} \tag{11}$$

If the current bounds matrix does not satisfy Equation (11) (i.e., $u_{ij} > u_{ik} + u_{kj}$), then $u_{ij}$ is decreased to match the sum of $u_{ik}$ and $u_{kj}$. This procedure is applied to all sets of three atoms until no further alterations can be made to the upper bounds.

A similar inverse triangle inequality can be applied to the lower bounds, enabling them to be adjusted upward until no further alterations are possible.[213,251] A more computationally intensive tetragonal inequality can be applied to each set of four atoms to give tighter distance bounds if required.[253] After the boundary matrix has been smoothed, trial distances, which will be used to generate a starting set of atomic coordinates, must be chosen. The trial distances are chosen to lie between the upper and lower distance bounds, but there is no general agreement on how best to generate them; they can be picked randomly or fitted to some predetermined distribution function (more on this later). The trial distances then need to be converted into atomic coordinates. This process, known as embedding, proceeds via generation of a metric matrix from the trial distances using the cosine rule; three-dimensional coordinates are subsequently calculated using the three largest eigenvalues of this matrix and their associated eigenvectors.[213] Negative eigenvectors in embedded structures imply imaginary distances, and hence these structures are usually discarded.[213] The structures immediately following embedding are unlikely to satisfy all distance bounds and therefore the final step in the metric-matrix DG approach is optimising the distances to satisfy the upper and lower bounds.

Optimisation proceeds by way of an objective (or error) function that measures the difference (or "error") between the distances in the current structure and the set boundary conditions. The usual form of this error function $(E)$[213] is

$$E = \begin{cases} k_{dist}\left(d_{ij} - u_{ij}\right)^2 & \text{if } d_{ij} \geq u_{ij} \\ 0 & \text{if } l_{ij} \leq d_{ij} \leq u_{ij} \\ k_{dist}\left(l_{ij} - d_{ij}\right)^2 & \text{if } l_{ij} \geq d_{ij} \end{cases} \tag{12}$$

where $k_{dist}$ is a constant weighting factor and $d_{ij}$ is the current value of the distance at the time that $E$ is evaluated. A standard descent algorithm (e.g., conjugate gradient minimisation) is then applied to minimise $E$ until it falls below some predetermined value (the tolerance) or until the gradient of the optimisation routine drops below a preset value. Metric-matrix DG algorithms also include a chirality error function, which checks to see that the embedded structures have correct local chirality as well as correct global handedness (*i.e.*, the embed procedure can produce a mirror image of the molecule).[213]

Creation and smoothing of the bounds matrix is performed only once. A number of embedded structures are subsequently generated and optimised from this smoothed bounds matrix to give a final family of DG structures that conform with the input NMR-derived constraints.

### 3   Torsion-Space DG Algorithms

DISMAN[254] and its refined descendent, DIANA,[255] are DG programs that operate by minimising a variable target function in torsion-angle space. The programs begin with a random structure generated on the basis of the known sequence of the protein and standard bond lengths and angles. Thus, the starting structures have sensible covalent geometry, unlike the distorted structures produced by the metric-matrix-embedding procedure. The starting structure is refined by varying the torsion angles in order to minimise a variable target function. Since torsion angles are the only independent variables in these calculations, this approach uses only about one third as many variables as in the metric-matrix method, and hence, it requires less computer memory.

The target function used for minimisation is similar in form to that used in the metric-matrix algorithms. The part of the target function $T$ dealing with violations of upper-distance bounds in DIANA is[255]

$$T = w_u \cdot \Sigma \left[ \Theta_u \left( \frac{d_{ij}^2 - u_{ij}^2}{2u_{ij}} \right) \right]^2 \tag{13}$$

where $d_{ij}$ is the distance between atoms $i$ and $j$ in the current structure, $u_{ij}$ is the upper bound on this distance, $w_u$ is a weighting factor for upper-bound violations, and $\Theta_u$ is the Heaviside (step) function, which equals 0 if $d_{ij} \le u_{ij}$ or 1 if $d_{ij} > u_{ij}$. The target function contains similar terms for experimental lower-distance bounds and the van der Waals repulsion lower limits on interatomic distances; the latter term is essentially a "soft" model for the repulsive term in the Lennard–Jones 6–12 potential.[55] A more complicated term is used to account for violations of dihedral angle constraints.

The problem with trying to minimise the target function by simultaneously introducing all constraints between all atoms $i$ and $j$ is that the function will have many local minima. The *variable* target function approach was introduced by Braun and Gō[254] in an attempt to alleviate this problem. Instead of introducing all constraints simultaneously, one first optimises using only local (such as intraresidue and sequential) constraints, and then introduces sequentially more distant constraints until they have all been added into the calculation. This has the effect of optimising the local conformation prior to determining the overall polypeptide fold, and in this sense the approach is somewhat analogous to manual model building.

The rate at which new constraints are introduced (i.e., the number of optimisation steps), the number of iterations of the conjugate gradient minimiser at each optimisation step, and the weights on upper-distance, lower-distance, van der Waals, and dihedral-angle constraints ($w_u$, $w_l$, $w_v$, and $w_a$, respectively) are user-defined parameters. It is common practice to keep the weight on steric violations $w_v$ low relative to the weights on experimental violations in the early stages ($w_v \sim 0.2w_u$) in order to ensure that the structure conforms to the experimental constraints, and then increase this weight considerably toward the end of the calculation ($w_v \sim 2–3w_u$) in order to minimise steric overlaps.[255]

## 4 (Dis)advantages of Torsion-Angle vs. Metric-Matrix DG Algorithms

DG is generally considered the optimal method for rapidly and reliably calculating initial structures from NMR-derived constraints. However, each of the two DG approaches has potential pitfalls.

The success of the metric-matrix DG algorithm depends intimately on the choice of trial distances from the bounds matrix. In most applications of metric-matrix-based DG programs, trial distances have been chosen randomly between the upper and lower bounds. This assumes that an ensemble of structures with random conformations has a uniform distribution of distances between the upper and lower bounds, whereas polymer theory predicts that the distribution should be skewed toward the lower bounds for freely rotating chains.[256,257] The result is that metric-matrix-based DG algorithms tend to produce extended conformations with smaller root-mean-square deviations (RMSDs) than obtained with torsion-space DG algorithms, especially in regions of the protein where there are few NOE constraints. In other words, the standard implementation of the metric-matrix embed procedure seems to sample conformational space less well than the torsion-angle approach.[257-259] Because of the fixed order (N → C terminus) in which trial distances are chosen in the DISGEO program, the N-terminus of the protein tends to be more compact than the C-terminus.[259] The literature contains numerous examples of authors claiming good definition of certain regions of a protein for which there are very few NMR-derived structural constraints and for which their "classical" implementation of a metric-matrix DG program has produced unrealistic extended conformations with low RMSDs among the family of structures.

It has been shown, however, that these problems can be overcome by choosing trial distances using a random metrisation procedure, even when the distances are chosen according to a simple uniform distribution.[259,260] Metrisation enables the trial distances to be chosen in such a way as to give a self-consistent set of distances that obey the triangle inequality, while randomisation simply ensures that the trial distances are generated in random order.[259] Thus, when using the metric-matrix-based approach, it is important to consider the method by which trial distances are generated prior to embedding and the impact this will have on the calculated structures.

The torsion-space DG programs have a higher probability of giving an incorrect polypeptide fold (as opposed to a mirror image) as they work in "real" space rather than distance space. Generally, however, these structures are easily recognised from the high residual values of the target function.[254]

While the torsion-angle-based DG algorithms are more memory efficient, a comparison of the DISGEO and DISMAN programs showed they are similar in terms of overall CPU requirements.[258] It would be interesting to see a comparison of the latest generation of metric-matrix DG programs with DIANA, a fully vectorised torsion-space DG program.[255] Note, however, that the "hit rate" for good structures using the torsion-space approach is low (the multiple minima problem), whereas a high proportion of embedded metric-matrix structures will converge; thus, comparisons of CPU time per structure must be viewed with this in mind.

## C   ENERGY MINIMISATION AND RESTRAINED MOLECULAR DYNAMICS

DG-derived structures have unrealistically high molecular energies because they do not take account of nonbonded interactions such as van der Waals and Coulombic interactions or they do so in a simplified manner such as the low-level steric term in the DIANA target function. Consequently, DG structures need to be refined using dynamical simulation or simple energy minimization in a molecular dynamics force field. A typical physical force field or effective potential for a protein has the form[261]

$$V_{physical} = \sum_{bonds} \frac{1}{2} K_b \left(b - b_0\right)^2 + \sum_{angles} \frac{1}{2} K_\theta \left(\theta - \theta_0\right)^2 +$$

$$\sum_{\substack{improper \\ dihedrals}} \frac{1}{2} K_\zeta \left(\zeta - \zeta_0\right)^2 + \sum_{dihedrals} K_\varphi \left[1 + \cos\left(n\varphi - \delta\right)\right] +$$

$$\sum_{pairs(i,j)} \left[C_{12}(i,j)/r_{if}^{12} - C_6(i,j)/r_{ij}^6 + q_i q_j / 4\pi\varepsilon_0 \varepsilon_r r_{ij}\right] \quad (14)$$

where the $K$ terms are force constants. The first term is a harmonic potential representing covalent bond stretching along bond $b$; the force constant $K_b$ and minimum-energy bond length $b_0$ vary with the type of covalent bond. A similar term is used to describe bending of bond angles $\theta$. Two forms are used to describe distortions of dihedral angles: a harmonic term is used for dihedral angles $\zeta$ that are not allowed to make transitions (e.g., dihedral angles within aromatic rings), whereas a cosinusoidal term is used for dihedral angles $\varphi$ that may make 360° turns. The final term is a sum over all pairs of nonbonded interatomic interactions: the first part sums the van der Waals interactions (a typical Lennard–Jones 6–12 potential), and the second part sums all Coulombic interactions.

While there are numerous variants of this physical force field, including explicit inclusion of terms for hydrogen bonds, the overall approach to NMR structure refinement is the same. The general strategy is to add a restraining potential to the force field so that the structure can be refined against the physical terms in the force field (*i.e.*, covalent geometry and nonbonded interactions) while still adhering to the experimental constraints. Thus

$$V_{\text{total}} = V_{\text{physical}} + V_{\text{exp, restr.}} \tag{15}$$

The experimental restraint terms are generally square-well potentials, similar in form to those used in DG algorithms:[251, 262]

$$V_{\text{exp. restr.}} = V_{\text{NOE}} + V_{\text{dihedral}}$$

where

$$V_{\text{NOE}} = \begin{cases} k_{\text{NOE}}\left(d_{ij} - u_{ij}\right)^2 & \text{if } d_{ij} > u_{ij} \\ 0 & \text{if } l_{ij} \le d_{ij} \le u_{ij} \\ k_{\text{NOE}}\left(l_{ij} - d_{ij}\right)^2 & \text{if } l_{ij} > d_{ij} \end{cases}$$

and

$$V_{\text{dihedral}} = \begin{cases} k_{\text{dihedral}}\left(\varphi_{ij} - \varphi_{ij}''\right)^2 & \text{if } \varphi_{ij} > \varphi_{ij}'' \\ 0 & \text{if } \varphi_{ij}' \le \varphi_{ij} \le \varphi_{ij}'' \\ k_{\text{dihedral}}\left(\varphi_{ij}' - \varphi_{ij}\right)^2 & \text{if } \varphi_{ij}' > \varphi_{ij} \end{cases} \tag{16}$$

$k_{\text{NOE}}$ and $k_{\text{dihedral}}$ are force constants, which can be used to weight these experimental terms relative to one another and relative to the physical terms in the force field.

In some studies, the DG structures are refined by simple energy minimization in the expanded molecular dynamics force field.[263] The force constants $k_{NOE}$ and $k_{dihedral}$ are usually chosen so that some arbitrarily chosen small violation of the experimental constraints (*e.g.*, 0.2 Å for distance constraints and 5° for dihedral-angle constraints)[263] corresponds to an energy of $kT/2$, which is the average kinetic energy of an atom per degree of freedom. In other words, small violations are tolerated so that the molecule has considerable freedom to sample low-energy conformations. The problem with this simple approach is that the structures will fall into the nearest local energy minimum, which may not be the global energy minimum.

A more sophisticated approach involves performing a molecular dynamics simulation in the expanded force field using the DG structures as the starting points in the simulation. Due to the inclusion of $V_{exp.\ restr.}$ in the force field, this approach is known as *restrained* molecular dynamics (RMD). The simulation proceeds by numerical integration of Newton's equations of motion, Equations (17 and 18), using very small time steps;[261] this yields both the velocity of the atom following the time step and its displacement during the time step.

$$F_i = -\partial V_{total}(r_i, r_j, \ldots r_N)/\partial r_i \qquad (17)$$

$$d^2 r_i(t)/dt^2 = m_i^{-1} F_i \qquad (18)$$

Initial velocities $\mathbf{v}_i$ for all atoms are chosen from a Maxwellian distribution[55] corresponding to the desired temperature, and the temperature is kept constant by scaling the velocities after each time step or by coupling to some form of heat bath.[261] The time step $\Delta t$ must be smaller than the inverse of the highest-frequency motion, which is bond stretching; this typically limits $\Delta t$ to ~1 fs. However, bond lengths can often be constrained to their mean values by means of an algorithm called SHAKE[264] without significantly affecting the simulation, and this enables the time step to be increased to ~2 fs, thus saving considerable computation time.

The motion of the molecule is simulated for sufficient time (periods of 30–50 ps are common)[265] to enable it to sample large regions of conformational space, with the goal of converging on the structure with the global energy minimum or something close to it by the end of the simulation. Following the RMD simulation, the structures are energy minimised. It has been observed by numerous investigators that the mean RMSD across a family of DG-calculated structures generally increases following RMD refinement,[262] indicating that this process samples conformational space better than DG. It is therefore pertinent to ask whether the DG step is really necessary: could the structures be calculated from random starting structures using only RMD? The answer is yes, as was demonstrated some time ago with the protein crambin.[246] However, the drawback with such an approach is that enormous computation time is wasted in calculating atomic trajectories for structures that are far removed from those that will ultimately satisfy the experimental constraints. The structures derived via the comparatively rapid DG process, on the other hand, usually satisfy the large majority of experimental constraints, thus minimising the amount of computationally intensive RMD that is necessary to produce final refined structures.

## D    DYNAMICAL SIMULATED ANNEALING

Nilges and co-workers[266] have developed an ingenious method for structure calculation known as dynamical simulated annealing (DSA). While similar in approach to high-temperature RMD,[267,268] there are some subtle differences. In the DSA strategy, the van der Waals and Coulombic terms in the RMD force field, that is, the last term in Equation (14) above, are replaced with a single repulsion term, which models nonbonded interactions. This term $V_{repel}$ has the following form:

$$V_{repel} = \begin{cases} k_{repel} \left( s^2 d_{ij,min}^2 - d_{ij}^2 \right)^2 & \text{if } d_{ij} < sd_{ij,min} \\ 0 & \text{if } d_{ij} \geq sd_{ij,min} \end{cases} \quad (19)$$

where $d_{ij,min}$ is the sum of the van der Waals radii of atoms $i$ and $j$; $k_{repel}$ is an adjustable force constant; and $s$ is the van der Waals radius scaling factor, which is typically set to 0.8 to allow for the fact that atoms can approach slightly closer than the sum of their van der Waals radii due to the attractive component of the van der Waals interaction.[269]

While the DSA protocol can be varied considerably to suit particular proteins and their associated NMR datasets, a typical protocol might be as follows. The starting structures (usually generated by DG) are first energy minimised in the modified force field in order to improve their covalent geometry. The simulated annealing protocol then proceeds in several stages. The first stage is performed at 1000 K and comprises 50 MD steps, each of 75-fs duration. $k_{repel}$ and $k_{NOE}$ are initially set to very small values (typically 0.01 kcal mol$^{-1}$ Å$^{-4}$ and 0.1 kcal mol$^{-1}$ Å$^{-2}$, respectively), thus allowing atoms to pass "through", or very near to, each other (i.e., the force constants on all nonbonded interactions are initially very low). These values are incrementally adjusted at the beginning of each new MD step to reach final values of ~4 kcal mol$^{-1}$ Å$^{-4}$ and ~50 kcal mol$^{-1}$ Å$^{-2}$, respectively, at the end of the high-temperature dynamics. While raising the force constants has an effect similar to lowering the temperature, the former approach enables force constants to be altered differentially and obviates the need for a variable time-step integrator.[266,269]

Stage 2 involves 1.5 ps of MD at 300 K with $k_{NOE}$ and $k_{repel}$ set to their final values at the end of Stage 1. Finally, the structures are energy minimised in the full RMD-type force field, that is, the $V_{repel}$ term is replaced by the full Lennard–Jones and Coulombic terms given in Equation (14). The advantage of the DSA protocol over RMD is that the initial high temperature, combined with weak constraints on nonbonded interactions, enables the molecule to sample regions of conformational space that would be energetically inaccessible in the classical room-temperature RMD protocol. Thus, the molecules are more likely to reach the global energy minimum corresponding to a structure with good covalent geometry, favourable nonbonded interactions, and minimal violations of the experimental constraints.

While DSA can be used to calculate protein conformations from random starting structures,[270] the same argument applies as that applied to the RMD approach: much computation time is saved by beginning with a structure that is close to the final conformation, and therefore the most common approach is to generate starting structures using DG[271] or hybrid-DG[272] methods. However, the DSA computation time is reduced relative to RMD due to the simplified force field, and consequently several groups have found it profitable to generate final conformations from random starting structures using only DSA.[273]

## E  USE OF TIME-AVERAGED NMR CONSTRAINTS

NOEs and $J$-coupling constants are derived from the entire ensemble of protein conformations present in solution during the time of the NMR experiment. Despite this, implementation of these parameters as restraints in conventional structure calculations, as described in Sections V.A–C above, implicitly assumes that the protein has a fixed conformation that satisfies all restraints simultaneously.[274,275] This assumption will be valid only if the lifetime of one conformational substate of the protein is overwhelmingly greater than the time spent in any vastly different states, or if the protein populates several highly similar conformational substates such that the observed averaging of parameters is a fair representation of all members of the conformational ensemble.

Problems can occur in structure calculations when intermediate motion of a molecule gives rise to mutually inconsistent NMR-derived restraints. Intermediate motion is defined as motion that is sufficiently fast to cause chemical-shift averaging, but too slow to avoid modulation of NOE effects (i.e., $10^{-3}$ s $> \tau_{effective} > 10^{-8}$ s).[276] In such cases, NOEs from the major conformations will be observed simultaneously, and attempts to generate structures using the derived restraints would be unlikely to completely satisfy the NOE data without introducing unrealistic steric overlap and torsional strain. Kim et al.[276] and Kim and Prestegard[277] addressed the problem by proposing a finite number of discrete conformations prior to commencing structure calculations; an error function with a double minimum allowed structures to diverge into two classes. However, one does not generally have *a priori* knowledge of all possible conformations in a dynamic ensemble of structures, and consequently a generalised function is required that allows for the averaging of the NOE through time without prior knowledge of the fractional conformer populations.

The use of time-averaged distance restraints in MD simulations allows motional averaging to be incorporated into the structure-refinement process.[249] The molecule is allowed to sample conformational space such that internuclear distances *averaged over the time course of the simulation* are in agreement with the NOE data, thus obviating the need for the molecule to simultaneously satisfy all NOE-derived restraints. This is achieved by replacing the instantaneous interatomic distance, $d_{ij}$ in Equation (16) above, with a time-averaged distance, $\bar{d}_{ij}(t)$, given by[249,278]

$$\bar{d}_{ij}(t) = \left[\frac{1}{t}\int_0^t d_{ij}(t')^{-n} dt'\right]^{-1/n} \tag{20}$$

where the exponent $n$ is chosen to reflect the quantity (NOE intensity) that is measured in the NMR experiment. If the time scale of the MD simulation $t_{max}$ is short compared to the molecular correlation time $\tau_c$, then angular fluctuations can be ignored and the NOE should be treated as a function of $d_{ij}^{-3}$ rather than $d_{ij}^{-6}$[280] thus, $n$ is set to 3 if $t_{max} \ll \tau_c$.[251,278]

According to Equation (20), the time period over which the distances are averaged increases as the MD simulation progresses. Thus, the time-averaged distance becomes progressively less sensitive to the instantaneous state of the molecule. To obviate this shortcoming, Torda et al.[278] scaled $\bar{d}_{ij}(t)$ as follows:

$$\bar{d}_{ij}(t) = \left\{1/\tau\int_0^t \exp(-t'/\tau)\left[d(t-t')\right]^{-n} dt'\right\}^{-1/n} \tag{21}$$

where $\tau$ is a memory-decay constant that progressively dampens the influence of temporally distant structures in the simulation, thus ensuring that the system remains sensitive to the current state of the molecule.[278] Decreasing $\tau$ results in higher weighting for more recent values of $d_{ij}(t)$ relative to the values obtained at earlier times in the simulation. The choice of $\tau$ is critical: it must be large enough so as not to hinder motion (i.e., short values of $\tau$ will lead to insignificant time averaging of the distances), but at the same time it directly affects the rates of motion in the system and therefore the length of time necessary to observe proper averaging. As a compromise, Torda et al.[278] suggest that the simulation time should be about an order of magnitude longer than $\tau$.

A minor adjustment also needs to be made to the force calculation in the simulation. Taking the partial derivative of the pseudopotential obtained by substituting the time-averaged distance $\bar{d}_{ij}(t)$ into Equation (16) leads to a force with fourth-power terms with respect to $\bar{d}_{ij}(t)/d_{ij}(t)$ (if $n = 3$, or seventh power if $n = 6$!). This occasionally leads to very large forces in simulations of macromolecules, thus making the MD trajectories unstable. To obviate this problem, a pseudoenergy term is not actually defined, but a nonconservative pseudoforce of the following form is used in the simulation:[278,279,281]

$$
F_i(t) = \begin{cases} -k_{\text{NOE}}\left[\bar{d}_{ij}(t) - u_{ij}\right]\dfrac{d_{ij}(t)}{d_{ij}(t)} & \text{if } \bar{d}_{ij}(t) > u_{ij} \\ 0 & \text{otherwise} \end{cases} \tag{22}
$$

where $F_i(t)$ is the force on atom $i$ due to atom $j$ and $d_{ij} = d_i - d_j$. This form of the potential leads to forces being "turned on" most strongly for those distances that most severely violate their restraints.[278]

Since the experimentally derived NOE intensities are exact whereas the interproton distances derived from them are at best semiquantitative, it is better to refine directly against NOE intensities (see next section). This can be achieved in the current context by replacing the instantaneous distance $d_{ij}$ and time-averaged distance $\bar{d}_{ij}$ in Equation (20) with the instantaneous NOE intensity $I_{ij}$ and the time-averaged NOE intensity $\bar{I}_{ij}$ which are calculated from the molecular structures using a complete relaxation matrix analysis (see next section). This procedure has been implemented and applied to the protein crambin.[282] A pseudoenergy term has also been derived for the inclusion of time-averaged $J$-coupling constant constraints in RMD calculations.[283,284]

## F  DIRECT REFINEMENT AGAINST NOE INTENSITIES

Cross-relaxation during the mixing time $\tau_m$ of the NOESY experiment is described by the following equation:

$$
M(\tau_m) = a(\tau_m)M(0) = \exp(-R\tau_m)M(0) \tag{23}
$$

where $R$ is the matrix describing the complete dipolar relaxation network, $a$ is the matrix of mixing coefficients, $M(0)$ is the magnetization at zero mixing time, and $M(\tau_m)$ is the magnetization after the mixing time $\tau_m$. This exponential can be recast in the form of a Taylor series expansion:[247]

$$a\left(\tau_m\right) = \exp\left(-\mathbf{R}\tau_m\right) \approx 1 - \mathbf{R}\tau_m + \frac{1}{2}\mathbf{R}^2\tau_m^2 - \ldots + \frac{\left(-1\right)^n}{n!}\mathbf{R}^n\tau_m^n + \ldots \quad (24)$$

Most NMR studies implicitly assume truncation of this series following the linear term. This leads to the following approximation which, however, is valid only in the limit of short mixing times $(\tau_m \to 0)$:[247]

$$\dot{a}_{ij}\left(\tau_m \to 0\right) \propto \frac{J\left(\omega\right)}{d_{ij}^6} \quad (25)$$

where $J(\omega)$ is the spectral density function and $d_{ij}$ is the internuclear distance. The salient feature of this equation is that the mixing coefficients (and consequently the NOESY intensities) are inversely proportional to the sixth power of the internuclear distance.

This relationship is used in the vast majority of NMR studies to derive interproton distance constraints from NOESY cross-peak intensities. Some studies have used a modification of this equation that takes account of motional averaging and gives an inverse fifth-power relationship (the "uniform averaging model").[285] The problem with these approaches is that they assume that cross-relaxation in the protein occurs via isolated pairs of spins (the ISPA assumption; see Section IV.E.1), which is far removed from the real situation where there are likely to be multiple spin-relaxation pathways and numerous opportunities for spin diffusion.

Thus, methods based on complete relaxation matrix (RMA) analysis have been developed. These fall into two categories: (1) extraction of interproton distances by using experimentally derived NOESY cross-peak intensities to construct the relaxation matrix;[286,287] (2) iterative structure refinement based on a comparison of experimental NOESY cross-peak intensities with those predicted from the coordinates of a model structure using RMA.[287,288] The problem with the first approach is that it requires a reasonably complete set of NOEs to construct the relaxation matrix, and this is generally not possible for biopolymers because of the large number of unresolved peaks. Signal that is undetectable because it is beneath the spectral noise level also adversely affects this calculation.[287] While methods have been developed to circumvent the problem of missing intensities, this approach subsequently requires some other method (such as DG or RMD) to calculate structures once the distances have been extracted from the relaxation matrix. This inherently sacrifices some of the accuracy that is potentially gained from direct refinement of the structure against the NOE intensities.

Hence, considerable effort has been directed toward implementation of the second approach mentioned above, namely, using the relaxation matrix to directly refine the structure (rather than interproton distances) against the experimental NOE intensities. The problem with this approach is computational complexity. Banks and co-workers[289] attacked the problem by implementing an iterative refinement procedure, which started with a DG-derived model of the protein. The NOESY intensities *predicted* from this model were then calculated from the complete relaxation matrix derived using the model coordinates. These were then compared with the experimental intensities, and adjustments were made to the NOESY-derived distance constraints whenever there were significant discrepancies. New DG structures were calculated and the procedure was iteratively repeated until the final refined structure yielded a good match between the experimental NOE intensities and those predicted from the model coordinates.

This approach, however, requires considerable user intervention in modifying the distance constraints at each stage of the structure-refinement process. Nilges and co-workers[290] have developed a more direct, though computationally more demanding, DSA procedure for structure refinement using the NOE intensities. Referring back to Equations (15) and (16), these investigators replaced the $V_{\mathrm{NOE}}$ pseudoenergy term with a penalty function that compares the difference between the experimental NOE intensities and those derived from the current structure of the protein (via RMA) during the course of the DSA trajectory, *viz.*:

$$V_{\mathrm{total}} = V_{\mathrm{physical}} + w_{\mathrm{relax}} V_{\mathrm{relax}} \qquad (26)$$

$$V_{\mathrm{relax}} = \sum_{\mathrm{NOEs}} \left( I_{\mathrm{obs}}^{1/6} - k I_{\mathrm{calc}}^{1/6} \right)^2 \qquad (27)$$

where $w_{\mathrm{relax}}$ is a weighting factor, $I_{\mathrm{obs}}$ is the observed NOE intensity, $I_{\mathrm{calc}}$ is the NOE intensity calculated from the current model of the protein, and $k$ is an adjustable scaling factor used to minimise Equation (27). Thus, $V_{\mathrm{relax}}$ is used to drive the structure-refinement process, and hence $w_{\mathrm{relax}}$ must be chosen carefully. The relaxation matrix is calculated every time a hydrogen atom moves some predefined distance; values of 0.05–0.075 Å require the full matrix to be calculated about every 2–4 fs.[290] Consequently, this process is very computationally expensive, but it allows direct refinement against the NOE intensities in a single step, requiring no user intervention. Similar approaches have been implemented by other groups,[291] including a DG-based algorithm.[292]

The RMA approach, however, has a number of shortcomings. First, in most RMA-based refinements, the protein is modelled as a rigid body with a single correlation time. Internal motions, which substantially affect calculation of the relaxation matrix, are generally ignored.[215,294] Second, NOESY spectra often contain biased cross-peak intensities; systematic errors can arise from imperfect pulses, insufficient delay time between transients to allow reattainment of thermal equilibrium, and differential efficiency of magnetization transfer through one-bond scalar couplings in isotope-filtered NOESY experiments (see Section IV.E.1).[215,294]

The problem of internal motion can be addressed by calculating the relaxation matrix using a special form of the spectral-density function that was developed by Lipari and Szabo[295] in their "model-free" analysis of internal motion:

$$J(\omega) = \frac{2}{5}\left[\frac{S^2\tau_m}{1+\omega^2\tau_c^2} - \frac{(1-S^2)}{1+\omega^2\tau^2}\right] \tag{28}$$

where

$$\frac{1}{\tau} = \frac{1}{\tau_c} + \frac{1}{\tau_e} \tag{29}$$

Here, $S^2$ is a generalised order parameter, $\tau_c$ is the overall correlation time of the protein, and $\tau_e$ is an effective correlation time for internal motion. If the internal motion is much faster than the overall rotation of the molecule (i.e., $\tau_e \ll \tau_c$), the second term in the brackets in Equation (28) disappears and only the order parameter is needed to describe the internal motion. Different values of the order parameter can be used for different interproton vectors: in a recent RMA-based refinement of the Arc repressor structure, Bonvin et al.[296] calculated the order-parameter values from an unrestrained MD simulation of the protein (which started from a structure calculated using DG and RMD). Calculation strategies have been recently developed that allow any arbitrary model of internal motion to be introduced into the RMA calculations.[216]

## G  OPTIMAL FILTERING

In describing the optimal filtering method, Altman and Jardetzky[248] draw a distinction between structure-refinement methods based on an adjustment paradigm and those that use an exclusion paradigm. In the adjustment paradigm, which includes the DG strategies outlined above, the starting structure is incrementally adjusted until a good match is obtained between the experimental data (e.g., NOE intensities, NOE-derived distances, or dihedral angles estimated from coupling constants) and those predicted from the current model of the protein. By contrast, methods employing the exclusion paradigm generate starting structures systematically and then exclude only those deemed by some evaluation process to be incompatible with the experimental data.

The optimal filtering method proposed by Altman and Jardetzky[248] is based on the exclusion paradigm. The logic underpinning optimal filtering is that the solution structure of a protein is not validly described by a single set of atomic coordinates because of its intrinsic solution dynamics; rather, one should try to generate a spatial-distribution function for each atom which conveys a more realistic indication of the ensemble of conformations accessed by the protein. Altman and Jardetzky[248] suggest that such a spatial-distribution function (essentially a statistical description of the protein structure) is more readily generated by exclusion methods because they can systematically search conformational space in a less biased manner than "structure-adjustment" methods.

Because of the high computational cost of systematically searching the conformational space available to a large protein with hundreds or thousands of atoms, the optimal filtering process is sometimes preceded by a hierarchical model-building phase. First, the protein is subdivided into secondary structure elements by sampling the NMR data for pertinent information (NOEs, $^3J_{HN\alpha}$ coupling constants, amide-proton exchange rates), and then the coarse topology of these secondary structure elements in the folded structure is determined by coarse systematic sampling. The use of secondary structure elements reduces the number of "objects" whose positions need to be sampled systematically. Finally, the spatial distribution of atomic positions is refined in accordance with the exclusion paradigm using nonlinear Kalman filtering.[248] Kalman filtering enables incremental refinement of a probabilistic description of the protein; the procedure can be implemented in either Cartesian space, in which case the protein structure is defined by an accessible volume for each atom (i.e., mean position and associated uncertainty),[248] or torsion space, in which case the protein structure is defined by a set of mean dihedrals and their associated uncertainties.[297]

At the present time it is difficult to gauge the general applicability of this approach since, apart from validations using model datasets,[298] it appears to have been used only in the initial stages of structure refinement of the *trp* repressor protein, a 25-kDa dimer for which only relatively sparse NOE datasets were available.[299] However, we note that this is the largest protein to date whose complete three-dimensional structure has been solved using NMR spectroscopy.[300] Hence, as previously suggested, optimal filtering strategies may be especially applicable to relatively large proteins for which there is only a small set of relatively imprecise NOEs.[298,300] Trial calculations on a CRAY/YMP supercomputer indicated that, for a 46-residue polypeptide, 112 metric-matrix DG structures or 12 DSA structures could be generated in the same time that it takes to calculate a complete statistical description of the protein using torsion-space optimal filtering.[298]

## H   ASSESSING THE QUALITY OF THE CALCULATED STRUCTURE(S)

There is currently much conjecture about the most reliable method for assessing the quality of protein structures calculated from NMR data. Since most methods generate a family of structures that "satisfy" the NMR-derived structural constraints, a common practice has been to assess the quality of structures by measuring the RMSDs of individual structures from the mean structure. Clearly, however, this is a measure of the precision of the structures rather than of their accuracy.[215,293,294] The global RMSD is not a very good measure of precision as it does not discriminate between a structure that is poorly reproduced on average and one that is accurately reproduced except for a single ill-defined segment. Residue-by-residue or segment-by-segment RMSD comparisons are often better indicators of precision,[298] although they generally lack the visual impact of an overlay of a series of structures based on minimisation of the global RMSD.

An alternative procedure, which was introduced to avoid biasing the mean structure toward any single structure,[301] is to measure the RMSDs (globally or residue by residue) against a "canonical" structure obtained by inputting the root-mean-squared interatomic distances, calculated from the family of structures, into a metric-matrix DG embed-algorithm.[301] The same investigators introduced an angle-order parameter $S$ to describe how precisely each dihedral angle is defined; $S = 1.0$ indicates that the angle is exactly defined, while a completely random distribution of the angle gives $S = 0$.[301]

Measurement of the accuracy of NMR-derived structures is a much more difficult task than estimating their precision. Some studies have attempted to estimate the "best-possible" accuracy available from NMR studies by first measuring "experimental" interproton distance constraints from a model structure (to which random noise is added to simulate the typical precision available with real NMR data), and then attempting to calculate the model structure using these constraints. Comparison of the calculated and model structures gives an indication of the accuracy of typical NMR structure determinations. In some cases this has led to inflated estimates of the best-possible accuracy (0.25 Å RMSD for backbone atoms and 0.65 Å for all atoms)[215] due to biased choice of the model structure from which the distances were chosen.[294] A recent study, in which distance constraints were derived from a "target" crystal structure, suggests that the best-possible accuracy is ~1–2 Å RMSD for all-atom representations of the protein.[294]

An absolute measure of the accuracy of an NMR-derived structure is not possible in the absence of any knowledge about the "true" structure; in this case, it has to be measured by some statistic.[293] An advantage of RMA is that it enables an $R$ factor to be calculated from a comparison of the experimental NOESY intensities with those predicted from the calculated structure by RMA. This $R$ factor is analogous to the $R$ factor (or reliability index) used in crystallography, which is derived from a comparison of the observed and calculated structure-factor amplitudes.[302] The NMR $R$ factor is usually calculated using the following equation:[293,303]

$$R_{1/6} = \frac{\sum_{\text{NOEs}} \left| I_{\text{obs}}^{1/6} - I_{\text{calc}}^{1/6} \right|}{\sum_{\text{NOEs}} I_{\text{obs}}^{1/6}} \tag{30}$$

However, the magnitude of $R_{1/6}$ will depend on the value of $w_{\text{relax}}$ in Equation (26); $R_{1/6}$ will decrease as $w_{\text{relax}}$ is increased. Hence, the value of the $R$ factor is diminished unless a rule is specified for choosing $w_{\text{relax}}$;[293] in most cases, $w_{\text{relax}}$ is chosen empirically to ensure that the experimental constraints are reasonably satisfied without introducing intolerable "strain" in the molecule, as measured by mean RMSDs of bond lengths and angles.

A considerable problem with $R$ factors of this type (from both an NMR and a crystallographic perspective) is that they inevitably get smaller as the number of parameters used in the fitting process is increased, but this does not necessarily correspond to an increase in the accuracy of the structure. Several crystal structures have been incorrectly modelled as a result of introducing extra parameters in the fitting process on the basis of declining values of the $R$ factor.[304] A similar problem may well exist with NMR structures calculated using time-averaged distance and angle constraints (time averaging represents a large increase in the number of fitting parameters).

Brünger and co-workers have addressed this problem by introducing cross-validated (or "free") $R$ factors for both crystallographic[304] and NMR[293] structure refinement. While partial cross-validation is satisfactory for X-ray refinement because of the highly correlated nature of the reflections (i.e., each reflection contains information relating to the whole structure), a more complete cross-validation is necessary with NMR refinement because each NOE contains information relating to only a single interproton distance.[293] The cross-validation process is essentially a computer "experiment." The distance constraints are randomly partitioned into 10 "test" sets of approximately equal size. The 10 "working" datasets then correspond to the complete set of distance constraints minus each one of the test datasets. The structure is calculated using each of the working datasets, and then various measures of fit (such as the $R$ factor, distance-bound violations, etc.) are calculated for the corresponding test datasets (and then averaged). The rationale behind this cross-validation procedure is that the measures of fit calculated using the test datasets will be unbiased as these data have not been used in the refinement process.

While it might be envisaged that significant redundancy in the NMR dataset would be essential for this procedure to work well, Brünger et al.[293] have shown that it can be successful with as few as two distance constraints per residue. The cross-validated $R$ factor might prove very useful in assessing whether multiple-conformer models (such as those produced using time-averaged constraints) improve the information content relative to single-conformer models.[293]

Finally, it is important to check the stereochemical quality of the final structures as this can often reveal errors that have not been detected during the refinement process. The PROCHECK program was developed in the laboratory of Janet Thornton[305,306] specifically for this purpose. The program reports numerous measures of stereochemical merit, including quality of the Ramachandran plot, deviations of bond lengths, bond angles, and torsion angles from ideality, unfavourable side-chain $\chi$ angles, and bad nonbonded interactions. An added bonus is that the program "cleans" up the coordinate files for submission to the Brookhaven protein databank[7] by ensuring that the atom labels conform to IUPAC-IUB nomenclature and by performing some basic stereochemical checks on the file. Structures of high stereochemical quality may still be misfolded; for example, large (stereochemically correct) patches of hydrophobic residues may be exposed on the surface of the protein. Eisenberg's group have therefore developed a program[307] that checks to see whether each residue in a protein is found in an environment consistent with its known physical and chemical properties. The program calculates a 3D–1D profile score for each residue by comparing its local environment (i.e., the buried, solvent-inaccessible, surface area; fraction of the side chain covered by polar O and N atoms; and local secondary structure) with that expected on the basis of an analysis of 16 highly refined crystal structures. An overall 3D–1D profile score (i.e., the sum of each of the residue profile scores) gives an indication of the overall correctness of the protein structure, while the residue scores are good indicators of local misfolds.

# VI CONCLUSIONS AND FUTURE PROSPECTS

This year marks the 50th anniversary of the first demonstration of the NMR phenomenon.[308,309] During these 50 years, the field has been punctuated by a number of revolutionary advances, so much so that making predictions about its future prospects is always likely to be imprudent. Nevertheless, having just witnessed a number of major developments in the field, it seems an appropriate time to reflect upon the future application of NMR to protein structure determination.

The recent introduction of heteronuclear triple-resonance-assignment strategies by Bax, Clore, and co-workers[7,310] has effectively doubled the size of proteins for which structures can be determined using NMR spectroscopy; proteins as large as ~31 kDa have been studied using these techniques.[113] The major factor limiting the application of these experiments to even larger proteins is the rapid transverse-relaxation rates of the $^{13}C\alpha$ and $^{1}H\alpha$ resonances, which severely limit the sensitivity of any experiment that attempts to transfer magnetization via $J$ couplings involving these nuclei. Thus, crucial cluster-linking experiments such as the 3D HNCA and 3D HN(CO)CA become increasingly inefficient as the size of the protein increases.

Thus, many new experiments are aimed at ameliorating these problems; examples include the introduction of constant-time periods to reduce transverse relaxation losses by minimising dephasing and rephasing delays,[131] the use of composite-pulse $^{1}H$ decoupling (rather than 180° pulses) to modify the relaxation properties of magnetization that is chemical-shift labelled during the evolution period,[113] and coherence transfer by heteronuclear cross-polarisation rather than pulsed free precession.[157] However, despite these efforts, it is likely that the application of triple-resonance-assignment strategies will still be limited to proteins of molecular mass less than 35 kDa.

Further increases in the applicable molecular weight range will most probably rely on combining random fractional deuteration of the protein with uniform $^{15}N/^{13}C$-labelling. As outlined in Section II.E.3, random fractional deuteration can markedly reduce transverse-relaxation rates by limiting the network of $^{1}H$ dipolar couplings; for large proteins, the gain in intensity from the reduced resonance linewidths is likely to more than compensate for the intrinsic decrease in $^{1}H$ signal-to-noise ratio. Indeed, selective protein deuteration was a critical part of the strategy used to determine the solution conformation of a 37-kDa *trp* repressor-DNA complex, by far the largest macromolecular structure solved to date using NMR techniques.[311]

In summary, it can be anticipated that NMR spectroscopy will be able to provide high-resolution structures for proteins of up to *ca.* 40 kDa within the next five years. An increase in size limit beyond 40 kDa will require a further revolutionary advance in the field; at present, however, it is difficult to envisage what this might be. The other major limiting factor in the use of NMR as a structural tool for rational drug design is the time required to solve the structures — a significant easing of this bottleneck should come from the introduction of automated strategies for resonance assignment, which are currently under development. Finally, it should be noted that a great deal of useful information is available using NMR techniques without knowledge of a protein's high-resolution solution structure; such studies are described elsewhere in this book.

## ACKNOWLEDGMENTS

Work reported from this laboratory was supported by the Cooperative Research Centre for Molecular Engineering & Technology and grants to GFK from the Australian Research Council and the Australian National Health and Medical Research Council. We would like to thank Professor Philip Kuchel, Dr. Tony Weiss, Dr. Mitch Guss, and Dr. Graeme Shaw for proofreading various parts of the manuscript and for making numerous helpful suggestions. We would also like to thank our wives, Lindsey Mackay and Susan Rowland, for their patience, tolerance, and meticulous proofreading.

# REFERENCES

1. Bugg, C.E.; Carson, W.M.; Montgomery, J.A.; *Sci. Am.* 1993, December, 60–66.
2. von Itzstein, M.; Wu, W.-Y.; Kok, G.B.; Pegg, M.S.; Dyason, D.C.; Jin, B.; Phan, T.V.; Smythe, M.L.; White, H.F.; Oliver, S.W.; Colman, P.M.; Varghese, J.N.; Ryan, D.M.; Woods, J.M.; Bethell, R.C.; Notham, V.J.; Cameron, J.M.; Penn, C.R.; *Nature* 1993, 363, 418–423.
3. Kendrew, J.; *Science* 1963, 139, 1259–1266.
4. Perutz, M.; *Science* 1963, 140, 863–869.
5. Williamson, M.P.; Havel, T.F.; Wüthrich, K.; *J. Mol. Biol.* 1985, 182, 295–315.
6. Bernstein, F.C.; Koetzle, T.F.; Williams, G.J.B.; Meyer, E.F., Jr; Brice, M.D.; Rogers, J.R.; Kennard, O.; Shimanouchi, T.; Tasumi, M.; *J. Mol. Biol.* 1977, 112, 535–542.
7. Bax, A.; Grzesiek, S.; *Acc. Chem. Res.* 1993, 26, 131–138.
8. Lee, M.S.; Gippert, G.P.; Somain, K.V.; Case, D.A.; Wright, P.E.; *Science* 1989, 245, 635–637.
9. Junius, F.K.; Weiss, A.S.; King, G.F.; *Eur. J. Biochem.* 1993, 214, 415–424.
10. Kent, S.B.H.; *Annu. Rev. Biochem.* 1988, 57, 957–989.
11. Junius, F.K.; Mackay, J.P.; Bubb, W.A.; Jensen, S.A.; Weiss, A.S.; King, G.F.; *Biochemistry* 1995, 34, 6164–6174.
12. Old, R.W.; Primrose, S.B.; *Principles of Gene Manipulation: An Introduction to Genetic Engineering, 4th ed.*; Blackwell Scientific: Oxford, 1989.
13. Ausubel, F.M.; Brent, R.; Kingston, R.E.; Moore, D.D.; Seidman, J.G.; Smith, J.A.; Struhl, K.; Eds; *Current Protocols in Molecular Biology, Vols 1 and 2 and Suppls 1–21*; John Wiley & Sons: New York, 1993.
14. Sambrook, J.; Fritsch, E.F.; Maniatis, T.; *Molecular Cloning: A Laboratory Manual, Vols 1–3, 2nd ed.*; Cold Spring Harbor Laboratory Press: Cold Spring Harbor, NY, 1989.
15. Mullis, K.B.; Faloona, F.A.; *Methods Enzymol.* 1987, 155, 335–350.
16. Erlich, H.A., Ed.; *PCR Technology: Principles and Applications for DNA Amplification*; Stockton Press: New York, 1989.
17. Cease, K.B.; Potcova, C.A.; Lohff, C.J.; Zeigler, M.E.; *PCR Methods Appl.*, 1994, 3, 298–300.

18. Pedersen, S.; *EMBO J.* 1984, 3, 2895–2898.
19. Makoff, M.B.; Oxer, M.D.; Romanos, M.A.; Fairweather, N.F.; Ballantine, S.; *Nucleic Acids Res.* 1989, 17, 10192–10194.
20. Scorer, C.A.; Carrier, M.J.; Rosenberger, R.F.; *Nucleic Acids Res.* 1991, 19, 3511–3516.
21. Kane, J.F.; Violand, B.N.; Curran, D.F.; Staten, N.R.; Duffin, K.L.; Bogosian, G.; *Nucleic Acids Res.* 1992, 20, 6707–6712.
22. Martin, S.L.; Vrhovski, B.; Weiss, A.S.; *Gene* 1995, 159–166.
23. Riley, L.G.; Junius, F.K.; Swanton, M.K.; Vesper, N.A.; Williams, N.K.; King, G.F.; Weiss, A.S.; *Eur. J. Biochem.* 1994, 219, 877–886.
24. Goeddel, D.V.; Emr, S.D.; Gold, L.; Henner, D.J.; Levinson, A.D.; Eds.; *Gene Expression Technology*; Academic Press: New York, 1991, 185.
25. Luckow, V.A.; Summers, M.D.; *Bio/Technology* 1988, 6, 47–55.
26. Marston, F.A.O.; *Biochem. J.* 1986, 240, 1–12.
27. Fischer, B.; Sumner, I.; Goodenough, P.; *Biotechnol. Bioeng.* 1993, 41, 3–13.
28. Baron, M.; Norman, D.; Willis, A.; Campbell, I.D.; *Nature* 1990, 345, 642–646.
29. Barlow, P.N.; Baron, M.; Norman, D.G.; Day, A.J.; Willis, A.C.; Sim, R.B.; Campbell, I.D.; *Biochemistry* 1991, 30, 997–1004.
30. Hansen, A.P.; Petros, A.M.; Mazar, A.P.; Pederson, T.M.; Rueter, A.; Fesik, S.W.; *Biochemistry* 1992, 31, 12713–12718.
31. Kato, K.; Matsunaga, C.; Nishimura, Y.; Waelchli, M.; Kainosho, M.; Arata, Y.; *J. Biochem.* (Tokyo) 1989, 105, 867–869.
32. Wu, R., Ed.; Recombinant DNA (Part H); *Methods Enzymol.* 1993, 217.
33. Smith, D.B.; Johnson, K.S.; *Gene* 1988, 67, 31–40.
34. Driscoll, P.C.; Campbell, I.D.; Cyster, J.G.; Williams, A.F.; *Nature* 1991, 353, 762–5.
35. Kellerman, O.K.; Ferenci, T.; *Methods Enzymol.* 1982, 90, 459–463.
36. Lauritzen, C.; Tuchsen, E.; Hansen, P.E.; Skovgaard, O.; *Protein Expression Purif.* 1991, 2, 372–378, 1991.
37. Emerson, S.D.; Waugh, D.S.; Scheffler, J.E.; Tsao, K.L.; Prinzo, K.M.; Fry, D.C.; *Biochemistry* 1994, 33, 7745–7752.
38. Ford, C.F.; Suominen, I.; Glatz, C.E.; *Protein Expression Purif.* 1991, 2, 95–107.
39. Smith, M.C.; Furman, T.C.; Ingolia, T.D.; Pidgeon, C.; *J. Biol. Chem.* 1988, 263, 7211–7215.
40. Schein, C.H.; Noteborn, M.H.M.; *Bio/Technology* 1988, 6, 291–294.
41. Takagi, H.; Morinaga, Y.; Tsuchiya, M.; Ikemura, H.; Inouye, M.; *Bio/Technology* 1988, 6, 948–950.
42. Muchmore, D.C.; McIntosh, L.P.; Russell, C.B.; Anderson, D.E.; Dahlquist, F.W.; *Methods Enzymol.* 1989, 177, 44–73.
43. Markley, J.L.; Kainosho, M.; Stable isotope labelling and resonance assignments in larger proteins, in *NMR of Macromolecules*; Roberts, G.C.K., Ed.; IRL Press: Oxford, 1993; chap. 5.
44. Wang, J.; Hinck, A.P.; Loh, S.N.; Markley, J.L.; *Biochemistry* 1990, 29, 102–113.
45. Sørensen, P.; Poulsen, F.M.; *J. Biomol. NMR* 1992, 2, 99–101.
46. LeMaster, D.M.; *Methods Enzymol.* 1989, 177, 23–43.
47. Arrowsmith, C.H.; Pachter, R.; Altman, R.B.; Iyer, S.B.; Jardetzky, O.; *Biochemistry* 1990, 29, 6332–6341.
48. LeMaster, D.M.; Richards, F.M.; *Biochemistry* 1988, 27, 142–150.
49. Kay, L.E.; Ikura, M.; Tschudin, R.; Bax, A.; *J. Magn. Reson.* 1990, 89, 496–514.
50. McIntosh, L.P.; Wand, A.J.; Lowry, D.F.; Redfield, A.G.; Dahlquist, F.W.; *Biochemistry* 1990, 29, 6341–6362.

51. Morris, M.B.; Ralston, G.B.; Biophysical characterization of membrane and cytoskeletal proteins by sedimentation analysis, in *Physicochemical Methods in the Study of Biomembranes (Subcellular Biochemistry, Vol. 23)*; Hilderson, H.J. and Ralston, G.B., Eds.; Plenum Press: New York, 1994; pp. 25–82.

52. Mills, R.G.; Ralston, G.B.; King, G.F.; *J. Biol. Chem.* 1994, 269, 23413–23419.

53. Mikol, V.; Hirsch, E.; Giege, R.; *J. Mol. Biol.* 1990, 213, 187–95.

54. Dynapro-801 Operator's Manual: Protein Solutions, Charlottesville, VA, 1994.

55. Atkins, P.W.; *Physical Chemistry, 2nd ed.*; Oxford University Press: Oxford, 1982.

56. Anglister, J.; Grzesiek, S.; Ren, H.; Klee, C.B.; Bax, A.; *J. Biomol. NMR* 1993, 3, 121–126.

57. Stejskal, E.O.; Tanner, J.E.; *J. Chem. Phys.* 1965, 42, 288–292.

58. Kuchel, P.W.; Kirk, K., King, G.F.; NMR Methods for measuring membrane transport, in *Physicochemical Methods in the Study of Biomembranes (Subcellular Biochemistry, Vol. 23)*; Hilderson, H.J. and Ralston, G.B., Eds.; Plenum Press: New York, 1994; pp. 247–327.

59. Dingley, A.J.; Chapman, B.E.; Morris, M.B.; Kuchel, P.W.; Hambly, B.D.; King, G.F.; *J. Biomol. NMR*, 5, in press.

60. Villafranca, J.J.; *Methods Enzymol.* 1989, 177, 403–413.

61. Primrose, W.U.; Sample preparation, in *NMR of Macromolecules*; Roberts, G.C.K., Ed.; IRL Press: Oxford, 1993; chap. 2.

62. Kralicek, A.V.; Vesper, N.A.; Ralston, G.B.; Wake, R.G.; King, G.F.; *Biochemistry* 1993, 32, 10216–10223.

63. Bai, Y.; Milne, J.S.; Mayne, L.; Englander, S.W.; *Proteins Struct. Funct. Genet.* 1993, 17, 75–86.

64. Tappin, M.J.; Cooke, R.M.; Fitton, J.E.; Campbell, I.D.; *Eur. J. Biochem.* 1989, 179, 629–637.

65. Neuhaus, D.; Williamson, M.P.; *The Nuclear Overhauser Effect in Structural and Conformational Analysis*; VCH Publishers: New York, 1989; pp. 30–39.

66. Grzesiek, S.; Döbeli, H.; Gentz, R.; Garotta, G.; Labhardt, A.M.; Bax, A.; *Biochemistry* 1992, 31, 8180–8190.

67. Wüthrich, K.; *NMR of Proteins and Nucleic Acids*; John Wiley & Sons: New York, 1986.

68. Ernst, R.R.; Bodenhausen, G.; Wokaun, A.; *Principles of Nuclear Magnetic Resonance in One and Two Dimensions*; Clarendon Press: Oxford, 1987.

69. Aue, W.P.; Bartholdi, E.; Ernst, R.R.; *J. Chem. Phys.* 1976, 64, 2229–2246.

70. Piantini, U.; Sørensen, O.W.; Ernst, R.R.; *J. Amer. Chem. Soc.* 1982, 104, 6800–6801.

71. Kumar, A.; Ernst, R.R.; Wüthrich, K.; *Biochem. Biophys. Res. Comm.* 1980, 95, 1–6.

72. Jeener, J.; Meier, B.H.; Bachmann, P.; Ernst, R.R.; *J. Chem. Phys.* 1979, 71, 4546–4553.

73. Braunschweiler, L.; Ernst, R.R.; *J. Magn. Reson.* 1983, 53, 521–528.

74. Davis, D.G.; Bax, A.; *J. Amer. Chem. Soc.* 1985, 107, 2820–2821.

75. Zuiderweg, E.P.R.; Doren, S.R.V.; *Trends Anal. Chem.* 1994, 13, 24–36.

76. Brown, S.C.; Weber, P.L.; Mueller, L.; *J. Magn. Reson.* 1988, 77, 166–169.

77. Roberts, G.C.K., Ed.; *NMR of Macromolecules: A Practical Approach*; Oxford University Press: New York, 1993.

78. Cavanagh, J.; Chazin, W.J.; Rance, M.; *J. Magn. Reson.* 1990, 87, 110–131.

79. Bundi, A.; Wüthrich, K.; *Biopolymers* 1979, 18, 285–298.

80. Bax, A.; Davis, D.G.; *J. Magn. Reson.* 1985, 63, 207–213.

81. Englander, S.W.; Wand, A.J.; *Biochemistry* 1987, 26, 5953–5958.

82. Vuister, G.W.; Boelens, R.; Kaptein, R.; *J. Magn. Reson.* 1988, 80, 176–185.

83. Wijmenga, S.S.; Mierlo, C.P.M.V.; *Eur. J. Biochem.* 1991, 195, 807–822.
84. Boelens, R.; Vuister, G.W.; Koning, T.M.G.; Kaptein, R.; *J. Am. Chem. Soc.* 1989, 111, 8525–8526.
85. Vuister, G.W.; Boelens, R.; Padilla, A.; Kleywegt, G.J.; Kaptein, R.; *Biochemistry* 1990, 29, 1829–1839.
86. Bodenhausen, G.; Ruben, D.J.; *Chem. Phys. Lett.* 1980, 69, 185–189.
87. Morris, G.A.; Freeman, R.; *J. Am. Chem. Soc.* 1979, 101, 760–762.
88. Bax, A.; Griffey, R.H.; Hawkins, B.L.; *J. Am. Chem. Soc.* 1983, 105, 7188–7190.
89. Norwood, T.J.; Boyd, J.; Heritage, J.E.; Soffe, N.; Campbell, I.D.; *J. Magn. Reson.* 1990, 87, 488–501.
90. Bax, A.; Ikura, M.; Kay, L.E.; Torchia, D.A.; Tschudin, R.; *J. Magn. Reson.* 1990, 86, 304–318.
91. Messerle, B.A.; Wider, G.; Otting, G.; Weber, C.; Wüthrich, K.; *J. Magn. Reson.* 1989, 85, 608–613.
92. Zuiderweg, E.R.P.; Fesik, S.W.; *Biochemistry* 1989, 28, 2387–2391.
93. Marion, D.; Kay, L.E.; Sparks, S.W.; Torchia, D.A.; Bax, A.; *J. Amer. Chem. Soc.* 1989, 111, 1515–1517.
94. Fesik, S.W.; Zuiderweg, E.R.P.; *J. Magn. Reson.* 1988, 78, 588–593.
95. Marion, D.; Driscoll, P.C.; Kay, L.E.; Wingfield, P.T.; Bax, A.; Gronenborn, A.M.; Clore, G.M.; *Biochemistry* 1989, 6150–6156.
96. Fesik, S.W.; Zuiderweg, E.R.P.; *Q. Rev. Biophys.* 1990, 23, 97–131.
97. Gronenborn, A.M.; Bax, A.; Wingfield, P.T.; Clore, G.M.; *FEBS Lett.* 1989, 243, 93–98.
98. Ikura, M.; Kay, L.E.; Tschudin, R.; Bax, A.; *J. Magn. Reson.* 1990, 86, 204–209.
99. Kay, L.E.; Clore, G.M.; Bax, A.; Gronenborn, A.M.; *Science* 1990, 249, 411–414.
100. Clore, G.M.; Kay, L.E.; Bax, A.; Gronenborn, A.M.; *Biochemistry* 1991, 30, 12–18.
101. Fesik, S.W.; Eaton, H.L.; Olejniczak, E.T.; Zuiderweg, E.R.P.; McIntosh, L.P.; Dahlquist, F.W.; *J. Am. Chem. Soc.* 1990, 112, 886–888.
102. Bax, A.; Clore, G.M.; Gronenborn, A.M.; *J. Magn. Reson.* 1990, 88, 425–431.
103. Kay, L.E.; Ikura, M.; Bax, A.; *J. Am. Chem. Soc.* 1990, 112, 888–889.
104. Majumdar, A.; Wang, H.; Morshauser, R.C.; Zuiderweg, E.R.P.; *J. Biomol. NMR* 1993, 3, 387–397.
105. Olejniczak, E.T.; Xu, R.X.; Fesik, S.W.; *J. Biomol. NMR* 1992, 2, 655–659.
106. Bendell, M.R.; Pegg, D.T.; Doddrell, D.M.; Field, J.; *J. Am. Chem. Soc.* 1981, 103, 934–936.
107. Freeman, R.; Mareci, T.H.; Morris, G.A.; *J. Magn. Reson.* 1981, 42, 341–345.
108. Muto, Y.; Yamasaki, K.; Ito, Y.; Yajima, S.; Masaki, H.; Uozumi, T.; Wälchli, M.; Nishimura, S.; Miyazawa, T.; Yokoyama, S.; *J. Biomol. NMR* 1993, 3, 165–184.
109. McIntosh, L.P.; Wand, A.J.; Lowry, D.F.; Redfield, A.G.; Dahlquist, F.W.; *Biochemistry* 1990, 29, 6341–6362.
110. Derome, A.E.; *Modern NMR Techniques for Chemistry Research*; Pergamon Press: Oxford, 1987.
111. Kessler, H.; Mronga, S.; Gemmecker, G.; *Magn. Reson. Chem.* 1991, 29, 527–557.
112. Ikura, M.; Kay, L.E.; Bax, A.; *Biochemistry* 1990, 29, 4659–4667.
113. Grzesiek, S.; Bax, A.; *J. Magn. Reson.* 1992, 96, 432–440.
114. Bax, A.; Ikura, M.; *J. Biomol. NMR* 1991, 1, 99–104.
115. Clubb, R.T.; Thanabal, V.; Wagner, G.; *J. Biomol. NMR* 1992, 2, 203–210.

116. Clubb, R.T.; Wagner, G.; *J. Biomol. NMR* 1992, 2, 389–393.
117. Kay, L.E.; Ikura, M.; Bax, A.; *J. Magn. Reson.* 1991, 91, 84–92.
118. Clubb, R.T.; Thanabal, V.; Wagner, G.; *J. Magn. Reson.* 1992, 97, 213–217.
119. Kay, L.E.; Wittekind, M.; McCoy, M.A.; Friedrichs, M.S.; Mueller, L.; *J. Magn. Reson.* 1992, 98, 443–450.
120. Boucher, W.; Laue, E.D.; Campbell-Burk, S.L.; Domaille, P.J.; *J. Biomol. NMR* 1992, 2, 631–637.
121. Olejniczak, E.T.; Xu, R.X.; Petros, A.M.; Fesik, S.W.; *J. Magn. Reson.* 1992, 100, 444–450.
122. Grzesiek, S.; Bax, A.; *J. Magn. Reson.* 1992, 99, 201–207.
123. Wittekind, M.; Mueller, L.; *J. Magn. Reson. B* 1993, 101, 201–205.
124. Grzesiek, S.; Bax, A.; *J. Biomol. NMR* 1993, 3, 185–204.
125. Grzesiek, S.; Bax, A.; *J. Am. Chem. Soc.* 1992, 114, 6291–6293.
126. Logan, T.M.; Olejniczak, E.T.; Xu, R.X.; Fesik, S.W.; *FEBS Lett.* 1992, 314, 413–418.
127. Montelione, G.T.; Lyons, B.A.; Emerson, S.D.; Tashiro, M.; *J. Am. Chem. Soc.* 1992, 114, 10974–10975.
128. Lyons, B.A.; Montelione, G.T.; *J. Magn. Reson. B* 1993, 101, 206–209.
129. Grzesiek, S.; Bax, A.; *J. Magn. Reson. B* 1993, 102, 103–106.
130. Palmer, A.G., III; Fairbrother, W.J.; Cavanagh, J.; Wright, P.E.; Rance, M.; *J. Biomol. NMR* 1992, 2, 103–108.
131. Powers, R.; Gronenborn, A.M.; Clore, G.M.; Bax, A.; *J. Magn. Reson.* 1991, 94, 209–213.
132. Seip, S.; Balbach, J.; Behrens, S.; Kessler, H.; Flukiger, K.; deMeyer, R.; Erni, B.; *Biochemistry* 1994, 33, 7174–7183.
133. Remerowski, M.L.; Domke, T.; Groenewegen, A.; Pepermans, H.A.M.; Hilbers, C.W.; van der Ven, F.J.M.; *J. Biomol. NMR* 1994, 4, 257–278.
134. Yamazaki, T.; Forman-Kay, J.D.; Kay, L.E.; *J. Am. Chem. Soc.* 1993, 115, 11054–11055.
135. Wittekind, M.; Metzler, W.J.; Mueller, L. *J. Magn. Reson. B* 1993, 101, 214–217.
136. Kraulis, P.J.; Domaille, P.J.; Campbell-Burk, S.L.; van Aken, T.; Laue, E.D.; *Biochemistry* 1994, 33, 3515–3531.
137. Stockman, B.J.; Nirmala, N.R.; Wagner, G.; Delcamp, T.J.; De Yarman, M.T.; Freisheim, J.H.; *Biochemistry* 1992, 31, 218–229.
138. Redfield, C.; Smith, L.J.; Boyd, J.; Lawrence, G.M.P.; Edwards, R.G.; Smith, R.A.G.; Dobson, C.M.; *Biochemistry* 1991, 30, 11029–11035.
139. Zhou, M.M.; Logan, T.M.; Theriault, Y.; van Etten, R.L.; Fesik, S.W.; *Biochemistry* 1994, 33, 5221–5229.
140. Powers, R.; Clore, G.M.; Bax, A.; Garret, D.S.; Stahl, S.J.; Wingfield, P.T.; Gronenborn, A.M.; *J. Mol. Biol.* 1991, 221, 1081–1090.
141. Clubb, R.T.; Thanabal, V.; Fejzo, J.; Ferguson, S.B.; Zydowsky, L.; Bake, C.H.; Walsh, C.T.; Wagner, G.; *Biochemistry* 1993, 32, 6391–6401.
142. Abeygunawardana, C.; Webe, D.J.; Frick, D.N.; Bessman, M.J.; Mildvan, A.S.; *Biochemistry* 1993, 32, 13071–13080.
143. Lyons, B.A.; Tashiro, M.; Cedergren, L.; Nilsson, B.; Montelione, G.T.; *Biochemistry* 1993, 32, 7839–7845.
144. Archer, S.J.; Vinson, V.K.; Pollard, T.D.; Torchia, D.A.; *Biochemistry* 1993, 32, 6680–6687.
145. Bagby, S.; Harvey, T.S.; Kay, L.E.; Eagle, S.G.; Inouye, S.; Ikura, M.; *Biochemistry* 1994, 33, 2409–2421.
146. Metzler, W.J.; Constantine, K.L.; Friedrichs, M.S.; Bell, A.J.; Ernst, E.G.; Lavoie, T.B.; Mueller, L.; *Biochemistry* 1993, 32, 13818–13829.

147. Grdadolnik, G.; Eberstadt, M.; Gemmecker, G.; Kessler, H.; Buhr, A.; Erni, B.; *Eur. J. Biochem.* 1994, 219, 945–952.

148. Werner, J.M.; Breeze, A.L.; Kara, B.; Rosenbrock, G.; Boyd, J.; Soffe, N.; Campbell, I.D.; *Biochemistry* 1994, 33, 7184–7192.

149. Constantine, K.L.; Goldfarb, V.; Wittekind, M.; Friedrichs, M.S.; Anthony, J.; Ng, S.-C.; Mueller, L.; *J. Biomol. NMR* 1993, 3, 41–54.

150. Sørensen, O.W.; *J. Magn. Reson.* 1990, 89, 210–216.

151. Morris, P.G.; *NMR Imaging in Medicine and Biology*; Oxford University Press: Oxford, 1986.

152. Roemer, P.B.; Edelstein, W.A.; Hickey, J.S.; *Proceedings of the 5th Annual Meeting of the Society for Magnetic Resonance in Medicine* 1986, Montreal, Quebec, p. 1067.

153. Wider, G.; Wüthrich, K.; *J. Magn. Reson. B* 1993, 102, 239–241.

154. Bax, A.; Pochapsky, S.; *J. Magn. Reson.* 1992, 99, 638–645.

155. John, B.K.; Plant, D.; Hurd, R.E.; *J. Magn. Reson. A* 1993, 101, 113–117.

156. Majumdar, A.; Zuiderweg, E.R.P., *J. Magn. Reson. B* 1993, 102, 241–244.

157. Zuiderweg, E.R.P.; Majumdar, A., *Trends Anal. Chem.* 1994, 13, 73–80.

158. Vuister, G.W.; Boelens, R.; Kaptein, R.; Hurd, R.E.; John, B.; VanZihl, P.C.M., *J. Am. Chem. Soc.* 1991, 113, 9688–9690.

159. Vis, H.; Boelens, R.; Mariani, M.; Stroop, R.; Vorgias, C.E.; Wilson, K.S.; Kaptein, R., *Biochemistry* 1994, 33, 14858–14870.

160. Zhang, O.; Kay, L.E.; Oliver, J.P.; Forman-Kay, J.D.; *J. Biomol. NMR* 1994, 4, 845–858.

161. Piotto, M.; Saudek, V.; Sklenár, V.; *J. Biomol. NMR* 1992, 2, 661–665.

162. Hurd, R.E.; *J. Magn. Reson.* 1990, 87, 422–428.

163. Grzesiek, S.; Bax, A.; *J. Am. Chem. Soc.* 1993, 115, 12593–12594.

164. Nagayama, K.; Kumar, A.; Wüthrich, K.; Ernst, R.R.; *J. Magn. Reson.* 1979, 40, 321–334.

165. Davis, A.L.; Keeler, J.; Laue, E.D.; Moskau, D.; *J. Magn. Reson.* 1992, 98, 207–216.

166. Boyd, J.; Soffe, N.; John, B.; Plant, D.; Hurd, R.; *J. Magn. Reson.* 1992, 98, 660–664.

167. Palmer, A.G., III; Cavanagh, J.; Wright, P.E.; Rance, M.; *J. Magn. Reson.* 1991, 93, 151–170.

168. Cavanagh, J.; Palmer, A.G., III; Wright, P.E.; Rance, M.; *J. Magn. Reson.* 1991, 91, 429–433.

169. Kay, L.E.; Keifer, P.; Saarinen, T.; *J. Am. Chem. Soc.* 1992, 114, 10663–10665.

170. Muhandiram, D.R.; Xu, G.Y.; Kay, L.E.; *J. Biomol. NMR* 1993, 3, 463–470.

171. Schleucher, J.; Schwendinger, M.; Sattler, M.; Schmidt, P.; Schedletsky, O.; Glaser, S.J.; Sørensen, O.W.; Griesinger, C.; *J. Biomol. NMR* 1994, 4, 301–306.

172. Levitt, M.H.; Freeman, R.; Frenkiel, T.; *J. Magn. Reson.* 1983, 50, 157–160.

173. Shaka, A.J.; Lee, C.J.; Pines, A.; *J. Magn. Reson.* 1988, 77, 274–293.

174. Shaka, A.J.; Keeler, J.; Freeman, R.; *J. Magn. Reson.* 1983, 53, 313–340.

175. Kadkhodaie, M.; Rivas, O.; Tan, M.; Mohebbi, A.; Shaka, A.J.; *J. Magn. Reson.* 1991, 91, 437–443.

176. Hartmann, S.R.; Hahn, E.L.; *Phys. Rev.* 1962, 128, 2042.

177. Gerstein, B.C.; Dybrowki, C.R.; *Transient Techniques in NMR of Solids*; Academic Press: London, 1985.

178. Zuiderweg, E.R.P.; *J. Magn. Reson.* 1990, 89, 533.

179. Ernst, M.; Griesinger, C.; Ernst, R.R.; Bermel, W.; *Mol. Phys.* 1991, 74, 219–252.

180. Bearden, D.W.; Brown, L.R.; *Chem. Phys. Lett.* 1989, 163, 432–436.

181. Richardson, J.M.; Clowes, R.T.; Boucher, W.; Domaille, P.J.; Hardman, C.H.; Keeler, J.; Laue, E.D.; *J. Magn. Reson. B* 1993, 101, 223–227.

182. Sørensen, O.W.; *J. Magn. Reson.* 1990, 89, 210–216.
183. Farmer, B.T., II; *J. Magn. Reson.* 1991, 93, 635–641.
184. Boelens, R.; Burgering, M.; Fogh, R.H.; Kaptein, R.; *J. Biomol. NMR* 1994, 4, 201–213.
185. Schmieder, P.; Stern, A.S.; Wagner, G.; Hoch, J.C.; *J. Biomol. NMR* 1993, 3, 569–576.
186. Robin, M.; Delsuc, M.-A.; Guittet, E.; Lallemand, J.-Y.; *J. Magn. Reson.* 1991, 92, 645–650.
187. Barna, J.C.J.; Laue, E.D.; Mayger, M.R.; Skilling, J.; Worrall, S.J.P.; *J. Magn. Reson.* 1987, 73, 69–77.
188. Gull, S.F.; Daniell, G.J.; *Nature* 1978, 272, 686–690.
189. Hodgkinson, P.; Mott, H.R.; Driscoll, P.C.; Jones, J.A.; Hore, P.J.; *J. Magn. Reson. B* 1993, 101, 218–222.
190. Laue, E.D.; Skilling, J.; Staunton, J.; Sibisi, S.; Brereton, R.G.; *J. Magn. Reson.* 1985, 62, 437–452.
191. Stephenson, D.S.; *Prog. NMR Spectrosc.* 1988, 20, 515–626.
192. Olejniczak, E.T.; *J. Magn. Reson.* 1990, 87, 628–632.
193. Gesmar, H.; Led, J.J.; Abildgaard, F.; *Prog. NMR Spectrosc.* 1990, 22, 255–288.
194. Zhu, G.; Bax, A.; *J. Magn. Reson.* 1990, 90, 405–410.
195. Zhu, G.; Bax, A.; *J. Magn. Reson.* 1992, 98, 192–199.
196. Chylla, R.A.; Markley, J.L.; *J. Biomol. NMR* 1993, 3, 515–533.
197. Meadows, R.P.; Olejniczak, E.T.; Fesik, S.W.; *J. Biomol. NMR* 1994, 4, 79–96.
198. Garrett, D.S.; Powers, R.; Gronenborn, A.M.; Clore, G.M.; *J. Magn. Reson.* 1991, 95, 214–220.
199. Johnson, B.A.; Blevins, R.A.; *J. Biomol. NMR* 1994, 4, 603–614.
200. Kjær, M.; Andersen, K.V.; Shen, H.; Ludvigsen, S.; Windekilde, D.; Sørensen, B.; Poulsen, F.M.; PRONTO, in *NATO ASI Series A*; Hoch, J.C.; Hoch, F. M.; Poulsen, Redfield, C., Eds; Plenum Press: New York, 1991; pp 291–302.
201. Bernstein, R.; Cieslar, C.; Ross, A.; Oschkinat, H.; Freund, J.; Holak, T.A.; *J. Biomol. NMR* 1993, 3, 245–251.
202. Friedrichs, M.S.; Mueller, L.; Wittekind, M.; *J. Biomol. NMR* 1994, 4, 703–726.
203. Hare, B.J.; Prestegard, J.H.; *J. Biomol. NMR* 1994, 4, 35–46.
204. Olson, Jr, J.B.; Markley, J.L.; *J. Biomol. NMR* 1994, 4, 385–410.
205. Clore, G.M.; Gronenborn, A.M.; *Crit. Rev. Biochem. Mol. Biol.* 1989, 24, 479–563.
206. Eccles, C.; Güntert, P.; Billeter, M.; Wüthrich, K.; *J. Biomol. NMR* 1991, 1, 111–130.
207. Güntert, P.; Berndt, K.D.; Wüthrich, K.; *J. Biomol. NMR* 1993, 3, 601–606.
208. De Marco, A.; Llinás, M.; Wüthrich, K.; *Biopolymers* 1978, 17, 637–650.
209. Clore, G.M.; Gronenborn, A.M.; *Science* 1991, 252, 1390–1399.
210. Burgering, M.J.M.; Boelens, R.; Gilbert, D.E.; Breg, J.N.; Knight, K.L.; Sauer, R.T.; Kaptein, R.; *Biochemistry* 1994, 33, 15036–15045.
211. Gronenborn, A.M.; Clore, G.M.; *Prog. NMR Spectrosc.* 1985, 17, 1–32.
212. Barsukov, I.L.; Lian, L.-Y.; Structure Determination from NMR data I, in *NMR of Macromolecules*; Roberts, G.C.K., Ed.; Oxford University Press: New York, 1993; pp 315–357.
213. Kuntz, I.D.; Thomason, J.F.; Oshiro, C.M.; *Methods Enzymol.* 1989, 177, 159–204.
214. Wüthrich, K.; Billeter, M.; Braun, W.; *J. Mol. Biol.* 1983, 169, 949–961.
215. Clore, G.M.; Robien, M.A.; Gronenborn, A.M.; *J. Mol. Biol.* 1993, 231, 82–102.
216. Dellwo, M.J.; Wand, J.; *J. Biomol. NMR* 1993, 3, 205–214.
217. Bystrov, V.F.; *Prog. NMR Spectrosc.* 1976, 10, 44–81.

218. Karplus, M.; *J. Am. Chem. Soc.* 1963, 85, 2870–2871.

219. Pardi, A.; Billeter, M.; Wüthrich, K.; *J. Mol. Biol.* 1984, 180, 741–751.

220. Richardson, J.; *Adv. Prot. Chem.* 1981, 34, 167–339.

221. Marion, D.; Wüthrich, K.; *Biochem. Biophys. Res. Commun.* 1983, 113, 967–974.

222. Neuhaus, D.; Wagner, G.; Vasak, M.; Kägi, J.H.R.; Wüthrich, K.; *Eur. J. Biochem.* 1985, 151, 257–273.

223. Neri, D.; Otting, G.; Wüthrich, K.; *J. Am. Chem. Soc.* 1990, 112, 3663–3665.

224. Billeter, M.; Neri, D.; Otting, G.; Qian, Y.Q.; Wüthrich, K.; *J. Biomol. NMR* 1992, 2, 257–274.

225. Kay, L.E.; Bax, A.; *J. Magn. Reson.* 1990, 86, 110–126.

226. Griesinger, C.; Sørensen, O.W.; Ernst, R.R.; *J. Am. Chem. Soc.* 1985, 107, 6394–6396.

227. Mueller, L.; *J. Magn. Reson.* 1987, 72, 191–196.

228. Clore, G.M.; Bax, A.; Gronenborn, A.M.; *J. Biomol. NMR* 1991, 1, 13–22.

229. Forman-Kay, J.D.; Clore, G.M.; Wingfield, P.T.; Gronenborn, A.M.; *Biochemistry* 1991, 30, 2685–2698.

230. Dyson, H.J.; Gippert, G.P.; Case, D.A.; Holmgren, A.; Wright, P.E.; *Biochemistry* 1990, 29, 4129–4136.

231. Montelione, G.T.; Winkler, M.E.; Rauenbuehler, P.; Wagner, G.; *J. Magn. Reson.* 1989, 82, 198–204.

232. Xu, R.X.; Olejniczak, E.T.; Fesik, S.W.; *FEBS Lett.* 1992, 305, 137–143.

233. Bax, A.; Max, D.; Zax, D.; *J. Am. Chem. Soc.* 1992, 114, 6924–6925.

234. Vuister, G.W.; Wang, A.C.; Bax, A.; *J. Am. Chem. Soc.* 1993, 115, 5334–5335.

235. Vuister, G.W.; Delaglio, F.; Bax, A.; *J. Am. Chem. Soc.* 1992, 114, 9674–9675.

236. Nilges, M.; Clore, G.M.; Gronenborn, A.M.; *Biopolymers* 1990, 29, 813–822.

237. Curley Jr, R.W.; Panigot, M.J.; Hansen, A.P.; Fesik, S.W.; *J. Biomol. NMR* 1994, 4, 335–340.

238. Hvidt, A.; Neilsen, S.O.; *Adv. Prot. Chem.* 1966, 21, 287–386.

239. Englander, S.W.; Kallenbach, N.R.; *Q. Rev. Biophys.* 1983, 16, 521–655.

240. Molday, R.S.; Englander, S.W.; Kallen, R.G.; *Biochemistry* 1972, 11, 150–158.

241. Wishart, D.S.; Richards, F.M.; Sykes, B.D.; *Biochemistry* 1992, 31, 1647–1651.

242. Spera, A.; Bax, A.; *J. Am. Chem. Soc.* 1991, 113, 5490–5492.

243. Wishart, D.S.; Sykes, B.D.; *J. Biomol. NMR* 1994, 4, 171–180.

244. Havel, T.; Wüthrich, K.; *Bull. Math. Biol.* 1984, 46, 673–698.

245. Kaptein, R.; Zuiderweg, E.R.P.; Scheek, R.M.; Boelens, R.; van Gunsteren, W.F.; *J. Mol. Biol.* 1985, 182, 179–182.

246. Brünger, A.T.; Clore, G.M.; Gronenborn, A.M.; Karplus, M.; *Proc. Natl. Acad. Sci. USA* 1986, 83, 3801–3805.

247. James, T.L.; Borgias, B.; Bianucci, A.M.; Zhou, N.; Solution structure refinement using complete relaxation matrix analysis of 2D NOE experiments: DNA fragments, in *NMR and Biomolecular Structure*; Bertini, I.; Molinari, H.; Niccolai, N., Eds; VCH Publishers: Weinheim, Germany, 1991; chap. 4.

248. Altman, R.B.; Jardetzky, O.; *Methods Enzymol.* 1989, 177, 218–246.

249. Torda, A.E.; Scheek, R.M.; van Gunsteren, W.F.; *Chem. Phys. Lett.* 1989, 157, 289–294.

250. Blumenthal, L.M.; *Theory and Applications of Distance Geometry*; Chelsea: New York, 1970.

251. Sutcliffe, M.J.; Structure determination from NMR data II, in *NMR of Macromolecules*; Roberts, G.C.K., Ed.; IRL Press: Oxford, 1993; chap. 11.

252. Némethy, G.; Pottle, M.S.; Scheraga, H.A.; *J. Phys. Chem.* 1983, 87, 1883–1887.

253. Crippen, G.M.; Havel, T.F.; *Distance Geometry and Molecular Conformation*; Research Studies Press: Letchworth, UK, 1988.
254. Braun, W.; Gō, N.; *J. Mol. Biol.* 1985, 186, 611–626.
255. Güntert, P.; Braun, W.; Wüthrich, K.; *J. Mol. Biol.* 1991, 217, 517–530.
256. Flory, P.J.; *The Statistical Mechanics of Chain Molecules*; Wiley-Interscience: New York, 1969.
257. Metzler, W.J.; Hare, D.; Pardi, A.; *Biochemistry* 1989, 28, 7045–7052.
258. Wagner, G.; Braun, W.; Havel, T.F.; Schaumann, T.; Gō, N.; Wüthrich, K., *J. Mol. Biol.* 1987, 196, 611–639.
259. Havel, T., *Biopolymers* 1990, 29, 1565–1585.
260. Kuszewski, J.; Nilges, M.; Brünger, A.T., *J. Biomol. NMR* 1992, 2, 33–56.
261. van Gunsteren, W.F.; Berendsen, H.J.C., *Angew. Chem. Int. Ed. Engl.* 1990, 29, 992–1023.
262. Scheek, R.M.; van Gunsteren, W.F.; Kaptein, R., *Methods Enzymol.* 1989, 177, 204–218.
263. Güntert, P.; Qian, Y.Q.; Otting, G.; Müller, M.; Gehring, W.; Wüthrich, K.; *J. Mol. Biol.* 1991, 217, 531–540.
264. Ryckaert, J.P.; Ciccotti, G.; Berendsen, H.J.C.; *J. Comput. Chem.* 1977, 23, 327.
265. van Nuland, N.A.J.; Hangyi, I.W.; van Schaik, R.C.; Berendsen, H.J.C.; van Gunsteren, W.F.; Scheek, R.M.; Robillard, G.T.; *J. Mol. Biol.* 1994, 237, 544–559.
266. Nilges, M.; Clore, G.M.; Gronenborn, A.M.; *FEBS Lett.* 1988, 229, 317–324.
267. Brünger, A.T.; Clore, G.M.; Gronenborn, A.M.; Karplus, M.; *Protein Eng.* 1987, 1, 399–406.
268. Moore, J.M.; Peattie, D.A.; Fitzgibbon, M.J.; Thomson, J.A.; *Nature* 1991, 351, 248–250.
269. Clore, G.M.; Nilges, M.; Gronenborn, A.M., Determination of three dimensional structures of proteins in solution by dynamical simulated annealing with interproton distances derived from nuclear magnetic resonance spectroscopy, in *Computer-Aided Molecular Design*; Graham, W.G., Ed.; IBC Technical Services: London, 1989; chap. 17.
270. Nilges, M.; Clore, G.M.; Gronenborn, A.M.; *FEBS Lett.* 1988, 239, 129–136.
271. Mills, R.G.; O'Donoghue, S.I.; Smith, R.; King, G.F.; *Biochemistry* 1992, 31, 5640–5645.
272. Clore, G.M.; Wingfield, P.T.; Gronenborn, A.M.; *Biochemistry* 1991, 30, 2315–2323.
273. Norman, D.G.; Barlow, P.N.; Baron, M.; Day, A.J.; Sim, R.B.; Campbell, I.D.; *J. Mol. Biol.* 1991, 219, 717–725.
274. Havel, T.F.; *Prog. Biophys. Molec. Biol.* 1991, 56, 43–78.
275. Sherman, S.A.; Johnson, M.E.; *Prog. Biophys. Molec. Biol.* 1993, 59, 285–339.
276. Kim, Y.; Ohlrogge, J.B.; Prestegard, J.H.; *Biochem. Pharmacol.* 1990, 40, 7–13.
277. Kim, Y.; Prestegard, J.H.; *Biochemistry* 1989, 28, 8792–8797.
278. Torda, A.E.; Scheek, R.M.; van Gunsteren, W.F.; *J. Mol. Biol.* 1990, 214, 223–235.
279. Torda, A.E.; van Gunsteren, W.F.; *Comput. Phys. Commun.* 1991, 62, 289–296.
280. Kessler, H.; Griesinger, C.; Lautz, J.; Müller, A.; van Gunsteren, W.F.; Berendsen, H.J.C.; *J. Am. Chem. Soc.* 1988, 110, 3393–3396.
281. Pearlman, D.A.; *J. Biomol. NMR* 1994, 4, 1–16.
282. Bonvin, A.M.J.J.; Boelens, R.; Kaptein, R.; *J. Biomol. NMR* 1994, 4, 143–149.
283. Torda, A.E.; Brunne, R.M.; Huber, T.; Kessler, H.; van Gunsteren, W.F.; *J. Biomol. NMR* 1993, 3, 55–66.

284. Pearlman, D.A.; *J. Biomol. NMR* 1994, 4, 279–299.
285. Braun, W.; Bösch, C.; Brown, L.R.; Gō, N.; Wüthrich, K.; *Biochim. Biophys. Acta* 1981, 667, 377–396.
286. Olejniczak, E.T.; Gampe, R.T., Jr.; Fesik, S.W.; *J. Magn. Reson.* 1986, 67, 28–41.
287. Borgias, B.A.; James, T.L.; *J. Magn. Reson.* 1990, 87, 475–487.
288. Yip, P.; Case, D.A.; *J. Magn. Reson.* 1989, 83, 643–648.
289. Banks, K.M.; Hare, D.R.; Reid, B.R.; *Biochemistry* 1989, 28, 6996–7010.
290. Nilges, M.; Habazettl, J.; Brünger, A.T.; Holak, T.A.; *J. Mol. Biol.* 1991, 219, 499–510.
291. Bonvin, A.M.J.J.; Boelens, R.; Kaptein, R.; *J. Biomol. NMR* 1991, 1, 305–309.
292. Mertz, J.E.; Güntert, P.; Wüthrich, K.; Braun, W.; *J. Biomol. NMR* 1991, 1, 257–269.
293. Brünger, A.T.; Clore, G.M.; Gronenborn, A.M.; Saffrich, R.; Nilges, M.; *Science* 1993, 261, 328–331.
294. Zhao, D.; Jardetzky, O.; *J. Mol. Biol.* 1994, 239, 601–607.
295. Lipari, G.; Szabo, A.; *J. Am. Chem. Soc.* 1982, 104, 4546–4559.
296. Bonvin, A.M.J.J.; Vis, H.; Breg, J.N.; Bergering, M.J.M.; Boelens, R.; Kaptein, R.; *J. Mol. Biol.* 1994, 236, 328–341.
297. Koehl, P.; Lefévre, J.-F.; Jardetzky, O.; *J. Mol. Biol.* 1992, 223, 299–315.
298. Liu, Y.; Zhao, D.; Altman, R.; Jardetzky, O.; *J. Biomol. NMR* 1992, 2, 373–388.
299. Arrowsmith, C.; Pachter, R.; Altman, R.; Jardetzky, O.; *Eur. J. Biochem.* 1991, 202, 53–66.
300. Zhao, D.; Arrowsmith, C.H.; Jia, X.; Jardetzky, O.; *J. Mol. Biol.* 1993, 229, 735–746.
301. Hyberts, S.G.; Goldberg, M.S.; Havel, T.F.; Wagner, G.; *Protein Science* 1992, 1, 736–751.
302. Woolfson, M.M.; *An Introduction to X-Ray Crystallography*; Cambridge University Press: Cambridge, 1970.
303. Thomas, P.D.; Basus, V.J.; James, T.L.; *Proc. Natl. Acad. Sci. USA* 1991, 88, 1237–1241.
304. Brünger, A.T.; *Nature* 1992, 355, 472–475.
305. Morris, A.L.; MacArthur, M.W.; Hutchinson, E.G.; Thornton, J.M.; *Proteins Struct. Funct. Genet.* 1992, 12, 345–364.
306. Laskowski, R.A.; MacArthur, M.W.; Moss, D.S.; Thornton, J.M.; *J. Appl. Cryst.* 1993, 26, 283–291.
307. Lüthy, R.; Bowie, J.U.; Eisenberg, D.; *Nature* 1992, 356, 83–85.
308. Purcell, E.M.; Torrey, H.C.; Pound, R.V.; *Phys. Rev.* 1946, 69, 37–38.
309. Bloch, F.; Hansen, W.W.; Packard, M.; *Phys. Rev.* 1946, 69, 127.
310. Clore, G.M.; Gronenborn, A.M.; *Protein Science* 1994, 3, 372–390.
311. Zhang, H.; Zhao, D.; Revington, M.; Lee, W.; Jia, X.; Arrowsmith, C.; Jardetzky, O.; *J. Mol. Biol.* 1994, 238, 592–614.

# CHAPTER 5

# CONFORMATIONAL ANALYSIS OF DRUG MOLECULES

*Jerzy W. Jaroszewski*

## CONTENTS

I   Introduction ............................................................................ 201

II   Neuroactive Drugs ................................................................ 203

III   Other Compounds ................................................................ 206

IV   Conclusions ........................................................................ 208

References ................................................................................ 209

## I   INTRODUCTION

There is a multitude of ways by which NMR methods can assist in the development of drugs.[1] As illustrated in the earlier chapters, the rational design of drugs that have well-defined macromolecular target molecules will benefit especially from knowledge of the exact molecular geometry of ligand–receptor complexes. For this reason, NMR and crystallographic investigations of receptor proteins and their complexes with ligands provide an exciting and highly promising new aspect of modern pharmacology.[2-4]

0-8493-7824-9/96/$0.00+$.50
© 1996 by CRC Press, Inc.

However, structure determination of macromolecular complexes is difficult, and there are currently only a limited number of examples of such structures. The macromolecular targets of most drugs are still inaccessible for studies at the molecular level because of problems with their isolation in a functional state, purification difficulties, or molecular size which makes the structural study beyond current capabilities. Not infrequently, the macromolecular target for a drug is unknown. In such cases, structure–activity studies involving the three-dimensional structure of the ligand are the only possibility. They are also essential with drugs exhibiting a balanced action by several mechanisms.

Conformational information about drug molecules can be derived from NMR spectra at various levels of sophistication. At the elementary level, there is no sharp division between the application of NMR to chemical structure determination and extraction of basic conformational information, since even a single interproton coupling constant can give general hints about the preferred conformation or population of conformations in solution. Likewise, simple NMR experiments are frequently used to prove whether a solution conformation of a drug molecule is similar or dissimilar to that found in the solid state by X-ray crystallography. At an advanced level, the full repertoire of NMR parameters, including $J$ couplings, NOE effects, relaxation times, their quantitative interpretation, and their temperature and solvent dependence, can be exploited to derive a largely complete picture of the conformational and motional properties of a drug molecule. Such investigations should preferably involve a series of compounds (in order to compare the conformational properties, derived from NMR, with biological activity) and will usually benefit from support by computational methods of conformational analysis. This kind of investigation is necessary to derive meaningful information relevant to drug action because, in the case of flexible molecules, the receptor is likely to alter the solution conformation upon binding. Therefore, the relevance of information about a single preferred conformation of a drug molecule in solution to the conformational requirements of the receptor site may not be clear.

Another reason for caution originates from the fact that for molecules that populate several conformations in fast exchange on the NMR time scale, experimental NMR parameters will be time averaged. If a certain molecular geometry is derived from such averaged parameters, it may have no physical significance, that is, it may not correspond to any of the actual conformers present in the solution. This problem and possible ways of circumventing it have been discussed in detail elsewhere.[5] For small drug molecules the problem can be conveniently solved by searching conformational space by computational methods and using the information about likely conformers to assist interpretation of NMR data.

A full description of the pharmacological significance of NMR results cannot be given without a discussion of biological data and results from the complementary techniques of conformational analysis. This is beyond the scope of the present chapter. Instead, the purpose is to provide an overview of the applications of NMR to conformational studies of a variety of small drug molecules, with emphasis on CNS-active drugs. Nucleotides, nucleosides, saccharides, and their oligomers are not included. The important field of peptides is covered extensively in Chapter 6.

---

# II  NEUROACTIVE DRUGS

The majority of drugs that act on the central or peripheral nervous system show a pronounced dependence of their action on seemingly minor changes of molecular shape, and, in many cases, considerable knowledge has been accumulated about structure–activity relationships. Accordingly, conformational investigations have been an integral part of pharmacological studies of neuroactive drugs.

Analogues of natural neurotransmitters constitute a large and diverse group of compounds, the development of which has benefited from NMR results. Acetylcholine has been studied extensively by NMR, including an examination of [1]H NMR spectra as a function of hydration.[6] Motional parameters of the molecule from molecular dynamics were found to be in good agreement with correlation times derived from NMR data.[7] The conformations of nicotine[8,9] and muscarine[10] and various nicotinic and muscarinic agonists and antagonists have been studied using mainly vicinal interproton couplings.[11-19]

Numerous N-methyl-D-aspartate, γ-aminobutyric acid, and glutamic acid analogues and other compounds interacting with their receptors have been synthesized and their conformations in solution assessed using $^3J_{HH}$ coupling information, usually in conjunction with molecular mechanics and X-ray crystallography.[20-25] The influence of ionic environment on the aspartate conformation has also been studied.[26] Rotamer populations in various neurotransmitter amino acid analogues can be estimated from limiting values of $^3J_{HH}$ in various rotamers.[27]

Antipsychotic drugs act by blocking dopamine receptors, and NMR spectroscopy has made significant contributions to the understanding of structural and conformational requirements of the antipsychotic pharmacophores.[28] Many sterically restricted dopamine analogues, such as derivatives of aminotetralins and related compounds, have been investigated mainly using vicinal interproton couplings,[29-36] with additional information derived from NOE[30,35,36] and low-temperature NMR studies.[32]

(R)-Apomorphine and (+)-butaclamol (**1**) were the first structures used to model the binding site of the neuroleptic agents.[28] NMR studies on butaclamol[37-39] were carried out to compare the solution structure to the crystal structure and to assess conformational mobility of the compound in solution. Molecular mechanics calculations identified[38] four low-energy conformations of protonated butaclamol, with a chair conformation of the E ring, but with either a *trans* (torsion angle HNCH4a close to 180°) or *cis* (torsion angle HNCH4a of 50°) junction of the D and E rings, and either of two possible conformations of the ethylene bridge connecting the A and C rings, differing in the torsion angle about the C8–C9 bond; one of the *trans* conformers was found in the crystal.[38]

**1** Butaclamol

NMR data suggested that butaclamol hydrochloride exists as a single conformer in chloroform. After spectral assignment using homo- and heteronuclear 2D techniques, vicinal interproton couplings were measured, or, in the case of complex patterns, obtained from *J*-resolved spectra or derived by iterative simulation of the spin systems.[38] The $^3J_{HH}$ couplings thus obtained were converted to conformational information using Karplus equations. The magnitude of the couplings to H4a demonstrated the presence of *trans* annulation of the D and E rings, with corroborative evidence obtained from qualitative NOE measurements.[38] The presence of several significantly populated conformations in fast exchange could be excluded because a number of the vicinal couplings that were observed approached limiting values. Analysis of couplings and NOEs within the cycloheptane ring strongly indicated a predominance of only one of the two possible conformations of the ethylene bridge. Additional evidence about the limited flexibility of the ethylene bridge was obtained from $^{13}C$ $T_1$ relaxation measurements, supported by a computational assessment of the dynamics of this part of the molecule, which indicated restricted flexing motions.[38] Also, the presence of the chair form of the E ring was suggested by the NMR data.

On the other hand, the spectrum of butaclamol hydrochloride in DMSO showed the presence of two conformers in slow exchange, as indicated by the presence of two distinct NH resonances in a ratio of 4:1.[37,39] Analysis of couplings revealed that the major component was identical to that observed in chloroform, whereas the minor component had a *cis* junction between the D and E rings.[39] The possibility that the chloroform spectrum was an averaged spectrum was excluded by the inability to freeze out any minor conformation in spectra recorded at $-60°C$ in $CDCl_3$ or $-95°C$ in $CD_2Cl_2$. The conformational behaviour of the hydrochloride in the latter solvents was distinctly different from that of the free butaclamol base, for which two conformations could be observed below $-70°C$, with the coalescence temperature corresponding to free-energy of activation of 10 kcal/mol.[39] The presence of slow exchange was further demonstrated by selective saturation transfer experiments,[39] and the conformational features of the *cis* conformation could be derived from $^3J_{HH}$ coupling data. The different conformational behaviour of butaclamol hydrochloride in $CDCl_3$ and DMSO is presumably due to the pronounced hydrogen-bond acceptor basicity of the latter solvent.

Studies of this kind provide an important insight into the energetics of conformational interconversions of drug molecules, unavailable from X-ray studies, and show the value of computational approaches when used in conjunction with experimental data. They emphasize that even for molecules having apparently limited flexibility it may be inappropriate to refer to a single biologically active conformation. Furthermore, such studies have the potential to identify a set of conformations available for receptor binding, and they demonstrate the pronounced effects of protonation and molecular environment on conformational behaviour. Such effects may be highly relevant to the receptor binding event and to subsequent effects caused by that binding.

The role of NMR in studying molecular dynamics of drugs has been further demonstrated with several other classes of CNS molecules, including antidepressants. $^{13}C$ $T_1$ measurements were used to examine internal molecular flexibility of imipramine and related tricyclic antidepressants.[40] Benzodiazepines have been studied using a variety of NMR techniques.[41-47] A study of barbiturates[48] provides a rare example of application of $^3J_{HC}$ coupling constants measured with $^{13}C$-enriched drugs; this study disclosed a largely unconstrained conformational mobility of the barbiturate side chain, providing evidence against an earlier hypothesis that conformational side-chain differences could distinguish convulsant and anticonvulsant activities. Interproton coupling constants and relaxation times have been used extensively to assess the conformation of flexible arylethylamine side chains in many dopaminergic, histaminergic, and other CNS-active compounds.[49-55]

Opiate agonists and antagonists are of profound importance because of their therapeutic applications as analgesics, as well as their connection with drug abuse; they have been the subject of intensive conformational studies in which NMR has played an important role. Although morphine (2) is a relatively rigid molecule, the piperidine ring has some flexibility, which affects the nitrogen position and the orientation of the N-substituent. The equatorial conformation of the latter substituent and the chair conformation of the piperidine ring, disclosed by X-ray studies, have provided a basis for speculation on the nature of the opiate receptor.[56] However, [1]H NMR studies of morphine salts have demonstrated the existence of methyl group inversion, which is slow on the NMR time scale,[56] with conformer populations corresponding to an energy difference of 1 kcal/mol, consistent with theoretical estimates.[56] Further support for the influence of hydrogen-bonding and crystal-packing forces on the conformation of crystalline morphine was obtained from solid-state [13]C NMR;[57,58] the resonances of C2, C7, C11, C15, and C16 changed chemical shift between aqueous solution and the solid, indicating a conformational change of the piperidine ring.[58] The crystal structure thus cannot be assumed to be the receptor-active conformation.

**2** Morphine

Further studies on morphine and derivatives, including solvation effects and hydrogen bonding, have been reported.[59,60] Agonist–antagonist relations were discussed in terms of motional properties of the nitrogen substituents derived from $T_1$ relaxation data,[61] averaging of [1]H NMR parameters,[62] hydrogen bond formation, and dissociation equilibria at the hydrated nitrogen.[59] NMR studies involving analysis of coupling constants and NOEs with a new class of κ opioid analgesics, characterized by the presence of the benzenacetamide system, have also been reported.[63-65]

Finally, NMR studies of anaesthetics,[66,67] analgesics,[68] ergot alkaloids,[69-71] various histaminergic compounds,[72-76] and cannabinoids[77-80] should be mentioned. Conformational mobility of aryl methoxy groups can be determined from [13]C $T_1$ relaxation times.[28,81]

# III  OTHER COMPOUNDS

The conformations of many other classes of drugs have been studied in solution using NMR methods, and some will be mentioned in this section. Various [1]H NMR investigations of cardiotonic and cardiovascular drugs[81-86] and of calcium channel blockers[87-92] have been reported. These include measurements of selective NOEs from $^1H$ to $^{13}C$ and selective $^1H$ $T_1$ relaxation times in diltiazem (**3**), and their interpretation in terms of dipolar cross-relaxation rates, from which interproton distances were derived and used for the construction of a molecular model. This was found to correspond well to the structure found in the solid state.[89] Similar techniques were used to obtain effective $^{13}C$ correlation times and interproton cross-relaxation rates for verapamil (**4**) in DMSO.[90] The solution structure of verapamil and its calcium complex in acetonitrile was derived from the measurement of NOESY cross-peak integrals.[92]

**3** Diltiazem (top)        **4** Verapamil (bottom)

Studies of antiinflammatory agents[93-96] include evaluation of reorientational rates of CH bond vectors.[95] Motional parameters of prostaglandins were evaluated from the magnetic field and temperature dependence of $^1H$ relaxation data,[97] allowing segmental motions to be detected. Prostaglandins and leukotrienes were also studied using interproton couplings, NOE, and selective and nonselective proton relaxation rates.[98-101] Adrenoceptor blockers have been studied using $^3J_{HH}$.[50,52,102-105]

Taxol (**5**) is a recent example of a clinically useful chemotherapeutic agent of plant origin. Considerable interest in this compound results from its unique mechanism of action on microtubules and the possibility of the development of second-generation drugs based on its structure. The assignment of taxol resonances was accomplished by homo- and heteronuclear 2D methods. Measurements of initial ROE buildup rates in

**5** Taxol

chloroform enabled derivation of interproton distances using a geminal proton pair as a reference distance.[107] The results were compatible with the presence of a rigid tetracyclic core, with an indication of preferred orientation of side chains. In another study, a conformational search on the chloroform- or water-solvated A-ring side chain of taxol that was performed with model compounds identified a number of low-energy structures.[108] From calculations, there appeared to be no conformational preference for the CH-NH torsion angle, which was confirmed by the observed $^3J_{CHNH}$ coupling, for which a fully averaged value (as compared to values calculated for single rotamers) was observed. Other interproton couplings within the side chain were used to identify preferred conformations. NOESY spectra and couplings observed in various solvents (water/DMSO mixtures, chloroform) were used to identify solvent-dependent conformational changes, mainly in the A-ring side chain and in the B ring. In chloroform, the apolar phenyl groups were exposed to the solvent, whereas in the aqueous solvents a greater exposure of the amide portion was observed.[108] Further data on taxol were obtained from a quantitative evaluation of NOESY cross-peak buildup rates using the spin-pair approximation;[109] the NMR-derived distances were compared with calculated data and a model X-ray structure. Conclusions from the conformational investigations, including the role of solvent effects, provided enough information for the construction of a qualitative model for the binding to tubulin.[109]

## IV   CONCLUSIONS

Although NMR techniques are being extensively used for the assessment of drug conformations in solution, a minority of the investigations reported in the literature go beyond simple application of interproton coupling constants or qualitative NOE observations. The relative absence of measurements giving insight into molecular mobility is especially problematic in the case of flexible molecules, because a so-called preferred average conformation may in reality reflect the existence of several widely different conformations in fast exchange, with only one of them represented in the bound state at the receptor site. Investigations of conformational equilibria, energy differences, and barriers between the conformers by relaxation studies and dynamic NMR techniques, supported by computational results, provide a basis for more meaningful conclusions about the conformations available for the receptor. Such studies often disclose the potential complexity of interactions between drugs and their macromolecular sites.

# REFERENCES

1. Jaroszewski, J. W.; Schaumburg, K.;  Kofod, H., Eds.; *NMR Spectroscopy in Drug Research*; Munsgaard: Copenhagen, 1988.
2. Fesik, S. W.; *J. Med. Chem.* 1991, 34, 2937-2945.
3. Erickson, J. W.; Fesik, S. W.; *Ann. Rep. Med. Chem.* 1992, 27, 271-289.
4. Feeney, J.; *Biochem. Pharmacol.* 1990, 40, 141-152.
5. Jardetzky, O.; *Biochim. Biophys. Acta* 1980, 621, 227-232.
6. Harmon, K. M.; Akin, A. C.; Avci, G. F.; Nowos, L. S.; Tierney, M. B.; *J. Mol. Struct.* 1991, 244, 223-236.
7. Edvardsen, Ø.; Dahl, S. G.; *J. Neural. Transm. Gen. Sec.* 1991, 83, 157-170.
8. Pitner, T. P.; Edwards, W. B., III,; Bassfield, R. L.; Whidby, J. F.; *J. Am. Chem. Soc.* 1978, 100, 246-251.
9. Pinter, T. P.; Whidby, J. F.; Edwards, W. B., III; *J. Am. Chem. Soc.* 1980, 102, 5149-5150.
10. Mubarak, A. M.; Brown, D. M.; *Tetrahedron* 1982, 38, 41-43.
11. Carroll, F. I.; Abraham, P.; Mascarella, S. W.; Singh, P.; Moreland, C. G.; Sankar, S. S.; Kwon, Y. W.; Triggle, D. J.; *J. Med. Chem.* 1991, 34, 1436-1440.
12. Carroll, P. J.; De Amici, M.; De Micheli, C.; Toma, L.; *J. Med. Chem.* 1992, 35, 305.
13. Koskinen, A. M. P.; Rapoport, H.; *J. Med. Chem.* 1985, 28, 1301-1309.
14. McGroddy, K. A.; Oswald, R. E.; *Biophys. J.* 1993, 64, 314-324.
15. McGroddy, K. A.; Carter, A. A.; Tubbert, M. M.; Oswald, R. E.; *Biophys. J.* 1993, 64, 325-338.
16. Trigo, G. G.; Matrínez, M.; Gálvez, E.; *J. Pharm. Sci.* 1981, 70, 87-89.
17. Galvez, E.; Martinez, M.; Gonzalez, J.; Trigo, G. G.; Smith-Verdier, P.; Florencio, F.; Gárcia-Blanco, S.; *J. Pharm. Sci.* 1983, 72, 881-886.
18. Izquierdo, M. L.; Arias, M. S.; Galvez, E.; Rico, B.; Ardid, I.; Sanz, J.; Fonseca, I.; Orjales, A.; Innerarity, A.; *J. Pharm. Sci.* 1991, 80, 554-558.
19. Carroll, F. I.; Coleman, M. L.; Lewin, A. H.; *J. Org. Chem.* 1982, 47, 13-19.
20. Krogsgaard-Larsen, P.; Brehm, L.; Schaumburg, K.; *Acta Chem. Scand. Ser. B* 1981, 35, 311-324.

21. Jacobsen, P.; Labouta, I. M.; Schaumburg, K.; Falch, E.; Krogsgaard-Larsen, P.; *J. Med. Chem.* 1982, 25, 1157-1162.

22. Krogsgaard-Larsen, P.; Brehm, L.; Johansen, J. S.; Vinzents, P.; Lauridsen, J.; Curtis, D. R.; *J. Med. Chem.* 1985, 28, 673-679.

23. Madsen, U.; Schaumburg, K.; Brehm, L.; Curtis, D. R.; Kragsgaard-Larsen, P.; *Acta Chem. Scand. Ser. B* 1986, 40, 92-97.

24. Madsen, U.; Brehm, L.; Schaumburg, K.; Jørgensen, F. S.; Krogsgaard-Larsen, P.; *J. Med. Chem.* 1990, 33, 374-380.

25. Hays, S. J.; Novak, P. M.; Ortwine, D. F.; Bigge, C. F.; Colbry, N. L.; Johnson, G.; Lescosky, L. J.; Malone, T. C.; Michael, A.; Reily, M. D.; Coughenour, L. L.; Brahce, L. J.; Shillis, J. L.; Probert, A., Jr.; *J. Med. Chem.* 1993, 36, 654-670.

26. Esposito, G.; Motta, A.; Temussi, P. A.; *J. Neurochem.* 1983, 40, 903-907.

27. De Leeuw, F. A. A. M.; Altona, C.; *Int. J. Peptide Protein Res.* 1982, 20, 120-125.

28. Höngberg, T.; Norinder, U.; Theoretical and experimental methods in drug design applied on antipsychotic dopamine antagonists, in *A Textbook of Drug Design and Development*; Krogsgaard-Larsen, P. and Bundgaard, H., Eds.; Harwood Academic Publishers: Reading, MA, 1991; pp 55-91.

29. Nichols, D. E.; Jacob, J. N.; Hoffman, A. J.; Kohli, J. D.; Glock, D.; *J. Med. Chem.* 1984, 27, 1701-1705.

30. Karlén, A.; Johansson, A. M.; Kenne, L.; Arvidsson, L. E.; Hacksell, U.; *J. Med. Chem.* 1986, 29, 917-924.

31. Johansson, A. M.; Karlén, A.; Grol, C. J.; Sundell, S.; Kenne, L.; Hacksell, U.; *Mol. Pharmacol.* 1986, 30, 258-269.

32. Johansson, A. M.; Nilsson, J. L. G.; Karlén, A.; Hacksell, U.; Svensson, K.; Carlsson, A.; Kenne, L. Sundell, S.; *J. Med. Chem.* 1987, 30, 1135-1144.

33. Johansson, A. M.; Nilsson, J. L. G.; Karlén, A.; Hacksell, U.; Sanchez, D.; Svensson, K.; Hjorth, S.; Carlsson, A.; Sundell, S.; Kenne. L.; *J. Med. Chem.* 1987, 30, 1827-1837.

34. Mellin, C.; Björk, L.; Karlén, A.; Johansson, A. M.; Sundell, S.; Kenne, L.; Nelson, D. L.; Andén, N.-E.; Hacksell, U.; *J. Med. Chem.* 1988, 31, 1130-1140.

35. Karlén, A.; Helander, A.; Kenne, L.; Hacksell, U.; *J. Med. Chem.* 1989, 32, 765-774.

36. Höök, B. B.; Johansson, A. M.; Hjorth, S.; Sundell, S.; Hacksell, U.; *Chirality* 1993, 5, 112-119.

37. Maryanoff, B. E.; McComsey, D. F.; Inners, R. R.; Mutter, M.S.; Wooden, G. P.; Mayo, S. L.; Olofson, R. A.; *J. Am. Chem. Soc.* 1989, 111, 2487-2496.

38. Casarotto, M. G.; Craik, D. J.; Lloyd, E. J.; *J. Med. Chem.* 1991, 34, 2043-2049.

39. Casarotto, M. G.; Craik, D. J.; Lloyd, E. J.; Partridge, A.C.; *J. Med. Chem.* 1991, 34, 2036-2043.

40. Munro, S. L.; Andrews, P. R.; Craik, D. J.; Gale, D.J.; *J. Pharm. Soc.* 1986, 75, 133-141.

41. Romeo, G.; Aversa, M. C.; Giannetto, P.; Vigorita, M. G.; Ficarra, P.; *Org. Magn. Reson.* 1979, 12, 593-597.

42. Paul, H.-H.; Sapper, H.; Lohmann, W.; Kalinowski, H.-O.; *Org. Magn. Reson.* 1982, 19, 49-53.

43. Chakrabarti, J. K.; Hotten, T. M.; Morgan, S. E.; Pullar, I. A.; Rackham, D. M.; Risius, F. C.; Wedley, S.; Chaney, M. O.; Jones, N. D.; *J. Med. Chem.* 1982, 25, 1133-1140.

44. Kovar, K.-A.; Linden, D.; Breitmaier, E.; *Arch. Pharm. (Weinheim)* 1983, 316, 834-845.

45. Finner, E.; Zeugner, H.; Milkowski, W.; *Arch. Pharm. (Weinheim)* 1984, 317, 79-81.
46. Finner, E.; Zeugner, H.; Milkowski, W.; *Arch. Pharm. (Weinheim)* 1984, 317, 1050-1053.
47. Chidichimo, G.; Longeri, M.; Menniti, G.; Romeo, G.; Ferlazzo, A.; *Org. Magn. Reson.* 1984, 22, 52-54.
48. Carroll, F. I.; Lewin, A. H.; Williams, E. E.; Berdasco, J. A.; Moreland, C. G.; *J. Med. Chem.* 1984, 27, 1191-1195.
49. Migliaccio, G. P.; Shieh, T. L. N.; Byrn, S. R. B.; Hathaway, B. A.; Nichols, D. E.; *J. Med. Chem.* 1981, 24, 206-209.
50. Henkel, J. G.; Sikand, N.; Makriyannis, A.; Gianutsos, G.; *J. Med. Chem.* 1981, 24, 1258-1260.
51. De Jong, A. P.; Fesik, S. W.; Makriyannis, A.; *J. Med. Chem.* 1982, 25, 1438-1441.
52. Solmajer, P.; Kocjan, D.; Solmajer, T.; *Z. Naturforsch. C* 1983, 38, 758-762.
53. Weinstock, J.; Oh, H.-J.; DeBrosse, C. W.; Eggleston, D. S.; Wise, M.; Flaim, K. E.; Gessner, G. W.; Sawyer, J. L.; Kaiser, C.; *J. Med. Chem.* 1987, 30, 1303-1308.
54. Arvidsson, L.-E.; Karlén, A.; Norinder, U.; Kenne, L.; Sundell, S.; Hacksell, U.; *J. Med. Chem.* 1988, 31, 212-221.
55. Liu, Y.; Mellin, C.; Björk, L.; Svensson, B.; Csöregh, I.; Helander, A.; Kenne, L.; Andén, N.-E.; Hacksell, U.; *J. Med. Chem.* 1989, 32, 2311-2318.
56. Glasel, J. A.; *Biochem. Biophys. Res. Comm.* 1981, 102, 703-709.
57. Hexem, J. G.; Frey, M. H.; Opella, S. J.; *J. Am. Chem. Soc.* 1983, 105, 5717-5719.
58. Brown, C. E.; Roerig, S. C.; Fujimoto, J. M.; Burger, V. T.; *J. Chem. Soc. Chem. Commun.* 1983, 1506-1983.
59. Glasel, J. A.; Reiher, H. W.; *Magn. Reson. Chem.* 1985, 23, 236-241.
60. Neville, G. A.; Ekiel, I.; Smith, I. C. P.; *Magn. Reson. Chem.* 1987, 25, 31-35.
61. Pappalardo, G. C.; Radics, L.; Baldo, M.; Grassi, A.; *J. Chem. Soc. Perkin Trans 2* 1985, 955-959.
62. Perly, B.; Pappalardo, G. C.; Grassi, A.; *Z. Naturforsch. B* 1986, 41, 231-238.
63. Vecchietti, V.; Giordani, A.; Giardina, G.; Colle, R.; Clarke, G. D.; *J. Med. Chem.* 1991, 34, 397-403.
64. Vecchietti, V.; Clarke, G. D.; Colle, R.; Giardina, G.; Petrone, G.; Sbacchi, M.; *J. Med. Chem.* 1991, 34, 2624-2633.
65. Froimowitz, M.; DiMeglio, C. M.; Makriyannis, A.; *J. Med. Chem.* 1992, 35, 3085-3095.
66. Eaton, T. A.; Houk, K. N.; Watkins, S. F.; Fronczak, F. R.; *J. Med. Chem.* 1983, 26, 479-486.
67. McMaster, P. D.; Noris, V. J.; Stankard, C. E.; Byrnes, E. W.; Guzzo, P. R.; *Pharm. Res.* 1991, 8, 1013-1020.
68. Glaser, R. Cohen, S.; Donnell, D.; Agranat, I.; *J. Pharm. Sci.* 1986, 75, 772-774.
69. Pierri, L.; Pitman, I. H.; Rae, I. D.; Winkler, D. A.; Andrews, P. R.; *J. Med. Chem.* 1982, 25, 937-942.
70. Kidric, J.; Kocjan, D.; Hadzi, D.; *Croat. Chem. Acta* 1985, 58, 389-397.
71. Kidric, J.; Kocjan, D.; Hadzi, D.; *Experientia* 1986, 42, 327-328.
72. Sadek, M.; Craik, D. J.; Hall, J. G.; Andrews, P. R.; *J. Med. Chem.* 1990, 33, 1098-1107.
73. Ishida, T.; In, Y.; Shibata, M.; Doi, M.; Inoue, M.; Yanagisawa, I.; *Mol. Pharmacol.* 1987, 31, 410-416.

74. Arán, V. J.; Dávila, E.; Francés, M.; Goya, P.; Martinez, A.; Mylonakis, N.; Pardo, I.; *Arzneim.-Forsch.* 1990, 40, 1003-1007.

75. Donetti, A.; Bastiaans, H. M. M.; Kramer, K.; Bietti, G.; Cereda, E.; Dubini, E.; Mondoni, M.; Bast, A.; Timmerman, H.; *J. Med. Chem.* 1991, 34, 1772-1776.

76. Saran, A.; Srivastava, S.; Kulkarni, V. M.; Coutinho, E.; *Indian J. Biochem. Biophys.* 1992, 29, 54-64.

77. Tamir, I.; Mechoulam, R.; Meyer, A. Y.; *J. Med. Chem.* 1980, 23, 220-223.

78. Kane, V. V.; Martin, A. R.; Jaime, C.; Osawa, E.; *Tetrahedron* 1984, 40, 2919-2927.

79. Van der Schyf, C. J.; Mavromoustakos, T; Makriyannis, A.; *Life Sci.* 1988, 42, 2231-2239.

80. Kriwacki, R. W.; Makriyannis, A.; *Mol. Pharmacol.* 1989, 35, 495-503.

81. Knittel, J. J.; Makriyannis, A.; *J. Med. Chem.* 1981, 24, 906-909.

82. Robertson, D. W.; Beedle, E. E.; Swartsendruber, J. K.; Jones, N. D.; Elzey, T. K.; Kauffman, R. F.; Wilson, H.; Hayes, J. S.; *J. Med. Chem.* 1986, 29, 635-640.

83. Moos, W. H.; Humblet, C. C.; Sircar, I.; Rithner, C.; Weishaar, R. E. Bristol, J. A.; McPhail, A. T.; *J. Med. Chem.* 1987, 30, 1963-1972.

84. Toma, L.; Cignarella, G.; Barlocco, D.; Ronchetti, F.; *J. Med. Chem.* 1990, 33, 1591-1594.

85. Natale, N. R.; Triggle, D. J.; Palmer, R. B.; Lefter, B. J. Edwards, W. D.; *J. Med. Chem.* 1990, 33, 2255-2259.

86. Aulabaugh, A. E.; Crouch, R. C.; Martin, G. E.; Ragouzeos, A.; Shockor, J. P.; Spitzer, T. D.; Farrant, R. D.; Hudson, B. D.; Lindon, J. C.; *Carbohydr. Res.* 1992, 230, 201-212.

87. Wynn, H.; Ramesh, M.; Matowe, W. C.; Wolowyk, M. W.; Knaus, E. E.; *Drug Design Delivery* 1988, 3, 245-256.

88. Dei, S.; Romanelli, M. N.; Scapecchi, S.; Teodori, E.; Chiarini, A.; Gualtieri, F.; *J. Med. Chem.* 1991, 34, 2219-2225.

89. Gaggelli, E.; Maccotta, A.; Valensin, G.; *J. Pharm. Sci.* 1992, 81, 367-370.

90. Maccotta, A.; Scibona, G.; Valensin, G.; Gaggelli, E.; Botre, F.; Botre, C.; *J. Pharm. Sci.* 1991, 80, 586-589.

91. Dei, S.; Romanelli, M. N.; Scapecchi, S.; Teodori, E.; Gualtieri, A.; Voigt, W.; Lemoine, H.; *J. Med. Chem.* 1993, 36, 439-445.

92. Tetreault, S.; Ananthanarayanan, V. S.; *J. Med. Chem.* 1993, 36, 1017-1023.

93. Vigorita, M. G.; Previtera, T.; Basile, M.; Fenech, G.; De Pasquale, R. C.; Occhiuto, F.; Circosta, C.; *Farmaco Sci.* 1984, 39, 1008-1023.

94. Smeyers, Y. G.; Cuéllare-Rodriguez, S.; Galvez-Ruano, E.; Ariaz-Pérez, M. S.; *J. Pharm. Sci.* 1985, 74, 47-49.

95. Rossi, C.; Casini, A.; Picchi, M. P.; Laschi, F.; Calabria, A.; Marcolongo, R.; *Biophys. Chem.* 1987, 27, 255-261.

96. Smeyers, Y. G.; Hernandez-Laguna, A.; Munoz-Caro, C.; Aguilera, J.; Galvez-Ruano, E.; Ariaz-Perez, M. S.; *J. Pharm. Sci.* 1989, 78, 764-766.

97. Anderson, N. H.; Lin, B.-S.; Nguyen, K. T.; *Biochem. Biophys. Res. Comm.* 1984, 121, 702-709.

98. Andersen, N. H.; Lin, B.-S.; *Biochemistry* 1985, 24, 2338-2347.

99. Loftus, P.; Bernstein, P. R.; *J. Org. Chem.* 1983, 48, 40-44.

100. Sugiura, M.; Beierbeck, H.; Bélanger, P. C.; Kotovych, G.; *J. Am. Chem. Soc.* 1984, 106, 4021-4025.

101. Kawaki, H.; Beierbeck, H.; Kotowych, G.; *J. Biomol. Struct. Dyn.* 1985, 3, 161-171.

102. Zaagsma, J.; *J. Med. Chem.* 1979, 22, 441-448.

103. Balsamo, A.; Macchia, B.; Macchia, F.; Martinelli, A.; Tognetti, A.; Veracini, C. A.; *Mol. Pharmacol.* 1981, 20, 371-376.
104. Balsamo, A.; Ceccarelli, G.; Crotti, P.; Macchia, B.; Macchia, F.; Tognetti, P.; *Eur. J. Med. Chem. Chim. Ther.* 1982, 17, 471-478.
105. Epifani, E.; Lapucci, A.; Macchia, B.; Macchia, F.; Tognetti, P.; Breschi, M. C.; Del Tacca, M.; Martinotti, E.; Giovannini, L.; *J. Med. Chem.* 1983, 26, 254-259.
106. Thomas, W. A.; Whitcombe, I. W. A.; *J. Chem. Soc. Perkin Trans. 2* 1986, 747-755.
107. Hilton, B. D.; Chmurny, G. N.; Muschik, G. M.; *J. Nat. Prod.* 1992, 55, 1157-1161.
108. Williams, H. J.; Scott, A. I.; Dieden, R. A.; Swindell, C. S.; Chirlian, L. E.; Francl, M. M.; Heerding, J. M.; Krauss, N. E.; *Tetrahedron* 1993, 49, 6545-6560.
109. Dubois, J.; Guénard, D.; Guéritte-Voegelein, F.; Guedira, N.; Potier, P.; Gillet, B.; Beloeil, J.-C.; *Tetrahedron*, 1993, 49, 6533-6544.

# CHAPTER 6

# CONFORMATIONAL ANALYSIS OF PEPTIDES: APPLICATION TO DRUG DESIGN

*Horst Kessler, Robert K. Konat, and Wolfgang Schmitt*

## CONTENTS

I   Introduction ................................................................. 216

II   Special Considerations with Peptides ............................................. 219

III   General Scheme for Structure Determination ............................. 221
   A   Assignment of NMR Resonances to Molecular
     Constitution ........................................................ 222
   B   Extraction of Conformational Parameters ............................. 224
   C   Calculation of 3D Structure Using Experimental
     Restraints .......................................................... 228

IV   Dynamics ................................................................... 229

V   Complexed Molecules ............................................... 230
   A   Transferred NOE ................................................... 231
   B   Mimicking Membranes ............................................. 233
   C   Metal Complexes .................................................. 233

VI   Conformationally Derived Drug Design ............................... 235

0-8493-7824-9/96/$0.00+$.50

**VII** Outlook ................................................................................ 237

**References** ................................................................................ 238

---

# I  INTRODUCTION

Peptides and proteins are extremely important molecules, responsible for many functions, including cellular communication, biochemical responses, and regulation phenomena.[1] Hence, there is increasing research activity on the use of biologically active peptides as drugs or lead compounds for the development of nonpeptidic drugs (peptidomimetics).[2] To understand the biological activities of these molecules a knowledge of their three-dimensional (3D) structure is of great importance.

Peptides may be isolated from natural sources or derived from sequence and/or structural comparison of bioactive sequences. Recently, efficient ways to identify bioactive peptide sequences or analogue polymers by combinatorial methods have been developed.[3] Synthetic peptide libraries[4] or phage libraries[5] help to speed up the identification of bioactive structures dramatically. However, these normally involve flexible structures. This facilitates finding pharmacophoric groups, which are able to reach a large conformational space. Peptoids are good examples of this approach.[6] These flexible structures cannot be used as drugs directly, because their biological activity and receptor selectivity are not yet optimized. The more rigid a molecule is, the higher is its activity, provided the receptor bound conformation is matched. The mimetic approach in rational drug design offers a way to improve these properties. However, the major problem in the development of peptidomimetics is to identify the 3D structural requirements for a defined biological activity. Before topological mimetics can be applied in drug design, extensive studies on lead compounds must be performed (Figure 1).

Usually, peptides with fewer than 20 amino acids do not adopt one predominant conformation in solution.[7] Investigation of the 3D structures of conformationally constrained and bioactive peptides offers a mechanism to overcome this problem of flexibility and elucidate the relationship between molecular structure and biological activity.[8]

NMR spectroscopy has become one of the most important methods for structure determination,[9] and it is currently the only way to determine 3D structures in solution. The latter makes NMR especially important for biological systems, in particular for determining structures of drugs[10] or other biological substrates like peptides,[11] and structures of receptors and drug–receptor complexes.[12] However, there are also severe limitations on the application of NMR to solution structures:

# Rational Drug Design -
# indirect substrate based strategy

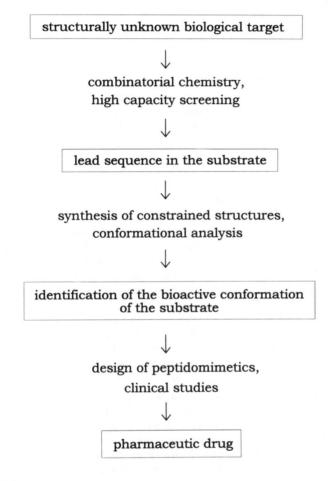

**structurally unknown biological target**

↓

combinatorial chemistry,
high capacity screening

↓

lead sequence in the substrate

↓

synthesis of constrained structures,
conformational analysis

↓

identification of the bioactive conformation
of the substrate

↓

design of peptidomimetics,
clinical studies

↓

**pharmaceutic drug**

**FIGURE 1**
Outline of the indirect approach to rational drug design applicable to peptides. This scheme is complementary to those described in Chapter 2 (Figure 1) and Chapter 3 (Figure 1), but in this case the structure of the receptor is unknown.

- The flexibility of molecules, especially peptides (see below) often does not allow a clear description of **the** solution conformation. Conformational equilibria of more than two structures in slow exchange are difficult to analyse and rapidly equilibrating structures cause averaged NMR parameters, which do not correspond to "mean" conformations (as NMR data are not linearly dependent on structural parameters).[13] This is also true of X-ray crystallographic analysis, although the picture of a single structure (or a few structures) "frozen" in the crystalline state gives the impression of a single, rigid, or at least dominant conformation. Flexible molecules are often difficult to crystallize, and different conformations are found in a single crystal and/or in different crystals.[14] Even in proteins, flexible regions (mainly on the surface and in loops) diffract poorly, and these regions are often modelled without experimental data, only for the purpose of presenting a reasonable X-ray picture.

- The upper limit of molecular size accessible to NMR spectroscopy is in the order of 30 kDa,[15] as outlined in Chapter 4. This limit is mainly caused by line broadening due to fast relaxation, which prohibits some of the sophisticated multidimensional NMR experiments required to obtain sufficient resolution of NMR signals. Molecules of this size also require uniform $^{13}C$, $^{15}N$, and sometimes partial deuterium labelling.[16] This limit may be extended a little in the near future, but NMR studies are currently restricted to very small receptors or receptor–substrate complexes. Alternatively, it is possible to study labelled drugs directly in the bound state by isotope-filtering methods.[17]

- NMR requires dissolved molecules that are tumbling fast and mainly isotropically in solution. This limitation, as well as that of size, is especially serious in studies of membrane-bound complexes such as G-protein-coupled receptors. Anisotropic orientation at membrane interfaces may be important for the structure of a peptidic hormone or drug itself.[18] Whereas vesicles tumble too slowly for high-resolution NMR studies, micellar solutions have been used as membrane mimics. Recently, new experiments have been developed to study membrane-bound peptides by solid-state techniques.[19] However, the information obtained is different than that obtained from high-resolution NMR and will not be discussed here.

- NMR is relatively insensitive. Concentrations of 1 m$M$ are typically the limit of detectability. Limited solubility of macromolecules can be a further obstacle to their structural analysis by NMR. In the case of a 30-kDa protein, it is necessary to dissolve at least 30 mg/ml to obtain a 1-m$M$ solution. Since this is much higher than physiological concentrations, aggregation phenomena often cause additional problems.

Nevertheless, the unique opportunity to investigate molecules in different environments (solvent, membrane, receptor) and of directly studying intermolecular interactions, as well as molecular dynamics, makes NMR, next to X-ray analysis, **the** method for structural studies of drugs.

The determination of molecular constitution and configuration is not the focus of this chapter. It is clear that NMR spectroscopy is well established among other physical and chemical methods in the verification of the molecular constitution of natural products, as well as synthetic drugs.

## II  SPECIAL CONSIDERATIONS WITH PEPTIDES

Backbone conformations of peptides are determined by the three dihedral angles φ, ψ, ω, as shown in Figure 2. The planar peptide bond strongly prefers the trans arrangement (ω = 180°), unless the amide nitrogen is *N*-alkylated (as in proline) or conformational strain (e.g., in small cyclic peptides)[20,21] forces the amide bond into the cis configuration.

There are also preferred dihedral angles for φ and ψ, but the energy difference is small and the interconversion of rotamers about these bonds is very fast (sp$^3$ vs. sp$^2$ centres generally exhibit small barriers of rotation). Conformational energies about φ and ψ of amino acids are mainly sterically controlled and are usually presented as "Ramachandran plots",[22] that is, energy as a function of φ and ψ. Whereas in proteins, φ and ψ angles are mostly, but not always,[23] found close to the calculated Ramachandran energetic minima (φ = −57°, ψ = −47° for α-helices, φ = −139°, ψ = 135° for antiparallel β-sheets), the situation is different for peptides, especially cyclic ones. Conformational strain caused by cyclization or insertion of peptidomimetic fragments into the peptide backbone can induce structural elements with dihedral angles in "forbidden" Ramachandran regions. Bearing in mind that Ramachandran energies were derived only for trans-peptide bond configurations, strong deviations are found especially in structures containing cis-peptide bonds.

Determination of the detailed spatial structures of bioactive peptides is made difficult because of their specific properties: peptides are relatively small molecules with a large surface-to-core ratio. This makes their

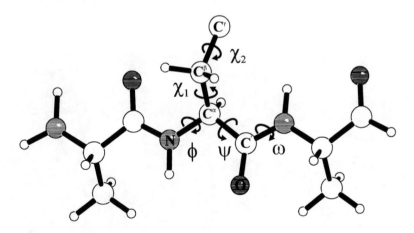

**FIGURE 2**
Model of a peptide backbone with dihedral angles according to IUPAC-IUB nomenclature.

conformations very sensitive to environmental effects. The solvent, membrane, or receptor interacting with the surface of the peptide can change the 3D structure dramatically. Hence, properties such as solubility or aggregation tendencies vary in an unpredictable way. A phenomenon known to every peptide chemist is the ability of a peptide to show dramatically different solubility, even compared to another peptide with a very similar sequence. The small size of peptides also has a direct impact on the availability of distance information. NOE-derived distances between protons provide the most important information for structure determination, but in general there are insufficient numbers of these, especially of the most important long-range NOEs. Protons at the surface can be localized only by distances to protons "inside" the molecule. This situation is very different in proteins, where protons in the core of a molecule are surrounded by many neighbours (Figure 3).

To overcome these problems, the following issues must be addressed:

- Use carefully determined distances. It is not sufficient to classify NOE intensities in peptides as strong, medium, and weak, as often done with proteins. In peptides the information from NOESY or ROESY must be quantified using known, fixed structural features as internal standards (e.g., geminal protons, 1.78 Å). It is also possible to start with an estimated distance as a reference for restrained molecular dynamics (MD) and adjust it iteratively to minimize the deviations between all observed and calculated distances.[24]

- Use diastereotopic assignment of protons (e.g., β-protons in aromatic amino acids) or groups (e.g., methyl groups in Val or Leu) to improve the structure significantly, as distance restraints can be set more precisely.[25]

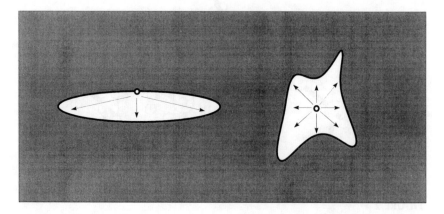

**FIGURE 3**
The large surface-to-core ratio in peptides yields limited NOE data. The position of a proton at the surface (*left*) is determined by distances in one direction only, whereas the proton in the core (*right*) is well determined by surrounding neighbours.

- Use as many parameters as possible to avoid underdetermined systems. The use of homo- and heteronuclear coupling constants[26,67] is necessary for accurate structural determination. Restraints derived from $J$ couplings should be used directly (from the full Karplus curve[27]) in the calculation.

- Use distance geometry (DG) calculations to create a starting structure. Alternatively, use different, manually built structures in restrained MD to avoid any bias. Since DG samples a larger conformational space, starting with DG and refining the structure with MD,[28] where interactions with the solvent can also be simulated,[29] is the recommended procedure.

- Use the same solvent for measurement and calculation. Due to various artifacts, calculating structures of peptides or analogues *in vacuo* is not recommended. It has been demonstrated several times that those structures can be far removed from reality.[30] Explicit force fields for solvents such as water,[31] methanol,[32] chloroform,[33] acetonitrile,[34] DMSO,[35] TFE,[36] and others are available.

- Use different solvents to check the stability of a "unique" conformation. If the structure is identical in different solvents, it is reasonable to assume relatively high conformational rigidity. Such a molecule cannot be transformed into a different conformation (e.g., during the receptor-binding process) without significant loss of energy; the transformation is thus improbable. [13]C spectra can be used to simply check conformational stability (see, e.g., Reference 37). The [13]C chemical shift is very sensitive to changes in configuration and conformation, but less dependent on the solvent. Different conformations usually give significantly different [13]C spectra.

- If possible, try to use cyclized or otherwise constrained peptides with strongly reduced conformational space.[8a]

- If necessary, use experimental conditions that help in structure formation: TFE,[38] micelles,[39] low temperature[40] (combined with cryomixtures[41]), etc. Low temperatures also make it easier to reach the slow tumbling limit, which is advantageous for NOE evaluation.[42]

# III   GENERAL SCHEME FOR STRUCTURE DETERMINATION

The general scheme for structure elucidation of peptides has been described[11,43] and will not be given in detail here. Instead, some techniques of special importance for each step of this procedure are emphasized:

- Assignment of NMR resonances to molecular constitution
- Extraction of conformational parameters

- Calculation of the 3D structure
- Refinement of the structure

## A   Assignment of NMR Resonances to Molecular Constitution

In most free peptides it is sufficient to assign only the proton and carbon resonances because the relatively small numbers of nitrogen atoms do not provide important structural parameters. Multidimensional NMR spectroscopy of free peptides can usually be performed without isotope labelling. However, when a peptide bound to a protein receptor is studied, isotope labelling[10a,44] and the use of heterofiltering techniques[45] are especially important.

The best way to identify the spin system of an amino acid is by a combination of TOCSY[46] and HMQC-COSY[47] or HMQC-TOCSY.[48] If an appropriate TOCSY mixing time is used (*ca.* 80 ms for amino acids), it is possible to identify the proton spin system of every single amino acid. By comparing these data with an HMQC-COSY spectrum, the proton and carbon resonances can be correlated. Here the carbon dimension is used to introduce more chemical-shift dispersion into the spectra, since a homonuclear COSY[49] is often difficult to analyse in crowded regions. An example is shown in Figure 4, which demonstrates the easy assignment of proline resonances in a cyclic peptide.

Isolated proton spin systems such as AM of the $H^N H^\alpha H^{\beta'} H^{\beta''}$ of aromatic amino acids and their sequential neighbours or aromatic protons can be connected using HMBC techniques.[50] The assignment of quaternary carbon resonances is obtained simultaneously. For example, the heteronuclear long-range coupling between the carbonyl carbon and the amide proton of the following amino acid is used to establish sequential assignments in peptides.[51] To avoid circular argumentation, it is recommended that dipolar coupling information (from NOEs) not be used for sequential-assignment purposes, if possible, because identification of connectivity **through bonds** (i.e., the chemical constitution) must be separated from connectivity **in space** (i.e., configuration and conformation). In particular, sequencing by the use of $H_{N_i}$–$H_{\alpha(i-1)}$ NOEs is often not reliable enough and may result in incorrect assignments, or even the wrong primary structure.[52]

Assignment of diasterotopic methylene protons or methyl groups can be achieved by quantitative analysis of coupling constants together with intraresidual NOEs.[53] This is found to be efficient for β-protons but more difficult for glycine α-protons, and sometimes also for the β-, γ-, and δ-protons of proline and the side chains of glutamine, arginine, and lysine. In these cases, a diasterotopic assignment is possible in many cases by

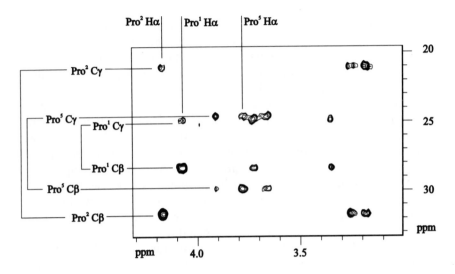

**FIGURE 4**

Part of an $^1$H–$^{13}$C HMQC-TOCSY spectrum of cyclo(–Pro$^1$–Pro$^2$–Tyr$^3$–Val$^4$–Pro$^5$–Leu$^6$–Ile$^7$–Ile$^8$–) in CDCl$_3$ at 300 K and 11.7 Tesla with a TOCSY mixing time of 66 ms. Cβ (at 32 ppm) and Cγ (at 21 ppm) can be unequivocally assigned to the Pro$^2$ spin system (Hα at 4.16 ppm), indicating a cis peptide bond configuration between Pro$^1$ and Pro$^2$. Note that a δ-proton in Pro$^5$ is located to low field from the α-proton. This assignment must be obtained from other spectra, for example, COSY. The sequential assignment also requires other experiments.

combined use of all interproton distances and coupling constants. Such a procedure is mainly used during structural refinement after a preliminary structure has been obtained.

In the case of large peptides, overlapping signals can become a serious problem, even for heteronuclear experiments. In particular, linear peptides, which do not show conformational preferences, exhibit small ranges of chemical shifts close to the values derived for the "random coil." Indeed, the chemical-shift dispersion of amide protons can be used as a first criterion of secondary structure formation in a peptidic compound.[8a]

Sometimes, even in relatively simple compounds, not all signals can be unequivocally assigned with the NMR experiments mentioned above. In the hinge-peptide of human G1 immunoglobulin, for example, a head-to-head dimer of the sequence Ac–Thr–Cys–Pro–Pro$^4$–Cys–Pro–Ala–Pro$^8$–NH$_2$ with two disulfide bridges, the proton and carbon signals of Pro$^4$ and Pro$^8$ show almost total overlap.[30a] Only a strongly folded HSQC spectrum[54] at 14.1 Tesla (600 MHz) yielded sufficient resolution to identify the spin systems.

Actual or apparent symmetry may also be the reason for a reduced number of observed NMR resonances. For example, cyclo(–Gly$_5$–), or cyclo(L–Ala–D–Ala)$_3$ yields only a single set of amino acid signals.[8a,55] Two alternatives may account for this fact: a highly symmetric conformation or rapidly exchanging, nonsymmetric conformations. Without the ability to freeze out the conformational equilibrium, it is not possible to discriminate between these two possibilities.

If more than one conformation is observed (see below) it is possible to prove conformational exchange by NOESY[56] or spin-locked experiments like ROESY or TOCSY. Since in a ROESY[57] spectrum, exchange cross-peaks can be recognized by their sign (exchange cross-peaks appear positive in contrast to negative signals from dipolar coupling),[58] ROESY is the ideal technique for this purpose. In most cases, cis-trans peptide bond isomerization is the main cause of the observed conformational exchange and, as the barriers are of the order of 70–80 kJ/mol, line broadening and coalescence due to exchange is observed in the range 0–1°C. To eliminate the assumption of peptide impurities, often formed by racemization or hydrolytic degradation, conformational exchange should be proven. This experimental proof of chemical exchange is a must for the statement: "Minor signals in the spectrum result from another conformation(s)." Such a statement is sometimes found in the literature without explicit investigation.

The low intensities of signals from minor conformers may prohibit a full assignment of their resonances. In these cases, it is often possible to make an assignment using exchange with signals of the major conformer once its assignments are known.[21b] This approach is one that also finds application in linking the assignments of free and bound ligands in the study of macromolecule–ligand binding interactions, as described in Chapters 8 and 12.

## B   EXTRACTION OF CONFORMATIONAL PARAMETERS

Three-dimensional molecular structures derived from NMR spectroscopy are based mainly on interproton distances and dihedral angles. Distances are obtained from cross-relaxation rates, which can be measured by the buildup rate of the NOE or ROE effect.[59] In the case of signal overlap, heteronuclear editing techniques (e.g., HMQC-NOESY[60], Figure 5) can also be used to identify the origin of an NOE via the adjacent carbon or nitrogen atom. We recently applied this technique successfully to discriminate βI/βII turns by quantitative evaluation of heteronuclear NOEs in a sample with $^{13}$C at natural abundance.[61] Selected characteristic NMR parameters for the most common reverse turns are shown in Figure 6.

Two- and three-dimensional NOE or ROE spectroscopy allows quantitative determination of interproton distances up to about 5 Å with an error of approximately 15%. This procedure has been described before and

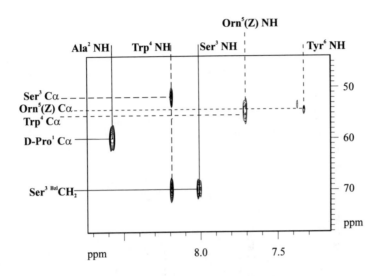

**FIGURE 5**

NH–Cα region of an $^1$H–$^{13}$C HMQC-NOESY spectrum of cyclo(–DPro–Ala–Ser(Bzl)–Trp–Orn(Z)–Tyr–) in $d^6$ DMSO at 300 K and 14.1 Tesla with a NOESY mixing time of 200 ms. The Hα signals of DPro$^1$, Ala$^2$, and Trp$^4$ are completely overlapping; hence it was not possible to identify the NOEs between the NH proton of Ala$^2$ and one of these three α-protons. Editing this NOE at the α-carbons clearly assigned the observed effect to the DPro$^1$ Hα, thus allowing the determination of a βII′ turn in this region. (Cα resonances: DPro$^1$ 59.8; Ala$^2$ 48.4, and Trp$^4$ 56.6 ppm). Integration of cross-peaks in this spectrum gave good agreement with homonuclear spectra, and additional NOEs have been identified.

will not be repeated here;[11] however, we would like to emphasize some important details for quantification of interproton distances:

- NOESY spectra with long mixing times (>400 ms) are often used because, in most cases, a larger number of NOE cross-peaks become available. Since interproton distances can only be correlated to the initial NOE buildup rate, a mixing time longer than 200 ms (at 300 K) should not be used if NOESY cross-peaks are to be quantified for use as interproton distance restraints. Due to spin diffusion, long mixing times cause significant errors in this very important structural parameter set. NOESY and ROESY techniques with long mixing times, however, can play an important role in analysis of conformational exchange processes (see above).[62]

- In ROESY spectra, TOCSY transfer can also be observed, especially when the carrier frequency is set between J-coupled nuclei, or for cross-peaks close to the diagonal. As the sign of these TOCSY signals is positive, this effect can lead to reduced intensity of ROESY cross-peaks[63] (e.g., for intraresidue Hα–Hβ peaks, which are very important for diastereotopic assignments and structural refinement). Due to these effects, NOESY spectra are preferable. It is often possible to lower the temperature and shift the system toward the slow tumbling limit, where

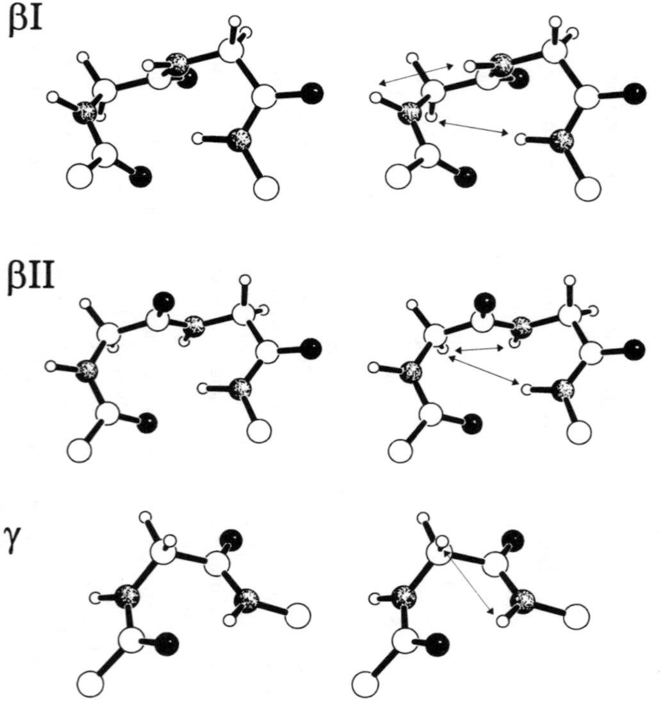

Turns with trans peptide bonds only
(all Hα - Hα distances over 400 pm)

| turn | | $\beta^I$ | $\beta^{II}$ | $\gamma$ |
|---|---|---|---|---|
| characteristic distance | | | | |
| NH(i+1) | NH(i+2) | 260 | 460 | 375 |
| $H_\alpha^R$(i+1) | NH(i+2) | 350 | 205 | 355 |
| $H_\alpha^S$(i+1) | NH(i+2) | 295 | 320 | 250 |
| $^3J_{CH}$ | coupling | | | |
| C'(i) | $H_\alpha^R$(i+1) | -0,8 | -0,8 | 11,3 |
| C'(i) | $H_\alpha^S$(i+1) | 12,6 | 12,6 | 1,1 |
| C'(i+1) | $H_\alpha^R$(i+2) | 2,1 | 11,3 | - |
| C'(i+1) | $H_\alpha^S$(i+2) | 9,8 | 1,1 | - |

βI

βII

γ

FIGURE 6

Stereoplots of the most common reverse turns in peptides chains. The βI′, βII′ and γ′ turns are mirror images in the paper plane of βI, βII, and γ turns, respectively. In these cases the characteristic data involving Hα^R and Hα^S have to be interchanged.

stronger (negative) NOEs will be found (giving positive cross-peaks in NOESY spectra). For example, low-temperature studies of antamanide[64] and cyclosporin A in $CDCl_3$[42] gave excellent NOESY spectra, and a large number of cross-peaks not found at room temperature could be identified. If ROESY spectra are to be analyzed quantitatively, a compensated ROESY is advantageous, and intensity corrections due to offset effects are necessary.[65]

Homo- and heteronuclear three-bond coupling constants yield dihedral angle information via Karplus-type equations.[66] For a quantitative determination of coupling constants from 1D spectra, only resonances that are baseline separated can deliver correct numeric values. For signals in crowded regions, and in the case of broad lines, two-dimensional techniques are necessary. (A recent review is given in Reference 67.) Coupling constants between amide protons and $\alpha$-protons can be obtained either from one-dimensional spectra directly or from COSY or TOCSY cross-peaks when the NH-protons are overlapped. However, in the latter case special attention must be paid to errors caused by partial overlap of antiphase multiplets.[68] There are different techniques to determine $^3J_{NH-H\alpha}$, the easiest of which is the processing of absorptive and dispersive patterns of COSY cross-peaks, and calculation of the coupling constants from peak maxima in the 90° phase-shifted signals.[69] Homonuclear coupling constants such as $^3J_{H\alpha-H\beta}$ may be determined from P.E.COSY spectra.[70] Heteronuclear $^3J_{NH-C\beta}$ coupling constants are easily determined from HETLOC[71] spectra. Analysis of couplings from protons to nuclei not bearing protons is possible using the Titman–Keeler technique[72] (a combination of a special HMBC spectrum and a homonuclear spectrum), which requires a good signal-to-noise ratio and suitable software and computational equipment.

The temperature dependence of NH chemical shifts in polar solvents or deuterium exchange rates can provide information on the orientation of amide protons. Solvent-accessible amide protons show fast deuterium exchange and a strong negative temperature gradient of chemical shift, while slowly exchanging NH-protons with small temperature shifts are shielded from the solvent, mainly by involvement in intramolecular hydrogen bonds.[8a,73]

In some cases, empirical rules allow direct interpretation of chemical shift data to obtain information about the orientation of a carbonyl group:

- A low-field shift of an H$\alpha$ to 5.0 (±0.2) ppm indicates that the preceding carbonyl bond and the C$\alpha$–H$\alpha$ bond are synperiplanar.[74]

- An increased $^{13}C$ chemical shift dispersion of C$\beta$ and C$\gamma$ in a proline residue ($\Delta\delta_{C\beta-C\gamma}$ = ca. 10 ppm) indicates that the preceding carbonyl is configured in a cis peptide bond, while a proline having the more common trans peptide bond shows significantly lower chemical shift dispersion ($\Delta\delta_{C\beta-C\gamma}$ = ca. 5 ppm).[8a,75]

## C   Calculation of 3D Structure Using Experimental Restraints

Distance geometry (DG)[76] calculations use interproton distances and/or *J*-coupling constants (according to the Karplus equations)[29,77] as experimental input and yield a set of 3D structures that are consistent with the NMR data. The initiation of structure calculations with DG as the first step is highly recommended because of its very good conformational sampling properties. Because of this sampling, and the simple geometrical force field, it is a fast and efficient method of generating a starting structure. These structures are then refined by molecular dynamics (MD)[29,78] calculations using a full force field, including explicit solvent. If only a few restraints are available, DG calculations will not converge and may lead to multiple conformations. In those cases, one must start directly with MD. However, even when high-temperature dynamics are used, it is often not possible to search the complete conformational space, and the calculation may be caught in a local minimum. The resulting structure must therefore be checked by performing MD with several, strongly differing, starting structures. The convergence of all these to one single, final structure is necessary for structural confidence. It is advisable to apply coupling constants directly as restraints in MD calculations.[26,27b] Due to the ambiguities of the Karplus curve — up to four possible angles for one *J*-value — this equation has to be used following the procedure of Kim and Prestegard.[27a]

Peptide conformations should not be calculated *in vacuo*. As pointed out above, the solvent strongly influences the conformation and should therefore be included in the form of explicit solvent molecules in MD.[78b] In our experience, the use of solvent mimics such as continuous electrostatic fields leads to unsatisfactory results. Force fields for solvents such as water,[31] methanol,[32] DMSO,[35] chloroform,[33] $CCl_4$[69] and others[34,36] are available, and modern computers allow sufficiently long trajectories (more than 200 ps) of simulations with solvent inclusion in reasonable time (*ca.* 40 h).

The final structure should be refined by carefully checking all measured data and assignments (including stereochemical ones). It must be remembered that differential internal mobility, neglect of conformational equilibria, disagreement in some parameters that have been carefully checked (distances, *J* values), and neglect of spin diffusion can produce misleading results. An additional check of accuracy of a structure can be performed by a long (at least 100 ps) trajectory of "free" MD (MD without any experimental restraints) in a solvent box.[80] If the appropriate force field is used, no further changes in the correct structure should occur. This calculation can provide important data about molecular mobility, averaged geometry, or solvent interactions from radial distribution functions (RDFs[81]). The refinement process is most time consuming, but distinguishes careful and reliable scientific research from lax, overinterpreted routine studies.

# IV DYNAMICS

Peptides containing proline or N-alkylated amino acids, as well as small cyclic peptides, often exist in several conformations due to cis/trans isomerism about amide bonds. The exchange is too fast to isolate these conformers at room temperature, but slow enough to give separate data sets in NMR spectra. In these cases, conformational analysis is especially difficult and may demand the most sophisticated techniques, as well as the highest magnetic field. Usually a conformational change at one peptide bond has a strong local effect, with the conformations of large parts of the molecule unchanged. Consequently, NMR chemical shifts for many residues are very similar. A reliable conformational analysis, however, requires exact assignment and integration of NOE cross-peaks, which may be difficult to obtain and which can be falsified by overlap with peaks of other conformations. The assignment procedure in these cases usually requires heteronuclear editing techniques (e.g., HMQC-NOESY[60]). Three-dimensional NMR spectroscopy with heteroatoms in natural abundance has even been successfully applied for this purpose.[82]

Small signals from minor conformers are much better represented in ROESY or NOESY spectra if temperature and mixing time are in the range where exchange occurs. Due to magnetization transfer into the "small" signal by conformational exchange, strong cross-peaks are observed in these cases. As noted earlier, ROESY is particularly important for this purpose because the different sign of exchange cross-peaks (positive with respect to diagonal signals) and ROE cross-peaks (negative) allows easy differentiation between signals from different conformations and between signals within each conformation.[58]

In terms of NMR spectroscopy, a process of structural interconversion is termed **slow** if multiple sets of signals are obtained for one compound. Often, in this case, exchange between different conformations can be observed via saturation transfer (ROESY, NOESY), as outlined in Chapter 3. A process is **fast** if only one set of signals (due to an averaged structure) is observed. If slow dynamics occurs, it is possible in favourable cases to determine the three-dimensional structures of all conformations populated to more than 10%. Of course, most of the less populated ones do not deliver the same number of structural parameters as the major conformer. Often, the most important long-range NOEs cannot be correctly quantified, and sometimes, they are not even observed due to the poorer signal-to-noise ratio. The determination of heteronuclear coupling constants also becomes more difficult. As previously mentioned, overlapping resonances can cause severe problems, as unambiguous assignment of all corresponding NOEs is not possible. Up to now, a mixture of three conformations has not been quantitatively analysed.

The kinetics of the exchange process can be estimated by varying the mixing time in ROESY experiments and examining the volume integrals of the exchange cross-peaks. A detailed analysis of conformational equilibria is much more difficult, and beyond the scope of this chapter.

Rapidly interconverting conformers can be identified indirectly when NOE restraints and coupling constant restraints do not converge to identical structures. Similarly, when a good NOE dataset shows significant violations in distinct parts of the molecule while other parts are well defined, molecular flexibility may be involved. Coupling constants that differ characteristically in the two (or more) states may be used to prove the assumption of a conformational equilibrium. These examples show that the different averaging properties of $J$ couplings and NOEs can be used to detect conformational averaging.[13] However, a good dataset (sufficient number of parameters to avoid an underdetermined system) is a prerequisite for this to apply. When restrained MD calculations are performed, the experimental restraints force the molecule to a single conformation, which may be different from one of the real structures in equilibrium. To overcome this problem and to allow for flexibility, time-dependent restraints (NOEs,[83] $J$ coupling restraints[84]) have been applied. When a good dataset is available, conformational equilibria can be readily identified with this procedure.[85] Restrained ensemble DG calculations can also be used to search the accessible conformational space of a molecule.[86]

Different motions of distinct molecular regions can sometimes be analysed via carbon spin–lattice relaxation rates and can show which parts of a peptide are more flexible than others.[87] However, as the overall tumbling rate of small molecules (cyclic pentapeptides) is of the same order as the internal flexibility, the Lipari–Szabo approach[88] (i.e., the "model-free" analysis of relaxation parameters by differentiation between overall molecular tumbling and internal mobility) has severe limitations. For large molecules (proteins), the Lipari–Szabo model can be successfully applied.

## V  COMPLEXED MOLECULES

Biological activity has its primary source in the interaction of a bioactive molecule (substrate) with a macromolecule (enzyme, receptor) to form a complex. The structural consequences of complex formation, which can be accompanied by conformational changes in both complexing partners, lead to modulation of properties delivering the specific signal (biological response). For drug design, it is therefore of the utmost importance to know the structure of the bioactive molecule in the bound state.[89] As these systems are significantly larger than free peptides, $^{13}C$ and $^{15}N$ labelling of the macromolecule is advantageous for several reasons:

- The heteronuclei allow for $^{13}C$ and $^{15}N$ editing of NMR signals in multidimensional spectra, greatly increasing the signal dispersion.

- Shorter relaxation times of larger molecules lead to very broad lines. Efficient coherence transfer via one-bond couplings that involve the heteronuclei helps to speed up the pulse sequences and allows for the use of multidimensional techniques.

- Heteronuclear editing allows separate detection of the signals from the receptor or substrate molecule, and allows intramolecular and intermolecular NOEs to be distinguished. Differently labelled receptors and ligands are required for this purpose.[45]

Up to now, only a few complexes of peptides with small receptors have been determined by NMR, including minor groove binders in DNA strands, which are described in Chapter 12.[12a] Other examples involving binding to proteins are given in Chapter 7. Pioneering studies have been reported by Fesik et al.[90] for enzyme-inhibitor complexes of pepsin. Recently, there has been considerable emphasis on studies of complexes of immunosuppressive drugs such as cyclosporin A (CsA), FK506, rapamycin (the structures of which are shown in Figure 7) and ascomycin (structure shown in Chapter 3) with their receptors (cyclophilins and FKBP).[17,91]

In the study of the CsA–cyclophilin complex, the ligand was uniformly labelled with $^{13}C$ and $^{15}N$. The interesting (and, for many researchers, unexpected) result was that the conformation in the bound state[17] is totally different from that found in lipophilic solvents[42,92] and in the crystal structure of CsA.[92b] A similar phenomenon was found for FK506: the crystal conformation[93] is changed when bound to the receptor FKBP (FK-binding protein).[94] In solution, FK506 exhibits two backbone conformations in slow exchange (amide bond isomers),[95] which are similar to the bound and crystal conformation, respectively. On the other hand, the dominant conformation of rapamycin in solution[96] is identical to the crystal structure[97] and the receptor-bound conformation. These studies suggest that induced fit and structural changes during the binding process may occur. As mentioned above, conformational restrictions can pin down these effects when no bound structures exist.

In cases where labelling of the ligand is not available due to (bio)synthetic difficulties, it is possible to use a $^{13}C$- and $^{15}N$-labelled receptor. In measurements of such peptide–receptor complexes, heterofiltering techniques to suppress the macromolecule signals allow the proton resonances of the peptide to be utilized for structural elucidation.

## A    Transferred NOE

Another approach to the study of bound conformation is by transferred NOE,[98] the theory of which is outlined in Chapter 3. For this method to work successfully, a fast equilibrium between bound and free molecules is required. The substrate is added in excess and the free

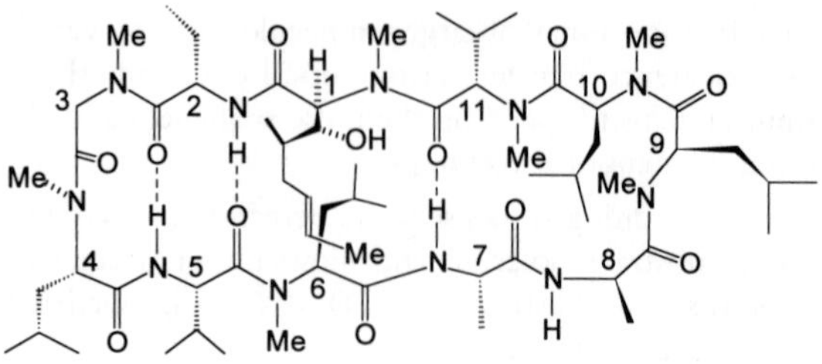

Cyclosporin A

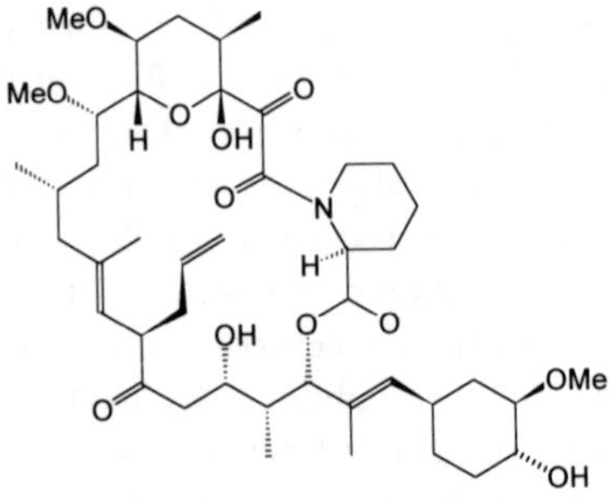

FK506

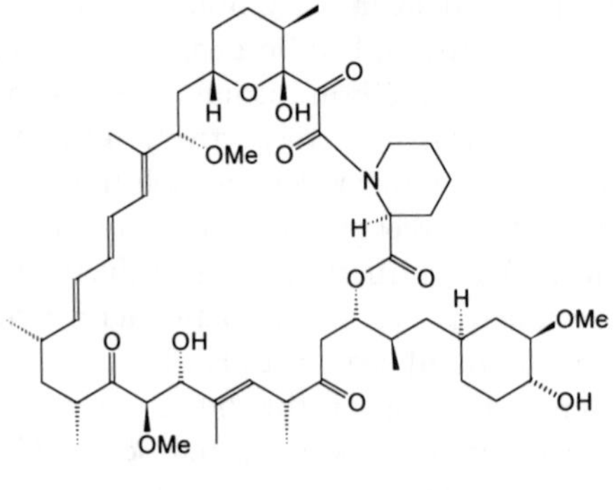

Rapamycin

**FIGURE 7**
Structures of cyclosporin A (CsA), FK506, and rapamycin. Bound and free conformations
of CsA are shown in Figure 7 of Chapter 7.

molecules (small entities) yield sharp signals, whereas the bound ones are
not detectable. In the bound state, the tumbling of the substrate is
significantly reduced, yielding strong negative NOE effects. These are
dominant, and as relaxation is slow compared to the exchange between
free and bound substrate, these negative NOEs are observed on the signals

from the free molecule. A structure calculated on the basis of such transferred NOEs shows the conformation in the **receptor-bound state**. Several examples of this approach are described in Chapter 7. A prerequisite for this procedure is that no nonspecific binding occurs, which is difficult to exclude.[99,100]

## B MIMICKING MEMBRANES

Many receptors are localized in cell membranes and, although their amino-acid sequences have in many cases been determined, few 3D structures are yet known. Among them are the G-protein-coupled receptors, which are targets for many peptide hormones (somatostatin, substance P, neurokinins, etc). So far, no direct study of functioning seven-helix bundles has been reported. Only isolated helical fragments of bacteriorhodopsin have been studied in isotropic media ($CDCl_3$, MeOH).[101]

Linear peptide hormones exhibit essentially random coil conformations in isotropic solvents ($H_2O$, DMSO). Wüthrich and co-workers have shown that in some cases these peptides exhibit specific long-range NOEs when studied in micellar solutions.[102a] The separation of polar and nonpolar phases induces a preferred orientation and conformation. Therefore, numerous NMR measurements of peptides in micelles (mainly SDS, which is relatively inexpensive) have been performed. For example, NMR data obtained for a bradykinin antagonist (HOE140, Figure 8) in SDS-micelles were recently used to calculate the conformation at the interface of a biphasic $CCl_4/H_2O$ system via molecular dynamics calculations with explicit inclusion of solvents.[102b] This demonstrates the information obtainable by combining high-resolution NMR (with micelles as mimics for membranes) with efficient computational techniques (with a two-solvent box as a mimic for membranes).

The structure obtained in this way shows new features compared with previous studies in isotropic media. This information can be used to design new constrained analogues with potential bradykinin-antagonistic activity. However, this structure can be used only as a pointer to new ideas for the synthesis of analogues because the structure at the interface may not be related to the receptor-bound conformation, and the same rearrangements as discussed above for CsA may occur in the process of receptor binding.

## C METAL COMPLEXES

A different situation is found if peptides act as ligands for metal ions. This coordination generally has very strong effects on the molecular conformation of peptides (see, e.g., Reference 103). In many proteins, metal ions are used to stabilize the secondary structure (e.g., the Zn-finger motif of DNA binding proteins). Additionally, the complexed peptides can

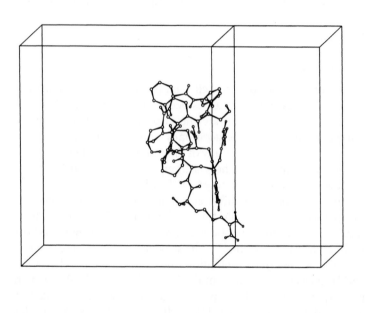

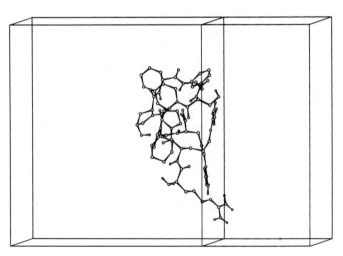

**FIGURE 8**

Stereoscopic view of HOE140 [H–DArg–Arg–Pro–Hyp–Gly–Thi–Ser–DTic–Oic–Arg–OH] calculated in a box of $H_2O$ (upper part) and $CCl_4$ (lower part) as a biphasic membrane mimetic. All guanidino groups of Arg residues and the Ser OH are oriented into the $H_2O$ phase, while Hyp OH forms an intramolecular hydrogen bond in the $CCl_4$ phase.

show dramatically different solution properties compared to the free peptide.[37,104] In the case of metal ions complexed by peptides, the use of NMR-active metal nuclei allows one to obtain additional structural parameters like metal-binding sites and the type of metal binding (ionic or covalent).[105] In the case of strong complexation, the adduct containing a desired metal ion can be easily detected (e.g., by FAB-MS). The complex field of metal-bound peptide conformations will not be discussed here.

# VI  CONFORMATIONALLY DERIVED DRUG DESIGN

The high flexibility of linear peptides prevents their use in conformation–activity relationships studies, especially if one takes into account the mutually induced fit of the ligand and its receptor. Cyclic peptides with drastically reduced conformational space are much better suited for this purpose.[8a] Cyclic peptides have the following advantages compared with their linear counterparts:

- They have higher metabolic stability due to slower enzymatic degradation.
- They have higher receptor selectivity as different receptors may bind different conformations.
- In the case of a matched receptor–ligand fit, binding should be stronger due to a lower loss of entropy.

A global constraint,[106] like cyclization, can be introduced into peptides by different strategies at different positions[8]: the C- and/or N-terminus, the side-chain groups, or even at Cα and the backbone nitrogen.[80,107] In small cyclic peptides (up to seven amino acids) conformational behaviour is dominated by local constraints (like chirality at the α-carbon or amide alkylation). As the size of the cycle is increased, the number of low-energy conformations tolerated by the global constraint is also increased. For example, in antamanide, a cyclic decapeptide, several amide plane rotations are found in chloroform solution.[108] Thus in large cyclic peptides, matrix effects (like polarity, ionic strength, or hydrogen donor and acceptor potential) have a major impact on conformational processes. Cyclosporin A, a cyclic undecapeptide mentioned several times in this chapter, which contains seven alkylated amide bonds, exhibits at least eight conformations in DMSO and at least four in methanol; in chloroform, however, one strongly dominant (>95%) conformation is found.

The backbone structures of small cyclic peptides have been studied extensively, and this experience can be used to force a distinct peptide sequence into a specific 3D arrangement. Chirality of the amino acids is of particular importance. In the case of cyclic penta- and hexapeptides, a series of scaffolds constructed from a set of D- and L-amino acids can be used. For example, in a cyclic penta- or hexapeptide with the sequence $c(\mathrm{DL}_n)$ [$n$ = 4,5], the D-amino acid always prefers the $i + 1$ position of a βII′ turn. Structure–activity studies have shown that the active sequence –Phe–Trp–Lys–Thr– of somatostatin seems to form a β-turn at the receptor. This is strongly supported by the fact that enhanced activity is observed with the sequence –Phe–DTrp–Lys–Thr–. Hence, cyclic structures of cyclo(–Xaa–Phe–DTrp–Lys–Phe–Ybb–) have almost the same somatostatin activity as the full molecule.[109]

This example shows how the concept of conformationally derived drug design has been applied to a series of peptides containing the active sequence of somatostatin (–Phe–Trp–Lys–Thr–) for optimization of the cytoprotective activity.[110] Another example relates to the sequence important for cell–cell and matrix–cell adhesion (–Arg–Gly–Asp–),[111] i.e., the so-called RGD sequence. By way of background, the relatively rigid backbone conformation found in the "side chain-free" stem peptide cyclo(–DAla¹–Ala–DAla³–Ala₂–) exhibits a βII′/γ conformation (Figure 9), with DAla³ in the $i + 1$ position of the βII′ turn and DAla¹ at the $i + 1$ position of the γ turn. This knowledge can be applied to generate different side-chain orientations in the cyclic pentapeptide –Arg–Gly–Asp–Phe–Val–. For example, incorporation of DPhe generates a cyclic peptide with backbone chirality analogous to that of the stem peptide above, since glycine can occupy the conformational space of either a D- or an L-amino acid. In this case DPhe occupies the $i + 1$ position of the βII′ turn (as for D-Ala³ in the stem peptide), and glycine

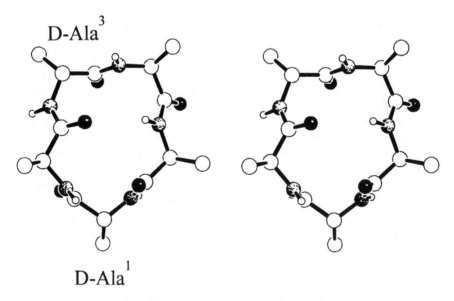

**D-Ala**³

**D-Ala**¹

**FIGURE 9**
Stereoview of cyclo(–DAla–Ala–DAla–Ala₂–).

D-Phe

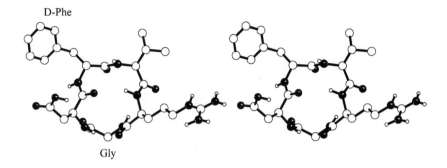

Gly

**FIGURE 10**
Stereoview of cyclo(-DVal–Arg–Gly–Asp–Phe–).

occupies the $i + 1$ position of the γ-turn, like DAla[1] in the stem peptide. The resulting peptide presents the RGD sequence with the side chains oriented as shown in Figure 10. This peptide is a very potent and selective inhibitor for the $\alpha_v\beta_3$ integrin,[111,112] which is important for inhibiting angiogenesis and inducing apoptosis in human tumour cells.[113]

Another way to achieve higher metabolic stability is the synthesis of retroinverso analogues, in which the peptide sequence is reversed, and at the same time, the chirality of each residue is inverted.[114] In these derivatives the orientations of the side chains (which represent "pharmacophoric groups") are similar to the parent peptide, if the hydrogen bonding of the amide groups in the backbone is disregarded. This first-order approximation is certainly not true for cyclic peptides, and it is not surprising to find different biological activities between "normal" cyclopeptides and their retroinverso analogues. Also, for cases when the amide bonds do participate in receptor binding, their reversal results in a loss of activity. The retroinverso concept, however, does allow the design of peptide backbones with a high D-amino acid content and similar side-chain orientations, or it can provide an additional variety of possible 3D arrangements of side-chain orientations.

The modification, or even replacement, of peptide bonds by analogues (e.g., thioamides), and side-chain cyclization, can provide increased enzymatic stability. With knowledge of the spatial orientation of the pharmacophore, it is possible to find nonpeptidic scaffolds (e.g., via the computer program CAVEAT[115]), which may eventually be developed into an orally active drug. This overall concept has been successfully used,[2b,116] and the field of peptidomimetics is certainly an open one for future drug research.

# VII OUTLOOK

Presently, more and more chemists are trying not only to generate new structures but also to design compounds with higher biological activity, higher (receptor/tissue) selectivity and higher bioavailability in well-defined biological systems. As peptides and proteins play a key role in biological processes, peptide-derived drugs are a major goal in drug design, as was indicated in Chapter 1. The use of peptides offers a very flexible and modular approach since almost all of the more than 2000 known amino acids can be used for synthesis. NMR spectroscopy combined with appropriate computational methodology for structural elucidation, together with X-ray crystallography, constitute the best method for the development of structure–activity relationships (SAR) in drug design. A major drawback of peptidic drugs, however, is their low bioavailability and low metabolic stability. The rational approach involving the design of peptidomimetics is one way to overcome these problems. The same procedure also becomes more important with modern screening via combinatorial techniques (e.g., peptide libraries), which yield peptides or other oligomers with high receptor-binding affinities. The approach to designing real drugs from these "active sequences" is similar to that outlined above. In the near future, when the number of known biological receptors increases, rational drug design based on SAR will become much more efficient.

# REFERENCES

1. Ward, D.J., Ed.; *Peptide Pharmaceuticals*; Open University Press: Milton Keynes, UK, 1991.
2. (a) Olson, G.L.; Bolin, D.R.; Bonner, M.P.; Bos, M.; Cook, C.M.; Frey, D.C.; Graves, B.J.; Hatada, M.; Hill, D.E.; Kahn, M.; Madison, V.S.; Rusiecki, V.K.; Sarabu, R.; Sepinwall, J.; Vincent, G.P.; *J. Med. Chem.* 1993, 36, 3039-3049. (b) Giannis, A.; Kolter, T.; *Angew. Chem.* 1993, 32, 1244-1267. (c) Liskamp, R.M.J.; *Recl. Trav. Chim. Pays-Bas* 1994, 113, 1-19.
3. (a) Kurth, M.J.; Ahlberg-Randall, L.A.; Chen, C.; Melander,C.; Müller, R.B.; *J. Org. Chem.* 1994, 59, 5862-5864. (b) Felder, E.R.; *Chimia* 1994, 48, 531-541.
4. (a) Lam, K.S.; Salomon, S.E.; Hersh, E.M.; Hruby, V.J.; Kazimierski, W.M.; Knapp, R.J.; *Nature* 1990, 354, 82-84. (b) Houghton, R.J.; Pinilla, C.; Blondelle, S.E.; Appel, J.R.; Dooley, C.T.; Cuervo, J.H.; *Nature* 1990, 354, 84-86. (c) Jung, G.; Beck-Sickinger, A.G.; *Angew. Chem. Int. Ed. Engl.* 1992, 31, 367-383.
5. (a) Parmley, S.F.; Smith, G.P.; *Gene* 1988, 73, 305-318. (b) Cull, M.G.; Miller, J.F.; Schatz, P.J.; *Proc. Natl. Acad. Sci. USA* 1991, 89, 1865-1869. (c) Brenner, S.; Lerner, R.A.; *Proc. Natl. Acad. Sci. USA* 1992, 89, 5381-5383. (d) Burton, D.R.; *Acc. Chem. Res.* 1993, 26, 405-411.
6. (a) Kessler, H.; *Angew. Chem. Int. Ed. Engl.* 1993, 32, 543-544. (b) Simon, R.J.; Kania, R.S.; Zuckermann, R.N.; Huebner, V.D.; Jewell, D.A.; Tan, R.; Frankel, A.D.; Santi, D.V.; Cohen, F.E.; Bartlett, P.A.; *Proc. Natl. Acad. Sci. USA* 1992, 89, 9367-9371.
7. Dyson, H.J.; Rance, M.; Houghton, R.A.; Lerner, R.A.; Wright, P.E.; *J. Mol. Biol.* 1988, 201, 161-200.
8. (a) Kessler, H.; *Angew. Chem. Int. Ed. Engl.* 1982, 21, 512-523. (b) Hruby, V.; *Life Sci.* 1982, 31, 189-199. (c) Gilon, C.; Halle, D.; Chorev, M.; Selinger, Z.; Byk, G.; *Biopolymers* 1991, 31, 745-750.

9. Wüthrich, K.; *NMR of Proteins and Nucleic Acids*; John Wiley & Sons: New York, 1986.

10. (a) Zuiderwe.g., E.R.P.; van Doren, S.R.; Kurochkin, A.V.; Neubig, R.R.; Majumdar, A.; *Perspectives in Drug Discovery and Design* 1993, 1, 391-417. (b) Jaroszewki, J.W.; Schaumburg, K.; Kofod, H., Eds; *NMR Spectroscopy in Drug Research;* Munksgaard: Copenhagen, 1988.

11. Kessler, H.; Seip, S.; NMR of peptides, in *Two-Dimensional NMR Spectroscopy: Applications for Chemists and Biochemists*; Croasmun, W.R.; Carlson, R., Eds; VCH Publishers: New York, 1994; pp. 619-654.

12. (a) Embrey, K.J.; Searle, M.S.; Craik, D.J.; *Eur. J. Biochem.* 1993, 211, 437. (b) Thériault, X.; Logan, T.M.; Meadows, R.; Yu, L.; Olejniczak, E.T.; Holzman, T.F.; Simmer, R.L.; Fesik, S.; *Nature* 1993, 361, 88-91. (c) Petros, A.M.; Gampe, R.T.; Gemmecker, G.; Neri, P.; Holzman, T.F.; Edalji, R.; Hochloewski, J.; Jackson, J.; McAlpin, J.; Luly, J.R.; Pilotmatias, T.; Pratt, S.; Fesik, S.W.; *J. Med. Chem.* 1991, 34, 2925-2928.

13. Jardetzky, O.; *Biochim. Biophys. Acta* 1980, 621, 227-232.

14. (a) Flippen-Anderson, J.L.; Deschamps, J.R.; Ward, K.B.; George, C.; Houghten, R.; *Int. J. Peptide Protein Res.* 1994, 44, 97-104. (b) Doi, M.; Ishibe, A.; Shinozaki, H.; Urata, H.; Inoue, M.; Ishida, T.; *Int. J. Peptide Protein Res.* 1994, 43, 325-331.

15. Wagner, G.; *J. Biomol. NMR* 1993, 3, 375-385.

16. Grzesiek, S.; Anglister, J.; Ren, H.; Bax, A.; *J. Am. Chem. Soc.* 1993, 115, 4369-4370.

17. (a) Weber, C.; Wider, G.; von Freyberg, B.; Traber, R.; Braun, W.; Widmer, H.; Wüthrich, K.; *Biochemistry* 1991, 30, 6563-6574. (b) Fesik, S.W.; Gampe, R.T.; Eaton, H.L.; Gemmecker, G.; Olejniczak, E.T.; Neri, P.; Holzman, T.F.; Egan, D.A.; Edalji, R.; Simmer, R.; Helfrich, R.; Hochloewski, J.; Jackson, M.; *Biochemistry* 1991, 30, 6574-6583.

18. (a) Schwyzer, R.; *Natural Products and Biological Activities*; Imura, H.; Gato, T.; Murachi, T.; Nakajima, T., Eds.; Tokyo Press, Elsevier: Tokyo, 1986; pp. 197-207. (b) Schwyzer, R. *Biopolymers* 1991, 31, 785-792.

19. (a) Creuzet, F.; McDermott, A.; Gebhard, R.; van der Hoef, K.; Spijker-Assink, M.B.; Herzfeld, J.; Lugtenburg, J.; Levitt, M.H.; Griffin, R.G.; *Science* 1991, 251, 783-786. (b) Griffiths, J.M.; Lakshmi, K.V.; Bennet, A.E.; Raap, J.; van der Wielan, C.M.; Lugtenburg, J.; Herzfeld, J.; Griffin, R.G.; *J. Am. Chem. Soc.* 1994, 116, 10178-10181. (c) Ketchem, R.R.; Hu, W.; Tian, F.; Cross, T.A.; *Structure* 1994, 2, 699-701.

20. (a) Kessler, H.; Krämer, P.; Krack, G.; *Israel J. Chem.* 1980, 20, 188-195. (b) Kato, T.; Tone, Y.; Lee, S.; Shimohigashi, Y.; Izumiya, N.; *Chem. Lett.* 1985, 1209-1212, (c) Terada, Y.; Kawai, M.; Rich, D.H.; *Int J. Peptide Protein Res.* 1989, 33, 3-10.

21. (a) Mierke, D.F.; Yamazaki, T.; Said-Nejad, O.E.; Felder, E.R.; Goodman, M.; *J. Am. Chem. Soc.* 1989, 111, 6847-6849. (b) Kessler, H.; Anders, U.; Schudok, M.; *J. Am. Chem. Soc.* 1990, 112, 5908-5916.

22. Ramachandran, G.N.; Sassekharan, V.; *Adv. Protein Chem.* 1968, 28, 283-438.

23. (a) Ludwigsen, S.; Poulsen, F.M.; *J. Biomol. NMR* 1992, 2, 227-233. (b) Nicholson, H.; Söderlind, E.; Tronrud, D.E.; Matthews, B.W.; *J. Mol. Biol.* 1989, 210, 181-193. (c) Overington, J.; Johnson, M.S.; Sali, A.; Blundell, T.L.; *Proc. Roy. Soc. Lond. B* 1990, 241, 132-145.

24. Kessler, H.; Kerssebaum, R.; Klein, A.; Obermeier, R.; Will, M.; *Liebigs Ann. Chem.* 1989, 269-294.

25. Günthert, P.; Braun, W.; Billeter, M.; Wüthrich, K.; *J. Am. Chem. Soc.* 1989, 111, 3997-4004.

26. (a) Mierke, D.F.; Kessler, H.; *Biopolymers* 1993, <u>33</u>, 1003-1017. (b) Eberstadt, M.; Mierke, D.F.; Köck, M.; Kessler, H.; *Helv. Chim. Acta* 1992, <u>75</u>, 2583-2592. (c) Mierke, D.F.; Golic-Grdadolnik, S.; Kessler, H.; *J. Am. Chem. Soc.* 1992, <u>114</u>, 8283-8284.

27. (a) Kim, Y.; Prestegard, H.; *Proteins: Struc. Function Genet.* 1990, <u>8</u>, 377-385. (b) Mierke, D.F.; Kessler, H.; *Biopolymers* 1992, <u>32</u>, 1277-1282.

28. Lautz, J.; Kessler, H.; Blaney, J.M.; Scheek, R.M.; van Gunsteren, W.; *Int. J. Peptide Protein Res.* 1989, <u>33</u>, 281-288.

29. van Gunsteren, W.F.; Berendsen, H.J.C.; *Angew. Chem. Int. Ed. Engl.* 1990, <u>29</u>, 992-1023.

30. (a) Kessler, H.; Mronga, S.; Müller, G.; Moroder, L.; Huber, R.; *Biopolymers* 1991, <u>31</u>, 1189-1204. (b) Kurz, M.; Mierke, D.F.; Kessler, H.; *Angew. Chem. Int. Ed. Engl.* 1992, <u>31</u>, 210-212..

31. Berendsen, H.J.C.; Postma, J.P.M.; van Gunsteren, W.F.; Hermans, J.; in *Intermolecular Forces*; Pullman, B., Ed; Reidel: Dordrecht, 1981.

32. (a) Jorgensen, W.L.; *J. Am. Chem. Soc.* 1980, <u>102</u>, 543-549. (b) Jorgensen, W.L.; *J. Phys. Chem.* 1986, <u>90</u>, 1276-1284.

33. (a) Jen, M.; Lide, D.R.; *J. Chem. Phys.* 1962, <u>36</u>, 2525-2526. (b) Jorgensen, W.L.; Briggs, J.M.; Contreras, M.L.; *J. Phys. Chem.* 1990, <u>94</u>, 1683-1686.

34. (a) Jorgensen, W.L.; Briggs, J.M.; *Molec. Phys.* 1988, <u>63</u>, 547-558. (b) Maroncelli, M.; *J. Chem. Phys.* 1991, <u>94</u>, 2084-2103.

35. (a) Allinger, N.L.; Kao, J.; *Tetrahedron* 1976, <u>32</u>, 529-536. (b) Itoh, S.; Ohtaki, H.; *Z. Naturforsch.* 1987, <u>42a</u>, 858-862. (c) Rao, B.G.; Singh, U.C.; *J. Amer. Chem. Soc.* 1990, <u>112</u>, 3803-3811; (d) Kessler, H.; Mierke, D., *J. Am. Chem. Soc.* 1991, <u>113</u>, 9466–9470.

36. De Loof, H.; Nilsson, L.; Rigler, R.; *J. Am. Chem. Soc.* 1992, <u>114</u>, 4028-4035.

37. Kessler, H.; Gehrke, M.; Lautz, J.; Köck, M.; Seebach, D.; Thaler, A.; *Biochem. Pharmacol.* 1990, <u>40</u>, 169-173.

38. (a) Nelson, J.W.; *Biochemistry* 1989, <u>28</u>, 5256-5261. (b) Storrs, R.W.; Truckses, D.; Wimmer, D.E.; *Biopolymers* 1992, <u>32</u>, 1695-1702.

39. Lee, K.H.; Fitton, J.E.; Wüthrich, K.; *Biochim. Biophys. Acta* 1987, <u>911</u>, 144-153.

40. (a) Kopple, K.D.; Baures, P.W.; Bean, J.W.; D'Ambrosio, C.A.; Hughes, J.L.; Peishoff, C.E.; Egglestone, D.E.; *J. Am. Chem. Soc.* 1992, <u>114</u>, 9615-9623. (b) Bean, J.W.; Kopple, K.D.; Peishoff, C.E.; in *Peptides 1992*; Schneider, C.H; Eberle, A.N., Eds; ESCOM Science Publishers: Leiden, 1993; pp. 545-546.

41. (a) Fesik, S.W.; Olejniczak, E.T.; *Magn. Reson. Chem.* 1987, <u>25</u>, 1046-1048. (b) Motta, A.; Picone, D.; Tancredi, T.; Temussi, P.A.; *J. Magn. Reson.* 1987, <u>75</u>, 364-370. (c) Temussi, P.A.; Picone, D.; Saviano, G.; Amodeo, P.; Motta, A.; Tancredi, T.; Salvadori, S.; Tomatis, R.; *Biopolymers* 1990, <u>32</u>, 367-372.

42. Kessler, H.; Köck, M.; Wein, T.; Gehrke, M.; *Helv. Chim. Acta* 1990, <u>73</u>, 1818-1832.

43. (a) Hermans, J., Ed.; *Molecular Dynamics and Protein Structure*; Polycrystal Bookservice: Western Springs, IL, 1985. (b) McCammon, J.A.; Harvey, S.C.; *Dynamics of Proteins and Nucleic Acids*; Cambridge University Press: Cambridge, 1987. (c) Case, D.A.; Wright, P.E.; in *NMR of Proteins*; G.M. Clore, A.M. Gronenborn, Eds; Macmillan Press Ltd: London, 1993; pp. 53-91. (d) Barsukov, I.L.; Lian, L-Y.; *NMR of Macromolecules, A Practical Approach*; Roberts, G.C.K., Ed.; Oxford University Press: Oxford, 1993; pp. 315-357. (e) Sutcliffe, M.J.; *NMR of Macromolecules, A Practical Approach*; Roberts, G.C.K., Ed.; Oxford University Press: Oxford, 1993; pp. 359-390. (f) Kessler, H.; Eberstadt, M.; Schmitt, W.; in *NMR of Biological Macromolecules*; Stassinopoulou, C.I., Ed.; NATO ASI Ser., Vol. H87; Springer-Verlag: Berlin, 1994; pp. 171-188.

44. (a) Clore, G.M.; Gronenborn, A.M.; *Progr. NMR Spectrosc.* 1991, 23, 43-92. (b) Oschkinat, H.; Müller, T.; Diekmann, T. *Angew. Chem. Int. Ed. Engl.* 1994, 32, 277-294.
45. (a) Otting, G.; Wüthrich, K.; *Q. Rev. Biophys.* 1990, 23, 39-96. (b) Fesik, S.W.; *J. Biomol. NMR* 1993, 3, 261-269.
46. (a) Braunschweiler, L.; Ernst, R.R.; *J. Magn. Reson.* 1983, 53, 521-528. (b) Bax, A.; Byrd, R.A.; Aszalos, A.; *J. Am. Chem. Soc.* 1984, 106, 7632-7633. (c) Bax, A.; Davis, D.G.; *J. Magn. Reson.* 1985, 65, 355-360. (d) Griesinger, C.; Otting, G.; Wüthrich, K.; Ernst, R.R.; *J. Am. Chem. Soc.* 1988, 110, 7870-7872.
47. Clore, G.M.; Gronenborn, A.M.; *Crit. Rev. Biochem. Mol. Biol.* 1989, 24, 479-564.
48. Lerner, A.; Bax, A.; *J. Magn. Reson.* 1986, 69, 375-380.
49. (a) Aue, W.P.; Bartholdi, V.; Ernst, R.R.; *J. Chem. Phys.* 1976, 64, 2229-2246. (b) Nagayama, N.; Kumar, A.; Wüthrich, K.; Ernst, R.R.; *J. Magn. Reson.* 1980, 40, 321-334. (c) Piantini, U.; Sørensen, O.W.; Ernst, R.R.; *J. Am. Chem. Soc.* 1982, 104, 6800-6801. (d) Rance, M.; Sørensen, O.W.; Bodenhausen, G.; Wagner, G.; Ernst, R.R.; Wüthrich, K.; *Biochem. Biophys. Res. Commun.* 1983, 117, 458-479.
50. Bax, A.; Summers, M.F.; *J. Am. Chem. Soc.* 1986, 108, 2093-2094.
51. (a) Kessler, H.; Griesinger, C.; Zarbock, J.; Loosli, R.; *J. Magn. Reson.* 1984, 57, 331-336. (b) Kessler, H.; Griesinger, C.; Lautz, J.; *Angew. Chem. Int. Ed. Engl.* 1984, 23, 444-459. (c) Griesinger, C.; Bermel, W.; Wagner, K.; *J. Magn. Reson.* 1989, 83, 223-232. (d) Kessler, H.; Schmieder, P.; Köck, M.; Kurz, M.; *J. Magn. Reson.* 1990, 88, 615-618.
52. Konat, R.K.; Mathä, B.; Winkler, J.; Kessler, H.; *Liebigs Ann.* 1995, 765-775.
53. (a) Kessler, H.; Griesinger, C.; Wagner, K.; *J. Am. Chem. Soc.* 1987, 109, 6927-6933. (b) Kuo, M.C.; Gibbons, W.A.; *Biochemistry* 1979, 26, 5855-5867.
54. Bodenhausen, G.; Ruben, D.J.; *Chem. Phys. Lett.* 1980, 69, 185-189.
55. Unpublished data from authors' laboratory.
56. Jeener, J.; Meier, B.H.; Bachmann, P.; Ernst, R.R.; *J. Chem. Phys.* 1979, 71, 4546-4553.
57. (a) Bothner-By, A.A.; Stevens, R.L.; Lee, J.; Warren, C.D.; Jeanloz, R.W.; *J. Am. Chem. Soc.* 1984, 106, 811-813. (b) Bax, A.; Davis, D.G.; *J. Magn. Reson.* 1985, 63, 207-213. (c) Kessler, H.; Griesinger, C.; Kerssebaum, R.; Wagner, K.; Ernst, R.R.; *J. Am. Chem. Soc.* 1987, 109, 607-609.
58. (a) Kessler, H.; Gehrke, M.; Griesinger, C.; *Angew. Chem. Int. Ed. Engl.* 1988, 27, 490-536. (b) Bax, A.; Davis, D.G.; *J. Magn. Reson.* 1985, 64, 533-535.
59. Kumar, A.; Wagner, G.; Ernst, R.R.; Wüthrich, K.; *J. Am. Chem. Soc.* 1981, 103, 3654-3658.
60. (a) Fesik, S.W.; Zuiderweg, E.R.P.; *J. Magn. Reson.* 1988, 78, 583-593. (b) Gronenborn, A.M.; Bax, A.; Wingfield, P.T.; Clore, G.M.; *FEBS Lett.* 1989, 243, 93-98.
61. Matter, H.; Gemmecker, G.; Kessler, H.; *Int. J. Peptide Protein Res.* 1995, 45, 430-440.
62. Mierke, D.F.; Dürr, H.; Kessler, H.; Jung, G.; *Eur. J. Biochem.* 1992, 206, 39-48.
63. Cavanagh, J.; Keeler, J.; *J. Magn. Reson.* 1988, 80, 186-194.
64. Kessler, H.; Bats, J.W.; Lautz, J.; Müller, A.; *Liebigs Ann. Chem.* 1989, 913-928.
65. (a) Griesinger, C.; Ernst, R.R.; *J. Magn. Reson.* 1987, 75, 261-271. (b) Bax, A.; *J. Magn. Reson.* 1988, 77, 134-147.
66. (a) Bystrov, V.F.; *Progr. NMR Spectrosc.* 1976, 10, 41-81. (b) Kopple, K.D.; Wiley, G.R.; Tauke, R.; *Biopolymers* 1973, 12, 527-636.

67. Eberstadt, M.; Gemmecker, G.; Mierke, D.F.; Kessler, H.; *Angew. Chem. Int. Ed. Engl.* 1995, 34, 2001-2025.

68. Kessler, H.; Müller, A.; Oschkinat, H.; *Magn. Reson. Chem.* 1985, 23, 844-852.

69. Kim, Y.; Prestegard, J.H.; *J. Magn. Reson.* 1989, 84, 9-13.

70. Mueller, L.; *J. Magn. Reson.* 1987, 72, 191-196.

71. (a) Kurz, M.; Schmieder, P.; Kessler, H.; *Angew. Chem. Int. Ed. Engl.* 1992, 30, 1329-1331. (b) Schmieder, P.; Kessler, H.; *Biopolymers* 1992, 32, 435-440.

72. (a) Titman, J.J.; Neuhaus, D.; Keeler, J.; *J. Magn. Reson.* 1989, 85, 111-131. (b) Richardson, J.M.; Titman, J.J.; Keeler, J.; *J. Magn. Reson.* 1991, 93, 533-553.

73. (a) Ovchinnikov, Y.; Ivanov, V.T.; *Tetrahedron* 1975, 31, 2177-2209. (b) Llinas, M.; Klein, M.P.; *J. Am. Chem. Soc.* 1975, 97, 4731-4737. (c) Bara, Y.A.; Friedrich, A.; Kessler, H.; Molter, M.; *Chem. Ber.* 1978, 111, 1045-1057.

74. Rich, D.H.; Bhatnagar, P.K.; *J. Am. Chem. Soc.* 1978, 100, 2212-2218.

75. Deber, C.M.; Madison, V.; Blout, V.; *Acc. Chem. Res.* 1976, 9, 106-113.

76. (a) Crippen, G.M.; Havel, T.F.; *Distance Geometry and Molecular Conformation*; John Wiley & Sons: New York, 1988. (b) Braun, W.; *Q. Rev. Biophys.* 1987, 19, 115-157. (c) Havel, T.F.; Wüthrich, K.; *J. Mol. Biol.* 1985, 182, 281-294.

77. Mierke, D.F.; Geyer, A.; Kessler, H.; *Int. J. Peptide Protein Res.* 1994, 44, 325-331.

78. (a) Brünger, A.T.; Karplus, M.; *Acc. Chem. Res.* 1991, 24, 54-61. (b) Karplus, M.; Petsk, G.A.; *Nature* 1990, 347, 631-639. (c) Brooks, C.L., II; Karplus, V.; Pettitt, B.M.; *Advances in Chemical Physics*; John Wiley & Sons: New York, 1988.

79. Rebertus, D.W.; Berne, B.J.; Chandler, D.J.; *J. Chem. Phys.* 1979, 70, 3395-3400.

80. (a) Saulitis, J.; Mierke, D.F.; Byk, G.; Gilon, C.; Kessler, H.; *J. Am. Chem. Soc.* 1992, 114, 4818-4827. (b) Golic-Grdadolnic, S.; Mierke, D.F.; Byk, G.; Zeltser, L.; Gilon, C.; *J. Med. Chem.* 1994, 37, 2145-2152.

81. Allen, M.P.; Tildsely, D.J.; *Computer Simulation of Liquids*; Clarendon Press: Oxford, 1987.

82. Seebach, D.; Ko, S.Y.; Kessler, H.; Köck, M.; Reggelin, M.; Schmieder, P.; Walshinshaw, M.D.; Bölsterli, J.J.; Bevec, D.; *Helv. Chim. Acta* 1991, 74, 1953-1990.

83. (a) Torda, A.E.; Scheek, R.M.; van Gunsteren, W.F.; *J. Mol. Biol.* 1990, 214, 223-235. (b) Torda, A.E.; Scheek, R.M.; van Gunsteren, W.F.; *Chem. Phys. Lett.* 1989, 157, 289-294.

84. (a) Torda, A.E.; Brunne, R.M.; Huber, T.; Kessler, H.; *J. Biomol. NMR* 1993, 3, 55-66. (b) Mierke, D.F.; Huber, T.; Kessler, H.; *J. Comp. Aided Mol. Design* 1994, 8, 29-40.

85. Kessler, H.; Matter, H.; Gemmecker, G.; Kottenhahn, M.; Bats, J.W.; *J. Am. Chem. Soc.* 1992, 114, 4805-4818.

86. (a) Mierke, D.F.; Kurz, M.; Kessler, H.; *J. Am. Chem. Soc.* 1994, 116, 1042-1049. (b) Mierke, D.F.; Scheek, R.M.; Kessler, H.; *Biopolymers* 1994, 34, 559-563.

87. (a) Clore, G.M.; Driscoll, P.C.; Wingfield, P.T.; Gronenborn, A.M.; *Biochemistry* 1990, 29, 7387-7401. (b) Kay, L.E.; Tordia, D.A.; Bax, A.; *Biochemistry* 1989, 28, 8972-8979.

88. (a) Lipari, G.; Szabo, A.; *J. Am. Chem. Soc.* 1982, 104, 4546-4559. (b) Lipari, G.; Szabo, A.; *J. Am. Chem. Soc.* 1982, 104, 4559-4570.

89. Craik, D.J.; Higgins, K.A.; *Annu. Rep. NMR Spectrosc.* 1989, 22, 61-138.

90. (a) Fesik, S.W.; Luly, J.R.; Ericson, J.W.; Abad-Zapatero, C.; *Biochemistry* 1988, 27, 8297-8301. (b) Fesik, S.W.; Zuiderweg, E.R.P.; *J. Am. Chem. Soc.* 1989, 111, 5013-5015.

91. (a) Rosen, M.K.; Schreiber, S.L.; *Angew. Chem. Int. Ed. Engl.* 1992, 31, 384-400. (b) Petros, A.M.; Gemmecker, G.; Neri, P.; Olejniczak, E.T.; Nettesheim, D.; Xu, R.X.; Gubbins, E.; Smith, H.; Fesik, S.W.; *J. Med. Chem.* 1992, 35, 2467-2473. (c) Meadows, R.P.; Nettesheim, D.G.; Xu, R.X.; Olejniczak, E.T.; Petros, M.; Holzman, T.F.; Severin, J.; Gubbins, E.; Smith, H.; Fesik, S.W.; *Biochemistry* 1993, 32, 754-765.

92. (a) Kessler, H.; Loosli, H.R.; Oschkinat, H.; *Helv. Chim. Acta* 1985, 68, 661-681. (b) Loosli, H.R.; Kessler, H.; Oschkinat, H.; Weber, H-P.; Petcher, T.J.; Widmer, A.; *Helv. Chim. Acta* 1985, 68, 682-704.

93. Tanaka, H.; Kuroda, A.; Marusawa, H.; Hatanaka, H.; Kino, T.; Goto, T.; Hashimoto, M.; *J. Am. Chem. Soc.* 1987, 109, 5031-5033.

94. Van Dyne, G.; Standaert, R.F.; Karplus, P.A.; Schreiber, S.L.; Clardy, J.C.; *Science* 1991, 252, 839-842.

95. Mierke, D.F.; Schmieder, P.; Karuso, P.; Kessler, H.; *Helv. Chim. Acta* 1991, 74, 1027-1047.

96. Kessler, H.; Haessner, R.; Schüler, W.; *Helv. Chim. Acta* 1993, 76, 117-130.

97. Swindells, D.C.; White, P.S.; Findlay, J.A.; *Can. J. Chem.* 1978, 56, 2491-2493.

98. (a) Balaram, P.; Bothner-By, A.A.; Dadok, J.; *J. Am. Chem. Soc.* 1972, 94, 4015-4017. (b) Balaram, P.; Bothner-By, A.A.; Breslow, E.; *J. Am. Chem. Soc.* 1972, 94, 4017-4018. (c) Clore, G.M.; Gronenborn, A.M.; *J. Magn. Reson.* 1983, 53, 423-442. (d) London, R.E.; Perlman, M.E.; Davis, D.G.; *J. Magn. Reson.* 1992, 97, 79-98.

99. Behling, R.W.; Yamane, T.; Navon, G.; Jelinsky, L.W.; *Proc. Natl. Acad. Sci. USA* 1988, 85, 6721-6725.

100. Bushweller, J.H.; Bartlett, P.A.; *Biochemistry* 1991, 30, 8144-8151.

101. (a) Pervushin, K.V.; Orekhov, V.Y.; Popov, I.; Musina, L.Y.; Arseniev, A.S.; *Eur. J. Biochem.* 1994, 219, 571-583. (b) Orekhov, V.Y.; Pervushin, K.V.; Arseniev, A.S.; *Eur. J. Biochem.* 1994, 219, 887-896. (c) Barsukov, I.L.; Nolde, D.E.; Lomize, A.L.; Arseniev, A.S.; *Eur. J. Biochem.* 1992, 206, 665-672. (d) Orekhov, V.Y.; Abdulaeva, G.V.; Musina, L.Y.; Arseniev, A.S.; *Eur. J. Biochem.* 1992, 210, 223-229.

102. (a) Wider, G.; Lee, K. H.; Wüthrich, K.; *J. Mol. Biol.* 1982, 155, 367–388. (b) Guba, W.; Haessner, R.; Breipohl, G.; Henke, S.; Knolle, J.; Santagada, V.; Kessler, H.; *J. Am Chem. Soc.* 1994, 116, 7532-7540.

103. Köck, M.; Kessler, H.; Seebach, D.; Thaler, A.; *J. Am. Chem. Soc.* 1992, 114, 2676-2686.

104. Miller, S.A.; Griffiths, S.L.; Seebach, D.; *Helv. Chim. Acta* 1993, 76, 563-595.

105. (a) Summers, M.F., *Coord. Chem. Rev.* 1988, 86, 43. (b) South, T.L.; Kim, B.; Summers, M.F., *J. Am. Chem. Soc.* 1989, 111, 395-396.

106. Rizo, J.; Gierasch, L.M., *Ann. Rev. Biochem.* 1992, 61, 387-418.

107. Gilon, C.; Halle, D.; Chorev, M.; Selinger, Z.; Byk, G., *Biopolymers* 1991, 31, 745-750.

108. (a) Kessler, H.; Batz, J.W.; Lautz, J.; Müller, A., *Liebigs Ann. Chem.* 1989, 903-912. (b) Schmidt, J. M.; Ernst, R. R.; Aimoto, S., Kainosho, M.; *J. Biol. NMR* 1995, 5, 95–105.

109. (a) Veber, D.F.; Strachan, R.G.; Bergstrand, S.J.; Holly, F.W.; Homick, C.; Hirschmann, R., *J. Am. Chem. Soc.* 1976, 98, 2367-2369. (b) Bauer, P.; Brimer, U.; Doepfner, W.; Haller, R.; Huguenin, R.; Marbach, P.; Petcher, T.J.; Pless, J., *Life Sci.* 1982, 31, 1133-1145 .

110. Kessler, H.; Haupt, A.; Will, M.; in *Computer-Aided Drug Design Methods and Applications*; Perun, T.J.; Propst, C.L., Eds.; Marcel Dekker: New York, 1989; pp. 461-484.

111. (a) Aumailley, M.; Gurrath, M.; Müller, G.; Calvete, J.; Timpl, R.; Kessler, H.; *FEBS Lett.* 1991, 291, 50-54. (b) Gurrath, M.; Müller, G.; Kessler, H.; Aumailley, M.; Timpl, R.; *Eur. J. Biochem.* 1992, 210, 911-921. (c) Müller, G.; Gurrath, M.; Kessler, H.; *J. Comp. Aided Mol. Des.* 1994, 8, 709-730.

112. Pfaff, M.; Tangemann, K.; Müller, M.; Gurrath, M.; Müller, G.; Kessler, H.; Timpl, R.; *J. Biol. Chem.* 1994, 269, 20233-20238.

113. Brooks, P.C.; Montgomery, A.M.P.; Rosenfeld, M.; Reisfeld, R.A.; Hu, T.; Klier, G.; Chersh, D.A.; *Cell* 1994, 79, 1157-1164.

114. (a) Shemyakin, M.M.; Ovchinnikov, Y.A.; Ivanov, V.T.; *Angew. Chem. Int. Ed. Engl.* 1969, 8, 492-498. (b) Goodman, M.; Chorev, M.; *Acc. Chem. Res.* 1979, 12, 1-7. (c) Freidinger, R.M.; Veber, D.F.; *J. Am. Chem. Soc.* 1979, 101, 6129-6131. (d) Chorev, M.; Goodman, M.; *Acc. Chem. Res.* 1993, 26, 266-273.

115. Lauri, G.; Bartlett, P.; *J. Comp. Aided Mol. Design* 1994, 8, 51-66.

116. (a) Adang, A.E.P.; Hermkens, P.H.H.; Linders, J.T.M.; Ottenheijm, H.C.J.; van Staveren, C.J.; *Recl. Trav. Chim. Pays-Bas* 1994, 113, 63-67. (b) Moore, G.J.; *TiPS* 1994, 15, 124-129. (c) Olson, L.G.; Bolin, D.R.; Bonner, M.P.; Bös, M.; Cook, C.M.; Fry, D.C.; Graves, G.J.; Hatada, M.; Hill, D.E.; Kahn, M.; Madison, V.S.; Rusiecki, V.K.; Sarabu, R.; Sepinwall, J.; Vincent, G.P.; Voss, M.E.; *J. Med. Chem.* 1993, 36, 3041-3049.

# CHAPTER 7

# Protein–Ligand Interactions: Examples in Drug Design

*Robert M. Cooke*

## CONTENTS

I   Introduction ................................................................................. 246

II  Low Affinity Binding ................................................................... 247
    A   Transferred NOEs ................................................................. 248
        1   Introduction ................................................................. 248
        2   Examples ..................................................................... 249
    B   Paramagnetic Labels ............................................................ 255
        1   Introduction ................................................................. 255
        2   Examples ..................................................................... 256

III High Affinity Binding ................................................................. 257
    A   Rare Nuclei ........................................................................ 259
        1   Introduction ................................................................. 259
        2   Examples ..................................................................... 259
    B   Isotope Filters .................................................................... 262
        1   Introduction ................................................................. 262
        2   Examples ..................................................................... 263

IV  Other NMR Studies ..................................................................... 269

0-8493-7824-9/96/$0.00+$.50
© 1996 by CRC Press, Inc.

**245**

V   Integration into a Drug Discovery Program .............................. 269

Acknowledgments ................................................................................. 270

References  ........................................................................................... 270

---

# I    INTRODUCTION

One of the fundamental questions in a drug discovery program is, *how is a compound of interest binding to its target?* This is present at all stages of the process, whether the compound derives from a substrate, a known effector, a novel lead from a screening program or has been designed *ab initio.* Most of the pharmaceuticals currently on the market have been developed with extremely limited information as to the interaction between the drug and its target, relying mainly on exhaustive medicinal chemistry. From this has evolved the concept of a structure–activity relationship (SAR), with a further advance made by considering the "bioactive conformation" of a molecule. A key component in many drug discovery programs now is the structure of a drug–target complex, allowing understanding of the potency of a molecule. Affinity may thus be improved, and if related complexes are also examined, selectivity may be designed.

Structures of several proteins, with actions of interest in therapeutic areas, have been solved by NMR,[1-3] and the potential to determine the structures of proteins that could form targets for intervention with small molecules has now been realised.[4,5] The use of NMR in determining the structure and conformation of small molecules has a much longer history. The limitations of drug design based on the solution conformations of molecules are, however, well recognised — this conformation may be totally distinct from the conformation adopted when bound to the target. (The case of cyclosporin described in the preceding chapter is an example of a situation where this is true.) This is particularly so in the case of intrinsically flexible molecules, where the "solution conformation" is merely an average of several, and is possibly meaningless. In this context, recent NMR advances that enable the visualization of a drug–target complex or of the drug in its bound form have revolutionised the role of the technique in the pharmaceutical industry. In this chapter we are concerned with the contributions NMR can make to the understanding of how a ligand binds to its target. These can range from understanding the mechanism of binding, to distinguishing between postulated binding modes, to selective visualisation of the bound ligand, to a detailed view of the ligand–target complex.

The choice of NMR experiments is largely dictated by the nature of the system. A high affinity for the target (dissociation constant in the nanomolar range), characteristic of most drugs, puts the system into the slow–exchange limit of the NMR time scale; separate resonances are observed for the free and complexed components. The size of complexes usually makes significant resonance assignments impossible unless an X-ray structure is available, isotope labels are employed, or the ligand is spectroscopically benevolent. While a subnanomolar dissociation constant is a common goal in drug design, this is usually developed from compounds displaying much weaker binding, placing the system in the fast-exchange limit of the NMR time scale. In such cases transferred NOE experiments often provide the first indication of the conformation adopted by a ligand when bound.

The questions to be answered also determine the choice of NMR experiment. The benefit may range from providing any information on a poorly characterised system to distinguishing between proposed modes or mechanisms of binding, to answering precise questions as to the geometry of a binding pocket or specific interactions within a complex. The questions usually become more specific as a drug discovery program progresses, and they require constant revision of the strategy of the NMR investigation.

# II  LOW AFFINITY BINDING

In cases of low affinity (dissociation constants above micromolar), resonances of the ligand are usually observed in fast exchange between free and bound forms. This can simplify the spectrum dramatically, and resonances of the ligand can be observed almost exclusively, if a significant excess over protein is used. Low concentrations of protein can be used, which is a great advantage if the solubility or supply is limited. The NMR parameters observed for the ligand are population-weighted averages for those of the free and bound forms. For parameters such as chemical shifts or coupling constants, the contribution from each free and bound species can be of a similar magnitude, the observed average value is dominated by the excess of ligands in the free state, and little information as to the bound state can be derived from these parameters. For relaxation processes, however, the contribution from the bound forms can dominate the observed value. This can be observed via NOEs, which build up far more quickly in the bound state, or paramagnetic relaxation, if the ligand is exposed to the paramagnetic centre only when it is bound.

## A  TRANSFERRED NOEs

### 1  Introduction

The transferred NOE (tNOE) experiment has become highly valuable in defining the conformation of the bound form of the ligand, which is particularly important in the case of flexible species such as small peptides or oligosaccharides. The principles of nuclear Overhauser enhancements have been described in several texts,[6,7] and in Chapter 3. The tNOE arises from the dependence of the NOE sign and magnitude on the correlation time of a molecule. Magnetisation that gives rise to the NOE may be transferred between two spins by two pathways: zero-quantum and double-quantum relaxation. Each displays a different dependence on the correlation time. For small molecules with short correlation times the double-quantum pathway dominates and NOEs are positive. For large molecules with longer correlation times the zero-quantum pathway is dominant and NOEs are negative. At the crossover point the pathways balance each other and no net NOE results. This typically occurs for molecules of molecular weight approximately 1000. When small molecules with intrinsically positive, zero, or small negative NOEs are bound to a large molecule with a much longer correlation time, large negative NOEs can be produced. In the limit of very slow exchange, the ligand is essentially part of the macromolecule: its resonances and their NOEs are likely to be poorly resolved. As the exchange rate increases, however, the ligand may dissociate from the macromolecule before the magnetisation transferred by the Overhauser effect has decayed completely. By this process the NOE generated by the bound form of the ligand is transferred to the free form and can be detected via the resonances of the latter. A large excess of ligand over macromolecule is normally employed, enabling NOEs arising from the ligand to be readily distinguished. These can be assigned to the bound form of the ligand by comparison of NOE intensities with those from spectra of the ligand in isolation, or in cases where the ligand conformation changes upon binding, by their absence in spectra of the isolated ligand.

The transferred NOE experiment offers several advantages over complete structural studies of proteins. First, the size limit for the receptor is far higher than if it were the subject of complete structure determination, and tNOEs represent a rare case where better quality data are obtained from larger systems. Second, the concentration of receptor can be quite low, on the micromolar level, which is of particular importance where sample is limited or is of limited solubility. Third, it is not essential to have a highly pure sample of protein, as long as the impurities do not interfere in the experiment.

Although most transferred NOEs reported arise from fast-exchange situations, they may be generated in a slow-exchange situation, provided the exchange rate is still faster than relaxation of the magnetisation.

Likewise, most studies concentrate on NOEs between resonances of the ligand, but it is possible to detect NOEs between resonances of the ligand and the protein. Transferred NOEs were originally observed in one-dimensional (1D) NMR spectra, and an appropriate theoretical analysis was developed,[8] but most studies are now conducted using two-dimensional (2D) NOESY experiments. The theory has been extended to the 2D situation,[9] highlighting several salient differences from the 1D analysis. In particular, the dependence on concentrations of the components, affinity, and NOE buildup times are quite different for 1D steady-state NOEs and 2D NOESY spectra. The importance of recording spectra at low ratios of macromolecule to ligand is emphasised, increasing the mixing time of the experiment if sensitivity is low. In our labs we have found that reasonable tNOEs can be observed with a ligand:protein ratio of approximately 1000:1.

Most researchers use the tNOE information in a qualitative fashion, although cases where conversion of tNOE intensities into reasonably precise distance restraints have been reported, using comparison of cross-peak intensities with those for known proton separation,[10] relying on measuring buildup rates as a function of mixing time to assess whether the two-spin approximation holds.[11]

We have found that it is possible to measure the dissociation constant for a complex using the intensities of tNOEs.[12] Spin diffusion observed via tNOEs was used to estimate the rate constants for the dissociation of two disaccharides from ricin B-chain to be 50 $s^{-1}$ and 300 $s^{-1}$.[13] The $^{19}F$ coupling observed in a $^{1}H$ NOESY spectrum was combined with the expected transition probability of the fluorine nucleus, to estimate a dissociation constant for a disaccharide–antibody complex of approximately 100 $s^{-1}$.[14] Some resonances of a peptide derived from the thrombin receptor were found to be in slow exchange between the free form and that complexed with thrombin.[15] Exchange broadening of the resonances enabled an estimate of the dissociation rate for the complex to be approximately 250–310 $s^{-1}$ at 25°C.

## 2   Examples

The exchange-rate requirement for tNOEs usually restricts cases where they are observed to those of low to moderate affinity (dissociation constants micromolar or greater). Some leads identified from screens will be of higher affinity than this, and tNOEs are often used for defining the binding mode of a natural ligand. Rapid improvements in affinity will follow, it is hoped, taking the system out of the tNOE regime. A particularly attractive feature of the tNOE experiment is the ability to distinguish a bound conformation of the ligand from a solution ensemble, but it is important to note that the requirement for low affinity cannot be met by having a very small proportion of a high-affinity form amid an ensemble of nonbinding forms as the rate limitations apply on a microscopic level, that is, the species that binds must do so with low affinity.

Many of the early reports of NOEs focussed on nucleotides binding to proteins,[16-18] but they have since diverged to cover systems such as hormones and proteins,[11] substrates and enzymes,[10,19] peptides and antibodies,[20,21] sugars and antibodies,[14] sugars and lectins,[13,22] and peptides from protein–protein interfaces.[23,24]

Transferred NOE studies of nucleotide–protein interactions have usually concentrated on distinguishing between a discrete number of possible conformations, for example, the sugar ring pucker and the orientation of the glycosidic link in the bound nucleotides.[16,18] The adenosine ribose pucker and the nicotinamide glycosidic conformation of $NAD^+$ bound to lactate dehydrogenase were observed to change upon binding of an allosteric effector.[25] These changes were also observed when $NAD^+$ was bound to chemically activated enzyme.[26] Similarly, tNOEs were used to define the relative disposition of the nicotinamide and dihydrofolate rings bound to plasmid derived dihydrofolate reductases (DHFRs), demonstrating that this was the opposite to that observed in chromosomal DHFRs;[27] the differences are therapeutically significant, as the plasmid-derived enzyme is believed to be responsible for resistance to the antibacterial agent trimethoprim. Chapter 7 describes in detail other examples involving DHFR as a drug target.

The conformations of Mg-ATP when bound to a nucleotidyl transferase, (methionyl tRNA synthetase) and a phosphoryl transferase (pyruvate kinase) were examined via 1D transient NOEs.[28] Buildup rates were analysed by a complete relaxation matrix to account for the effect of exchange on NOE intensities; incorporation of the data into molecular mechanics calculations produced similar conformations for the bound nucleotide in each case. The authors acknowledge that these calculations are dominated by the *in vacuo* force field and they were not able to estimate the effects of the protein on the NOE buildup or the energy of the bound nucleotide.

The conformation of a tetrapeptide bound to porcine pancreatic elastase was examined with transferred NOEs.[10] Intramolecular tNOEs were used in a molecular dynamics refinement of the peptide conformation. Exemplifying the fact that the information from tNOEs is usually restricted to the conformation of the ligand, electron density for part of the bound ligand in an X-ray structure was used to locate the ligand in the active site. Rather than bridging the active site as expected, the inhibitor occupies the S' sites of the enzyme. The variability in binding modes made it difficult to predict the structure of one inhibited complex from another, justifying the use of NOEs for a number of inhibitors. In a subsequent study the conformation of a slowly hydrolysing substrate was examined by tNOEs and X-ray diffraction, providing information as to a likely Michaelis complex.[19]

A complete structure of oxytocin bound to neurophysin was reported from a distance geometry and molecular dynamics analysis of tNOEs.[11] As in many NMR studies of globular proteins the oxytocin backbone was far better defined than the side chains, and a tripeptide extension to the cyclic core was particularly ill defined. In this study, it was necessary to define a conformation from a limited number of precise NOEs, which is opposite to the prevailing school of thought in structure determination by NMR. The bound structure was found to be quite different from the X-ray structure of oxytocin, in both the rupture of hydrogen bonds between backbone residues and the adoption of a nonminimal conformation for a tyrosine side chain. As in many other tNOE studies, it is unfortunate that the protein residues responsible for stabilising a seemingly high-energy conformation of the ligand cannot be visualised or included in structure calculations.

Recognition of a high-energy substrate conformer by an enzyme has been demonstrated for a catalytic antibody, which binds its substrate, chorismate, in a diaxial conformation as opposed to the diequatorial form that predominates in solution.[29] In this study tNOEs were used to identify the bound conformation shown in Figure 1. This was anticipated from its similarity to the postulated transition state and the transition-state analogue used to generate the antibody. Additional tNOEs observed were attributed to spin diffusion or the fact that the substrate is not totally restrained when bound to the enzyme.

The power of transferred NOEs to distinguish between the bound conformation of a ligand and the average solution conformation has been demonstrated for oligosaccharides. The coupling constants and Overhauser enhancements across a glycosidic linkage were found to be inconsistent with a single solution conformation for a disaccharide, and several rapidly exchanging conformations were predicted.[14] Transferred NOEs were used to predict two possible bound conformations, that could not be discriminated between, neither of which resembled the constituents of the "solution conformation". Similarly, a 1–6 linked disaccharide appears to exist in at least two conformations in solution, but careful fitting of the buildup rates for tNOEs showed that in this case the major component preferentially binds to its receptor.[22] This study was complicated by the fact that the receptor, the ricin B-chain, contains two binding sites for the ligand. We have used tNOEs to demonstrate a conformational change of the sialyl Lewis X ligand upon binding to its receptor, E-selectin.[12] While a core trisaccharide structure could be defined by tNOEs, a terminal glycosidic link was characterised by their absence. A "bound" conformation was selected from a series of low-energy species as the only one that could fit the tNOE criteria.

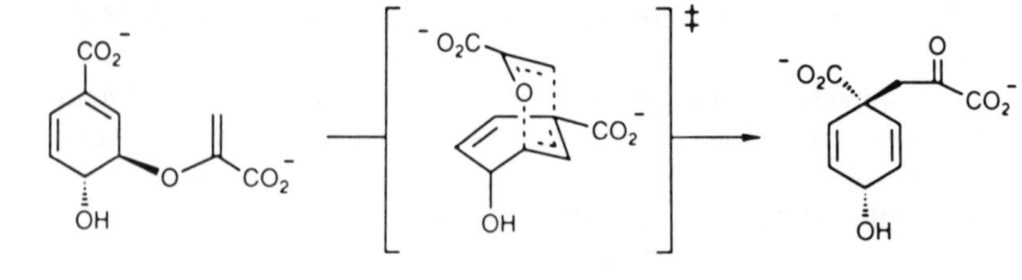

**FIGURE 1**

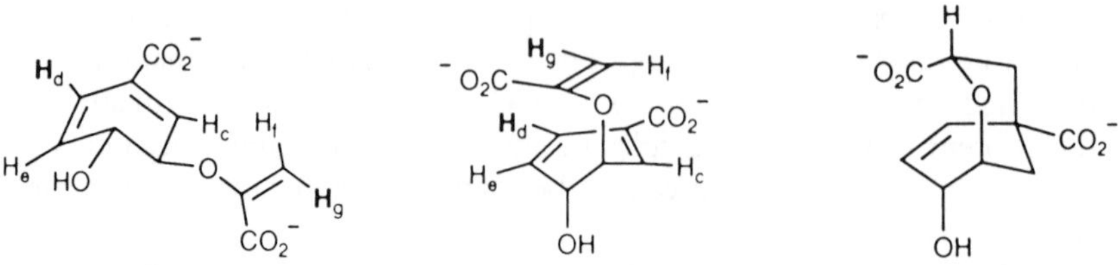

The conversion of chorismate to prephenate is believed to proceed via the constrained transition state **1**. While the diequatorial conformer of chorismate **2** is preferred in solution, tNOEs demonstrate that the diaxial form **3** is recognised by a catalytic antibody raised against the transition state analogue **4**. (From Campbell, A.P., et al., *Proc. Natl. Acad. Sci. USA*, 90, 8663–8667, 1993. With permission. Copyright National Academy of Sciences USA.)

Disruption of the interaction between the subunits of ribonucleotide reductase (RNR) is seen as a viable means of intervention in herpes simplex virus (HSV) infections. Interaction with the B1 subunit of RNR is believed to be dominated by the C-terminus of the B2 subunit, and peptides corresponding to the last nine residues of B2 are known inhibitors of HSV-1. The interactions of peptides from the C-terminus of the B2 subunit of *Escherichia coli* RNR with the B1 subunit were probed via tNOEs.[23] Interaction with B1 was not observed with a peptide corresponding to the effective sequence from HSV-1; rather a peptide corresponding to an adjacent sequence was observed to interact via tNOEs, which further highlighted a cluster of hydrophobic residues from the peptide when bound to B1.

Phospholipase $A_2$ (PLA$_2$) is a well-characterised target for intervention in inflammatory and cardiovascular diseases.[30] Cobra venom PLA$_2$ is viewed as a reasonable model of the human enzymes, and the binding of nonhydrolysable thioether amide substrate analogues has been characterised by NMR.[31] The analogue of phosphatidylethanolamine (IC$_{50}$ 8 m$M$) and the analogue of phosphatidylcholine (IC$_{50}$ 90 m$M$) both inhibit the enzyme, and tNOEs are observable. A sample of protein chemically modified at the active site was used to demonstrate the specificity of the tNOEs. ROESY spectra showed no evidence for a preferred conformation for either ligand in solution, but 25 and 27 tNOEs respectively, were observed for each inhibitor in the presence of $PLA_2$. In each case, five of these NOEs were to an aromatic spin system, which was assigned to Phe 5 by comparison with spectra from porcine pancreatic $PLA_2$. The intensities of the tNOEs developed steadily with mixing time, but concern about the effects of exchange on the measurements prompted the authors to use broad classes of distance restraints rather than precise ones. Enzyme-bound conformations for the inhibitors were generated by two means: (1) manually docking extended models of the inhibitors into an X-ray structure of the protein, followed by minimisation and dynamics with the tNOE-derived restraints; and (2) calculating the bound inhibitor conformation initially in the absence of the protein using intramolecular tNOEs, then docking into the protein followed by refinement using all tNOEs. Both protocols gave similar results (Figure 2). For neither inhibitor was there sufficient NMR information to define the conformation of the head group in the docked structures, which relies heavily on additional restraints to the calcium ion and the strength of the force field.

Inhibition of the blood-coagulation enzyme thrombin is a widely recognised therapeutic goal in cardiovascular disease.[32] Thrombin proteolytically activates fibrinogen and other proteins in the coagulation cascade, as well as its receptor on platelets, and can be inhibited by the leech protein hirudin. Each of these interactions represents a potential point for therapeutic intervention. The thrombin-bound conformation of a decapeptide corresponding to the recognition sequence in fibrinogen was characterised by transferred NOEs.[33] The tNOEs immediately indicated that the peptide bent back on itself, explaining the conservation of residues sequentially distant from the cleavage site. The NOEs were converted into maximum distance restraints, which along with inferred hydrogen bonds and minimum distance restraints deduced from the absence of tNOEs, were analysed by a distance geometry method. A set of reasonably well-converged structures was produced, in which the first few residues, of the decapeptide adopt a helical conformation, followed by a sequence of multiple turns. This clustered a group of hydrophobic residues, which were postulated to contact the enzyme in the bound state. Following the determination of the X-ray structure of thrombin, the predicted structure of the fibrinogen peptide was modified in the light of docking attempts and comparison with the trypsin-BPTI complex.[34] A pseudopeptide was synthesised incorporating a bicyclic ring system to mimic a proposed Gly–Gly reverse turn in the fibrinogen peptide. This resulted in a potent inhibitor, and the determination of its structure

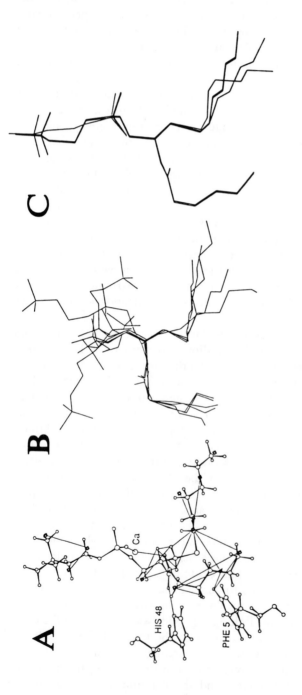

**FIGURE 2**

The conformation of a thioether amide phosphatidyl choline bound to cobra phospholipase A2. (A) The tNOE-derived distance constraints. (B) Initial structures generated by molecular dynamics using intramolecular distance constraints. (C) Structures produced after initial ones were docked into the protein, followed by further molecular dynamics with additional distance restraints to the protein and calcium. (From Plesniak, L.A., et al., *Biochemistry*, 32, 5009–5016, 1993. With permission. Copyright [1993] American Chemical Society.)

complexed to thrombin by X-ray diffraction showed that the binding model, derived from tNOE data, was essentially correct.[35]

The bound conformation of a decapeptide from hirudin, which inhibits thrombin by binding remote from the site of catalysis, was also determined via tNOEs.[36] The first part of the peptide is extended but the last four residues form a distorted $\alpha$-helix. This results in an amphiphilic disposition of residues, creating a hydrophobic surface that was predicted to form the binding site with the enzyme. The subsequently reported X-ray structure of thrombin complexed with hirudin confirmed these findings.[37] The enzyme-bound structure of a dodecapeptide corresponding to residues of the thrombin receptor preceding the cleavage site was characterised by tNOEs.[15] In this case only the final four residues of the peptide were found to be structured, but well-converged structures for these amino acids were produced by distance geometry.

Given that a large proportion of the world's pharmaceuticals act against membrane receptors, the almost complete absence of information as to the structures of these receptors is a testament to the difficulties associated with this field. A significant breakthrough, however, was made with the conformation of a peptide from the a subunit of the G protein transducin bound to rhodopsin.[38] Photoactivation of the rhodopsin produced changes in the NOESY spectrum, in both the resonances producing cross-peaks and their intensities, suggesting a conformational change in the complex. Enough tNOEs were identified in each case for restrained molecular dynamics simulations of the structures of the peptide in the two complexes.

## B  PARAMAGNETIC LABELS

### 1  Introduction

The use of paramagnetic labels has a long history in the study of protein structure by NMR.[39] The shift or broadening properties of certain paramagnetic nuclei allowed resonances from neighbouring groups to be identified at what are now modest field strengths, well before the introduction of multidimensional techniques. Well after the establishment of NOEs as the predominant input for the determination of protein structures by NMR, the value of paramagnetic shift information is still recognised.[40] Several proteins utilise metals in their interactions with ligands. If the metal is paramagnetic or can be substituted by a paramagnetic analogue, NMR information specific to the ligand and/or its binding site can be readily obtained. The presence of a paramagnetic centre may change the chemical shift of a resonance and/or alter its longitudinal $T_1$ and transverse $T_2$ relaxation times. Whether the paramagnetic centre acts as a shift or a broadening reagent is determined primarily by the relaxation time of the electron spin and the anisotropy of the electronic $g$ tensor values.

### 2   Examples

Paramagnetic shifts or broadening can be observed in cases of slow exchange, monitoring the resonances of the complex directly, but the majority of recent reports arise from cases of fast exchange, where the altered relaxation rate is measured via resonances of the bulk ligand.

The coordination of ATP and ADP to $Mg^{2+}$ within arginine kinase were examined through $Mn^{2+}$- and $Co^{2+}$-induced relaxation of $^{31}P$ resonances of the bound nucleotides.[41] It was found that for the $Mn^{2+}$ complex the broadening was not field dependent, was characterised by a high activation energy (10–11 kcal/mol), and displayed a discontinuity with temperature. The authors interpreted this as representing relaxation dominated by exchange between the diamagnetic enzyme–nucleotide complex and the paramagnetic enzyme–nucleotide–$Mn^{2+}$ complex, thus making any distance estimation invalid. The $Co^{2+}$ complex, however, displayed none of these problems, and direct coordination between the metal and all phosphate groups of ATP and ADP was deduced. The study was extended to $^1H$ resonances of arginine in equlibrium with the enzyme–$Co^{2+}$–ADP complex, allowing a preliminary view of its disposition within the active site.

The 200-kDa enzyme tyrosine hydroxylase was modified by replacing its cofactor with an inactive analogue, replacing tyrosine with the weaker binding phenylalanine to produce a fast-exchange situation, and replacing the normal $Fe^{2+}$ cation with $Co^{2+}$ to induce relaxation.[42] Distances between protons and the metal in the complex were determined from the broadening of the phenylalanine resonances. As the protons on opposite sides of the phenyl ring are magnetically equivalent in the unbound form, it is impossible to separate the contributions to relaxation from the individual resonances of the bound form. Hence, two limiting cases were considered: the paramagnetic effect is experienced by only one resonance from each equivalent pair, or each of the two resonances experiences an equal paramagnetic effect. Distances derived from paramagnetic relaxation were combined with transferred NOEs in a distance geometry calculation of the metal–phenylalanine conformation. The resulting proximity of the metal to the aromatic ring is consistent with its possible role in the transfer of oxygen.

A stable, exchange-inert metal nucleotide analogue, Cr(III)ATP, was used to examine ligand binding to phosphoglycero kinase.[43] The broadening of $^{31}P$, $^1H$, and $^{13}C$ resonances of 3-phosphoglycerate suggested that, unlike the situation in the X-ray structure, the distance between the nucleotide and substrate is small enough for phospho transfer. The distance was slightly longer in the presence of sulphate, consistent with the allosteric effect of this anion.

The nucleic acid hydrolysing enzyme staphylococcal nuclease binds $Ca^{2+}$, but this can be replaced by $Mn^{2+}$, $Co^{2+}$, and $La^{3+}$, yielding an inactive enzyme. The increased $T_1$ and $T_2$ relaxation for $^1H$ and $^{31}P$ resonances of the dinucleoside substrate dTdA in exchange with $Co^{2+}$ substituted enzyme were analysed to produce a set of seven metal–ligand distances.[44] These were combined with 17 transferred NOEs determined for the diamagnetic $La^{3+}$ complex to produce a narrow range of bound dTdA conformations. These exhibited an extended conformation with no base stacking, precluding A-, B-, or Z-DNA as the recognised conformation, although the authors acknowledged the limitation of studying inactive complexes. The bound conformation differed significantly from that determined using tNOEs for the binary dTdA–enzyme complex. Subsequently 2D NOESY and HMQC and 3D NOESY-HMQC experiments with $^{15}N$–labelled protein and $Ca^{2+}$ or $La^{3+}$ present were used to assign resonances of aromatic residues around the active site.[45] NOEs between dTdA and the enzyme were identifed, and the bound conformation of the ligand was docked into the X-ray structure of the enzyme followed by energy minimisation. This gave a high-resolution view of the substrate-bound complex, enabled rationalisation of the effects of a number of known mutations, and explained why the inhibitor thymidine 3′,5′-diphosphate binds with 1400-fold greater affinity. A similar protocol was used to dock this inhibitor into the enzyme.[46] This resulted in a structure for the complex significantly different from that determined by X-ray diffraction (Figure 3). The X-ray structure was considered to be less likely to occur in solution as it is affected by crystal-packing restraints, and mutational data supports the NMR binding mode.[47]

---

## III   HIGH AFFINITY BINDING

As mentioned in the introduction most, if not all, useful drugs will form high-affinity complexes with their target. From the NMR viewpoint, this takes the system into the slow-exchange regime, and resonances of the complex can be observed directly. Sensitivity considerations will normally require a higher concentration of the complex, although some experiments are run over extended periods. The fact that the ligand is observed as a complex can cause problems in $^1H$ resonance assignment, due to the abundance and limited dispersion of $^1H$ resonances. Even for systems within the generally accepted size limits for complete proton assignment (approximately 15 kDa, or 25 kDa with $^{13}C$ and $^{15}N$ labels), a significant level of assignment can take months. Fortuitous cases exist, such as that where a pair of phospholipase $A_2$ ($PLA_2$) inhibitors was selected for study based on the presence of a vinyl group, which was expected to place resonances from the ligand in a "window" away from resonances of the protein.[48] This did indeed occurred (Figure 4), and with the assistance of

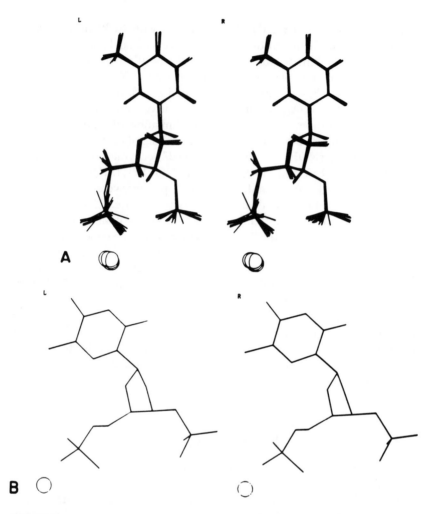

**FIGURE 3**
(A) An overlay of 10 structures of 3′,5′-pdTp bound to staphylococcal nuclease, produced by distance geometry from NMR data. (B) The structure as seen by X-ray crystallography. The metal ion is represented by a sphere. (From Weber, D.J., et al., *Proteins Struct. Function Genet.,* 17, 20–35, 1993. With permission of John Wiley & Sons. Copyright 1993 Wiley-Liss, Inc.)

a good X-ray structure for the protein, NOEs between the protein and the inhibitor could be assigned. Using just four NOEs, the ligand could be docked into the X-ray structure of the protein in a restrained molecular dynamics simulation. Such cases are unfortunately rare, and other intervention is required. Two general ways have been developed to circumvent the overlap of $^1$H resonances: the incorporation of rare nuclei to observe

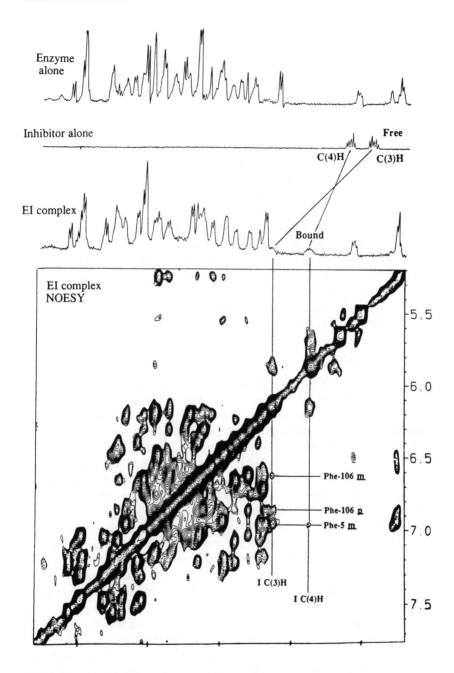

**FIGURE 4**

1D and 2D ¹H spectra of a substrate analogue inhibitor of phospholipase A₂. Although resonances of the ligand shift upon binding, they are still distinct from those of the protein, enabling intermolecular NOEs to be identified. (Reproduced with permission from Dr. W. Primrose.)

their resonances directly, and the incorporation of $^{13}$C and/or $^{15}$N labels into part of the system to enable selective observation of neighbouring $^{1}$H resonances.

## A  RARE NUCLEI

### 1  Introduction

Specific information concerning binding can be obtained quickly with the introduction of rare isotopes into the system. Popular nuclei are $^{19}$F, $^{31}$P, $^{13}$C, and $^{15}$N. All are reasonably sensitive; the first two are rare but exist almost exclusively as the magnetically active isotopes, while the last two represent common elements that are rare as these isotopes. While $^{13}$C and $^{15}$N have been incorporated into specific sites in proteins,[49] this is far from trivial, and incorporation of $^{19}$F and $^{31}$P is restricted to aromatic residues or Ser/Thr residues.[50,51] Introduction of the label via the ligand has a longer history, and has the advantage of placing the label directly in the region of interest. Many natural ligands contain $^{31}$P, and $^{19}$F may be viewed as a synthetically accessible replacement for $^{1}$H.

### 2  Examples

The type of NMR information obtainable from these studies is usually quite limited, being restricted to basic NMR parameters such as chemical shifts, intensities, relaxation times and coupling constants. NOEs between resonances of the heteronucleus and surrounding protons are considered possible,[7] but with the exception of some $^{19}$F–$^{1}$H studies,[52] actual reports are few and far between (except of course for directly bonded protons, which provide little structural insight). The basic NMR parameters can provide useful information in the right experiment. They may be used to probe the difference between binding to related enzymes, which could be exploited in designing selectivity. In many cases an X-ray structure or a good model is available for the target, and NMR can be used to distinguish between postulated modes of binding. Alternatively, the ligand may undergo a reaction with the target, and the spectral parameters may be compared with those for a series of model compounds to distinguish between possible structures for the complex.

Heteronuclear NMR has played a vital role in defining the nature of intermediates in enzymatic catalysis, information that is vital if mimetics of intermediates or transition states are sought as inhibitors. In particular, the $^{13}$C shift of trigonal and tetrahedral centres differs by about 100 ppm, a fact that was exploited in demonstrating the existence of a tetrahedral intermediate in the serine protease reaction pathway.[53] Previously $^{13}$C shifts had been used to demonstrate that pepstatin analogues, in which the statine alcohol is replaced by a carbonyl, formed tetrahedral intermediates when bound to pepsin.[54]

The nature of the interactions between ligands and dihydrofolate reductase (DHFR) has been the subject of exhaustive NMR studies for many years. These are described in detail by Feeney in the following chapter and so just a few examples are given now for comparison with other studies described in this chapter. DHFR utilises NADH to reduce dihydro- to tetrahydrofolate and is the target for the antibacterial agent trimethoprim, the antimalarial agent pyrimethamine and the antitumour agent methotrexate. Although high-quality X-ray diffraction structures are available, these cannot answer all the questions as to the modes of ligand binding. Using the *Lactobacillus casei* enzyme and (3-carboxamido $^{13}$C) NADP[+], multiple forms of the DHFR–folate–NADP[+] complex were demonstrated by $^{13}$C NMR;[55] the relative proportions of the components varied with pH. The multiplicity was observed only for resonances from the nicotinamide ring, not for $^{31}$P resonances of the adenine pyrophosphate or the diphosphate linker. A later study used $^{15}$N-labelled folate to demonstrate heterogeneity in the binary DHFR–folate and ternary DHFR–NADP[+]–folate complexes.[56] Multiplicity was observed for the DHFR–trimethoprim–NADP[+] complex using $^{13}$C- and $^{15}$N-labelled ligands,[17] and the rate of interconversion between forms of bound trimethoprim was estimated from the separation of $^{13}$C resonances.[57] More detailed analyses of $^{13}$C relaxation times and linewidths were used to characterise the rate of flip of the phenyl ring of trimethoprim, demonstrating that the rate decreased approximately by a factor of 10 upon binding of NADPH.[58] $^1$H, $^{13}$C, and $^{31}$P NMR were used to characterise the effect of mutations of the enzyme on the relative stability of each form.[59] Although the heteronuclear studies could demonstrate multiplicity and measure interconversion, $^1$H assignments around the active site were required to orient accurately the forms within the enzyme.[60] The conformation of folate was similar in two of the complexes to that of the inhibitor methotrexate, while the third involved a ring flip of 180° to form a productive complex. Similarly, $^{19}$F NMR was used to demonstrate multiple binding modes for analogues of pyrimethane, related by rotation between the biphenyl rings,[61] but $^1$H NOEs were needed to orient the forms in the active site. Spectra of bovine DHFR and $^{13}$C- and $^{15}$N-labelled folate demonstrated a single bound ligand form, and chemical shifts indicated no protonation at N5 of folate.[62] A single conformation for folate bound to *E. coli* DHFR was reported from $^1$H and $^{15}$N NMR studies of the binary DHFR–folate and ternary DHFR–folate–NADP+ complexes.[63,64] The DHFR–methotrexate complex was seen to consist of two species,[64] which were attributed to two forms of the protein fold.[65]

In our laboratories $^{19}$F has been used to distinguish quickly between possible binding modes of a series of dimeric penicillin inhibitors of the

HIV-1 protease.[66] The series, which had been identified by screening, had been modelled to bind in three possible modes, two symmetric and one asymmetric. In order to answer whether the mode of binding was symmetric or asymmetric, fluorine groups were introduced into symmetrically disposed postions. [19]F NMR spectra of the complex with HIV-1 protease were characterised by a single resonance for the bound species. This was interpreted as demonstrating a symmetric mode of binding, and the medicinal chemistry strategy could be focussed accordingly. Subsequently, the demands of pharmacokinetics directed research toward smaller compounds, which were achieved with monomeric penicillin inhibitors. At this stage, through the similar shift upon binding of [19]F resonances, the monomeric inhibitors were demonstrated to bind in a manner similar to half of a dimer.[67]

## B   ISOTOPE FILTERS

### 1   Introduction

The development of isotope filters has paralleled that of uniform isotope labelling, both of which utilise [15]N and/or [13]C nuclei to extend the size limit for detailed [1]H resonance assignment. While the latter utilises the increased spectral dispersion offered by heteronuclei as well as the opportunities for additional spectral dimensions, the former relies primarily on the presence of heteronuclei in a specific part of the system to select [1]H magnetisation from adjacent groups. Incorporation of the label within the ligand makes it possible for [1]H NMR studies to be performed in which the bound ligand and its environs are viewed selectively. Thus the same NMR techniques used to study small molecules in solution can be applied to the bound form of the ligand (although decreased relaxation times can prove a limitation), and of the general classes of techniques described in this chapter, this has the potential to provide the most detailed information. Chemical shifts, coupling constants, and NOEs characterise the bound conformation. In addition intermolecular NOEs, identification of hydrogen bonds through slow exchange of amide protons, and analysis of secondary chemical shifts can allow visualisation of the ligand within its binding site, at high precision if the structure of the target is already known.

Labelling parts of a system with [15]N or [13]C to observe resonances of attached [1]H selectively was first proposed in the mid-1980s,[68-71] and since then two main methods of selective observation have evolved. One relies on creating single or multiple quantum coherence between the protons and heteronuclei.[72] The phase cycling can select for [1]H resonances, which have evolved through single or multiple quantum coherence only, thus removing resonances from [1]H attached to [12]C or [14]N. The other method discriminates between protons bound to $^{15}$N or $^{13}$C and those bound to $^{14}$N or $^{12}$C by putting the $^1$H magnetisation through a defocus–refocus period.[73] When the refocussing $^1$H pulse is combined with a $^{15}$N or $^{13}$C 180° pulse, $^1$H magnetisation from nuclei attached to $^{15}$N or $^{13}$C will refocus with the opposite phase to that which is not. Spectra are recorded with and without the heteronuclear 180° pulse; subtraction or addition of these will leave only resonances from protons attached to the heteronucleus or not attached to the heteronucleus, respectively. It is thus possible to select for or filter out resonances depending on their attached nuclei. These "half filters" can be applied individually to each dimension of a 2D experiment, selecting, for example, protons attached to $^{13}$C in one dimension and protons attached to $^{12}$C in the other (Figure 5).[74]

It is not clear whether one form of the experiment is superior to the other, and so far both forms have been widely used. While the half filters offer the possibility of observing both the labelled and unlabelled parts of the complex separately, the HMQC/HSQC experiments have been reported to be more sensitive.[75]

## 2 Examples

A series of tripeptide inhibitors of the aspartyl protease pepsin were synthesised with incorporation of $^{15}$N, $^{13}$C, and $^2$H at two leucine residues, and isotope-filtered NOESY experiments were performed on the peptide/pepsin complexes.[76] Intramolecular $^1$H–$^1$H NOEs were used to determine the conformation of the bound peptide, and a number of NOEs with resonances of the protein were observed. These were assigned to specific sites with the aid of a partially refined X-ray structure of pepsin with a similar inhibitor, which allowed a rough model of the inhibitor within the active site to be constructed (Figure 6).

$^{13}$C half filters were used to select $^1$H resonances from labelled 1,3-diacetyl-chloramphenicol bound to the 75-kDa enzyme chloramphenicol acetyltransferase (CAT),[77] which is the main means by which chloramphenicol resistance is mediated in bacteria. As CAT functions in both directions, diacetylchloramphenicol is a weak substrate; therefore, to facilitate study by NMR, the enzyme activity was reduced by a Ser to Ala mutation. NOEs were observed between the methyl resonances of the ligand and an aromatic spin system of the enzyme. Examination of the X-ray structure of the enzyme complexed with chloramphenicol identified four possible residues that could be involved; mutation of each of these demonstrated that the NOEs arose from Tyr 25. Incorporation of the NOE data with the X-ray structure of the chloramphenicol/CAT complex enabled a rough model of the 1,3-diacetylchloramphenicol/CAT complex to be constructed.

Peptides specifically $^{13}$C labelled at alanine methyl groups or uniformly throughout the molecule were synthesised to make possible study of their

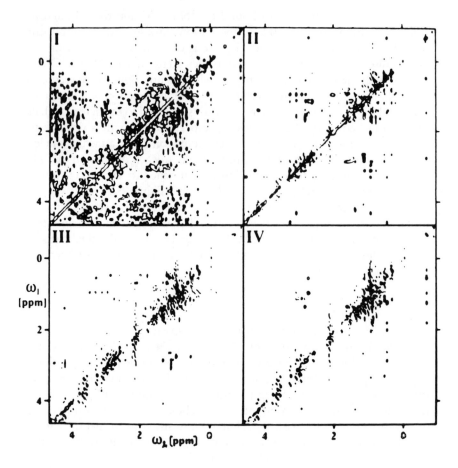

**FIGURE 5**

Editing of ¹H NOESY spectra of ¹³C-labelled cyclosporin A bound to unlabelled cyclophilin. (I) ¹³C filtered in both dimensions. (II) ¹³C selected in both dimensions. (III) ¹³C selected in $F_1$ and filtered in $F_2$. (IV) ¹³C filtered in $F_1$ and selected in $F_2$. (From Wider, G., et al., *J. Am. Chem. Soc.,* 112, 9015–9016, 1990. With permission. Copyright [1990] American Chemical Society.)

interaction with class II major histocompatability complex (MHC).[78] Differential line broadening in HMQC spectra of the complex enabled residues of the bound peptide to be classified as solvent exposed or buried. HMQC-NOESY spectra identified contacts between residues of the peptide and the MHC. The data clearly indicate that the first 4 residues of the peptide were outside the binding groove, while the last 11 were bound. The authors highlight the limitations of this technique in studying a 70-kDa complex when compared with smaller systems, due chiefly to linewidth and overlap of resonances with those from the natural abundance of ¹³C in mobile regions of the protein.

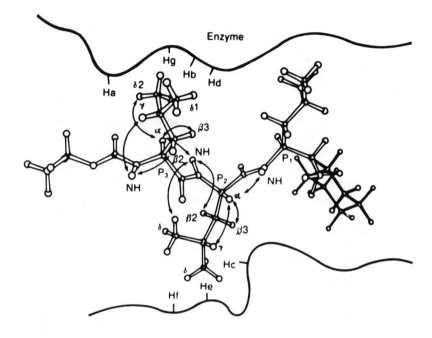

**FIGURE 6**

A model of a bound pepsin inhibitor generated using NMR data from isotope-edited spectra with ¹³C-, ¹⁵N- and ²H-labelled ligands. Arrows indicate NOEs. (From Fesik, S.W., et al., *Biochemistry*, 27, 8297–8301, 1988. With permission. Copyright [1988] American Chemical Society.)

Perhaps the most striking example of the use of NMR in visualising receptor–ligand interactions is that of the immunosuppressants and immunophilins.[79] The cyclic undecapeptide cyclosporin A (CsA) is a well-established immunosuppressant of key importance in organ transplant operations. It is known to bind to cyclophilin (CyP), a peptidyl-prolyl isomerase (or rotamase). X-ray diffraction and NMR studies of CsA in nonpolar solvents produced similar structures: an antiparallel β-sheet pairing two sides of the molecule with intramolecular hydrogen bonds, a type II′ β-turn at one end and a loop containing a *cis* peptide at the other. The presence of the *cis* peptide was deemed to be essential for binding to cyclophilin, and this formed a basis for the design of more potent immunosuppressants.

The first evidence that the bond was not *cis* when CsA was complexed with cyclophilin was provided by NMR.[80] CsA was uniformly ¹³C labelled to distinguish its ¹H resonances from those of the cyclophilin. Following assignment of the ¹³C and ¹H resonances of CsA, the ¹H–¹H NOESY was found not to contain a cross-peak between the αCH resonances of residues 9 and 10, which would be expected for a *cis* peptide; instead an NOE was observed betwen the *N*-methyl resonance of residue 10 and the αCH resonance of residue 9, characteristic of an extended backbone conformation with a *trans* peptide.

Complete descriptions of the bound conformations of CsA were subsequently reported.[81,82] Using [13]C- and [15]N-labelled CsA (in separate samples), [1]H resonances of CsA were identified using isotope filters in one or both dimensions of 2D spectra and were sequentially assigned using slight variations from the established procedures.[81] The presence of the heteronuclei gave the additional option of avoiding overlaps in the [1]H spectrum of the ligand by labelling resonances with the heteronuclear frequency prior to observing [1]H–[1]H correlations. NOEs between proton resonances were combined with [3]JNH–αCH coupling constants as input for structure determination via distance geometry calculations. Well-converged structures resulted, which demonstrated drastic changes from the structures calculated for CsA in isolation (Figure 7). All peptide bonds were *trans,* and no β-sheet or intramolecular H bonds were found. Using the isotope filters in only one dimension of 2D NOESY spectra, it was possible to identify NOEs between resonances of CsA and cyclophilin. Thus the residues of CsA in contact with its receptor could be identified, and these agreed with those predicted from the differences in shifts of resonances between the free and bound CsA. Similar results were obtained using [13]C-labelled CsA only.[82] HMQC, [13]C TOCSY-REVINEPT, and [13]C–[13]C COSY experiments were used to assign [1]H resonances, exploiting the large [13]C–[13]C coupling constants. Rather than labelling the CsA with [15]N, the cyclophilin was labelled instead, and its NH resonances were removed by a variation on the half-filter technique. A 3D HMQC-NOESY spectrum was combined with [13]C half filters to generate datasets with intramolecular CsA NOEs only and intermolecular CsA–cyclophilin NOEs only. This also provided a conformation of bound CsA and highlighted the residues involved in intermolecular contacts. The burial of these residues was subsequently confirmed by their reduced susceptibility to the paramagnetic relaxation agent HyTEMPO.[83] The bound conformation of cyclosporin was also studied using unlabelled CsA and fully deuterated cyclophilin.[84] The removal of most of the resonances from the spectrum is dramatic (Figure 8), and it enabled full sequential assignment and structure generation using standard homonuclear techniques. Recording spectra in 90% $H_2O$-restored amide protons to the cyclophilin, and NOEs from their resonances enabled buried residues of CsA to be identified.

The information as to the bound conformation of CsA and the portions of its structure involved in intermolecular contacts were combined with X-ray structures of cyclophilin to generate a model of the CsA–cyclophilin complex.[85] Following the discovery that the immuno-suppressant effects arise from the binding of the CsA/CyP complex to

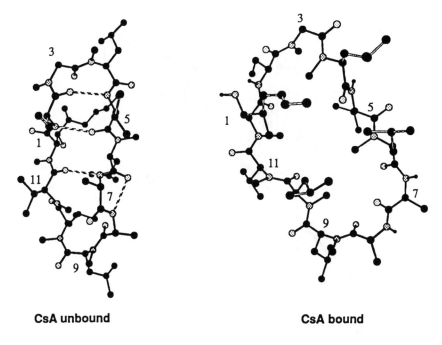

**CsA unbound**                                    **CsA bound**

**FIGURE 7**
Unbound and cyclophilin-bound conformations of cyclosporin A. (From Jorgensen, W.L., *Science,* 254, 954–955, 1991. With permission. Copyright 1991 by the AAAS.)

another protein, calcineurin, it was realised that it is not just the residues of CsA in contact with CyP that are important, but also many of the remaining residues that probably interact with calcineurin. NMR has now been used to define the complete structure of the CsA/CyP complex.[86] Interestingly, this was achieved using differential [15]N and [13]C labelling to distingush NOEs within each component and between the two components.

Recently, an NMR study of CsA in DMSO and water[87] demonstrated a similar conformation to CsA bound to CyP, suggesting that most of the differences reported earlier do not occur upon receptor binding but are due to the nature of the solvent. Chapter 6 contains a description of the complex array of conformations that may be populated in CsA solutions. While the evidence for an induced-fit mode of binding is greatly diminished, the importance of studying a ligand when complexed remains.

Another example of an immunosuppressant is FK506, which like CsA, binds to an intracellular prolyl-peptidyl isomerase, FKBP, and the immunosuppressant effects arise from the binding of this complex to calcineurin. FK506 was reported to contain a *cis* peptide bond in its free

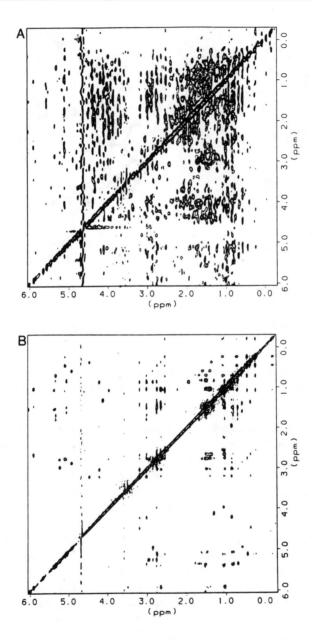

**FIGURE 8**

[1]H NOESY spectra of cyclophilin–cyclosporin A complexes. (A) Both components are protonated. (B) Cyclosporin is protonated and cyclophilin is deuterated. (From Hsu, V.L., and Armitage, I.M., *Biochemistry*, 31, 12778–12784, 1992. With permission. Copyright [1992] American Chemical Society.)

form, although it was observed to be *trans* in the X-ray diffraction structure of the FK506/FKBP complex.[88] The $^1$H spectrum of FK506 complexed with FKBP was assigned using $^{13}$C labelling and a combination of $^{13}$C–$^{13}$C COSY, HSQC, HMQC-TOCSY, and HSQC-NOESY spectra.[75] The authors comment that the HSQC-NOESY spectrum provided more intramolecular NOEs than the double half-filtered NOESY spectrum. For most of the prochiral pairs of resonances, stereospecific assignments could be obtained. NOE restraints were fed into distance geometry, and molecular dynamics algorithms and well-converged structures resulted. Overall these closely resembled the X-ray structure, but the allyl side chain appeared far less well defined. As it is likely that the allyl group interacts with calcineurin in the ternary complex, care should be taken in interpreting its structure from the binary complex alone. The $^{13}$C-labelled FK506 complexed to FKBP also provided the means for correlating the mobility of groups, via $^{13}$C–$^1$H NOEs, with their solvent exposure, by the sensitivity of longitudinal relaxation to paramagnetic HyTEMPO added to the solvent.[89] The mobility generally correlated with solvent exposure, with the exception of the macrocycle, which was found to be relatively immobile.

# IV OTHER NMR STUDIES

While the examples described above have concentrated on ligand–protein interactions, NMR has also made significant contributions to the understanding of drug–nucleotide interactions (see, e.g, References 90–93 and the final two chapters of this book). In addition, the use of solid-state NMR to define the conformations of bound ligands represents an exciting development, particularly for systems that are presently unapproachable by solution-state methods.[94-95]

# V INTEGRATION INTO A DRUG DISCOVERY PROGRAM

Although the examples described above demonstrate the power of several NMR techniques to study ligands in their bound form, it is clear that NMR does not have all the answers. The time pressures associated with drug discovery usually ensure that the means by which a protein–ligand structure is analysed are selected on the basis of efficiency. In many pharmaceutical research establishments, NMR studies are conducted in parallel with several other spectroscopic and diffraction techniques. While

NMR may comprise overall the most detailed information of the spectro-scopic methods, circumstances do exist where alternative techniques, such as fluorescence or ESR, can provide information more useful to the drug-optimisation process. The close reliance of several of the studies described above on X-ray structures of the target (or a model derived from an X-ray structure) is also significant. X-ray diffraction is still seen as providing the most precise information about the structure of a complex; the argument that it is much slower than NMR studies does not apply once a structure is solved, as complexes with the protein can usually be examined on a time scale of a month or two.

A great advantage that NMR has in such a field is its adaptability; the examples described above range from a detailed description of the structure of a complex to an indication of multiplicity of binding modes. Experiments can be designed appropriate to the nature of the system and the questions pending in the drug-optimisation program. This often requires imaginative production of suitable ligands or proteins to facilitate the NMR process. New developments in NMR technology are rapidly incorporated; a recent example is the demonstration of water displacement from an inhibitor complex of HIV protease,[96] as is further discussed in Chapter 10. The progression of NMR over the past two decades now makes it an automatic option when structures of complexes are being examined.

In summary, the past has been exciting and the future will be even more so.

---

## ACKNOWLEDGMENTS

I wish to thank Chun-wa Chung, Mike Hann, and Malcolm Weir for their helpful comments and suggestions.

# REFERENCES

1. Clore. G.M.; Apella, E.; Yamada, M.; Matsushima, K.; Gronenborn, A.M. *Biochemistry* 1990, 29, 1689-1696.
2. Clore. G.M.; Wingfield, P.T.; Gronenborn, A.M. *Biochemistry* 1991, 30, 2315-2323.
3. Smith, L.J.; Redfield, C.; Boyd, J.; Lawrence, G.M.P.; Edwards, R.G.; Smith, R.A.G.; Dobson, C.M. *J. Mol. Biol.* 1992, 224, 899-904.
4. Booker, G.W.; Breeze, A.L.,; Downing, A.K.; Panayotou, G.; Gout, I.; Waterfield, M.D.; Campbell, I.D. *Nature* 1992, 358, 684-687.
5. Yu, H.; Rosen, M.K.; Shin, T.B.; Seidel-Dugan, C.; Brugge, J.S.; Schreiber, S.L. *Science* 1992, 258, 1665-1668.

6. Noggle, J.H.; Schirmer, R.E. *The Nuclear Overhauser Effect*; Academic Press: New York, 1971.

7. Neuhaus, D.; Williamson, M.P. *The Nuclear Overhauser Effect in Structural and Conformational Analysis*; VCH Publishers: New York, 1989.

8. Clore G.M.; Gronenborn, A.M. *J. Magn. Reson.* 1983, 48, 402-417.

9. Campbell, A.P.; Sykes, B.D. *Ann. Rev. Biophys. Biomol. Struct.* 1993, 22, 99-122.

10. Clore, G.M.; Gronenborn, A.M.; Carlson, G.; Meyer, E.F. *J. Mol. Biol.* 1986, 190, 259-267.

11. Lippens, G.; Hallenga, K.; Van Belle, D.; Wodak, S.J.; Nirmala, N.R.; Hill, P.; Russell, K.C.; Smith D.D.; Hruby, V.J. *Biochemistry* 1993, 32, 9423-9434.

12. Cooke, R.M.; Hale, R.S.; Lister, S.G.; Shah, G.; Weir, M.P. *Biochemistry* 1994, 33, 10591-10596.

13. Bevilacqua, V.L.; Thomson, D.S.; Prestegard, J.H. *Biochemistry* 1990, 29, 5529-5537.

14. Glaudermans, C.P.J.; Lerner, L.; Daves, G.D.; Kovac, P.; Venable, R.; Bax, A. *Biochemistry* 1990, 29, 10906-10911.

15. Ni, F.; Ripoli, D.R.; Martin, P.D.; Edwards, B.F.P. *Biochemistry* 1992, 31, 11551-11557.

16. Gronenborn, A.M.; Clore, G.M.; Brunori, M.; Giardina, B.; Falcioni, G.; Perutz, M.F. *J. Mol. Biol.* 1984, 178, 731-742.

17. Birdsall, B.; Bevan, A.W.; Pascual, C.; Roberts, G.C.K.; Feeney, J.; Gronenborn, A.; Clore, G.M. *Biochemistry* 1984, 23, 4733-4742.

18. Banerjee, A.; Levy, H.R.; Levy, G.C.; Chan, W. W.-C. *Biochemistry* 1985, 24, 1593-1598.

19. Meyer, E.F.; Clore, G.M.; Gronenborn, A.M.; Hansen, H.A.S. *Biochemistry* 1988, 27, 725-730.

20. Zilber, B; Scherf, T.; Levitt, M.; Anglister, J. *Biochemistry* 1990, 29, 10032-10041.

21. Cung, M.T.; Demange, P.; Marraud, M.; Tsikaris, V.; Sakarellos, C.; Papadouli, I.; Tzartos, S.J. *Biopolymers* 1991, 31, 769-776.

22. Bevilacqua, V.L.; Kim, Y.; Prestegard, J.H. *Biochemistry* 1992, 31, 9339-9349.

23. Bushweller, J.H; Bartlett, P.A. *Biochemistry* 1991, 30, 8144-8151.

24. Landry, S.J.; Gierasch, L.M. *Biochemistry* 1991, 30, 7359-7362.

25. Machida M.; Yokoyama, S.; Matsuzawa, H.; Miyazawa, T.; Ohta, T. *J. Biol. Chem.* 1985, 260, 16143-16147.

26. Koide, S.; Yokoyama, S.; Matsuzawa, H.; Miyazawa, T.; Ohta, T. *J. Biol. Chem.* 1989, 264, 8676-8679.

27. Brito, R.M.; Rudolph, F.B.; Rosevear, P.R. *Biochemistry* 1991, 30, 1461-1469.

28. Landy, S.B.; Ray, B.D.; Plateau, P.; Lipkowitz, K.B.; Nageswara Rao, B.D. *Eur. J. Biochem.* 1992, 205, 59-69.

29. Campbell, A.P.; Tarasow, T.M.; Massefski, W.; Wright, P.E.; Hilvert, D. *Proc. Natl. Acad. Sci. USA* 1993, 90, 8663-8667.

30. Pruzanski, W.; Vadas, P. *Immunology Today* 1991, 12, 143-146.

31. Plesniak, L.A.; Boegeman, S.C.; Segelke, B.W.; Dennis, E.A. *Biochemistry* 1993, 32, 5009-5016.

32. Poller, L., Ed.; *Recent Advances in Blood Coagulation No. 5*; Churchill Livingstone: Edinburgh, 1991.

33. Ni, F.; Meinwald, C.; Vasquez, M.; Scheraga, H.A. *Biochemistry* 1989, 28, 3094-3105.

34. Nakanishi, H.; Chrusciel, R.A.; Shen, R.; Bertenshaw, S.; Johnson, M.E.; Rydel, T.J.; Tulinsky, A.; Kahn, M. *Proc. Natl. Acad. Sci. USA* 1992, 89, 1705-1709.

35. Wu, T.-P.; Yee, V.; Tulinsky, A.; Chrusciel, R.A.; Nakanishi, H.; Shen, R.; Priebe, C.; Kahn, M. *Prot. Eng.* 1993, 6, 471-478.
36. Ni, F.; Konishi, Y.; Scheraga, H.A. *Biochemistry* 1990, 29, 4479-4489.
37. Rydel, T.J.; Ravichandran, K.G.; Tulinsky, A.; Bode, W.; Huber, R.; Roitsch, C.; Fenton, J.W. *Science* 1990, 249, 277-280.
38. Dratz, E.A.; Furstenau, J.E.; Lambert, C.G.; Thireault, D.L.; Rarick, H.; Schepers, T.; Pakhlevaniants, S.; Hamm, H.E. *Nature* 1993, 263, 276-280.
39. Wüthrich, K. *Struct. Bond.* 1970, 8, 53-121.
40. Gao, Y.; Veitch, N.C.; Williams, R.J.P. *J. Biomol. NMR* 1991, 1, 457-471.
41. Jarori, G.K; Ray, B.D.; Nageswara Rao, B.D. *Biochemistry* 1989, 28, 9343-9350.
42. Martinez, A.; Abeygunawardana, C.; Haavik, J.; Flatmark, T.; Mildvan, A.S. *Biochemistry* 1993, 32, 6381-6390.
43. Gregory, J.D.; Serpesu, E.H. *J. Biol. Chem.* 1993, 268, 3880-3888.
44. Weber, D.J.; Mullen, G.P.; Mildvan, A.S. *Biochemistry* 1991, 30, 7425-7437.
45. Weber, D.J.; Gittis, A.G.; Mullen, G.P.; Abeygunawardana, C.; Lattman, E.E.; Mildvan, A.S. *Proteins Struct. Function Genet.* 1992, 13, 275-287.
46. Weber, D.J.; Serpescu, E.H.; Gittis, A.G.; Lattman, E.E.; Mildvan, A.S. *Proteins Struct. Function Genet.* 1993, 17, 20-35.
47. Chuang, W.J.; Weber, D.J.; Gittis, A.G.; Mildvan, A.S. *Proteins Struct. Function Genet.* 1993, 17, 36-48.
48. Bennion, C.; Connolly, S.; Gensmantel, N.P.; Hallam, C.; Jackson, C.G.; Primrose, W.U.; Roberts, G.C.K.; Robinson, D.H.; Slaich, P.K. *J. Med. Chem.* 1992, 35, 2939-2951.
49. Griffey, R.H.; Redfield, A.G.; Loomis, R.E.; Dahlquist, F.W. *Biochemistry* 1985, 24, 817-822.
50. Peersen, O.B.; Pratt, E.A.; Truong, H.-T.N.; Ho, C.; Rule, G.S. *Biochemistry* 1990, 29, 3256-3262.
51. Vogel, H.J.; Bridger, W.A. *Biochemistry* 1982, 21, 5825-5831.
52. Hammond, S.J. *J. Chem. Soc. Chem. Commun.*, 1984, 712-713.
53. Malthouse, J.P.G.; Mackenzie, N.E.; Boyd, A.S.F.; Scott, A.I. *J. Am. Chem. Soc.* 1983, 105, 1685-1686.
54. Rich, D.H.; Bernatowicz, M.S.; Schmidt, P.G. *J. Am. Chem. Soc.* 1982, 104, 3535-3536.
55. Birdsall, B.; Gronenborn, A.; Hyde, E.I.; Clore, G.M.; Roberts, G.C.K.; Feeney, J.; Burgen, A.S.V. *Biochemistry* 1982, 21, 5831-5838.
56. Birdsall, B.; De Graw, J.; Feeney, J.; Hammond, S.; Searle, M.S.; Roberts, G.C.K.; Colwell, W.T.; Crase, J. *FEBS Letts.* 1987, 217, 106-110.
57. Cheung, H.T.A.; Searle, M.S.; Feeney, J.; Birdsall, B.; Roberts, G.C.K.; Kompis, I.; Hammond, S. *Biochemistry* 1986, 25, 1925-1931.
58. Searle, M.S.; Forster, M.J.; Birdsall, B.; Roberts, G.C.K.; Feeney, J.; Cheung, H.T.A.; Kompis, I.; Geddes, A.J. *Proc. Natl. Acad. Sci. USA* 1998, 85, 3787-3791.
59. Birdsall, B.; Andrews, J.; Ostler, G.; Tendler, S.J.B.; Feeney, J.; Roberts, G.C.K.; Davies, R.W.; Cheung, H.T.A. *Biochemistry* 1989, 28, 1353-1362.
60. Birdsall, B.; Feeney, J.; Tendler, S.J.B.; Hammond, S.J.; Roberts, G.C.K. *Biochemistry* 1989, 28, 2297-2305.
61. Birdsall, B.; Tendler, S.J.B.; Arnold, J.R.P.; Feeney, J.; Griffin, R.J.; Carr, M.D.; Thomas, J.A.; Roberts, G.C.K.; Stevens, M.F.G. *Biochemistry* 1990, 29, 9660-9667.
62. Selinsky, B.S.; Perlman, M.E.; London, R.E.; Unkefer, C.J.; Mitchell, J.; Blakley, R.L. *Biochemistry* 1990, 29, 1290-1296.

63. Falzone, C.J.; Benkovic, S.J.; Wright, P.E. *Biochemistry* 1990, 29, 9667-9677.
64. Huang, F.-Y.; Yang, Q.-X.; Huang, T.-H. *FEBS Letts.* 1991, 289, 231-234.
65. Falzone, C.J.; Wright, P.E.; Benkovic, S.J. *Biochemistry* 1991, 30, 2184-2191.
66. Wonacott, A.; Cooke, R.; Hayes, F.R.; Hann, M.M.; Jhoti, H.; McMeekin, P.; Mistry, A.; Murray-Rust, P.; Singh, O.M.P.; Weir, M.P. *J. Med. Chem.* 1993, 36, 3113-3119.
67. Jhoti, H.; Singh, O.M.P.; Weir, M.P.; Cooke, R.; Murray-Rust, P.; Wonacott, A. *Biochemistry* 1994, 33, 8417-8427.
68. Griffey, R.H.; Jarema, M.A.; Kunz, S.; Rosevear, P.R.; Redfield, A.G. *J. Am. Chem. Soc.* 1985, 107, 711-712.
69. Worgotter, E.; Wagner, G.; Wüthrich, K. *J. Am. Chem. Soc.* 1986, 108, 6162-6167.
70. Weis, M.A.; Redfield, A.G.; Griffey, R.H. *Proc. Natl. Acad. Sci. USA* 1986, 83, 1325-1329.
71. Otting, G.; Senn, H.; Wagner, G.; Wüthrich, K. *J. Magn. Reson.* 1986, 70, 500-505.
72. Griffey, R.H.; Redfield, A.G. *Quart. Rev. Biophys.* 1987, 19, 51-82.
73. Otting, G.; Wüthrich K. *Quart. Rev. Biophys.* 1990, 23, 39-96.
74. Wider, G.; Weber, C.; Traber, R.; Widmer, H.;, Wüthrich K. *J. Am. Chem. Soc.* 1990, 112, 9015-9016.
75. Lepre, C.A.; Thomson, J.A.; Moore, J.M. *FEBS Lett.* 1992, 302, 89-96.
76. Fesik, S.W.; Luly, J.R.; Erickson, J.W.; Abad-Zapatero, C. *Biochemistry* 1988, 27, 8297-8301.
77. Derrick, J.P.; Lian, L.-Y.; Roberts, G.C.K.; Shaw, W.V. *Biochemistry* 1992, 31, 8191-8195.
78. Driscoll, P.C.; Altman, J.D.; Boniface, J.J.; Sakaguchi, K.; Reay, P.A.; Omichinski, J.G.; Apella, E.; Davis, M.M. *J. Mol. Biol.* 1993, 232, 342-350.
79. Schreiber, S.L. *Science* 1991, 251, 283-287.
80. Fesik, S.W.; Gampe, R.T.; Holzman, T.F.; Egan, D.A.; Edalji, R.; Luly, J.R.; Simmer, R.; Helfrich, R.; Kishore, V.; Rich, D.H. *Science* 1990, 250, 1406-1409.
81. Weber, C.; Wider, G.; von Freyberg, B.; Traber, R.; Braun, W.; Widmer, H.; Wüthrich, K. *Biochemistry* 1991, 30, 6563-6574.
82. Fesik, S.W.; Gampe, R.T.; Eaton, H.L.; Gemmecker, G.; Olejniczak, E.T.; Neri, P.; Holzman, T.F.; Egan, D.A.; Edalji, R.; Simmer, R.; Helfrich, R.; Hochlowski, J.; Jackson, M. *Biochemistry* 1991, 30, 6574-6583.
83. Fesik, S.W.; Gemmecker, G.; Olejniczak, E.T.; Petros, A.M. *J. Am. Chem. Soc.* 1991, 113, 7080-7081.
84. Hsu, V.L.; Armitage, I.M. *Biochemistry* 1992, 31, 12778-12784.
85. Spitzfaden, C.; Weber, H.-P.; Braun, W.; Kallen, J.; Wider, G.; Widmer, H.; Walkinshaw, M.D.; Wüthrich, K. *FEBS Letts.* 1992, 300, 291-300.
86. Theriault, Y.; Logan, T.M.; Meadows, R.; Yu, L.; Olejniczak, E.T.; Holzman, T.F.; Simmer, R.L; Fesik, S.W. *Nature* 1993, 361, 88-91.
87. Wenger, R.M.; France, J.; Bovermann, G.; Walliser, L.; Widmer, A.; Widmer, H. *FEBS Lett.* 1994, 340, 255-259.
88. Van Duyne, G.D.; Standaert, R.F.; Karplus, P.A.; Schreiber, S.L.; Clardy, J. *Science* 1991, 252, 839-842.
89. Lepre, C.A.; Cheng, J.-W.; Moore, J.M. *J. Am. Chem. Soc.* 1993, 115, 4929-4930.
90. Gao, X.; Patel, D.J. *Biochemistry* 1989, 28, 751-762.
91. Banville, D.L.; Keniry, M.A.; Shafer, R.H. *Biochemistry* 1990, 29, 9294-9304.
92. Searle, M.S.; Bicknell, W.; Wakelin, L.P.; Denny, W.A. *Nucleic Acids Res.* 1991, 19, 2897-2906.

93. Kumar, S.; Joseph, T.; Singh, M.P.; Bathini, Y.; Lown, J.W. *J. Biomol. Struct. Dyn.* 1992, 9, 853-880.
94. McDermott, A.E.; Creuzet, F.; Griffin, R.G.; Zawadzke, L.E.; Ye, Q.-Z.; Walsh, C.T. *Biochemistry* 1990, 29, 5767-5775.
95. Christensen, A.M.; Schaefer, J. *Biochemistry* 1993, 32, 2868-2873.
96. Grzesiek, S.; Bax, A.; Nicholson, L.K.; Yamazaki, T.; Wingfield, P.; Stahl, S.J.; Eyermann, C.J.; Torchia, D.A.; Hodge, C.N.; Lam, P.Y.S.; Jadhav, P.K.; Chang, C.-H. *J. Am. Chem. Soc.* 1994, 116, 1581-1582.

## CHAPTER 8

# NMR Studies of Ligand Binding to Dihydrofolate Reductase and Their Application in Drug Design

*J. Feeney*

## CONTENTS

I Introduction ................................................................................ 276

II Enzymatic Reduction of Substrates by DHFR ............................ 278

III Assignment of NMR Resonances ................................................ 281
   A Protein-Resonance Assignments .............................................. 281
   B Ligand-Resonance Assignments ............................................... 285

IV Detection Of Specific Interactions ............................................. 288
   A Determination of Ionization States ......................................... 288
   B Interactions Involving the Glutamic Acid Moiety of
     Folate Analogues ..................................................................... 290

V Rational Design of Inhibitors ..................................................... 291

VI Multiple Conformations ............................................................. 294
   A DHFR–Trimethoprim–NADP⁺ Complexes ............................. 295

0-8493-7824-9/96/$0.00+$.50
© 1996 by CRC Press, Inc.

B  Conformational Selection of Rotational Isomers of
   Pyrimethamine Analogues Bound to *L. casei* DHFR .............. 296
C  DHFR Complexes with the Substrate Folate ......................... 301
D  *Escherichia coli* DHFR Complex with Methotrexate ............... 306

VII  Dynamic Processes in DHFR–Ligand Complexes ........................ 306

VIII  Conclusion ................................................................................ 308

Acknowledgments ................................................................................ 308

References ........................................................................................ 308

# I    INTRODUCTION

For several years dihydrofolate reductase (DHFR) has been the focus of intense study, stimulated largely by pharmacological interest in the enzyme because of its importance as a target for antifolate drugs. This enzyme catalyses the reduction of dihydrofolate (and folate with lower efficiency) to tetrahydrofolate using NADPH as coenzyme.[1]

$$\text{Folate} + \text{NADPH} + \text{H}^+ \rightleftarrows 7,8\text{-dihydrofolate} + \text{NADP}^+$$

$$7,8\text{-Dihydrofolate} + \text{NADPH} + \text{H}^+ \rightleftarrows 5,6,7,8\text{-tetrahydrofolate} + \text{NADP}^+$$

The product of the reaction, tetrahydrofolate, is a required cofactor in several biosynthetic processes involved in synthesis of purines, pyrimidines, and some amino acids. Because the enzyme is essential in all cells, it provides an excellent target for agents that selectively inhibit the enzyme in parasitic or malignant cells. Antifolate drugs such as trimethoprim **1** (antibacterial), methotrexate **2** (antineoplastic), and pyrimethamine (antimalarial) all act by inhibiting the enzyme.

**1** Trimethoprim          **2** Methotrexate

A considerable amount of ligand-binding and structural data has been acquired for DHFRs from several sources. Binding studies of inhibitors and coenzyme to DHFR have revealed examples of both positive and negative cooperative binding.[2,3] X-ray crystal structures have been determined for several DHFR complexes.[4-14] Because the enzyme is fairly small (18,000–25,000 Da in most species), it is also amenable to NMR studies aimed at probing its interactions, conformations, and dynamics in solution.[15-20] There have also been numerous studies involving DHFR variants prepared by site-directed mutagenesis in order to address specific questions relating to the enzyme catalysis or ligand binding.[21-25] Structures of complexes of DHFR with ligands have also been modelled using quantum energy calculations.[26,27]

The availability of high-quality X-ray crystal structures for several complexes of DHFR from various sources has provided the major impetus for rational design of DHFR inhibitors. By using such structural information in combination with molecular graphics and molecular-modelling methods, several inhibitors of DHFR have been designed.[28-38] While X-ray structural information on DHFR complexes has been available for more than a decade, it is only relatively recently that NMR spectroscopy has been able to provide comparable information for proteins of this size. Detailed information about the structures of DHFR complexes from NMR studies is now emerging, and the next two or three years should see the full determination of the structures of several DHFR–ligand complexes in solution. NMR has already shown that the overall structures of DHFR–ligand complexes in solution are similar to those in the crystal state.[39,40]

NMR has been able to make several useful contributions to the inhibitor design process. For example, it has proved to be good at defining specific interactions between the protein and ligand, especially where these involve groups capable of existing in different protonation states. NMR can sometimes be used to monitor whether or not a predicted interaction has been formed in a complex, and it has proved to be a useful tool for monitoring inhibitor design. It can also be used to detect conformational differences between protein–ligand complexes formed with related inhibitors. Thus, it can report on whether a particular chemical modification to an inhibitor has introduced or removed a specific protein–ligand interaction, and also whether there has been any accompanying change in conformation. These factors will clearly affect the energetics of the interactions. NMR can also be used for detecting multiple conformations in protein–ligand complexes. These are difficult to study using other methods, such as X-ray crystallography. We have detected several examples of flexible ligands that occupy essentially the same binding site but bind in different conformational states. It is important to be aware of the various options for occupying the binding site, since each of these can provide a different starting point for the design of novel inhibitors. NMR also provides useful information about dynamic processes within the protein–ligand complex. While these dynamic processes may not have a large effect on the energetics of the equilibrium binding in the protein–ligand complex, they can influence the kinetics of binding. These processes could have important consequences in cases where it is the rate of ligand binding that controls the response to receptor binding.

A limited amount of NMR work has also been carried out on R-67 DHFR, the R-plasmid-encoded protein that confers clinical resistance to trimethoprim.[41] This enzyme is a tetramer of 33,720 Da with no homology to chromosomal DHFR.

---

## II  ENZYMATIC REDUCTION OF SUBSTRATES BY DHFR

NMR has made several important contributions to the understanding of the enzymatic reduction of substrates by DHFR. Although a full understanding has still not been reached, the knowledge currently available provides useful background information for assisting in inhibitor design.

DHFR reduces folate (3) first to 7,8-dihydrofolate (4) and then to 5,6,7,8-tetrahydrofolate (5), the first step being 100 times slower than the second for the *L. casei* enzyme reaction.[42] The stereochemistry of the reduction has been determined by using a combination of X-ray and NMR data. Previous work has shown that reduction of 7,8-dihydrofolate at C6 involves transfer of the 4-pro-R hydrogen of NADPH.[43,44]

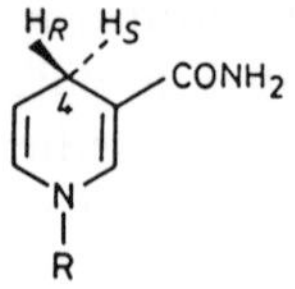

We have used NMR to examine the 5,6,7,8-tetrahydrofolate produced by reducing folate with *Lactobacillus casei* DHFR and selectively deuterated NADPH ((4R)-[4-²H]NADPH). Comparison of the ¹H spectrum of the deuterated tetrahydrofolate with nondeuterated tetrahydrofolate could show that the deuterons transferred to the C6 and C7 positions are both added on the same face of the pterin ring[45,46] (see Structure 5).

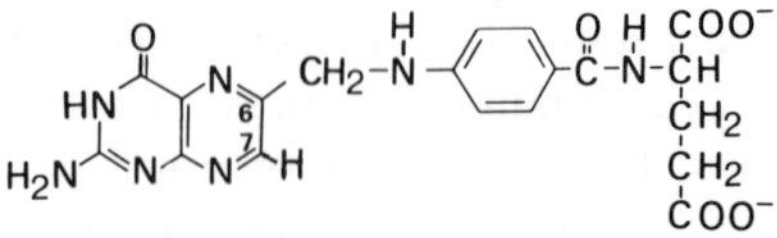

3 Folate

**4** Dihydrofolate

**5** Tetrahydrofolate

The assignments of the proton signals were based on considerations of the $^3J_{HH}$ vicinal coupling constants. Earlier X-ray crystallographic studies on a tetrahydrofolate had established the absolute configuration of the hydrogen at the 6 position as 6S (see Structure **5**).[47,48] Thus, the NMR result gives the configuration of the added proton at the 7 position as 7S, that is, on the same face as 6S. In the X-ray structure of the complex of methotrexate (MTX) with NADPH and DHFR, the "transferred" proton $4\text{-}H_R$ of NADPH was seen to be near the face of the pteridine ring, which is opposite to that which receives the protons in folate reduction.[3,28,45-47] Thus, although folate and methotrexate have similar structures, it is clear that the pteridine ring of methotrexate binds to DHFR in a different orientation to that for 7,8-dihydrofolate[5,28,47] and folate.[45,46] Subsequent X-ray[49] and NMR NOE data[50] confirmed that the pterin ring in the folate–DHFR complex is turned over by ~180° compared to its orientation in the methotrexate–DHFR complex. The finding that such similar molecules can bind in very different ways emphasizes the value of carrying out detailed structural studies in evaluating inhibitor design.

One aspect of the reduction that is still not fully understood is the mechanism of protonation of N8 (for folate) and N5 (for dihydrofolate) as the first stage of each reduction step. Selinsky and co-workers[51] have examined binary complexes of bovine DHFR with folate and dihydrofolate (labelled with $^{15}N$ at N5 and $^{13}C$ at C6) and shown that N5 is not protonated in any of the complexes. Site-directed mutagenesis studies have indirectly implicated a conserved Asp (or Glu) residue in the enzymatic reduction: in *L. casei* dihydrofolate reductase the only ionizable group close to the active site is Asp 26 (equivalent to Asp 27 in *E. coli* and Glu 30 in human DHFR). It is clear from the X-ray structure[49] that this residue is not sufficiently close to either N8 or N5 to be involved in direct protonation. The carboxyl group of the conserved Asp residue is hydrogen bonded to the 2-NH$_2$ group and to N3 of the folate,[52,53] and protonation schemes for N8 and N5 have been proposed in which the Asp residue promotes the formation of a protonated enolic form of the pteridine ring as an intermediate prior to reduction at N5. However, studies of binary complexes of [13]C- and [15]N-labelled folates show that bound folate exists in the keto form for human and bacterial enzymes.[52-55] Blakley et al.[53] have also shown that the N3 proton is retained, even at pH 9.5, in the folate complex with human DHFR. They concluded that the predominance of the imino-keto form of bound folate strongly suggests that protonation schemes involving the enolic forms are unlikely to be correct. Blakley et al.[53] could find no evidence for a change in ionization of the Glu 30 carboxylate over the pH range 5 to 7, and this led them to suggest that ionization of Glu 30 is unlikely to be the origin of the observed pH dependence of hydride transfer (apparent pKa ~ 6.0). In the crystal-structure studies of the human DHFR-folate complex, Oefner et al.[49] detected a bound water molecule near to N5, which was suggested as a likely candidate for mediating a proton transfer from Glu 30 to N5. We have recently used 3D [15]N/[1]H ROESY-HMQC and NOESY-HMQC experiments to detect two long-lived water molecules in the active site of the *L. casei* DHFR-MTX-NADPH complex.[56] One of these is near to the Trp 21 indole NH and corresponds to the water molecule implicated in the proton transfer in the human DHFR-FOLATE complex (see Figure 1). The fact that this is a long-lived water molecule in solution supports its possible involvement in the proton transfer to N5.

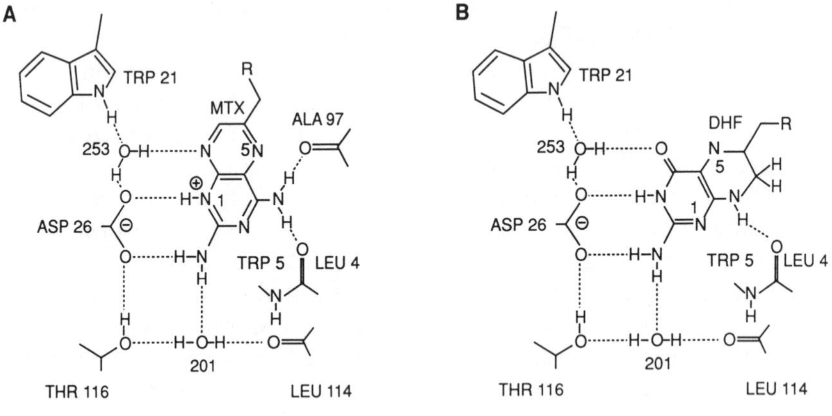

**FIGURE 1**

Schematic diagrams showing the location of water molecules 201 and 253 in the (A) methotrexate-binding site of the *L. casei* DHFR–MTX–NADPH complex as determined by X-ray crystallography,[4] and (B) proposed dihydrofolate (DHF) binding site.[4] (Trp 5 has been incorporated into the original figure from Bolin et al.[4]) (From Bolin, J.T., et al., *Biol. Chem. J.*, 257, 13650–13662. With permission.)

Extensive kinetic studies on various DHFRs have been reported from the laboratories of Benkovic[57,136] and Blakley.[58] For example, Andrews and co-workers[57] have shown that for the *L. casei* enzyme, the dissociation of the product is the rate-limiting step for the steady-state turnover at low pH, with tetrahydrofolate dissociating from the enzyme after NADP[+] is replaced by NADPH.

---

# III   ASSIGNMENT OF NMR RESONANCES

In order to obtain detailed structural information about protein–ligand complexes from their NMR spectra, it is first necessary to assign the protein and ligand resonances. As outlined in Chapter 4, 2D and 3D (even 4D) NMR methods in combination with $^2$H-, $^{13}$C-, and $^{15}$N-labelled proteins can now provide complete assignments for proteins of MW ~ 20 kDa.[59,60] Sets of signal assignments have been reported for several complexes of DHFR from bacterial (*L. casei*,[39,40] *E. coli*[54]) and mammalian (human[61]) species.

## A   PROTEIN-RESONANCE ASSIGNMENTS

In our own studies of *L. casei* DHFR complexed with methotrexate, the backbone (NH and αCH) and side-chain resonance assignments have been obtained for almost all 162 amino acids using multidimensional NMR techniques on a sample of DHFR uniformly labelled with $^{15}$N and $^{13}$C.[39,40] The 3D TOCSY-HMQC, NOESY-HMQC,[62] HMQC-NOESY-HMQC,[63,64] and HNCA[62,65] experiments were the most useful for making the backbone resonance assignments, while the 3D HCCH-COSY and HCCH-TOCSY[66,67] experiments provided most of the side-chain resonance assignments. In the 3D $^{13}$C/$^1$H HCCH-COSY and HCCH-TOCSY spectra of the uniformly $^{13}$C-labelled *L. casei* DHFR complexed with methotrexate, the through-bond $^1$H–$^1$H correlations are characterized by $^1$H and $^{13}$C chemical shifts of the proton/carbon pair from which the magnetization originates and also by the $^1$H chemical shift of the proton to which the magnetization is transferred.[40] The spectra can be considered as a series of 2D $^1$H COSY[68,69] or TOCSY[70,71] slices ($^1$H(F$_1$)/$^1$H(F$_3$)) at different $^{13}$C chemical shifts (F$_2$). The COSY and TOCSY slices can be used to distinguish between cross-peaks from direct and relayed connectivities. Figure 2 shows a series of F$_1$/F$_3$ strips from the HCCH-TOCSY spectrum of the complex taken at the $^{13}$C chemical shifts (F$_2$) of the δ-carbons of the five Ile residues in *L. casei* DHFR. The $^1$H–$^1$H through-bond correlations for all protons along the side chains could be detected and assigned. Similar results were found for side chains from

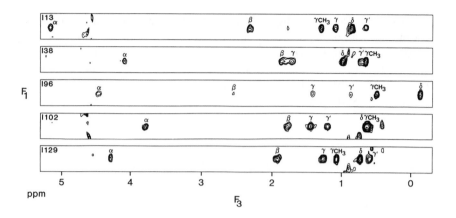

**FIGURE 2**

A series of $F_1/F_3$ strips from the HCCH-TOCSY spectrum of the *L. casei* DHFR–MTX complex taken at the δ-carbon shifts $F_2$ of I13 (15.11 ppm), I38 (16.23 ppm), I96 (11.20 ppm), I102 (10.64 ppm) and I129 (16.79 ppm). The labelled cross-peaks correspond to through-bond correlations spanning the full length of the isoleucine side chains from the δ-methyl protons $F_1$ to γ-methyl, γ-, γ*-, β-, and α-protons $F_3$. (From Soteriou, A., et al., *J. Biomol. NMR*, 3, 535–546, 1993. With permission.)

other residues in DHFR, and most of the side-chain ¹H and ¹³C assignments could be made in this way.

Once the assignments had been made for one complex of *L. casei* DHFR, it proved relatively easy to transfer the assignments to related complexes because of the similarities in the connectivity patterns seen in the 2D spectra of the different complexes. Assigned resonances of *L. casei* DHFR have been used to monitor ionization changes, to characterize conformational mixtures and to provide conformational information from NOE measurements for various complexes of ligands with DHFR.

Stockman and co-workers[61] have reported detailed signal assignments for the complex of human DHFR with methotrexate using 2D and 3D methods with ¹⁵N-enriched protein. By measuring intermolecular NOEs between the ligand and the protein, they have shown that the orientation of the methotrexate pteridine ring in solution is the same as that found in crystal studies.

For large proteins, where sequential-assignment methods are sometimes difficult to apply, assignments can often be made by using NOE measurements to correlate resonances from nuclei known to be close to each other in the crystal structure of the complex. Many of the early assignments for complexes of *L. casei* DHFR were made in this way, and all have proved to be in complete agreement with the sequential assignments made subsequently.[39,40,72] Obviously, for this approach to succeed, the solution and crystal structures need to be similar; frequently, this appears to be the case. Falzone and co-workers[54,73] have used this method to obtain signal assignments for the complexes of *E. coli* DHFR in complexes with methotrexate and folate. They also made many assignments for important residues near to or in the active site by using site-directed mutagenesis studies. By examining variants with a specific amino acid replaced, they could detect the absence of the appropriate signals in the spectrum of the complex with the normal DHFR. Based on these assignments, they were able to determine the orientation of the pterin ring of folate and show it to be similar to that of the productive dihydrofolate complex. Folate was found to bind in a single conformational form to *E. coli* DHFR.[73]

Selective isotope labelling can also be used to simplify spectra and assist in spectral assignments. Selective deuterated proteins can be prepared by biosynthetic incorporation of deuterated amino acids; by comparing spectra of the nondeuterated and selectively deuterated samples, it is possible to detect and assign those $^1$H signals that are present in the former and absent in the latter.[74-79] This is a particularly useful method for assigning signals to a particular type of amino acid. By examining 2D COSY spectra from DHFR containing γ-Me-deuterated valine[75,76] and α-deuterated valine,[77] it was possible to assign the protons normally at the deuterated sites. This approach is also useful for making stereospecific assignments. We have prepared *L. casei* DHFR containing [4-Pro-*R*-CH$_3$]-deuterated leucine,[78] and, by examining the $^1$H COSY spectra (see Figure 3) of deuterated and nondeuterated samples, have made stereospecific assignments for 12 of the 13 Leu residues (one of the leucines had methyl groups with degenerate chemical shifts). The sequential assignments of the signals to specific leucines had been made earlier using the 2D and 3D sequential assignment methods discussed above.[39]

In some experiments, *L. casei* DHFR samples containing several deuterated amino acids have been examined.[76,79] This is a particularly useful approach for examining aromatic amino acid signals and their NOE connections. One of the samples examined containing fully deuterated tryptophan and partially deuterated Tyr, Phe, and His. This mixture of deuterated residues was chosen in order to remove enough protons to simplify the spectra while retaining sufficient protons to give useful NOE information.

We have also incorporated various fluorine-containing amino acids (3-F-Tyr, 3-F-Phe, 6-F-Trp) into *L. casei* DHFR and studied the $^{19}$F spectra to see which residues are influenced by ligand binding.[80,81] It is usually difficult to quantitate the results in structural terms. In complexes formed with *L. casei* DHFR containing 6-F Trp, the fluorine substituents in two of the Trp residues (Trp 5 and Trp 133) are sufficiently close together to show through-space $^{19}$F–$^{19}$F scalar coupling.[81]

Cocco and co-workers[82] have introduced selectively $^{13}$C-labelled arginine, tryptophan and methionine into *Streptococcus faecium* DHFR and used $^{13}$C NMR to monitor various protein–ligand complexes. In $^{13}$C

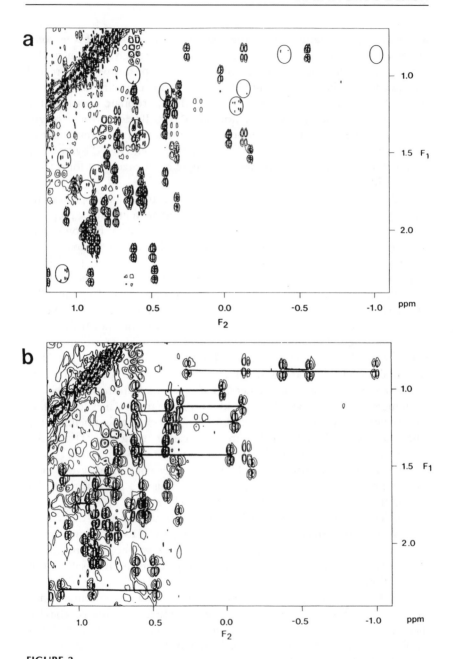

**FIGURE 3**
The high-field "aliphatic" region of the 2D DQFCOSY $^1H$ contour plot for the *L. casei* DHFR–MTX complex recorded at 308 K (a) selectively deuterated enzyme incorporating $(2S,4R)[5,5,5-^2H_3]$leucine, and (b) nondeuterated enzyme. The positions of the leucine cross-peaks involving the 4-pro-R methyl group are circled in (a), and the methyl pairs from each leucine are joined with a line in (b). (From Ostler, G., et al., *FEBS Lett.,* 318, 177–180, 1993. With permission.)

spectra from [guanidino-$^{13}$C] Arg samples they noted different chemical shifts, which allowed the residues to be divided into two classes, one having shifts similar to free Arg corresponding to accessible residues and the other with different shifts corresponding to inaccessible residues. Differences in relaxation times were also noted, with the values for the former class indicating Arg residues with higher mobility. In complexes with NADPH or coenzyme fragments, specific shifts were seen for some Arg signals, indicating interactions between the corresponding Arg residues and the coenzyme phosphate groups. Studies of the $^{13}$C spectra of *S. faecium* DHFR labelled with [3-$^{13}$C]-Trp in the absence of ligands indicated the presence of two conformations.[82] However, in the complex with 3′,5′-dichloromethotrexate the protein was shown to take up a single conformational form.[82]

## B LIGAND-RESONANCE ASSIGNMENTS

Assignments of ligand resonances are particularly important because ligand nuclei, of necessity, are well placed to provide direct information about the binding site in the complex. For complexes with weak binding ligands ($K_a < 10^3$ M$^{-1}$), fast-exchange behaviour is usually observed, and the chemical shifts of the bound ligand can be calculated from the analysis of the binding curves.[83,84] In inhibitor design studies there is usually more interest in studying very tightly binding ligands. The signals from such bound ligands ($K_a > 10^9$ M$^{-1}$) are more difficult to assign. The usual method is to examine isotopically labelled analogues ($^2$H, $^3$H, $^{15}$N, $^{13}$C) in combination with various experimental procedures. For example, deuterated ligands can assist $^1$H assignments by producing differences between $^1$H spectra of complexes formed with deuterated and nondeuterated ligands.[85,86] Another method is to selectively label the ligand with tritium ($^3$H) and then to observe the $^3$H spectra of the complexes; for example, by examining [7,3′,5′-$^3$H]folate in its complex with *L. casei* DHFR and NADP$^+$, it was possible to confirm the presence of three different conformational states by using $^3$H NMR to monitor the assigned tritium resonances for the 7,3′,5′-tritium nuclei.[87] Experiments have also been carried out with [7,3′,5′-$^3$H]methotrexate bound to DHFR.[87]

Complexes formed with $^{15}$N- or $^{13}$C-labelled ligands can be examined directly by using $^{15}$N or $^{13}$C NMR. Only the signals from nuclei at the enriched positions are observed, and thus the assignment problem is usually trivial. Several studies of this type involving isotopically labelled folate,[88,89] methotrexate,[90] and trimethoprim[91-93] have been carried out in our laboratory. Blakley and co-workers[53] have also used this approach to examine [2-amino, 3-$^{15}$N]- and [2-$^{13}$C]folate bound to human DHFR, and Huang and co-workers have likewise studied *E. coli* DHFR complexes containing isotopically labelled folate and trimethoprim.[94,129] Where protons are directly attached to $^{15}N$ or $^{13}C$, the opportunity arises for using isotope editing or filtering pulse sequences. Heteronuclear multiple quantum coherence (HMQC) experiments allow the attached protons to be detected selectively (they are then characterized by both the $^1H$ and $^{15}N$ (or $^{13}C$) frequencies, the X nuclei being detected indirectly). Fesik et al.[95] have shown how these experiments can be used to study protein–ligand complexes. A powerful extension of these experiments is the 3D NOESY-HMQC experiment: this allows selective detection of the NOEs from the ligand protons (on $^{13}C$ or $^{15}N$) to neighbouring protons in the protein and the observed NOESY cross-peaks to be dispersed over the X-chemical-shift frequency range. This considerably simplifies the NOESY spectrum at any particular X frequency and is very important for examining complexes involving large proteins, since the normal NOESY spectrum containing all the ligand–protein and protein–protein NOEs is often too complex to analyse.[62]

We have used 2D HMQC-NOESY $^1H/^{13}C$ experiments to examine complexes of *L. casei* DHFR with [4,7,8a,9-$^{13}C$]methotrexate (see Figure 4): the edited NOEs between MTX H7 and the methyl protons of Leu 19 and 27 indicate that the pteridine ring has the same orientation in the solution and crystal states[50] (see Section VI.C). We have also examined complexes of *L. casei* DHFR with [1,3,2-amino-$^{15}N$]- and [7,4'-OCH$_3$-$^{13}C$]trimethoprim using these approaches and have been able to define details of the trimethoprim binding site from the measured NOEs.[96] This involves docking the ligand into the crystal structure coordinates taken from a related complex by using energy minimization procedures that take into account the distance constraints obtained from the NOEs.

For complexes formed using less tightly binding ligands ($K_a \sim 10^6\ M^{-1}$), the spectra can show slow-exchange behaviour on the chemical-shift time scale, giving separate signals for bound and free species, but the dissociation rate constants can be sufficiently large to allow transfer of saturation or 2D exchange methods to be used to connect the resonances of the bound and free species. Because the assignments in the free ligand are usually known with certainty, the assignments of the connected signals from the bound species can be made. The transfer-of-saturation method has proved useful for assigning signals from NADP$^+$,[97] trimethoprim,[98] and pyrimethamine[99] analogues bound to *L. casei* DHFR.

$^{31}P$ NMR can be used to examine complexes formed with ligands containing phosphorus. In the $^{31}P$ spectrum of NADPH bound to *L. casei* DHFR, the two pyrophosphate $^{31}P$ nuclei could be assigned unequivocally by using heteronuclear correlation experiments.[100] The $^{31}P$ studies provided detailed information about the ionization states and conformations in the bound coenzyme.[101-103]

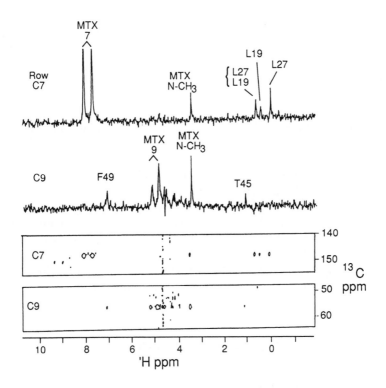

**FIGURE 4**

Part of the two-dimensional $^1H/^{13}C$ HMQC-NOESY spectrum of the binary complex of *L. casei* DHFR with [4,7-8a,9-$^{13}C$]methotrexate at 308 K and pH 6.5 showing the regions containing C7 and C9. The upper traces are the rows at the frequency of C7 and C9 showing the connections to their attached protons and NOEs to signals of nearby residues. The H7 signal appears as a doublet because no $^{13}C$ decoupling in $F_2$ was used. (From Cheung, H.T.A., et al., *FEBS Lett.*, 312, 147–151, 1992. With permission.)

When fluorine-containing ligands are available, $^{19}F$ NMR measurements can be used to examine their complexes with DHFR. The assignments of $^{19}F$ signals from the ligand are often straightforward, since usually only one or two sites are labelled. We have examined complexes of *L. casei* DHFR formed with fluorine containing pyrimethamines; their simple $^{19}F$ spectra proved ideal for monitoring multiple conformations and dynamic processes in the complexes.[99,104]

Once the detailed assignments of the resonances are known, one can measure and compare the NMR parameters for the various nuclei in the free and bound species in a protein–ligand complex or series of related complexes. Changes in chemical shifts, spin-coupling constants, and relaxation behaviour (including nuclear Overhauser effects) have all been monitored to provide information about interactions, conformations, and dynamic processes in the complexes. Chemical-shift changes can sometimes be used for determining ionization states or hydrogen-bonding states where there is a well-documented difference in chemical shift between the two states. Studies of nuclei other than $^1$H can be very useful in this regard; for example, the $^{15}$N chemical shift of a pyrimidine N1 ring nitrogen changes by 80 ppm on protonation.[91]

Measurements of coupling constants in the bound ligand can provide localized conformational information by utilizing the well-established relationships between three-bond vicinal coupling constants and dihedral torsion angles. Surprisingly, few examples of such studies on protein–ligand complexes have been reported,[101,105] probably because of the difficulties of obtaining good coupling-constant data from poorly resolved multiplets detected in their spectra. By far the most direct method of obtaining conformational information is by measuring protein–ligand intermolecular NOEs from a 2D or 3D NOESY spectrum of the complex. Using this approach, spatial information within the binding site can be obtained and details of the specific interactions deduced.

---

# IV  DETECTION OF SPECIFIC INTERACTIONS

## A  DETERMINATION OF IONIZATION STATES

NMR is particularly useful for determining the ionization states of ionizable groups in either the ligand or the protein, and for monitoring how these are perturbed on forming the protein–ligand complex. For example, Cocco et al.[106] examined the $^{13}$C spectrum of [2-$^{13}$C]-methotrexate bound to *S. faecium* DHFR, and by measuring the characteristic $^{13}$C shift of the C2 carbon, showed that the adjacent N1 is protonated in the complex and remains protonated, even at pH 10. Consideration of the crystal structure data of Matthews and co-workers[4-6] indicates that the pteridine protonated N1 would be sufficiently close to a carboxylate oxygen of the conserved Asp 27 in the binding site to form a hydrogen bond. Thus, a combination of NMR (to give the protonation state) and X-ray (to indicate the interacting partner [Asp 27]) gives a more complete picture of this particular interaction. Experiments of the same type have been carried out with wild-type *E. coli* DHFR[107] and also with two mutant enzymes in which Asp 27 was replaced by asparagine and serine. While the pKa of methotrexate is greater than 10 in the complex with the wild-type enzyme, the pKa value is less than 4 in complexes with the mutant enzymes. Similar experiments have been carried out on *L. casei* DHFR.[50]

Similar experiments using [2-$^{13}$C]trimethoprim have been carried out to show that N1 is protonated in trimethoprim bound to *L. casei*

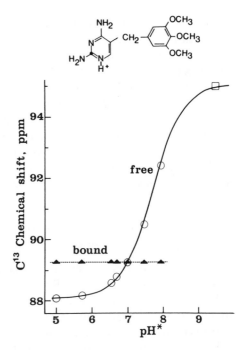

**FIGURE 5**
The pH titration curves of the $^{13}C$ chemical shifts of [2-$^{13}C$]trimethoprim (O) free (▲) in its complex with *L. casei* dihydrofolate reductase. The solid line is calculated for a pKa 7.70 and a shift difference between protonated and unprotonated forms of 7.09 ppm. The enzyme is unstable above pH*8; the data point at pH*9.2 (□) for free trimethoprim was obtained in the absence of enzyme. (From Roberts, G.C.K., et al., *FEBS Lett.*, 131, 85–88, 1981. With permission.)

DHFR.[91,108] Figure 5 shows the titrations of the $^{13}C$ chemical shifts of the C2 resonances in bound and free trimethoprim as a function of pH.[91] The chemical shift of the bound species is seen to be near that for the free protonated N1 species, and the pKa of the bound trimethoprim is decreased by at least 3 pKa units. For the trimethoprim complex with the *L.casei* DHFR, the N1 protonation state could also be measured directly by carrying out $^{15}N$ NMR experiments on a complex of [1,3,2-amino $^{15}N$]-trimethoprim with the enzyme. As mentioned earlier, the $^{15}N$ chemical shift of N1 changes by 80 ppm on protonation, which facilitates detection of the protonated state. In this case, it is also possible to detect the directly bonded proton by observation of its proton signal (it appears at 14.4 ppm from DSS and has a 90-Hz splitting characteristic of $J_{NH}$ coupling).[91] The linewidth of the N1 proton signal changes with temperature because of exchange with protons in the solvent water. At 298 K, the rate of exchange is 34 s$^{-1}$: this represents the minimum rate of breaking and of re-forming the hydrogen bond between N1 proton and the carboxylated oxygen of Asp 26 (equivalent to Asp 27 in *E. coli*).[91]

In the ternary complex of [2-$^{13}C$]-trimethoprim with the *E. coli* DHFR Asp 27/Ser mutant and NADPH, the bound trimethoprim has a pKa of 7.6, which is similar to that of free trimethoprim: in the presence of excess trimethoprim, three signals were observed corresponding to free trimethoprim, bound protonated trimethoprim, and bound unprotonated trimethoprim.[107]

Blakley and co-workers[53] have used $^{15}N$ chemical-shift measurements to show that the N3 atom of [2-amino,3-$^{15}N$]-folate bound to human DHFR exists as the protonated un-ionized form, even at pH 9.5. In earlier experiments on complexes of [2-$^{13}C$]-folate with *S. faecium* DHFR, it was found that the bound folate exhibited the same protonation behaviour as free folate.[106]

Ionization states of phosphate groups can be conveniently measured via $^{31}P$ chemical-shift measurements. For example, the 2′-phosphate groups of NADP$^+$ and NADPH have been shown to exist in their dianionic forms when bound to DHFR (for *L. casei* and *E. coli*) with the pKa of the 2′-phosphate in the bound coenzyme group being decreased by at least three units compared to its pKa in the free species.[101,102]

## B    INTERACTIONS INVOLVING THE GLUTAMIC ACID MOIETY OF FOLATE ANALOGUES

In the crystal structure studies of Matthews and co-workers[4-6] on the ternary complex of *L. casei* DHFR with methotrexate and NADPH, the α-carboxylate of the glutamic acid moiety was located such that it could form an ion pair with the guanidine group of the conserved Arg 57, while the γ-carboxylate group could interact with the imidazole ring of His 28 as shown in Figure 6. In previous NMR studies of the histidine imidazole C2 proton signals in complexes of the DHFR with methotrexate (or other ligands containing the glutamic acid moiety), the pKa of His 28 was found to be ~1 pKa higher than its value in the apoenzyme.[109,110] This change in pKa clearly reflects the interaction of the His 28 with the MTX γ-carboxylate group.[111] These effects have proved useful in studies of complexes of *L. casei* DHFR with the α- and γ-amide analogues of methotrexate (**6** and **7**).[112]

Methotrexate binds an order of magnitude more tightly to *L. casei* DHFR than does its γ-amide analogue and two orders of magnitude more tightly than the α-amide analogue. For the γ-amide MTX complex with

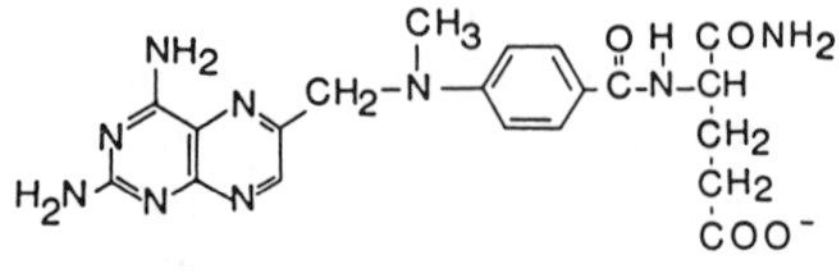

**6** α-amide methotrexate

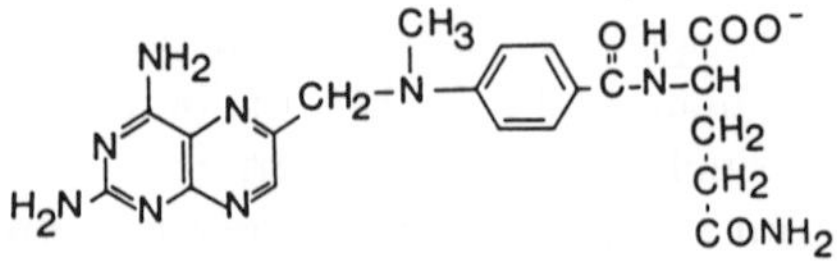

**7** γ-amide methotrexate

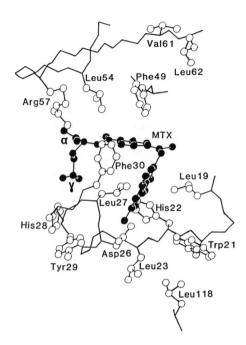

**FIGURE 6**
Part of the crystal structure of the *L. casei* DHFR–MTX–NADPH complex (from the data of Matthews and co-workers[4-6]) showing residues around the methotrexate binding site. (From Hammond, S.J., et al., *Biochemistry*, 26, 8585–8590, 1987. With permission.)

DHFR, the NMR spectrum indicates that the pKa of His 28 was not perturbed from its value in the apoenzyme, showing that the ion-pair interaction is no longer present: the 2D-COSY ¹H spectrum indicated that there was very little other structural change compared with the enzyme–methotrexate complex.[112] Surprisingly, the NMR spectrum of the α-amide MTX complex with DHFR also showed that the pKa of His 28 was not perturbed. Thus, modifying the α-carboxylate not only prevents the Arg 57 interaction, but also perturbs the overall structure such that the available free γ-carboxylate can no longer form an ion pair with His 28. In the 2D COSY spectrum of the DHFR complex with the α-amide MTX, ¹H signals from several residues close to the benzoyl ring (e.g., methyl protons of Leu 19, Leu 27, and Leu 54) are shifted compared to their frequencies in the spectrum of the methotrexate–DHFR complex. The shielding of all these protons is sensitive to the ring-current shielding effects of the benzoyl ring. Thus, the observed shift differences indicate that the removal of the α-$CO_2$-interaction with Arg 57 is accompanied by a change in orientation of the benzoyl ring, resulting in the observed changes in chemical shift of neighbouring protons.[112]

# V RATIONAL DESIGN OF INHIBITORS

The availability of detailed structural information for complexes of dihydrofolate reductase with various inhibitors from both X-ray crystallography[4-14] and NMR spectroscopy[15-20] provides a basis for the rational design of improved inhibitors. These techniques also provide methods for monitoring whether or not novel inhibitors are binding in the predicted manner.

In attempts to achieve improved inhibitor binding to DHFR, analogues of trimethoprim have been prepared with side chains on the benzyl ring aimed at making additional interactions with protein residues involved in substrate binding but not used for trimethoprim binding. Crystal structure studies of trimethoprim and methotrexate complexes of the *E. coli* and chicken liver enzymes and NMR studies of the complexes with the *L. casei* enzyme[86,97,98,113-116] indicate that the 2,4-diaminopyrimidine ring of trimethoprim binds in the same binding site as the corresponding part of the pteridine ring of methotrexate. If we examine the model for trimethoprim (or brodimoprim [**8**]) in its complex with the *L. casei* enzyme, it is seen that the trimethoprim (or brodimoprim), unlike folate or methotrexate, cannot make any direct interactions with Arg 57 and His 28 (see Figures 6 and 7). In collaboration with colleagues from Hoffmann-La Roche, we have synthesized several analogues of brodimoprim, which were designed to have improved binding to the enzyme by making additional interactions with Arg 57 and/or His 28.[117] Computer graphics and molecular modelling techniques were used to assist in designing side chains at the 3'-O-position of brodimoprim aimed at making these interactions (see Table 1).

The measured inhibition constants for the various analogues (Table 1) provide estimates of their improved binding. NMR was used to monitor the pKa values of His 28 residues in the various complexes with DHFR in order to assess whether the side chains were binding in the predicted manner. It was found that the 4,6-dicarboxylate analogue (**9**) binds three orders of magnitude more tightly to DHFR than does the parent molecule and provides a ~1 pKa unit shift in the pKa of His 28, indicating that the carboxylate–His 28 interaction (see Figure 7) has been made. Interestingly,

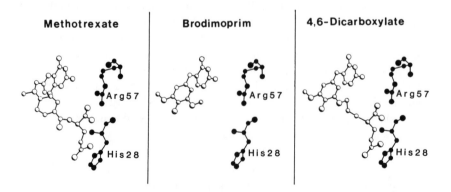

**Methotrexate**            **Brodimoprim**            **4,6-Dicarboxylate**

Arg57    Arg57    Arg57

His28    His28    His28

**FIGURE 7**

Conformations of methotrexate, brodimoprim, and the 4,6-dicarboxylate analogue of brodimoprim in their complexes with *L. casei* DHFR. (From Birdsall, B., et al., *J. Med. Chem.*, 27, 1672–1676, 1984. With permission.)

**TABLE 1**

Inhibition Constants ($K_i$) and His-28 Dissociation Constants ($pK$ Values) for Complexes of *L. casei* Dihydrofolate Reductase with Brodimoprim and Its Derivatives[117]

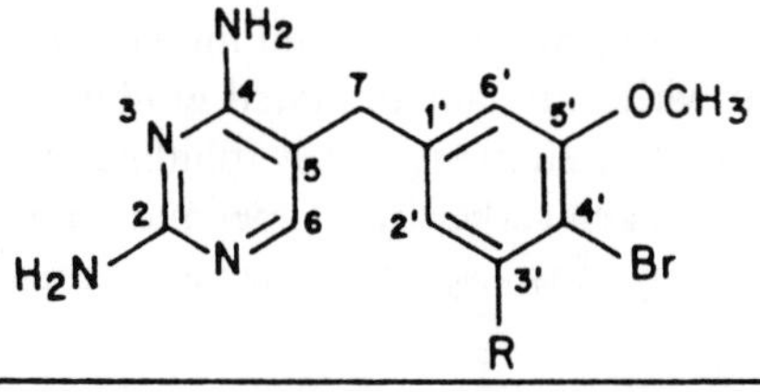

| R | $K_i$, nM | $pK$ His-28 |
|---|---|---|
| OCH$_3$ | 11.3 | 6.80 |
| 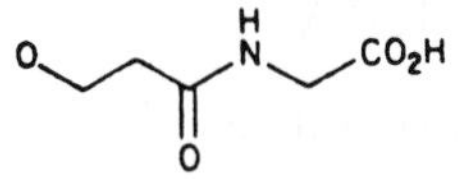 (structure) | 4.1 | 6.71 |
| 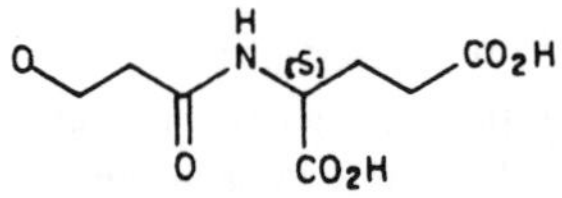 (structure) | 1.7 | 7.12 |
| 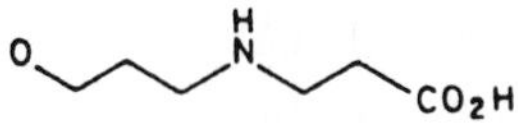 (structure) | 5.3 | 6.71 |
| 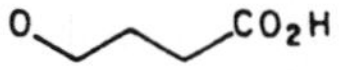 (structure) | 0.9 | |
| 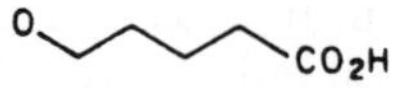 (structure) | 0.2 | 6.83 |
| 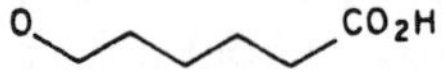 (structure) | 0.4 | |
| 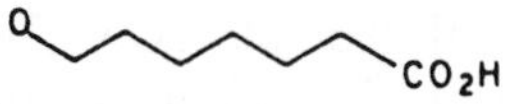 (structure) | 0.6 | 6.80 |
| 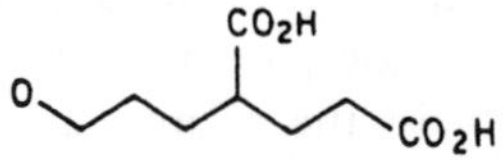 (structure) | <0.01 | 7.80 |

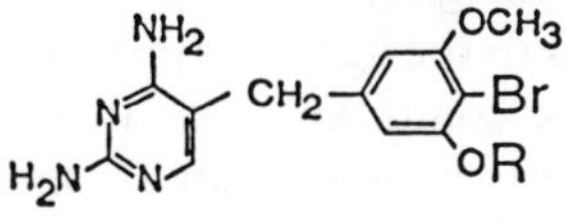

**8** R = CH$_3$

R = (structure)

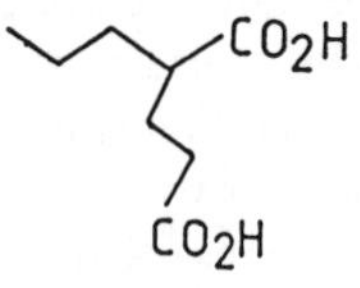

**9**

**8** Brodimoprim and **9** its 4,6-dicarboxylate analogue.

the 6-monocarboxylate analogue (see Table 1), which is modelled to achieve the carboxylate–His 28 interactions, does not perturb the pKa value of His 28, even though it binds fairly tightly. Thus, although the 6-carboxylate analogue can reach His 28, it appears to prefer to bind at some alternative site, possibly Arg 57. For these complexes, NMR provides a convenient method for assessing when predicted interactions are taking place in complexes formed with rationally designed inhibitors.[117]

A similar study aimed at designing tightly binding analogues of trimethoprim had been undertaken earlier by Kuyper and co-workers;[35] in that case X-ray crystallography was used to determine their mode of binding.

# VI MULTIPLE CONFORMATIONS

There have been numerous reports concerned with the existence of multiple conformations in complexes formed with DHFRs from several different sources. Early kinetic[118,119] and NMR studies[76,93,120-122,134] on E. coli, S. faecium, and L. casei DHFR pointed to the presence of multiple conformations in the enzyme. Early [1]H NMR experiments on the L. casei apoenzyme gave broad signals that were thought to be broadened by exchange processes between different conformational states.[72] More recent 2D NMR studies on the E. coli apoenzyme have identified two conformations (in slow exchange on the chemical-shift time scale) and have implicated differences in a mobile loop centred on residues 16–20.[12,123] NMR studies on complexes formed with the enzyme from various sources have provided direct evidence that several of the complexes exist as mixtures of conformations with lifetimes such that the individual conformations give separate [1]H spectra.[89,99,104,125-127] In these cases, intensity measurements of the NMR signals can be used to obtain the relative amounts of the different conformers in the equilibrium. The conformational equilibria can often be perturbed by changing the temperature or the pH, or by making structural modifications to the ligand or protein (the latter by site-directed mutagenesis). For some complexes, the rate of interconversion between the conformational states can be measured from analysis of the lineshapes. The existence of multiple conformations in a DHFR–ligand complex depends on the particular species of DHFR being examined. For example, L. casei DHFR in its complex with methotrexate gives an NMR spectrum containing a single set of signals corresponding to a well-defined single conformational form.[128] In contrast, the corresponding complex formed using E. coli DHFR exists as two forms.[73,90,94] However, for other ligands, such as folate, it is the complex with the L. casei enzyme[50,89,124] that shows multiple conformations, whereas that with the E. coli enzyme exists as a single form.[123] For other complexes, such as DHFR–trimethoprim–NADP$^+$

complexes, the *L. casei*[125-127] and *E. coli*[129] enzymes both exist in two different conformational states.

## A    DHFR–TRIMETHOPRIM–NADP+ COMPLEXES

The ternary complex formed by *L. casei* DHFR with trimethoprim and NADP+ has been shown to exist as a mixture of two conformations with almost equal populations (forms I and II).[125-127] The original observation of the two conformations was made in the [1]H spectrum of the complex where separate signals were detected for six of the seven histidine imidazole C2 protons in *L. casei* DHFR.[125,126] On raising the temperature, the histidine "doublets" coalesced into single lines in a manner typical of a two-site exchange process: a lineshape analysis at 314 K yielded the rate of interconversion ($18$ s$^{-1}$) between the two forms. Subsequent [13]C and [31]P studies confirmed the presence of two conformations (see the [13]C spectra in Figure 8). The [31]P spectra are particularly useful for estimating the amounts of the two conformations. Studies of complexes of analogues of TMP and NADP+ with DHFR indicated that the two conformations exist in many related complexes, the actual populations depending on the particular structures of the analogues. Such information provides an additional insight into

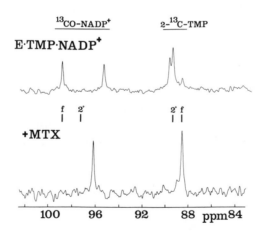

**FIGURE 8**

(Top) The 50.3-MHz [13]C NMR spectrum of the complex between *L. casei* dihydrofolate reductase, [carboxamide-[13]C]NADP+, and [2-[13]C]trimethoprim. The lower-field pair of resonances arise from NADP+ and the high-field pair from trimethoprim (there is also a signal at 88.5 ppm from a small amount of free trimethoprim). (Bottom) The same sample after addition of excess methotrexate. The "sticks" indicate the [13]C chemical shifts of NADP+ and trimethoprim free (f) and in their respective binary complexes (2°). (From Birdsall, B., et al., *Biochemistry*, 23, 4733–4742, 1984. With permission.)

structure-activity relationships. The structures of the two conformations, although different from each other, seem to be fairly similar in the complexes formed with different analogues, except that the populations of the conformational forms vary with the substituents. It is interesting that the two conformations also seen in the DHFR–trimethoprim–NADP+ complex formed with the *E. coli* enzyme[129] appear to be similar to those observed in the complex formed with the *L. casei* enzyme.[125-127]

A consideration of the measured chemical shifts, coupling constants, and NOEs indicates that the conformation of bound NADP+ is very different in the two forms; in form II the NADP+ nicotinamide ring extends out into solution, while in form I it is buried within the protein.[125,126] There are also conformational differences in the nicotinamide ribose ring and the pyrophosphate linkages between forms I and II, but the adenine ring and its ribose moiety bind similarly in the two forms. There is no major difference in the trimethoprim conformation between the two forms. Each is associated with a different protein conformation, and as mentioned above, these appear to be similar in complexes formed using different analogues of trimethoprim and NADP+. The differences in protein conformation between forms I and II are reflected in the widespread differences in the $^1$H chemical shifts between corresponding protons in the two forms. These differences are more pronounced than those noted for the protein signals observed in other complexes where the multiple conformations result from flexible ligands binding in essentially the same binding site but in different conformational states. Some examples of such complexes will now be considered.

## B  CONFORMATIONAL SELECTION OF ROTATIONAL ISOMERS OF PYRIMETHAMINE ANALOGUES BOUND TO *L. CASEI* DHFR

A flexible ligand that exists in solution in more than one conformational state can bind to the protein in different conformational forms. Such effects have been seen for DHFR complexes with pyrimethamine analogues, which

|    | R$'_4$ | R$'_3$ |
|----|--------|--------|
| 10 | Cl     | H      |
| 11 | F      | H      |
| 12 | F      | NO$_2$ |

have a biphenyl-like structure that can give rise to rotational isomers resulting from hindered rotation about the pyrimidine–phenyl bond.[99,104] This type of restricted rotation has been well characterized in ortho-substituted biphenyls, and ortho-substituted phenyl pyrimidines are expected to behave in a similar manner. NMR spectroscopy has been used to investigate such restricted rotation in complexes of *L. casei* DHFR with pyrimethamine and several of its analogues (**10-12**).[99,104] These analogues are of continuing therapeutic interest as both antimalarial[30] and potential antitumour agents.[130-132]

An analogue such as 3-nitro-4-fluoropyrimethamine (**12**), containing an asymmetrically substituted aromatic ring, can exist as a mixture of two rotational isomers (an enantiomeric pair). In the [19]F NMR spectrum of the 3-nitro-4-fluoropyrimethamine–DHFR complex, two separate [19]F signals were detected for the bound ligand (spectrum not shown),[99] showing that two different conformational states exist in the complex. The populations of the two forms (designated A and B) are different, the A:B intensity ratio being 0.6:0.4 in the binary complex. Addition of $NADP^+$ to this complex caused the preference for binding to be reversed, with the A:B ratio in the ternary complex being 0.3:0.7. However, these results do not in themselves provide direct evidence that the two observed conformations are related to different rotameric states involving the pyrimidine–phenyl bond.[99,104] In order to obtain more information about the different bound forms, [1]H NMR studies of the complexes were carried out. All three pyrimethamine analogues (**10–12**) bind tightly to *L. casei* DHFR ($K_a > 5 \times 10^5\ M^{-1}$) and the exchange between the bound and free species is slow on the NMR chemical-shift time scale such that separate NMR spectra are observed for the bound and free species in each case. Two-dimensional exchange [1]H NMR spectroscopy can be used to connect the signals from the bound species with their corresponding signals in the free ligand for complexes of DHFR formed with ligands **10–12**.

In the complex where the ligand has a symmetrically substituted phenyl ring, such as pyrimethamine (**10**), four signals were observed for the four aromatic protons, indicating that each is shielded differently. This clearly indicated the presence of hindered rotation about the phenyl–pyrimidine bond, with the phenyl taking up a fixed position within its binding site such that each of the four phenyl protons is in a different shielding environment in the protein. Had there been rapid interconversion between the different rotamers, then only a single average signal would have been detected for each of the pairs of protons on opposite sides of the ring (H2′, H6′ and H3′, H5′) as a result of the ring flipping.[104]

In the case of the other symmetrically substituted pyrimethamine analogue, fluoropyrimethamine (**11**), again four signals for the nonequivalent aromatic protons were detected, and the corresponding protons in the two complexes (with **10** and **11**) have very similar shielding contributions resulting from the binding. This indicates that the phenyl ring is binding in a similar environment in each complex.

DHFR complexes containing pyrimethamine analogues with asymmetrically substituted phenyl rings, such as 3-nitro-4-fluoropyrimethamine (**12**), showed two complete sets of signals (form A and form B) for the phenyl protons in the bound ligands. This is illustrated in Figure 9, which shows the aromatic region of the 2D exchange spectrum of the 3-nitro-4-fluoropyrimethamine-DHFR complex in the presence of free ligand. The aromatic proton signals of the free ligand are labelled in the 1D spectrum, and the two sets of cross-peaks for the two bound species are indicated with boxes in the 2D spectrum. By comparing the $^1$H chemical shifts of these protons in bound ligand (**12**) with those in the pyrimethamine–DHFR complex, it was possible to show that the phenyl ring protons in form A and form B are experiencing essentially the same protein environment in each of the two forms as that found for the corresponding protons in the pyrimethamine–DHFR complex. This can be the case only if forms A and B correspond to two rotational isomers which result from a ~180° rotation about the pyrimidine–phenyl bond, the 2,4-diaminopyrimidine ring being bound similarly in the two forms.

Kuyper et al.[35] have examined the crystal structure of a complex of pyrimethamine with *E. coli* DHFR and found that the 2,4-diamino-pyrimidine ring binds in essentially the same binding site as that occupied by the corresponding part of the methotrexate ring in its complex with *E. coli* DHFR[7] and that the phenyl ring is oriented at approximately 90° to the plane of the pyrimidine ring. Based on this information, Birdsall et al.[104] built a model of the *L. casei* DHFR-pyrimethamine complex and noted that a pair of aromatic ring protons on one side of the phenyl ring of bound pyrimethamine had substantial upfield shielding contributions that would be consistent with ring-current shifts from Phe 30 if these protons were on the side of the ring oriented toward this residue. NOE measurements[104] confirmed these assignments by showing connections between an ortho proton (H2' or H6') on the phenyl ring of bound pyrimethamine and the H4' and H3',5' aromatic protons of Phe 30.

The conformational preference for binding form A in the binary complex of 3-nitro-4-fluoropyrimethamine with DHFR can also be considered in terms of the model of the complex shown in Figure 10. In form A, the nitro substituent would be directed toward the vacant nicotinamide ring-binding site, and this could assist in favourable binding. Addition of the NADP+ to form the ternary complex that reverses the preference for form A would be consistent with the unfavourable steric interaction between the bulky nitro group and the nicotinamide ring of bound NADP+.[104]

It was mentioned earlier that NMR studies of the trimethoprim–NADP+–DHFR complex reveal two different conformations (forms I and II),[30,31] with the nicotinamide ring of NADP+ being bound differently in

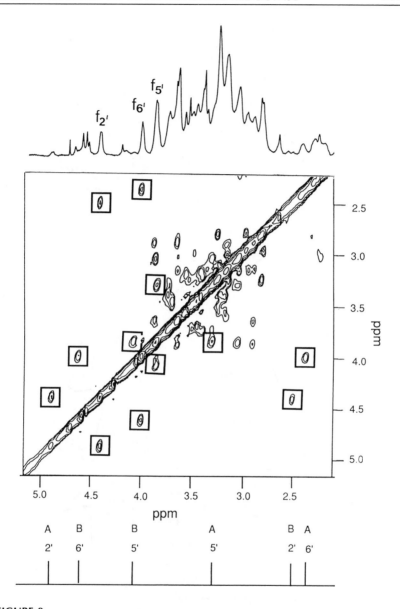

**FIGURE 9**

Aromatic region of the [1]H NOESY spectrum of the 3-nitro-4-fluoropyrimethamine *L. casei* DHFR complex in the presence of free 3-nitro-4-fluoropyrimethamine (500 MHz at 308 K and pH 6.5). The 2D exchange cross-peaks connecting aromatic signals in the two bound species with the corresponding signals in the free ligand (f) are labelled by boxes. The stick diagram below shows the positions of the bound signals in the two conformational states, A and B. (From Birdsall, B., et al., *Biochemistry,* 29, 9660–9667, 1990. With permission.)

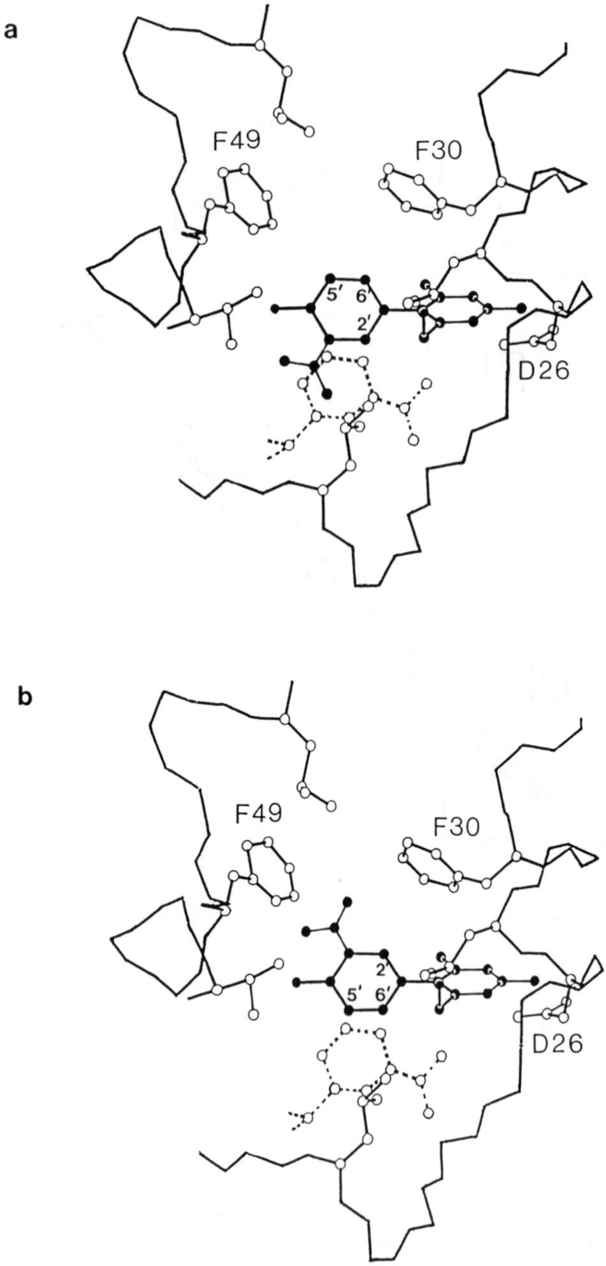

**FIGURE 10**

Model of the binding site in the 3-nitro-4-fluoropyrimethamine–DHFR complex for (a) form A and (b) form B. The position of the NADP+ nicotinamide ring-binding site is also indicated as a dotted-line structure. Modelling was carried out using QUANTA (Polygen, Inc.) on a Silicon Graphics IRIS 3130 incorporating crystallographic data from Matthews et al.[5] (From Birdsall, B., et al., *Biochemistry,* 29, 9660–9667, 1990. With permission.)

the two forms. Similar conformations have also been detected in ternary complexes of DHFR with pyrimethamine analogues and NADP+.[104] The two forms can be characterized quantitatively by measuring the relative intensities of the two different sets of pyrophosphate $^{31}$P signals corresponding to forms I and II. For the complex of 3-nitro-4-fluoropyrimethamine–NADP+–DHFR, such measurements indicate 65% form I and 35% ± 10% form II. For this complex it was also possible to measure the populations of the rotational isomeric bound forms A and B (30% and 70% ± 10%, respectively). These results raise the intriguing possibility that the two types of conformational states could be strongly correlated, with only forms IB and IIA populated. This would be consistent with a model with the nitro substituent oriented toward the vacant site for the nicotinamide ring binding in Form IIA and oriented away from the nicotinamide binding site in form IB (see Figure 10). However, one cannot exclude the alternative explanation that all four forms exist but that none of the detected NMR signals is affected by more than one of the different conformational states. It would be interesting to see if both rotational isomers of the pyrimethamine analogues bind in the presence of NADPH: the reduced coenzyme is known not to show the form I/form II type of equilibrium in complexes with DHFR and trimethoprim.

In summary, both rotational isomers of asymmetrically substituted pyrimethamine analogues have been shown to bind with comparable energy to *L. casei* DHFR. While *L. casei* DHFR is not a directly relevant target for these analogues, the results have general implications for design of modified pyrimethamines. Changes in the substituents will have different effects on the binding of the two rotational isomers: a proper understanding of the binding of new analogues of pyrimethamine to DHFR requires that the populations of the two bound rotamers be monitored.

## C DHFR COMPLEXES WITH THE SUBSTRATE FOLATE

Several NMR studies have shown that the *L. casei* DHFR–folate complex exists as a mixture of at least two conformations and that the enzyme–folate–NADP+ complex has three distinct conformational states, designated forms I, IIA, and IIB.[50,89,124,127] Figure 11 shows the multiple $^{13}$C signals seen for the three different forms in the $^{13}$C spectrum of the complex of *L. casei* DHFR with NADP+ and [4,6,8a-$^{13}$C]folate measured at various pH values. Similar multiple peaks are seen when the complexes formed with differently labelled ligands are examined. The populations of these conformational states are pH dependent. At pH 5.5 the ternary complex is almost exclusively in form I, for which NOE measurements clearly indicate that the H7 proton of folate is close to methyl group protons of Leu 19 and 27, as shown in Figure 12a. This defines the orientation of the pterin ring in form I as being very similar to that of

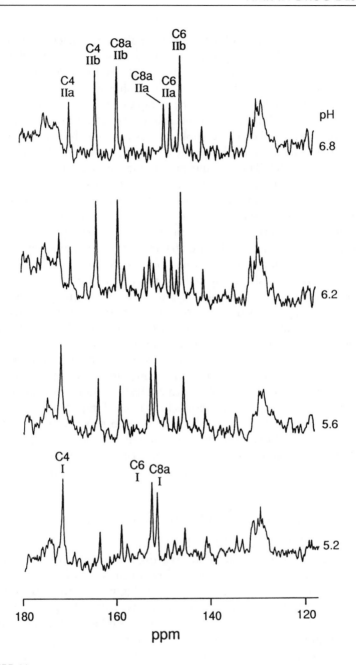

**FIGURE 11**

The low-field region of the 100.6-MHz $^{13}$C NMR spectra at 281 K of the ternary complex of *L. casei* DHFR and NADP$^+$ and [4,6,8a-$^{13}$C]folate at different pH values. Signals arising from the naturally occurring $^{13}$C in the protein are also observed (~130, 157, ~175 ppm). (From Cheung, H.T.A., *Biochemistry*, 32, 6846–6854, 1993. With permission.)

methotrexate in the DHFR–methotrexate complex. This orientation had previously been shown to be different from that of folate in catalytically active folate complexes (see Section II).[59] NOE data indicated that one of the other forms of the DHFR–folate–NADP+ complex (form IIB) does not have the same orientation of the pterin ring as in the methotrexate complex. In the 2D NOESY spectrum the H7 proton in form IIB showed an NOE connection to the Ala 97 methyl protons, indicating its proximity to those protons, but showed no NOEs to Leu 19 and 27 protons. More recently, these intermolecular NOE results have been confirmed by examining the 2D ¹H/¹³C HMQC-NOESY spectra of ¹³C-labelled folates

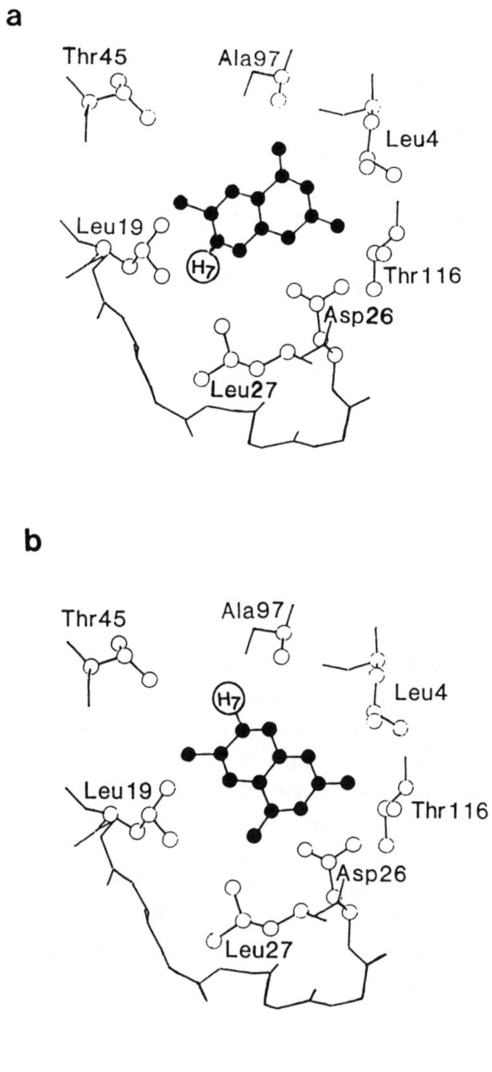

**a**

**b**

**FIGURE 12**

(a) Proposed conformation of the pterin ring in the folate–DHFR complex in forms I and IIA (based on crystal structure data of Matthews and co-workers[4] for the methotrexate complex, which has the same orientation of the pteridine ring). (b) Proposed conformation of the pterin ring in the folate–DHFR "productive" form IIB (turned over by ~180° compared to the other forms). (From Feeney, J., *Biochem. Pharmacol.*, 40, 141–152, 1990. With kind permission from Elsevier Science Ltd., The Boulevard, Langford Lane, Kidlington OX5 16B, UK.)

(structures **13** and **14**) bound to *L. casei* DHFR. Consideration of the crystal structure data of Bolin et al.[4] on the DHFR-MTX-NADPH complex indicates that a "turned-over" pteridine ring occupying essentially the same binding site would have its H7 proton ~3 Å from the methyl protons of Ala 97. Thus the major conformational difference between forms I and IIB is the different orientation of the pterin ring in the two forms, as illustrated in Figure 12. In these structures, forms I (and IIA) have the pterin ring orientation the same as in the methotrexate complex, and form IIB has the folate pterin ring turned over by 180° about an axis coincident with the ligand C2-NH$_2$ bond. Such an orientation would allow the catalytic reduction to proceed with the correct stereochemistry and can be considered as the "productive" conformation (Figure 12b). Forms I and IIA, with the methotrexate-like orientation of the pterin ring, would correspond to "nonproductive" conformations (Figure 12a). It is seen that the folate pterin ring occupies approximately the same binding site in the different forms.[50,124]

Attempts to measure the interconversion rate between forms I and IIB using multiple-site transfer of saturation experiments were not successful, indicating that this rate is low (<1 s$^{-1}$). It seems unlikely that such an interconversion will be directly implicated in the catalytic process. The similar COSY $^1$H spectra (not shown) observed at low pH (form I) and high pH (forms IIA and IIB) indicate that the protein conformation is not very different in the three forms.

The ionizable group responsible for the pH dependence of the equilibrium between the three forms has been estimated to have a pKa < 5 in states IIA and IIB, and pKa > 7 in state I. Site-directed mutagenesis studies involving Asp 26 have provided direct evidence that this is the residue involved in controlling the pH dependence of the conformational equilibrium.[127]

To summarize, in the complex of *L. casei* DHFR with folate, the bound ligand exists in different conformations, which occupy essentially the same binding site in the protein, with the conformation of the protein being largely unchanged. NMR can also provide useful information about the tautomeric states of bound folate. We have already seen that folate binds to *E. coli* DHFR and human DHFR in a single conformational form and in the keto tautomeric state.[54] A more complicated picture is seen for the folate complex with *L. casei* DHFR. In this case information on the tautomeric states of folate in its different bound conformational states has been obtained by considering the $^{13}$C chemical shifts of the labelled folates, **13** and **14**, complexed with the enzyme. Form IIB has $^{13}$C chemical shifts, which are very similar to free folic acid at pH 5.5, for which the structure is known to be in the 4-keto form with N1 unprotonated (see structure **15**).

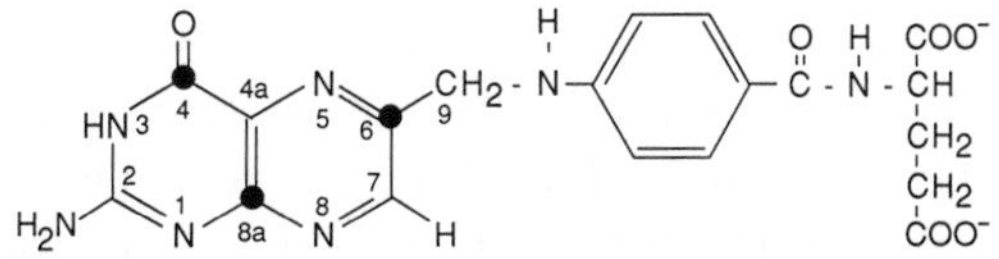

**13**   [4,6,8a-$^{13}$C] folate

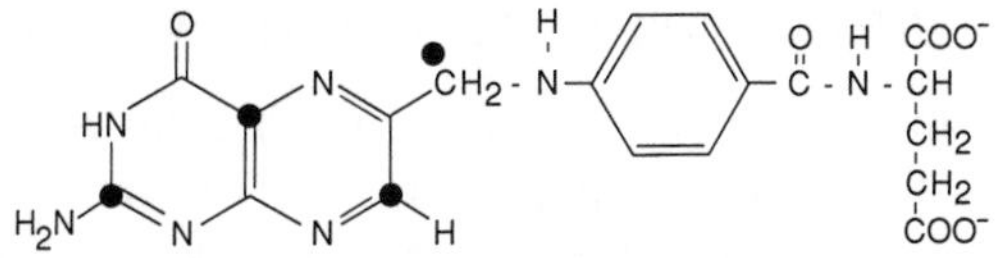

**14**   [2,4a,7,9-$^{13}$C] folate

In contrast, the C2 and C4 chemical shifts of bound folate in form IIA are very different to IIB, indicating a possible change in the tautomeric state or N1/N3 protonation states. We used model compounds to estimate the $^{13}$C chemical shifts for various tautomeric and ionization states of folate and compared them with the experimental data focusing on the pterin ring carbons. This comparison indicates that forms I and IIA exist as enolic forms (see structures **16** and **17**). $^1$H NMR studies suggest that

**15**   Keto Active form

**16**

**17**   Enolic Inactive forms 'Methotrexate-like'

R = p-aminobenzoyl-L-glutamate

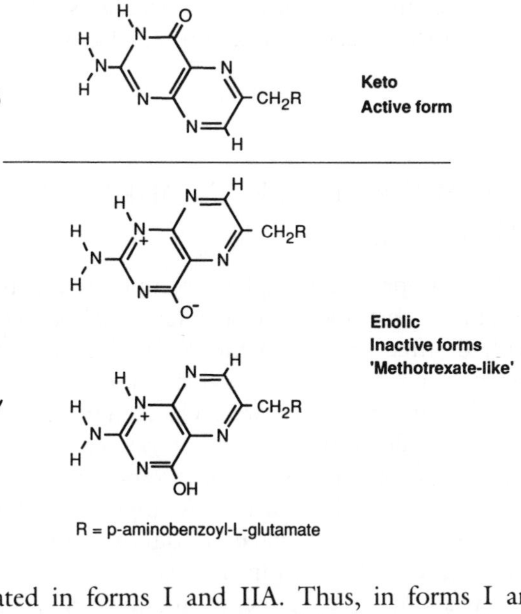

N1 is protonated in forms I and IIA. Thus, in forms I and IIA the tautomeric form and ionization state at N1 are very similar to those in methotrexate. Since the pterin ring has the same orientation as in the

methotrexate–DHFR complex, it is likely that the pterin ring of folate in forms I and IIA binds to residues in the protein that are similar to those involved in methotrexate binding. However, it should be emphasized that in form IIB, the "productive complex", the keto tautomeric state exists, as is the case in folate complexes with *E. coli* and human DHFR.

### D   ESCHERICHIA COLI DHFR COMPLEX WITH METHOTREXATE

Falzone and co-workers[73] have shown that this complex exists in two conformational forms with populations in the ratio 2:1. Two-dimensional exchange experiments indicated that the two forms were slowly interconverting at 323 K. The NOEs from the H7 protons of the pteridine ring of the bound methotrexate to protein protons showed the pteridine ring to have the same overall orientation in the two forms and to be similar to that in the crystal structure. The ternary complex DHFR–MTX–NADPH, in contrast, showed only a single conformational form in solution. Other workers have used $^{13}$C-labelled methotrexate to confirm these results.[74,75]

In summary, the detection of multiconformational states in several different complexes of dihydrofolate reductase suggests that this phenomenon may not be uncommon in other protein–ligand complexes. It seems likely that many examples of multiple conformations will be uncovered as more extensive NMR studies on other protein–ligand complexes are undertaken.

## VII   DYNAMIC PROCESSES IN DHFR–LIGAND COMPLEXES

Several dynamic processes in these complexes can be conveniently measured using NMR methods. In cases where the bound ligand is in slow exchange with the free species on the NMR time scale (each giving a separate spectrum), it is sometimes possible to use transfer of saturation or 2D exchange experiments to measure exchange rates between the bound and free species. Usually, if the dissociation rate constant is >1 s$^{-1}$, it can be measured by this approach: such measurements have been made for complexes of *L. casei* DHFR with trimethoprim, NADP$^+$, and folate. However, the dissociation rates for more tightly binding ligands such as methotrexate cannot be obtained in this way.

Information about rapid segmental motions in the enzyme–ligand complexes has been obtained by analysing $^{13}$C and $^{15}$N relaxation data. By analysing the $^{13}$C relaxation times of the C7-carbon in [7,4'-OCH$_3$-$^{13}$C$_2$]trimethoprim bound to *L. casei* DHFR, the overall correlation time was calculated to be 15.4 ns at 295 K. The 4'-OCH$_3$ carbon has a sixfold lower relaxation rate. This could be interpreted in terms of additional rapid motions affecting the 4'-OCH$_3$ carbon relaxation. Using a Lipari and Szabo[133] analysis of the data gave an effective correlation time of 4.3 ps for internal motion affecting the 4'-OCH$_3$ and also provided information on the order parameters relating to the C7-C1', C4'-O, and O-CH$_3$ bonds. The relaxation rate of the 4'-OCH$_3$ carbon cannot be explained simply by an additional rapid motion about the O-CH$_3$ bond. It was not possible to decide which of the other two bonds featured the additional subnanosecond motions, but their amplitudes would need to be up to ±35°.[73]

For several complexes of *L. casei* DHFR with ligands containing a symmetrically substituted aromatic ring, it has been possible to investigate rates of ring flipping of the aromatic ring. In some complexes, such as those with folate, the rate of flipping is fast enough to ensure that only a single signal is seen for the 2',6'-protons (and another for the 3',5'). It has not proved possible to detect the corresponding signals in the $^1$H spectrum of the DHFR–methotrexate complex, and this suggests line broadening of the signals due to intermediate rates of ring flipping. By examining $^{19}$F spectra of the complex of 3',5'-di-fluoromethotrexate with DHFR, it has been possible to characterize the ring flipping in detail. At 274 K, two separate signals are seen for the 3',5'-fluorine nuclei, and on increasing the temperature the signals broaden and eventually coalesce (at ~298 K). It was possible to analyse this classical two-site exchange behaviour to give the rate of ring flipping as $7 \times 10^3$ s$^{-1}$ at 298 K for the binary complex and $2 \times 10^4$ s$^{-1}$ at 298 K for the ternary complex with NADPH. Similar measurements have been used to characterize rates of ring flipping for the benzyl ring in DHFR complexes with trimethoprim analogues (a rate of 250 s$^{-1}$ at 298 K was determined for the binary DHFR–TMP complex).

It has already been mentioned that analysis of linewidths of NH-proton signals can give rates of proton exchange with the solvent and that these can sometimes be related to rates of breaking and re-forming hydrogen bonds (where this occurs as a required step before proton exchange can take place).[91] For the DHFR–TMP complex, the rate of breaking of the hydrogen bond between the trimethoprim N1-proton and the carboxylate oxygen of Asp 26 was estimated as 34 s$^{-1}$ at 298 K. Because the dissociation rate for the complex (2 s$^{-1}$) is much lower than the rates of ring flipping (250 s$^{-1}$) and hydrogen-bond breaking (34 s$^{-1}$), it is clear that protein–ligand interactions within the complex are being broken and reformed many times within the lifetime of the complex. While such effects are probably not important in controlling the overall equilibrium binding constants, they could influence the rates of association and dissociation of the complex. This could be important in cases where the response to ligand binding is kinetically controlled. However, this would not be the case for inhibitor binding to dihydrofolate reductase.

# VIII CONCLUSION

The advances made in NMR methodology over the last few years have opened up the possibility for detailed NMR structural studies on protein–ligand complexes. The most extensive studies made to date relating to drug–receptor complexes have concerned complexes formed by ligands binding to dihydrofolate reductase from several sources. Now that detailed structural studies are possible, these should increase our understanding of the specificity of ligand binding in these systems and contribute to drug design procedures. Applications relevant to drug–receptor interactions involving larger proteins will certainly increase as the NMR technology becomes more widely available.

## ACKNOWLEDGMENTS

I would like to acknowledge the contribution of many colleagues (particularly Berry Birdsall and Gordon Roberts) in the NMR studies on ligand complexes with *L. casei* DHFR. I would like to thank Berry Birdsall for her helpful comments on this article and Linda Dunphy for processing the manuscript.

# REFERENCES

1. Blakley, R.L., Chemistry and biochemistry of folates, in *Folates and Pterins*; R.L. Blakley, S.J. Benkovic, Eds.; John Wiley & Sons: New York, 1984; chap. 5, pp. 191-253.
2. Birdsall, B.; Hyde, E.I.; Burgen, A.S.V.; Roberts, G.C.K.; Feeney, J. *Biochemistry*, 1981, 20, 7186-7195.
3. Birdsall, B.; Burgen, A.S.V.; Roberts, G.C.K. *Biochemistry*,. 1980, 19, 3723-3731 and 3732-3737.
4. Bolin, J.T.; Filman, D.J.; Matthews, D.A.; Hamlin, R.C.; Kraut, J. *Biol. Chem. J.*, 1982, 257, 13650-13662.
5. Matthews, D.A.; Alden, R.A.; Bolin, J.T.; Filman, D.J.; Freer, S.T.; Hamlin, R.; Hol, W.G.J.; Kisliuk, R.L.; Pastore, E.J.; Plante, L.T.; Xuong, N.; Kraut, J. *J. Biol. Chem.*, 1978, 253, 6946-6954.
6. Matthews, D.A.; Alden, R.A.; Freer, S.T.; Xuong, N.; Kraut, J. *J. Biol. Chem.*, 1979, 254, 4144-4151.

7. Matthews, D.A.; Bolin, J.T.; Burridge, J.M.; Filman, D.J.; Volz, K.W.; Kaufman, B.T.; Beddell, C.R.; Champness, J.N.; Stammers, D.K.; Kraut, J. *J. Biol. Chem.*, 1985, 260, 381-399.

8. Filman, D.J.; Bolin, J.T.; Matthews, D.A.; Kraut, J. *J. Biol. Chem.*, 1982, 257, 13663-13672.

9. Champness, J.N.; Stammers, D.K.; Beddell, C.R. *FEBS Lett.*, 1986, 199, 61-67.

10. Davies J.F., II; Delcamp, T.J.; Prendergast, N.J.; Ashford, V.A.; Freisheim, J.H.; Kraut, J. *Biochemistry*, 1990, 29, 9467-9479.

11. Groom, C.R.; Thillet, J.; North, A.C.; Pictet, R.; Geddes, A.J. *J. Biol. Chem.*, 1991, 266, 19890-19893.

12. Bystroff, C.; Kraut, J. *Biochemistry*, 1991, 30, 2227-2239.

13. Cody, F.; Luft, J.R.; Ciszak, E.; Kalman, T.I.; Freisheim, J.H. *Anti-Cancer Drug Design*, 1992, 7, 483-491.

14. Baker, D.J.; Beddell, C.R.; Champness, P.J.; Norrington, F.E.A.; Smith, D.R.; Stammers, D.K. *FEBS Lett.*, 1981, 126, 49-53.

15. Feeney, J.; Birdsall, B., NMR studies of protein–ligand interactions, in *NMR of Macro-molecules: A Practical Approach*; Roberts, G.C.K., Ed.; Oxford University Press: Oxford, 1993; pp. 181-215.

16. Roberts, G.C.K., The interaction of substrates and inhibitors with dihydrofolate reductase, in *Chemistry and Biology of Pteridines*; Blair, J.A., Ed.; W. de Gruyter: Berlin, 1983; pp. 197-214.

17. Feeney, J. NMR studies of dynamic processes and multiple conformation in protein–ligand complexes, in *NMR and Biomolecular Structure*; Bertin, M.; Molinari, T.; Niccolai, A, Eds.; VCH Publishers: New York, 1991; pp. 198-205.

18. Feeney, J., *Biochem. Pharmacol.*, 1990, 40, 141-152.

19. Feeney, J., NMR studies of drug-receptor complexes: antifolate drugs binding to dihydrofolate reductase, in *NMR in Living Systems*; Axenrod, T.; Ceccarelli, G, Eds.; Reidel Publishing Co.: Amsterdam, 1986; pp. 347-366.

20. Birdsall, B., NMR spectroscopy and drug design: lessons from dihydrofolate reductase inhibitors, in *The Scientific Basis of Antimicrobial Chemotherapy*; Greenwood, D; O'Grady, F., Eds.; Cambridge University Press: Cambridge, 1985; pp. 267-281.

21. Benkovic S.J.; Fierke, C.A.; Naylor, A.M. *Science*, 1988, 239, 1105-1110.

22. Birdsall, B.; Andrews, J.; Ostler, G.; Tendler, S.J.B.; Davies, W.; Feeney, J.; Roberts, G.C.K.; Cheung, H.T.A. *Biochemistry*, 1989, 28, 1353-1362.

23. Benkovic, S.J.; Adams, J.A.; Fierke, C.A.; Naylor, A.M. *Pteridines and Folid Acid Derivatives*, 1989, 1, 37-43.

24. Thillet, J.; Absil, J.; Stone, S.R.; Pictet, R. *J. Biol. Chem.*, 198, 263, 12500-12508.

25. Villafranca, J.E.; Howell, E.E.; Voet, D.H.; Strobel, M.S.; Ogden, R.C.; Abelson, J.N.; Kraut, J. *Science*, 1983, 222, 782-788.

26. Fisher, C.L.; Roberts, V.A.; Hagler, A.T. *Biochemistry*, 1991, 30, 3518-3526.

27. Fleischman, S.H.; Brooks, C.I., III *Proteins Struct. Function Genet.*, 1990, 7, 52-61.

28. Hitchings, G.R.; Roth, B., Dihydrofolate reductases as targets for selective inhibitors, in *Enzyme Inhibitors as Drugs*; Sandler, M., Ed.; Macmillan: London, 1980; pp. 263-270.

29. Hitchings, G.H. *In-Vitro Cellular and Developmental Biology*, (Nobel Lecture in Physiology or Medicine). 1989, 25, 303-310.

30. Roth, B.; Cheng, C.C. *Prog. Med. Chem.*, 1982, 19, 1-58.

31. Seeger, D.R.; Cosulich, D.B.; Smith, J.M.; Hultquist, M.E. *J. Am Chem. Soc.*, 1949, 71, 1753-1758.

32. Ohemeng, K.A.; Roth, B. *J. Med. Chem.*, 1991, 30, 3518-3526.

33. Selassie, C.D.; Fang, Z.X.; Li, R.L.; Hansch, C.; Debnath, G.; Klein, T.E.; Langridge, R.; Kaufman, B.T. *J. Med. Chem.*, 1989, 32, 1895-1905.

34. Roth, B. *Fed. Proc., Design of dihydrofolate reductase inhibitors from X-ray crystal structures.* 1986, 45, 2765-2772.

35. Kuyper, L.F.; Roth, B.; Baccanari, D.P.; Ferone, R.; Beddell, C.R.; Champness, J.N.; Stammers, D.K.; Dann, J.G.; Norrington, F.E.; Baker, D.J.; Goodford, P.J. *J. Med. Chem.*, 1982, 25, 1120-1122.

36. Hansch, C. *Drug Intell. Clin. Pharm.*, 1982, 16, 391-396.

37. Roth, B.; Aig, E. *J. Med. Chem.*, 1987, 30, 1998-2004.

38. Breckenridge, R.J. *Experientia*, 1991, 147, 1148-1161.

39. Carr, M.D.; Birdsall, B.; Jimenez-Barbero, J.; Polshakov, V.I.; Bauer, C.J.; Frenkiel, T.A.; Roberts, G.C.K.; Feeney, J. *Biochemistry*, 1991, 30, 6330-6341.

40. Soteriou, A.; Carr, M.D.; Frenkiel, T.A.; McCormick, J.E.; Bauer, C.J.; Sali, D.; Birdsall, B.; Feeney, J. *J. Biomol. NMR*, 1993, 3, 535-546.

41. Nichols, R.; Weaver, C.D.; Eisenstein, E.; Blakley, R.L.; Appleman, J.; Huang, T.H.; Huang, F.Y.; Howell, E.E. *Biochemistry*, 1993, 32, 1695-1706.

42. Dann, J.G.; Ostler, G.; Bjur, R.A.; King, R.W.; Scudder, P.; Turner, P.C.; Roberts, G.C.K.; Burgen, A.S.V. *Biochem. J.*, 1976, 157, 559-571.

43. Pastore, E.J.; Friedkin, M. *J. Biol. Chem.*, 1962, 237, 3002-3010.

44. Lorenson, M.Y.; Maley, G.F.; Maley, F. *J. Biol. Chem.*, 1967, 242, 3332-3344.

45. Charlton, P.A.; Young, D.W.; Birdsall, B.; Feeney, J.; Roberts, G.C.K. *J. Chem. Soc. Chem. Commun.*, 1979, 922-924.

46. Charlton, P.A.; Young, D.W.; Birdsall, B.; Feeney, J.; Roberts, G.C.K. *J. Chem. Soc. Perkin Trans. II*, 1985, 1349-1353.

47. Fontecilla-Camps, J.C.; Bugg, C.E.; Temple, C.; Rose, J.D.; Montgomery, J.A.; Kisliuk, R.L., X-ray crystallography studies of the structure of 5,10-methenyltetrahydrofolic acid, in *Chemistry and Biology of Pteridines*; Kisliuk, R.L.; Brown, G.M., Eds.; Elsevier: New York, 1979; pp. 235-240.

48. Fontecilla-Camps, J.C.; Bugg, C.E.; Temple, C.; Rose, J.D.; Montgomery, J.A.; Kisliuk, R.L. *J. Am. Chem. Soc.*, 1979, 101, 6114-6115.

49. Oefner, C.; D'Arcy, A.; Winkler, F.K. *Eur. J. Biochem.*, 1988, 174, 377-385.

50. Cheung, H.T.A.; Birdsall, B.; Frenkiel, T.A.; Feeney, J. *Biochemistry*, 1993, 32, 6846-6854.

51. Selinsky, B.S.; Perlman, M.E.; London, R.E.; Unkefer, C.J.; Mitchell, J.; Blakley, R.L. *Biochemistry*, 1990, 29, 1290-1296.

52. Bystroff, C.; Oatley, S.J.; Kraut, J. *Biochemistry*, 1993, 29, 3263-3277.

53. Blakley, R.L.; Appleman, J.R.; Freisheim, J.H.; Jablonsky, M.J. *Arch. Biochem. Biophys.*, 1993, 306, 501-509.

54. Falzone, C.J.; Benkovic, S.J.; Wright, P.E. *Biochemistry*, 1990, 29, 9667-9677.

55. Stockman, B.J.; Nirmala, N.R.; Wagner, G.; Delcamp, T.J.; De Yarman, M.T.; Freisheim, J.H. *Biochemistry*, 1992, 31, 218-229.

56. Gerothanassis, I.P.; Birdsall, B.; Bauer, C.J.; Frenkiel, T.A.; Feeney, J. *J. Mol. Biol.*, 1992, 204, 549-554.

57. Andrews, J.; Fierke, C.A.; Birdsall, B.; Ostler, G.; Feeney, J.; Roberts, G.C.K.; Benkovic, S.J. *Biochemistry*, 1989, 28, 5743-5650.

58. Maharaj, G.; Selinsky, B.S.; Appleman, J.R.; Perlman, M.; London, R.E.; Blakley, R.L. *Biochemistry*, 1990, 29, 4554-4560.

59.  Wüthrich, K.; *NMR of Proteins and Nucleic Acids*; John Wiley and Sons: New York, 1986.
60.  Clore, G.M.; Gronenborn, A.M. *Science*, 1991, 252, 1390.
61.  Stockman, B.J.; Nirmala, N.R.; Wagner, G.; Delcamp, T.J.; De Yarman, M.T.; Freisheim, J.H. *FEBS Lett.*, 1991, 2, 267-269.
62.  Ikura, M.; Kay, L.E.; Bax, A. *Biochemistry*, 1990, 29, 4659-4667.
63.  Frenkiel, T.; Bauer, C.J.; Carr, M.D.; Birdsall, B.; Feeney, J. *J. Magn. Reson.*, 1990, 90, 420-425.
64.  Ikura, M.; Bax, A.; Clore, G.M.; Gronenborn, A.M. *J. Am. Chem. Soc.*, 1990, 112, 9020-9022.
65.  Kay, L.E.; Ikura, M.; Tschudin, R.; Bax, A. *J. Magn. Reson.*, 1990, 89, 496-514.
66.  Bax, A.; Clore, G.M.; Driscoll, P.C.; Gronenborn, A.M.; Ikura, M.; Kay, L.E. *J. Magn. Reson.*, 1990, 87, 620-627.
67.  Fesik, S.W.; Zuiderweg, E.R.P. *Q. Rev. Biophys.*, 1990, 23(2), 97-131.
68.  Marion, D.; Wüthrich, K. *Biochem. Biophys. Res. Commun.*, 1983, 113(3), 967-974.
69.  Aue, W.P.; Bartholdi, E.; Ernst, R.R. *J. Chem. Phys.*, 1976, 64, 2229-2246.
70.  Braunschweiler, L.; Ernst, R.R. *J. Magn. Reson.*, 1983, 53, 521-528.
71.  Davis, D.G.; Bax, A.; *J. Am. Chem. Soc.*, 1985, 107, 2820-2821.
72.  Hammond, S.J.; Birdsall, B.; Searle, M.S.; Roberts, G.C.K.; Feeney, J. *J. Mol. Biol.*, 1986, 188, 81-97.
73.  Falzone, C.J.; Wright, P.E.; Benkovic, S.J. *Biochemistry*, 1991, 30, 2184-2191.
74.  Feeney, J.; Roberts, G.C.K.; Birdsall, B.; Griffiths, D.V.; King, R.W.; Scudder, P.; Burgen, A.S.V. *Proc. Roy. Soc. Lond. B*, 1977, 196, 267-290.
75.  Searle, M.S.; Hammond, S.J.; Birdsall, B.; Roberts, G.C.K.; Feeney, J.; King, R.W.; Griffiths, D.V. *FEBS Lett.*, 1986, 194, 165-170.
76.  Birdsall, B.; Feeney, J.; Griffiths, D.V.; Hammond, S.; Kimber, B.J.; King, R.W.; Roberts, G.C.K.; Searle, M.S. *FEBS Lett.*, 1984, 175, 364-368.
77.  Feeney, J.; Birdsall, B.; Ostler, G.; Carr, M.D.; Kairi, M. *FEBS Lett.*, 1990, 272, 197-199.
78.  Ostler, G.; Soteriou, A.; Moody, C.M.; Khan, J.A.; Birdsall, B.; Carr, M.D.; Young, D.W.; Feeney, J. *FEBS Lett.*, 1993, 318, 177-180.
79.  Birdsall, B.; Arnold, J.R.P.; Jimenez-Barbero, J.; Frenkiel, T.A.; Bauer, C.J.; Tendler, S.J.B.; Carr, M.D.; Thomas, J.A.; Roberts, G.C.K.; Feeney, J. *Eur. J. Biochem.*, 1990, 191, 659-668.
80.  Kimber, B.J.; Griffiths, D.V.; Birdsall, B.; King, R.W.; Scudder, P.; Feeney, J.; Roberts, G.C.K.; Burgen, A.S.V. *Biochemistry*, 1977, 16, 3492-3500.
81.  Kimber, B.J.; Feeney, J.; Roberts, G.C.K.; Birdsall, B.; Burgen, A.S.V.; Sykes, B.D. *Nature (Lond.)*, 1978, 271, 184-185.
82.  Cocco, L.; Blakley, R.L.; Walker, T.I.; London, R.E.; Matwiyoff, N.A. *Biochemistry*, 1978, 17, 4285-4290.
83.  Roberts, G.C.K.; Feeney, J.; Burgen, A.S.V.; Yuferov, V.; Dann, J.; Bjur, R. *Biochemistry*, 1974, 13, 5351-5357.
84.  Feeney, J.; Batchelor, J.G.; Albrand, J.P.; Roberts, G.C.K. *J. Magn. Reson.*, 1979, 33, 519-529.
85.  Birdsall, B.; Gronenborn, A.; Hyde, E.I.; Clore, G.M.; Roberts, G.C.K.; Feeney, J.; Burgen, A.S.V. *Biochemistry*, 1982, 21, 5831-5838.
86.  Cayley, J.; Albrand, J.P.; Feeney, J.; Roberts, G.C.K.; Piper, E.A.; Burgen, A.S.V. *Biochemistry*, 1979, 18, 3886-3895.
87.  Curtis, N.; Moore, S.; Birdsall, B.; Bloxidge, J.; Gibson, C.L.; Jones, J.R.; Feeney, J. *Biochem. J.*, 1994, 303, 401–405.

88. Cheung, H.T.A.; Chau, D.D.; Morrison, J.F.; Birdsall, B.; Feeney, J. *Pteridines*, 1992, 3, 103-104.

89. Birdsall, B.; De Graw, J.; Feeney, J.; Hammond, J.; Searle, M.S.; Roberts, G.C.K.; Colwell, W.T.; Crase, J. *FEBS Lett.*, 1987, 217, 106-110.

90. Cheung, H.T.A.; Birdsall, B.; Feeney, J. *FEBS Lett.*, 1992, 312, 147-151.

91. Bevan, A.W.; Roberts, G.C.K.; Feeney, J.; Kuyper, I. *Eur. Biophys. J.*, 1985, 11, 211-218.

92. Searle, M.S.; Forster, M.J.; Birdsall, B.; Roberts, G.C.K.; Feeney, J.; Cheung, H.T.A.; Kompis, I.; Geddes, A.J. *Proc. Natl. Acad. Sci. USA*, 1988, 85, 3787-3791.

93. Cheung, H.T.A.; Searle, M.S.; Feeney, J.; Birdsall, B.; Roberts, G.C.K.; Kompis, I.; Hammond, S.J. *Biochemistry*, 1986, 25, 1925-1931.

94. Huang, F.-Y.; Yang, Q.-X.; Huang, T.-H. *FEBS Lett.*, 1991, 289, 231-234.

95. Fesik, S.W.; Zuiderweg, E.R.P.; Olejniczak, E.T.; Gampe, R.T., Jr. *Biochem. Pharmacol.*, 1990, 40, 161-167.

96. Martorell, G.; Gradwell, M.J.; Birdsall, B.; Bauer, C.J.; Frenkiel, T.A.; Cheung, H.T.A.; Polshakov, V.I., Kuype, L.; Feeney, J., *Biochemistry*, 1994, 33, 12416–12426.

97. Hyde, E.I.; Birdsall, B.; Roberts, G.C.K.; Feeney, J.; Burgen, A.S.V. *Biochemistry*, 1980, 19, 3738-3746.

98. Birdsall, B.; Roberts, G.C.K.; Feeney, J.; Dann, J.G.; Burgen, A.S.V. *Biochemistry*, 1983, 22, 5597-5604.

99. Tendler, S.J.B.; Griffin, R.J.; Birdsall, B.; Stevens, M.F.G.; Roberts, G.C.K.; Feeney, J. *FEBS Lett.*, 1988, 240, 201-204.

100. Gerothanassis, I.P.; Birdsall, B.; Bauer, C.J.; Feeney, J. *Eur. J. Biochem.*, 1992, 204, 173-177.

101. Feeney, J.; Birdsall, B.; Roberts, G.C.K.; Burgen, A.S.V. *Nature*, 1975, 257, 564-566.

102. Cayley, P.J.; Feeney, J.; Kimber, B.J. *Int. J. Biol. Macromolecules*, 1980, 2, 251-255.

103. Birdsall, B.; Roberts, G.C.K.; Feeney, J.; Burgen, A.S.V. *FEBS Lett.*, 1977, 80, 313-316.

104. Birdsall, B.; Tendler, S.J.B.; Arnold, J.R.P.; Feeney, J.; Griffin, R.J.; Carr, M.D.; Thomas, J.A.; Roberts, G.C.K.; Stevens, M.F.G. *Biochemistry*, 1990, 29, 9660-9667.

105. Rodgers, P.; Roberts, G.C.K. *FEBS Lett.*, 1973, 36, 330-333.

106. Cocco, L.; Groff, J.P.; Temple, C., Jr.; Montgomery, J.A.; London, R.E.; Matwiyoff, N.S.; Blakley, R.L. *Biochemistry*, 1981, 20, 3972-3978.

107. London, R.E.; Howell, E.E.; Warren, M.S.; Kraut, J. *Biochemistry*, 1986, 25, 7229-7235.

108. Roberts, G.C.K.; Feeney, J.; Burgen, A.S.V.; Daluge, S. *FEBS Lett.*, 1981, 131, 85-88.

109. Birdsall, B.; Griffiths, D.V.; Roberts, G.C.K.; Feeney, J.; Burgen, A.S.V. *Proc. Roy. Soc. Lond. B*, 1977, 196, 251-265.

110. Gronenborn, A.; Birdsall, B.; Hyde, E.I.; Roberts, G.C.K.; Feeney, J.; Burgen, A.S.V. *Biochemistry*, 1981, 20, 1717-1722.

111. Wyeth, P.; Gronenborn, A.; Birdsall, B.; Roberts, G.C.K.; Feeney, J.; Burgen, A.S.V. *Biochemistry*, 1980, 19, 2608-2615.

112. Antonjuk, D.J.; Birdsall, B.; Burgen, A.S.V.; Cheung, H.T.A.; Clore, G.M.; Feeney, J.; Gronenborn, A.; Roberts, G.C.K.; Tran, W. *Br. J. Pharmacol.*, 1984, 81, 309-315.

113. Birdsall, B.; Feeney, J.; Roberts, G.C.K.; Burgen, A.S.V. *FEBS Lett.*, 1980, 120, 107-109.
114. Way, J.L.; Birdsall, B.; Feeney, J.; Roberts, G.C.K.; Burgen, A.S.V. *Biochemistry*, 1975, 14, 3470-3475.
115. Hyde, E.I.; Birdsall, B.; Roberts, G.C.K.; Feeney, J.; Burgen, A.S.V. *Biochemistry*, 1980, 19, 3746-3754.
116. Clore, G.M.; Roberts, G.C.K.; Gronenborn, A.; Birdsall, B.; Feeney, J. *J. Magn. Reson.*, 1981, 45, 151-161.
117. Birdsall, B.; Feeney, J.; Pascual, C.; Roberts, G.C.K.; Kompis, I.; Then, R.L.; Muller, K.; Kroehn, A. *J. Med. Chem.*, 1984, 27, 1672-1676.
118. Cayley, P.J.; Dunn, S.M.J.; King, R.W. *Biochemistry*, 1981, 20, 874-879.
119. Dunn, S.M.J., King, R.W. *Biochemistry*, 1980, 19, 766-773.
120. Birdsall, B.; Gronenborn, A.; Clore, G.M.; Hyde, E.I.; Roberts, G.C.K.; Feeney, J.; Burgen, A.S.V. *Pteridines and Folic Acid Derivatives*, 1982, 563-566.
121. Birdsall, B.; Gronenborn, A.; Clore, G.M.; Roberts, G.C.K.; Feeney, J.; Burgen, A.S.V. *Biochem. Biophys. Res. Commun.*, 1981, 101, 1139-1144.
122. Feeney, J.; Birdsall, B.; Roberts, G.C.K.; Burgen, A.S.V., Dihydrofolate reductase: interactions with the coenzyme NADPH, in *NMR in Biology*; Dwek, R.A., Ed.; Academic Press: London, 1977; pp. 111-124.
123. Li, L.; Falzone, C.J.; Wright, P.E.; Benkovic, S.J. *Biochemistry*, 1992, 31, 7826-7833.
124. Birdsall, B.; Feeney, J.; Tendler, S.J.B.; Hammond, S.J.; Roberts, G.C.K. *Biochemistry*, 1989, 28, 2297-2305.
125. Gronenborn, A.; Birdsall, B.; Hyde, E.I.; Roberts, G.C.K.; Feeney, J.; Burgen, A.S.V. *Nature*, 1981, 290, 273-274.
126. Birdsall, B.; Bevan, A.W.; Pascual, C.; Roberts, G.C.K.; Feeney, J.; Gronenborn, A.; Clore, G.M. *Biochemistry*, 1984, 23, 4733-4742.
127. Jimenez, M.A.; Arnold, J.R.P.; Andrews, J.; Thomas, J.A.; Roberts, G.C.K.; Birdsall, B.; Feeney, J. *Protein Eng.*, 1989, 2, 627-631.
128. Hammond, S.J.; Birdsall, B.; Feeney, J.; Searle, M.S.; Roberts, G.C.K.; Cheung, H.T.A. *Biochemistry*, 1987, 26, 8585-8590.
129. Huang, F.-Y.; Yang, Q.-X.; Huang, T.-H.; Gelbaum, L.; Kuyper, L.F. *FEBS Lett.*, 1991, 283, 44-46.
130. Hill, B.T.; Price, L.A. *Cancer Treat. Rev.* 1980, 95-112.
131. Bliss, E.A.; Griffin, R.J.; Stevens, M.F.G. *J. Chem. Soc. Perkin Trans. I*, 1987, 3317-2228.
132. Griffin, R.J.; Meek, M.A.; Schwalbe, C.H.; Stevens, M.F.G. *J. Med. Chem.*, 1989, 32, 2468-2474.
133. Lipari, G.; Szabo, A. *J. Am. Chem. Soc.*, 1982, 104, 4546-4558.
134. Groff, J.P.; London, R.E.; Cocco, L.; Blakley, R.L. *Biochemistry*, 1981, 20, 6169-6178.
135. London, R.E.; Groff, G.P.; Blakley, R.L. *Biochem. Biophys. Res. Commun.*, 1979, 86, 779-786.
136. Wagner, C.R.; Thillet, J., Benkovic, S.J. *Biochemistry*, 1992, 31, 7834-7840.

# CHAPTER 9

# STUDIES OF DRUG-CALMODULIN BINDING USING ISOTOPICALLY LABELLED PROTEIN

*David G. Reid, Andrew J. Edwards, and Patricia J. Sweeney*

## CONTENTS

I  Introduction ................................................................................. 316

II  Studies of Calmidazolium–Calmodulin Binding .......................... 319
   A  Proton NMR Approaches ......................................................... 319
      1  Calcium Dependence .......................................................... 319
      2  Calmidazolium Binding ...................................................... 321
      3  Temperature Dependence ..................................................... 321
      4  Two-Dimensional Experiments on [Phe-d$_5$]
         CaM–Calmidazolium .................................................... 326
   B  Multinuclear Approaches ......................................................... 329
   C  Modelling the Calmidazolium–CaM Complex ....................... 329

Acknowledgments ............................................................................. 331

**References** ..................................................................................... 334

# I   INTRODUCTION

Calmodulin (CaM) is a small, acidic protein, ubiquitous in eukaryotic organisms, which has been strongly conserved in evolution.[1] The protein is able to bind four calcium ions at two cooperative pairs of binding sites. One of these pairs, located in the C-terminal half, displays higher affinity for the cation than the other pair, in the N-terminal half. Calcium binding induces conformational changes, which cause the activation of a large number of intracellular enzymes, the list of which is lengthening rapidly. This activation appears to involve binding of the calcium–CaM complex to a recognition domain on the inactive or basally active target protein, which results in deinhibition. Direct, high-affinity interactions between synthetic putative CaM-binding domains, which generally have a strong propensity for α-helix formation, and the calcium-saturated protein have indeed been demonstrated by NMR.[2]

The physiological importance of CaM-regulated processes argues for a possible pharmacological role for compounds that can act as "calmodulin function inhibitors" or as "calmodulinomimetics." It remains to be established whether the modes of interaction of CaM with its various target proteins are sufficiently diverse to allow design of compounds that will discriminate between them. However, acute application of CaM antagonists may be beneficial in the treatment of conditions such as postmyocardial or cerebral ischaemic reperfusion injury, in which morbidity seems to be associated with abnormally elevated intracellular calcium activity. Several clinically effective and experimental calcium channel blockers also bind to calmodulin,[3] so that "mixed action" calcium antagonists that impede both calcium entry into the cytosol and its activation of calcium-CaM-triggered functions are quite conceivable.

X-ray studies of CaM crystallized from acidic media show it to be a "dumbbell"-shaped molecule, consisting of two globular domains of roughly equal size, each containing two Asp- and Glu-rich calcium-binding stretches, joined by an acidic, extended α-helical "linker."[4] This is, however, significantly distorted in solution, allowing the two domains to approach each other. Both domains bind simultaneously to the CaM binding sequence of myosin light chain kinase (MLCK),[5] and the large number of polar and hydrophobic interactions this allows contributes to the high stability of the interaction. There is a similarity with respect to general disposition of charged, polar, and hydrophobic side chains, although little marked formal homology, between the CaM-binding domains of CaM-activated enzymes. This fact encourages the notion that highly specific inhibitors of a given interaction, and thereby of a specific enzyme, may be attainable.

CaM's propensity to interact with diverse peptide sequences, its versatility in interactions with synthetic compounds, and the fact that CaM complexes are sufficiently small for atomic-level structural characterization, all suggest that the protein may represent a useful model system for the study of peptide–protein interactions and comparative studies of protein interactions with synthetic peptidomimetics. CaM's abundance and its propensity to bind to medicinal compounds may also be important in pharmacokinetics and toxicology. In general, compounds that possess one or more basic centres and flexible aromatic ring systems are likely candidates to bind to CaM.[4] Smaller synthetic compounds appear to bind to one or both of the two domains independently. However, higher-molecular-weight molecules, including peptides longer than about 20 amino acid residues, can contact groups on both domains simultaneously, probably by inducing large interdomain movements similar to those characterized for the MLCK peptide. These are most likely brought about by disruption of the linker between residues 74 to 82 of the protein.

The binding sites of drugs on their receptors can be studied by the observation of NOEs between protons or groups of protons on the two molecules. In practice, extensive overlap between signals from both molecular species often hampers this approach. The introduction of rare isotopes into one or both molecules provides several strategies for solving or mitigating these problems of spectral degeneracy. The availability of efficient bacterial expression systems for CaM, in fact, meant that it was one of the first proteins on which the most simple device for addressing this overlap problem was used. This consisted of the biosynthetic production of fully deuterated, spectroscopically "silent" protein.[6] Of course, this approach only enables nuclei from one of the two interacting species to be visualized and so excludes observation of intermolecular NOEs, but it can permit signals from this species to be identified unambiguously (not necessarily simple under conditions of slow exchange) and to be used in the determination of the receptor-bound conformation. An additional, and usually insurmountable, drawback of this approach is that the preparation of fully deuterated proteins places great demands on bacterial expression systems.

More general approaches to the use of isotopic labelling in studies of drug–receptor interactions are provided by the incorporation of $^{13}C$ or $^{15}N$, or both isotopes simultaneously, into one or the other of the interacting molecules. This enables the application of multinuclear NMR procedures, which discriminate in favour of, or against, the signals from protons that are $J$ coupled to either heteronucleus. Examples of these approaches were described in earlier chapters.

Calmodulin from the African trypanosome (*Trypanosoma brucei rhodesiense*, the parasite responsible for sleeping sickness in humans) differs from the mammalian protein by 17 residues out of a total of 148.[7]* This difference may be sufficient to make parasitic CaMs possible targets for antiprotozoal drugs.[8]**

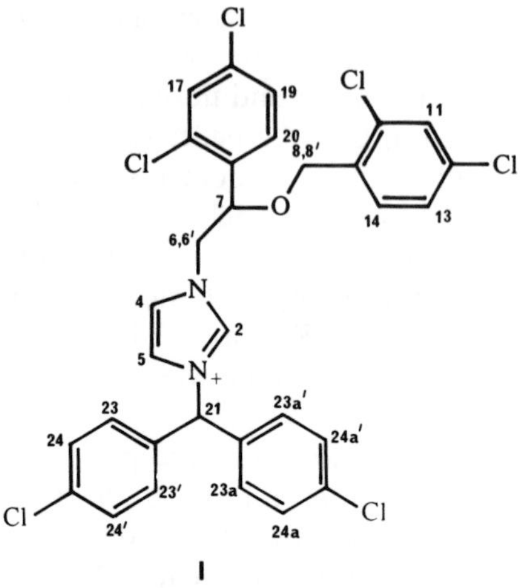

**1** Calmidazolium

Calmidazolium (R24571, **1**) is a potent inhibitor of CaM function,[9] with a dissociation constant (2 to 3 n$M$) that is comparable with those of high-affinity CaM-binding peptides. Its interactions with mammalian CaM have been studied by [1]H NMR.[10] The compound is in slow exchange with the protein on the [1]H chemical-shift time scale, and drug-induced perturbations of protein signals indicate that the bound calmidazolium contacts both lobes of the protein simultaneously. Severe overlap between drug and protein signals, however, makes it impossible to explore the drug-binding site on the protein using intermolecular NOEs. Nevertheless, as calmidazolium is high in aromatic functionalities, it is relatively simple to eliminate much of the overlap in the proton NMR spectrum of its 1:1 complex with CaM by growing a CaM-expressing strain of *Escherichia coli*

---

* Trypanosome CaM differs from mammalian CaM with respect to the following 17 mutations: T5-S5; E6-N6; A10-S10; A57-Q57; N60-S60; M71-L71; K77-Q77; T79-S79; R86-K86; N97-D97; Y99-F99; V108-I108; I130-V130; V136-I136; Q143-K143; T146-M146; and A147-S147.

---

** Drosophilia CaM, also extensively studied by NMR, differs from mammalian CaM with respect to three mutations: Y99-F99; Q143-T143; and A147-S147.

on minimal medium supplemented with phenylalanine in which all the aromatic protons have been replaced by deuterons [Phe-d$_5$]. The same expression system can also be used for the preparation of CaM that is uniformly enriched in $^{13}$C and $^{15}$N, offering opportunities for studies of drug–CaM interactions based on multinuclear isotope-editing and -filtering techniques.

## II STUDIES OF CALMIDAZOLIUM–CALMODULIN BINDING

### A PROTON NMR APPROACHES

#### 1 Calcium Dependence

In view of the considerable differences between trypanosome CaM and the more extensively characterized CaMs from higher species, it is important to confirm that the protozoal protein behaves similarly with respect to its interactions with calcium. Calmodulin from higher organisms binds calcium in two distinct phases. Changes in the $^1$H NMR spectrum of the protein are consistent with both the domain (C- or N-terminal), and the kinetics — slow exchange (high affinity ) or fast exchange (low affinity) — with which the interaction takes place. Thus, in the first stages of a titration of CaM with calcium, in which two calcium ions are bound cooperatively in the C-terminal domain, resonances from residues in this domain gradually diminish in intensity, being replaced by resonances at new chemical-shift positions characteristic of the calcium-bound C-terminal domain. This slow-exchange behaviour clearly reflects the high affinity of the two C-terminal binding sites for calcium. This behaviour is evident for a number of the signals observed in Figure 1, most strikingly so for the low-field singlet at 8.15 ppm in Figure 1A due to the H2 proton of the single histidine residue, His 107. After the addition of one mole equivalent of calcium (II), which produces half an equivalent of dicalcium-CaM and half an equivalent of calcium-free CaM because of the cooperativity between the binding sites, this signal is split into two components, corresponding to each form of the two coexistent species (Figure 1B). After the addition of another equivalent (Figure 1C) only the higher field of the two His-107 H2 signals is evident at about 8.0 ppm, corresponding to a preponderance of the dicalcium-bound form. Changes involving the binding of the second two equivalents of calcium (II) to the two N-terminal sites are less marked (Figure 1D and 1E). (Assignments shown in Figure 1 are based on mammalian CaM assignments and on considerations of homology between mammalian and trypanosome calmodulin.[11]) These

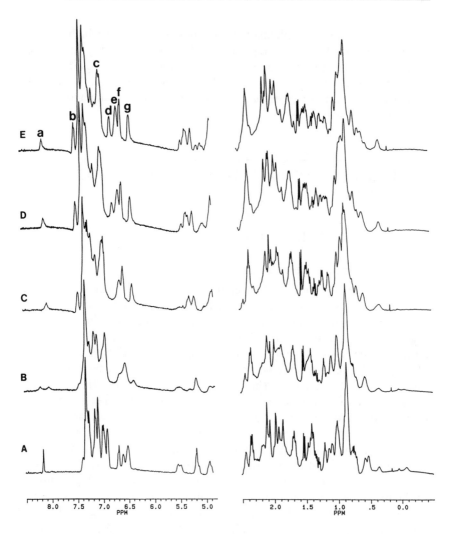

**FIGURE 1**

360-MHz $^1$H NMR spectra of *ca.* 20 mg trypanosome CaM at 37°C in $^2H_2O$ containing potassium phosphate and potassium chloride in (A) the absence of calcium chloride, and the presence of (B) 1, (C) 2, (D) 3, and (E) 4 equivalents of calcium chloride. Assignments shown in (E) are based on mammalian CaM assignments and on considerations of homology between mammalian and trypanosome calmodulin: (a) His 107 H2; (b) Phe 92 H3,5 and H4; (c) Phe 16 H3,5, Phe 89 H3,5 and H4, Phe 68 H2,6, Phe 141 H2,6; (d) Phe 16 H2,6, Phe 89 H2,6; (f) Tyr 138 H3,5; (g) Tyr 138 H2,6.

involve gradual changes in the chemical shifts of a few resonances that are proportional to the amount of added calcium and indicative of fast exchange. In displaying these biphasic calcium-binding properties, trypanosome CaM closely resembles mammalian CaM.[12]

## 2 Calmidazolium Binding

Figure 2 shows the results of titrating aliquots of calmidazolium into a solution of trypanosome CaM. Several of the changes, such as the appearance of new signals at 7.6 and 5.55 ppm during the course of the titration, are indicative of slow exchange of the protein between drug-bound and drug-free environments. Within the resolution limits of the experiment, this is a general observation. However, it is immediately obvious from the appearance of the spectrum of the 1:1 complex (Figure 2i) that overlap between protein and compound signals is so extensive as to prevent observation, or at least unambiguous interpretation, of inter-molecular NOEs. (It is interesting to note that differences between the spectra of the 1:1 complexes of calmidazolium and trypanosome CaM,[9] and calmidazolium and human CaM [Figure 2 of Reference 9] are considerable, although both proteins complex with high affinity.)

Figure 3 shows the dramatic increase in resolution of the signals from the bound drug produced by working with phenylalanine ring-deuterated protein. Figure 3a shows the downfield region of the spectrum of calcium-saturated [Phe-$d_5$] CaM; the only significant signals remaining in the aromatic region downfield of 6 ppm are due to the single tyrosine (138) of the trypanosome protein. Addition of aliquots of calmidazolium is accompanied by the appearance of signals downfield of 6.5 ppm. These can be confidently and unambiguously ascribed to the bound compound. Moreover, all the signals from the bound drug increase steadily in intensity in proportion to the amount of compound added, with no indication of any significant chemical-shift changes. This fact proves a slow-exchange interaction, consistent with a very high formation constant. Changes observed in the region of the spectrum upfield of the HOD signal are identical to those exerted on the isotopically normal protein (data not shown). Thus complete resolution of the aromatic signals of the bound drug from those of the protein has been achieved, although the five nonaromatic nonexchanging proton signals still overlap with protein signals.

## 3 Temperature Dependence

Insights into the stability and dynamical properties of ligand–receptor complexes can frequently be gained by observing the appearance of the spectrum over a range of temperatures (several examples are given in Chapters 3, 8, and 12). Figure 4 shows the downfield region of the 360-MHz spectrum of the [Phe-$d_5$] CaM:calmidazolium complex at various temperatures between 15 and 60°C. At the lower temperatures all signals are broad due to slow tumbling of the entire complex and resultant efficient $T_2$ relaxation. As the sample is warmed up to about 30°C, all the signals due to the drug in the aromatic region of the spectrum progressively sharpen as the correlation time of the complex decreases, with only

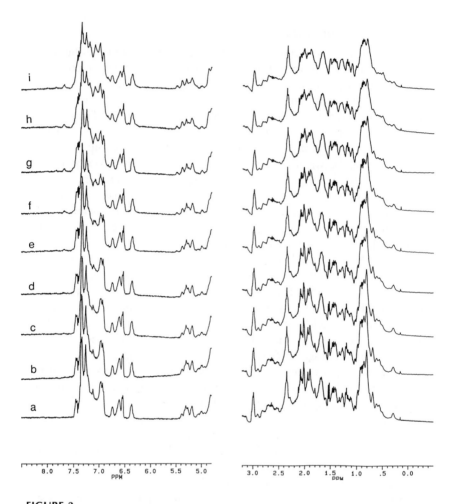

**FIGURE 2**

360-MHz $^1$H NMR spectra of isotopically normal trypanosome CaM at 30°C in the presence of the following number of equivalents of racemic calmidazolium: (a) 0, (b) 0.125, (c) 0.25, (d) 0.375, (e) 0.50, (f) 0.625, (g) 0.75, (h) 0. 875, and (i) 1.0.

negligible changes in chemical shift. This observation may be interpreted as the drug essentially experiencing only a single environment. At and above about 35°C, however, the reasonably well-resolved drug signals begin to broaden again. This is presumably due to an exchange process, intermediate on the 360-MHz proton chemical-shift time scale, becoming significant. Above about 50°C the drug signals sharpen again, possibly reflecting fast exchange between bound and free environments. Although changes are observed in the spectrum of the protein, it remains dispersed and broad at all temperatures, suggesting negligible denaturation. All

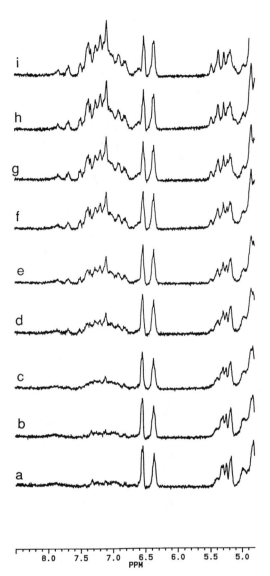

**FIGURE 3**
The downfield region of the 360-MHz ¹H NMR spectrum of ca. 20 mg [Phe-d5] CaM in the presence of increasing amounts of racemic calmidazolium. Lettering on traces corresponds to the same ratios as in Figure 2.

temperature-induced changes are rapidly and completely reversible. Further investigations of the complex were carried out in the lower-temperature, slow-exchange regime.

Because calmidazolium is virtually insoluble in water in the absence of CaM, NMR studies of its aqueous conformational properties are impossible. However, it gives rise to a good proton spectrum in methanol (Figure 5), which is interesting because of the high degree of dispersion in the aromatic region, in particular, the striking nonequivalence of the

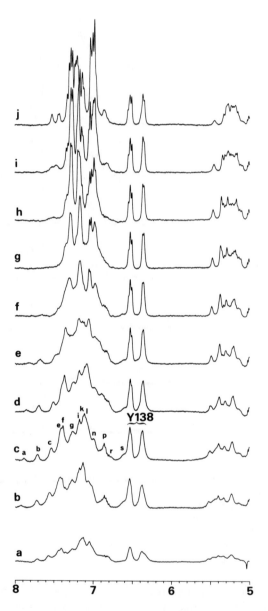

**FIGURE 4**

The downfield region of the 360-MHz spectrum of the [Phe-d₅] CaM–calmidazolium complex at (a) 15°C, (b) 20°C, (c) 25°C, (d) 30°C, (e) 35°C, (f) 40°C, (g) 45°C, (h) 50°C, (i) 55°C, and (j) 60°C.

two dichlorophenyl rings. The chemical shifts are also strongly dependent on temperature (results not shown). Both these facts argue for the

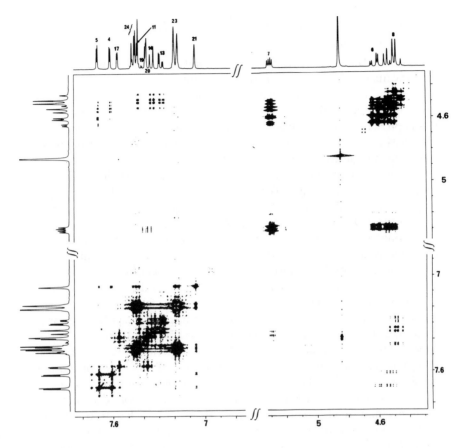

**FIGURE 5**

360-MHz double-quantum-filtered phase-sensitive COSY spectrum of ca. 45 mg calmidazolium in fully deuterated methanol (0.7 ml ) at 25°C showing resonance assignments. (H2 is observable at low field in the early stages of the experiment but rapidly exchanges with solvent deuterons.)

significant population of, and rapid interconversion between, conformational states that impose considerably different magnetic environments on each proton. Elucidation of rapidly exchanging conformations is notoriously difficult, and the free drug conformers are of only marginal interest in drug design anyway, so we have not pursued investigations in this area. However, the two-dimensional double-quantum filtered COSY spectrum,[13] besides enabling total (nonstereospecific) assignment, does show evidence of some long-range couplings between aromatic and neighbouring aliphatic protons, which should prove useful in assigning the spectrum of the CaM-bound compound with the use of through-bond-sensitive experiments like TOCSY.[14]

### 4   Two-Dimensional Experiments on [Phe-$d_5$] CaM–Calmidazolium

The availability of an isotopically manipulated CaM in which all the phenylalanine rings are spectroscopically silent offers considerable opportunities for the conformational analysis of bound drugs, and also for unambiguous ascription of NOEs to intermolecular contacts. (Of course, this approach does suffer from the drawback that any drug contacts with phenylalanine rings will not be observable. These will have to be established unambiguously by the use of $^{13}$C, $^{15}$N double-labelled protein.)

Figure 6 shows the aromatic regions of a total correlation (TOCSY) spectrum (above the diagonal) and a NOESY spectrum (below the diagonal) of the [Phe-$d_5$] CaM–calmidazolium complex. The mixing time $\tau_M$ used in the TOCSY experiment was 16.6 ms, a comparatively short value that would only be expected to delineate direct scalar (through-bond) interactions, and not those that are transmitted to distant members of a given spin system by homonuclear Hartmann–Hahn-type transfer via intervening mutual coupling partners. In other words, this mixing time produces information similar to that yielded by the familiar COSY experiment; the latter, however, is not so advantageously applied to large molecules in which efficient spin–lattice relaxation leads to broad resonances. The mixing time used in the NOESY experiment was 25 ms, also comparatively short and expected to elucidate contacts between protons within about 3 to 5 Å of each other without complications from the effects of spin diffusion, the indirect transfer of the NOE to more distant nuclei via intervening nuclei. Thus the top left-hand half of Figure 6 contains through-bond information, which is a function primarily, though not entirely, of the chemical structure of the compound, while the bottom right-hand half displays information that reflects both its chemistry and its conformation.

There is evidence in the one-dimensional spectrum of the complex in Figure 6 of compositional heterogeneity, as some of the better-resolved drug signals display fractional integrated intensities relative to the intensities of the two pairs of Tyr 138 protons. The simplest explanation for this is that the protein binds the two enantiomers of calmidazolium differently such that each gives rise to a different $^1$H NMR spectrum. (CaM has been shown by NMR to be able to discriminate between enantiomers of imidazole-containing medicinal compounds.[15]) Thus the drug–protein mixture may be thought of as consisting of two diastereomeric complexes between CaM and each drug enantiomer. Of course, equivalent protein nuclei in each diastereomer are not necessarily degenerate, and this could lead to "doubling" of protein as well as drug signals. We expect that considerable simplification of the drug–protein complex will result from using enantiomerically pure calmidazolium; preparation of both enantiomers has been achieved, but we have yet to perform the CaM-binding experiments.

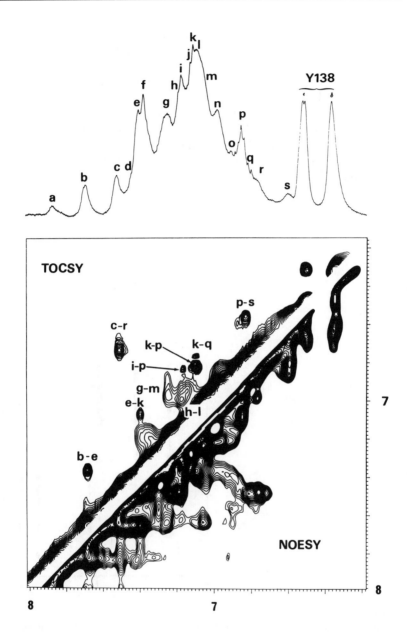

**FIGURE 6**
A composite display of the aromatic regions of 500-MHz TOCSY ($\tau_M = 16.6$ ms; *top left*) and NOESY ($\tau_M = 25$ ms; *bottom right*) spectra of the 1:1 [Phe-d$_5$] CaM–calmidazolium complex at 37°C accompanied by the same region of a 1D spectrum. Labels on the 2D spectrum signify through-bond connectivities between corresponding peaks in the 1D trace. Two-dimensional spectra shown in this and the subsequent figures were resolution enhanced using the Maximum Entropy deconvolution routine available in the NMRi processing software.

At longer NOESY mixing times a large number of NOEs become apparent between the drug aromatic protons, and higher field protein signals between 4 and 0 ppm. A representative example of a region of a 200-ms $\tau_M$ NOESY spectrum is shown in Figure 7. At this mixing time the large number of NOEs to the 0- to 2-ppm region of the protein makes the corresponding portion of the 2D matrix rather indigestible, and these interactions will have to be explored using intermediate $\tau_M$s. For this reason we have chosen to illustrate intermolecular effects by showing the region corresponding to protein chemical shifts between 1.9 and 3.6 ppm. The effects are highly specific to a few of the drug aromatic signals.

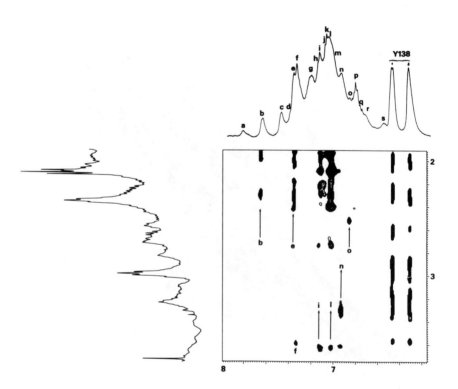

**FIGURE 7**

A region of a 200-ms $\tau_M$ NOESY spectrum of the 1:1 [Phe-d$_5$] CaM–calmidazolium complex showing some of the numerous NOEs observed between drug signals and signals in the aliphatic region of the protein spectrum. Vertical arrows in the 2D trace mark correspondences between NOE cross-peaks and the labelled features in the 1D plot of the drug spectrum. NOEs between specific drug signals and peaks in the region of the protein spectrum between 1.9 and ca. 2.2 ppm, containing some of the methionine methyl group signals, are particularly prominent.

## B   Multinuclear Approaches

The use of specifically deuterated protein probably represents the method of choice for conformational analysis of bound calmidazolium. However, a comprehensive understanding of how it interacts with the protein requires a detailed picture of the protein structure and that all the intermolecular NOEs be ascribed to specific amino acid residues in the sequence. To do this, assignments of the spectrum of the bound protein are essential. The molecular weight of CaM is about 16.8 kDa, and it is quite beyond the limits of total assignment and structure determination by homonuclear methods. Accordingly, CaM was prepared with total $^{13}$C and $^{15}$N incorporation. This allows a number of three- and multidimensional approaches (see Chapter 4) to be adopted for assignment and protein structure elucidation, and subsequent delineation of the drug-binding site.[16]

So far we have performed and are in the process of analysing several $^1$H-$^1$H-$^{15}$N TOCSY-HMQC and NOESY-HMQC experiments. These techniques use the chemical-shift dispersion of the $^{15}$N spectrum of the protein to "spread" the $^1$H spectrum out into a series of slices, each of which corresponds to a narrow range of $^{15}$N chemical shifts. The data are best visualized as a series of 2D $^1$H-$^1$H spectra, such as the two representative examples from a 100ms $\tau_M$ NOESY-HMQC spectrum shown in Figure 8. Signals from NH protons which have a $^{15}$N one-bond scalar coupled partner at the same ($^{15}$N) chemical shift appear on the "diagonal" near the bottom of each contour plot. Off-diagonal features correspond to NOE connectivities between these and other protons. Of course, the TOCSY analogue of this experiment contains information about scalar coupling systems that originate at the NH protons. The next step in our analysis will be to relate connectivities, delineated by NOE methods, between TOCSY-defined spin systems to the primary structure of the protein to obtain "sequence-specific" assignments. These will then be used in combination with $^{13}$C-based editing techniques to interpret drug–protein NOEs more specifically than has been possible using the partially deuterated protein alone.

## C   Modelling the Calmidazolium–CaM Complex

Although we have not yet assigned all the NOEs between CaM and calmidazolium protons to contacts between specific residues on the protein and functionalities on the drug, there is generalized evidence for the importance of intermolecular hydrophobic interactions in conferring stability on the complex. The majority of the intermolecular NOEs that are clear in the complex between calmidazolium and [Phe-$d_5$] CaM are between

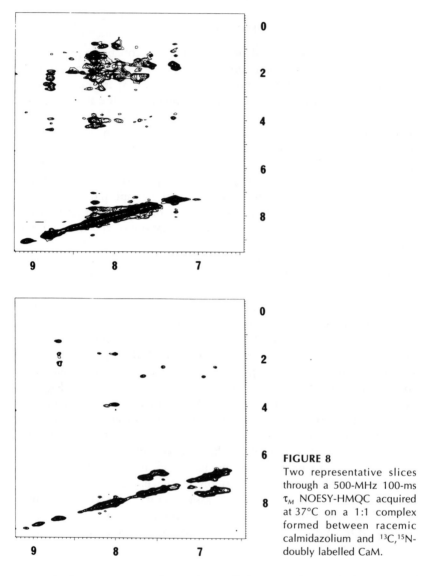

**FIGURE 8**
Two representative slices through a 500-MHz 100-ms $\tau_M$ NOESY-HMQC acquired at 37°C on a 1:1 complex formed between racemic calmidazolium and $^{13}C,^{15}N$-doubly labelled CaM.

aromatic drug protons and protein methyl groups, in particular those of methionines. The participation of these residues — which are extraordinarily abundant in CaM — in binding peptides and synthetic compounds has frequently been remarked upon.

Several attempts, implicating changes in the conformation of the "linker" helix joining the two domains,[17,18] have been made to model the way in which CaM complexes with its ligands. We have chosen the NMR structure of the CaM–MLCK peptide complex as a starting point for understanding how the protein forms its high-affinity complex with calmidazolium. Using the coordinates deposited in the Brookhaven protein structure database[19] and the Insight II macromolecular modelling package (Biosym), it was possible, by making only a very minor alteration to the relative orientation of the two hydrophobic surfaces on each protein globular domain (by changing the $\phi$ and $\phi$ angles of Ser 81 from –99 to –96 and from 55 to 51, respectively), to produce numerous hydrophobic contacts between CaM and the calmidazolium molecule. Arbitrarily the S-enantiomer of the compound was chosen for this exercise. The two *para*-chlorophenyl rings were docked with the C-terminal domain of CaM, and the "miconazole" moiety containing the two *ortho, para* -dichlorophenyl rings with the N-terminal domain. By imposing an extended conformation on the drug, one has little difficulty in achieving numerous van der Waals contacts between these groups and hydrophobic residues on the protein — Phe 12, Ala 15, Leu 18, Phe 19, Ala 35, Met 36, Ala 39, Phe 68, and Met 72 in the N-terminal domain, and Ala 88, Phe 92, Ile 100, Leu 105, Val 108, Met 109, Met 124, Phe 141, Met 144, and Met 145 in the C-terminus. Models of these interactions in the N- and C-terminal domains are presented in stereo in Figure 9.

It is clear that the flexible methionine side chains are important in allowing CaM to interact with a diverse range of ligands. Small changes in the side-chain torsion angles of these residues would enable each hydrophobic patch to accommodate a stereochemically varied range of lipophilic ligands as well as offering the opportunity of sulphur lone-pair interactions with aromatic groups. It was also evident in the course of the modelling that the chlorophenyl rings of the drug, especially the two *o,p*-dichlorophenyls of the miconazole moiety, could form ring-stacked "sandwich" structures with protein phenylalanines; the electron-withdrawing propensity of the chloro substituents could be important in helping to reduce repulsions between the aromatic *p*-electron clouds. In spite of the preponderance of negatively charged aspartate and glutamate residues on the protein, this "low-resolution" docking exercise failed to suggest any ion pair interaction with the positively charged imidazolium group of the drug. Overall views of the model are shown in heavy atom and ribbon representation in Figure 10.

# ACKNOWLEDGMENTS

We are grateful to Dr. Nabil Elshourbagy (SB Pharmaceuticals, Philadelphia) and Drs. Curtis L. Patton, Charles Eguagu and Jim Young (Yale University School of Medicine) for the *E. coli* expression system for trypanosome CaM. Much of this work was performed by Patricia Sweeney during the course of a jointly SERC/SB-funded CASE studentship, and

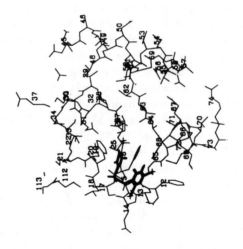

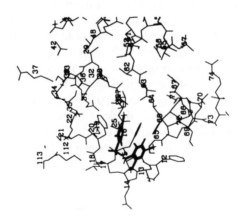

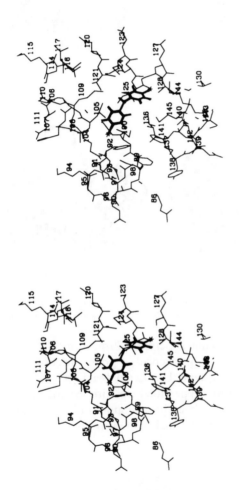

**FIGURE 9**

Stereo views of possible docking modes of (*top*) the "miconazole" and (*bottom*) the *bis*-(*p*-chlorophenyl) methine moieties of calmidazolium with the N- and C-terminal domain hydrophobic surfaces, respectively, of CaM.

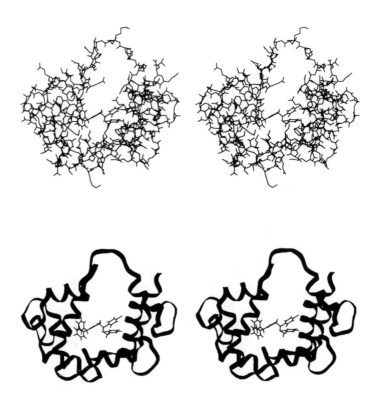

**FIGURE 10**
Stereo views of (*top*) the entire model of the CaM–calmidazolium complex, and (*bottom*) the same view simplified by imposing a ribbon representation on the protein.

all the support of her academic supervisor, Prof. John Walker, University of Hertfordshire, Division of Biosciences, is gratefully acknowledged. We are also indebted to our colleagues Drs. Lesley MacLachlan, Julia Hubbard, Martin Saunders, and Ted Pepper for help with experimental and data-processing aspects of this work, and for support and encouragement, and to Dr. Chris Southan for N-terminal sequencing of expressed CaM.

# REFERENCES

1. (a) Klee, C.B.; Vanaman, T.C. *Adv. Protein Chem.* 1982, 35, 213. (b) Forsen, S.; Vogel, H.J.; Drakenberg, T., in *Calcium and Cell Function*; Cheung, W.Y., Ed.; Academic Press: Orlando, FL, 1986; Vol. 6, pp. 113-157. (c) Klee, C.B., in *Molecular Aspects of Cellular Regulation*; Cohen, P. and Klee, C.B., Eds; Elsevier: New York, 1988; Vol. 5, pp. 35-56.

2. (a) Seeholzer, S.H.; Munier, H.; Mispeltre, J.; Barzu, O.; Craescu, C.T. *Biochemistry* 1992, 31, 229-236. (b) Roth, S.M.; Schneider, D.M.; Strobel, L.A.; VanBerkum, M.F.A.; Means, A.R.; Wand, A.J. *Biochemistry* 1991, 30, 10078-10084.

3. (a) Epstein, P.M.; Fiss, K.; Hachisu, R.; Adrenyak, D.M. *Biochem. Biophys. Res. Commun.* 1982, 105, 1142-1149. (b) Lugnier, C.; Follenius, A.; Gerard, D.; Stoclet, J.C. *Eur. J. Pharmacol.* 1984, 98, 157-158. (c) Zimmer, M.; Hoffmann, F. *Eur. J. Biochem.* 1987, 165, 411-420. (d) Bostrom, S-L.; Ljung, B.; Mardh, S.; Thulin, E. *Nature* 1981, 292, 777-778. (e) Andersson, A.; Drakenberg, T.; Thulin, E.; Forsen, S. *Eur. J. Biochem.* 1983, 134, 459-465. (f) Kubo, K.; Matsuda, Y.; Kase, H.; Yamada, K. *Biochem. Biophys. Res. Commun.* 1984, 124, 315-321.

4. Babu, Y.S.; Bugg, C.E.; Cook, W.J. *J. Molec. Biol.* 1988, 204, 191-204.

5. (a) Ikura, M.; Clore, G.M.; Gronenborn, A.M.; Zhu, G.; Klee, C.B.; Bax, A. *Science* 1992, 2256, 632-638. (b) Ikura, M.; Kay, L.E.; Krinks, E.; Bax, A. *Biochemistry* 1991, 30, 5498-5504.

6. Seeholzer, S.H.; Cohn, M.; Putkey, J.A.; Means, A.R.; Crespi, H.L. *Proc. Natl. Acad. Sci. USA* 1986, 83, 3634-3638.

7. (a) Ruben, L.; Engwuagu, C.; Patton, C.L. *Biochim. Biophys. Acta* 1983, 758, 104-113. (b) Ruben, L.; Strickler, J.E.; Egwuagu, C.; Patton, C.L. *Molec. Biol. Host-Parasite Interact.* 1984, 13, 267-278. (c) Ruben, L.; Patton, C.L. *Mol. Biochem. Parasit.* 1985, 17, 331-341. (d) Ruben, L.; Patton, C.L. *Methods Enzymol.* 1987, 139, 262-276.

8. Scheibel, L.W.; Colombani, P.M.; Hess, A.D.; Aikawa, M.; Atkinson, C.T.; Milhouse, W.K. *Proc. Natl. Acad. Sci. USA* 1987, 84, 7310-7314.

9. (a) Gietzen, K.; Wüthrich, K.; Bader, H. *Biochem. Biophys. Res. Commun.* 1981, 101, 418-425. (b) Wulfroth, P.; Petzelt, C. *Cell Calcium* 1985, 6, 295-310. Johnson, J.D.; (c) Wittenauer, L.A. *Biochem. J.* 1983, 211, 473-479. (d) Lee, G.L.; Hait, W.N. *Life Sci.* 1985, 36, 347-354.

10. Reid, D.G.; MacLachlan, L.K.; Gajjar, K.; Voyle, M.; King, R.J.; England, P.J. *J. Biol. Chem.* 1990, 265, 9744-9753.

11. Dalgarno, D.C.; Klevit, R.E.; Levine, B.A.; Williams, R.J.P.; Dobrowolski, Z.; Drabikowski, W. *Eur. J. Biochem.* 1984, 138, 281-289.

12. (a) Seamon, K.B. *Biochemistry* 1980, 19, 207-215. (b) Klevit, R.E.; Dalgarno, D.C.; Levine, B.A.; Williams, R.J.P. *Eur. J. Biochem.* 1984, 139, 109-114. (c) Krebs, J.; Carafoli, E. *Eur. J. Biochem.* 1984, 124, 619-627. (d) Ikura, M.; Hiraoki, T.; Hikichi, K.; Mikuni, T.; Yazawa, M.; Yagi, K. *Biochemistry* 1983, 22, 2573-2579.

13. (a) Rance, M.; Sorenson, O.W.; Bodenhausen, G.; Wagner, G.; Ernst, R.R.; Wüthrich, K. *J. Magn. Reson.* 1983, 113, 967-974. (b) Piantini, U.; Sorenson, O.W.; Ernst, R.R. *J. Am. Chem. Soc.* 1982, 104, 6800-6801.

14. (a) Braunschweiler, L.; Ernst, R.E. *J. Magn. Reson.* 1983, 53, 521-528. (b) Davis, D.G.; Bax, A. *J. Am. Chem. Soc.* 1985, 107, 2820-2821.

15. Reid, D.G.; MacLachlan, L.K.; Robinson, S.P.; Camilleri, P.; Dyke, C.A.; Thorpe, C.J. *Chirality* 1990, 2, 229-232.

16. (a) Petros, A.M.; Gemmecker, G.; Neri, P.; Olejniczak, A.T.; Nettesheim, D.; Xu, R.X.; Gubbin, E.G.; Smith, H.; Fesik, S.W. *J. Med. Chem.* 1992, 35, 2467-2473. (b) Fesik, S.W.; Grampe, R.T.; Eaton, H.L.; Gemmecker, G.; Olejniczak, E.T.; Neri, P.; Holzman, T.F.; Egan, D.A.; Edalji, R.; Simmer, R.; Helfrich, R.; Hochlowski, J.; Jackson, M. *Biochemistry* 1991, 30, 6574-6583. (c) Fesik, S.W.; Grampe, R.T., Jr.; Holzman, T.F.; Egan, D.A.; Edalji, R.; Luly, J.R.; Simmer, R.; Helfrich, R.; Kishore, V.; Rich, D.H. *Science* 1990, 250, 1406-1409.

17. Persechini, A.; Kretsinger, R.J. *J. Cardiovasc. Pharmacol. (S5)* 1988, 12, 1.
18. O'Neill, K.T.; De Grado, W.F. *Proteins* 1988, 6, 284.
19. (a) Bernstein, F.C.; Koetzle, T.F.; Williams, G.J.B.; Meyer, E.F., Jr.; Brice, J.B.; Rodgers, J.R.; Kennard, O.; Shimanouchi, T.; Tasumi, M. *J. Mol. Biol.* 1977, 112, 535-542. (b) Abola, E.E.; Bernstein, F.C.; Bryant, S.H.; Koetzle, T.F.; Weng, J., in *Crystallographic Databases - Information Content, Software Systems, Scientific Applications*; Allen, F.H.; Bergerhoff, R.; Sievers, G., Eds.; Commission of the International Union of Crystallography: Bonn, Germany; 1987, pp. 107-132.

CHAPTER 10

# FLEXIBILITY AND FUNCTION IN THE HIV-1 PROTEASE[*]

*Linda K. Nicholson, Chong-Hwan Chang, and C. Nicholas Hodge*

## CONTENTS

I  Introduction ................................................................................ 338

II  Elucidation of Protein Motions ....................................................... 339
   A  Molecular Motion and Nuclear Spin Relaxation ..................... 339
   B  A Physical Picture of Protein Motions ................................... 340
   C  Mathematical Description of Protein Motions ....................... 342
   D  NMR Measurements ............................................................. 344
      1  Relaxation Parameters ..................................................... 344
      2  The Influence of Chemical-Exchange Processes ............... 347
      3  Hydrogen–Deuterium Exchange as a Probe of
         Structural Stability ......................................................... 348

III  Application to the HIV-1 Protease ................................................ 348
   A  Targeting the HIV-1 Protease ............................................... 349
   B  Characterization of Backbone Flexibility in
      Protease/Inhibitor Complexes ............................................. 351
      1  Symmetry of the Dimer When Bound to
         Symmetric Inhibitors ..................................................... 351
      2  Comparison of Chemical Environments ........................... 351
      3  Comparison of Backbone Motions in the
         Two Complexes ............................................................... 354

* Adapted from Nicholson, L.K., et al., *Nature Structural Biology*, 1995, 2, 274–280.

4   Characteristics of Backbone Flexibility in
    Both Complexes ................................................................. 361
    a   Residues Undergoing Large-Amplitude, Fast
        Internal Motions ........................................................ 361
    b   Residues Affected by Chemical Exchange ................... 365

IV   Conclusions and Perspective ........................................... 370

Acknowledgments ................................................................... 373

References ............................................................................. 374

# I   INTRODUCTION

The assault of the AIDS epidemic has resulted in a focused research effort over the past decade to understand the life cycle of the human immunodeficiency virus (HIV) and to identify and attack vulnerable points in this cycle. Currently the only drugs that have been approved by the U.S. Food and Drug Administration (FDA) for general treatment of AIDS are nucleoside analogs that act by inhibiting the key viral replication enzyme, reverse transcriptase (RT). These compounds include AZT, ddI, ddC, and recently approved d4T. Although these drugs slow the spread of the virus, they fail to present a cure. Hence, attention is being given to other aspects of the viral life cycle for new angles of attack. The HIV-1 protease is currently the most promising of these aspects. Structure-based drug design has resulted in an array of compounds targeted against the active sites of the viral proteases that have been shown to effectively block the enzyme *in vitro*.[1-3] The small size of these compounds and their low toxicity make them promising candidates for clinical use. However, a myriad of difficulties can be encountered when taking the step between *in vitro* and *in vivo* effectiveness, including low bioavailability and rapid mutation of the viral protease that can impart drug resistance. Therefore, it is imperative to understand as much as possible about the biophysical basis of enzyme function and specificity, including the structural and dynamic details of the protein and its interactions with different inhibitors. Information about the structure and dynamics of the protease at the atomic level can be used to identify regions of an inhibitor where modifications can be made such that potency, bioavailability, and transport of the potential drug into the cell can be optimized. It is also important to identify all potential vulnerabilities of the protease to inhibition, which requires information about not only the active site, but also other regions of the enzyme that are essential for function.

As noted in the introductory chapters, most rational drug design approaches focus on the relationship between structure and function. Protein–ligand interactions are currently understood in terms of spatial relationships that place potential hydrogen bond, ionic, and hydrophobic partners within reach of one another. It is indeed necessary to know the molecular architecture in which highly specific chemical events take place. However, essentially all experimental techniques that are sensitive to dynamics have detected internal motions in proteins. In order to fully understand the forces that govern protein function, the effects of internal motions and the subsequent fluctuation of energy fields must be taken into account and incorporated into the drug design process. Investigation of the relationships between structure, dynamics, and function is the motivation for the work presented herein.

We report the results of NMR relaxation studies that represent the first experimental characterization of backbone dynamics in the HIV-1 protease, and present a comparative analysis of these motions in the presence of two different inhibitors, the cyclic urea DMP323, and the C-2 symmetric linear diol P9941.[2] These inhibitors, which differ in both size and inherent flexibility, have binding constants that differ by more than an order of magnitude. Hence, dynamics studies shed light on the entropic contribution of the protein backbone to the free energy of binding and to offer the opportunity to relate dynamic details to function. The importance of dynamics in the HIV-1 protease has been emphasized in a number of theoretical studies in which molecular dynamics simulations have predicted functionally relevant motions.[4-6] Hence, we have employed $^{15}N$ NMR relaxation techniques to investigate the flexibility of the protein backbone when bound to two different inhibitors in order to gain insight into what role, if any, backbone motions play in protease function and inhibitor binding. Through correlation of the dynamics results with structural details derived from both X-ray crystallography and NMR, and with functional results from site-directed mutagenesis, several important aspects of flexibility in this protein are elucidated.

## II  ELUCIDATION OF PROTEIN MOTIONS

### A  MOLECULAR MOTION AND NUCLEAR SPIN RELAXATION

Solution NMR is an extremely powerful technique for characterizing the detailed motions that occur within proteins. With this technique, a wide range of time scales can be probed, ranging from pico- to nanosecond time frames and slower. Recent advances in solution NMR now enable protein dynamics to be accurately measured relatively quickly. These advances include the rapid resonance assignment capabilities offered by newly developed heteronuclear multidimensional techniques[7,8] described in detail in Chapter 4, and the effective elimination of artifacts in the measurement of relaxation parameters.[9-13]

The relaxation of nuclear spin states provides a sensitive probe of both global tumbling of a protein and internal motions of individual bonds within the protein. The state of the nuclear spin system can be perturbed by application of radio frequency (rf) pulses, and the rate of return to equilibrium can be monitored. The rate of return to equilibrium, or relaxation rate, is directly related to molecular motions. As discussed in Chapter 3, the nuclear spin interactions that typically dominate relaxation of a nucleus include the chemical shift anisotropy (CSA) and the dipolar interactions, which are tensor quantities that express the perturbation of the local magnetic field at the nucleus due to circulating electrons and neighboring nuclei with magnetic dipoles, respectively. These nuclear spin interactions are directly dependent upon the orientation of the nucleus with respect to the applied static magnetic field. Hence, as a site undergoes motion, the local magnetic field at the nucleus fluctuates. From a classical viewpoint, these fluctuating magnetic fields associated with the chemical shift and dipolar interactions exert a torque on the nonequilibrium magnetization, causing the system to relax back to equilibrium. Hence, the rate of relaxation of a nuclear spin is directly dependent upon the amplitude and rate of motions experienced by its local environment.

## B   A Physical Picture of Protein Motions

From an NMR perspective, it is generally assumed that protein motions are random, stochastic, overdamped processes, including global tumbling of the molecule as well as internal motions of individual bonds. This is easily understood for global tumbling of a protein in solution by considering an ensemble of protein molecules, each undergoing random thermally driven collisions with solvent molecules and occasionally with each other. At any given point in time, some proteins within this sample will have just experienced a collision in which they gained kinetic energy and will be rapidly tumbling, while others will perhaps have undergone a collision in which they gave up kinetic energy and are moving very slowly. Hence, a distribution of frequencies will be present, rather than a single rotational rate. A similar situation can be used to visualize internal motions of bond vectors within the randomly tumbling protein. Although normal modes of vibration, torsion, and bending clearly govern the motions of bond vectors on the femto- to picosecond time frame, at any given instant in time various forces will be experienced by a given site within an ensemble of identical proteins, and a distribution of frequencies corresponding to different motional states will be present in the sample. This distribution will depend upon local environment and on specific structural features that either limit or enhance the ability of the given site to move. Since motions span a large range of frequencies, it is not meaningful to assign a single frequency of motion to describe the various aspects of protein dynamics. Instead, a mathematical description of random processes is employed.

To obtain a physical picture of how internal motions can be described, consider a protein represented by a sphere, and an NH bond within this sphere (Figure 1). If the fluctuation of the NH bond relative to a reference frame fixed in the laboratory is to be characterized, three pieces of information are necessary: (1) the rate of overall tumbling of the protein in solution, (2) the rate of internal motion of the NH bond, and (3) the amplitude of NH bond motion. Because of the random nature of these motions, amplitudes and rates must be described in terms of generalized order parameters and correlation times.[14,15] The rate of overall tumbling can be represented by the correlation time $\tau_m$, which roughly corresponds to the average time required for the protein to undergo rotation through 1 rad. Similarly, the rate of internal motion of the NH bond can also be described by an effective correlation time $\tau_e$, and the amplitude of this motion can be described by the order parameter $S^2$. The order parameter is a measure of the spatial restriction to motion, and is directly related to amplitude. A simple example is the specific model in which the NH bond

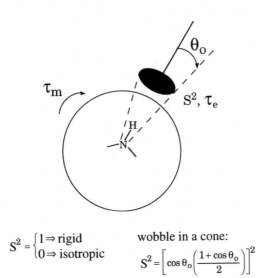

$$S^2 = \begin{cases} 1 \Rightarrow \text{rigid} \\ 0 \Rightarrow \text{isotropic} \end{cases}$$

wobble in a cone:

$$S^2 = \left[ \cos \theta_0 \left( \frac{1 + \cos \theta_0}{2} \right) \right]^2$$

**FIGURE 1**
Physical picture of protein motions. The protein is represented by a sphere, which tumbles isotropically in solution, with associated correlation time $\tau_m$. An individual NH bond vector within the protein undergoes rapid internal motions, with the amplitude of motion characterized by the order parameter $S^2$ ($0 < S^2 < 1$) and the time scale by the effective internal correlation time $\tau_e$. The direct relationship between $S^2$ and amplitude for a specific model of motion is illustrated for the case of wobble within a cone.

is restricted to wobble within a cone, where $S^2$ is an explicit function of the solid angle $\theta$ that describes the cone (Figure 1). The value of $S^2$ can range from 0 to 1, where a value of 1 corresponds to complete restriction (no motion, the site is completely rigid), and a value of 0 corresponds to absolutely no restriction to motion (all orientations are equally probable, the motion is isotropic).

## C    Mathematical Description of Protein Motions

Random protein motions can be mathematically described in terms of a correlation function $C(t)$ and its Fourier transform partner, the spectral density function $J(\omega)$. In order to gain a physical understanding of the correlation function, consider a hypothetical ensemble of vectors, which at time $t = 0$ are all pointing in the same direction (Figure 2). The vector sum over the ensemble along the initial direction of orientation at $t = 0$ represents the initial value of the correlation function $C(0)$. If a random force is applied, the vectors will reorient as a function of time, according to the restrictions to motion imposed by their environment. Depending upon these restrictions, the net sum of the vectors along the direction of initial alignment will decrease. Case A corresponds to a more highly restrictive environment, while case B corresponds to a less restrictive environment. For a purely stochastic, random process, the vector sum will decay in an exponential manner with a time constant $\tau$ (the correlation time) that is indicative of the rate of reorientation. As $\tau$ approaches $\infty$, the vector sum asymptotically approaches a characteristic value, which corresponds to the generalized order parameter $S^2$. As illustrated, the more highly restricted case, A, results in a larger $S^2$ value, corresponding to smaller amplitude. Hence, $S^2$ is a measure of the spatial restriction to motion, while $\tau$ indicates the time scale of motion.

The Fourier transform (FT) of the correlation function $C(t)$ into the frequency domain yields the spectral density function $J(\omega)$. The spectral density function represents the probability of a given frequency occurring, given a characteristic motion. Since the FT of an exponential function results in a Lorentzian function, $J(\omega)$ (for random motions) has a Lorentzian lineshape. The theoretical form of $J(\omega)$ for the case of isotropic molecular tumbling and internal motions in the extreme narrowing limit, that is $(\omega\tau_e)^2 \ll 1$, is given by[14]

$$J(\omega) = S^2\tau_m/[1 + (\omega\tau_m)^2] + (1 - S^2)\tau/[1 + (\omega\tau)^2] \qquad (1)$$

where $1/\tau = [1/\tau_m + 1/\tau_e]$, with $S^2$, $\tau_m$, and $\tau_e$ defined in the previous section. This function is plotted in Figure 3 on a semilog scale. A majority of motions within proteins are fit well by this formalism, and this approach, often referred to as the Lipari and Szabo formalism,[14] has been widely

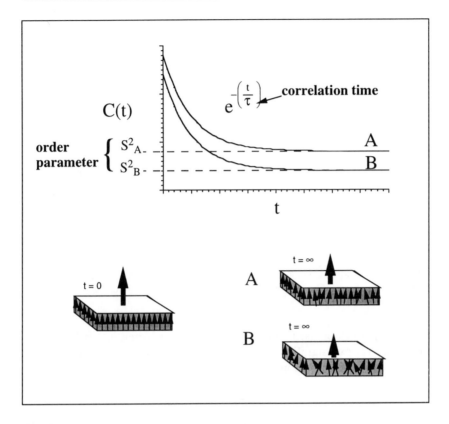

**FIGURE 2**
Physical interpretation of the correlation function $C(t)$ and its relationship to the associated parameters of motion $S^2$ and $\tau$.

applied to extract information about molecular motion. Note that there are three parameters that characterize the motions: the correlation time for overall tumbling of the molecule $\tau_m$, the order parameter for the internal motion $S^2$, and the effective correlation time for internal motion $\tau_e$. In order to describe the motion of a specific bond within a protein, three independent measurable quantities that depend explicitly on $S^2$, $\tau_m$, and $\tau_e$ are required. It should be noted that, under the assumption of isotropic overall tumbling, all individual sites within a protein will experience the same effects of global motion; hence, the overall correlation time is not a site-specific, but is rather a molecule-specific parameter. However, $S^2$ and $\tau_e$ are parameters that describe the internal motion of an individual bond vector. Thus, for $n$ individual NH groups in a protein, there will be $2n$ site-specific parameters ($S^2$ and $\tau_e$ for each NH group) and a single value of $\tau_m$, for a total of $(2n + 1)$ unknowns. If three experimental quantities can be measured for each site, then a total of $3n$ "knowns" for $(2n + 1)$ unknowns are available, and the fit is overdetermined. This allows for more complex

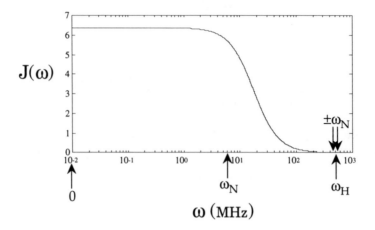

**FIGURE 3**

The spectral density function $J(\omega)$, corresponding to Equation (1), plotted as a function of frequency. The frequencies contributing to relaxation processes for a backbone amide $^{15}$N site are denoted by arrows.

forms of $J(\omega)$ to be used when necessary, such as when internal motions take place on two significantly different time scales. In this case, a useful and approximate extension of Equation 1 is given by[16]

$$J(\omega) = S^2\tau_m/[1 + (\omega\tau_m)^2] + (1-S_f^2)\tau_1/[1 + (\omega\tau_1)^2]$$
$$+ S_f^2(1-S_s^2)\tau_2/[1 + (\omega\tau_2)^2] \tag{2}$$

where $S^2 = S_f^2 S_s^2$, and $(S_f^2, \tau_1)$ and $(S_s^2, \tau_2)$ are order parameters and correlation times associated with the "fast" and "slow" (defined as outside the extreme narrowing limit) internal motions, respectively.

## D   NMR MEASUREMENTS

### 1   Relaxation Parameters

Three experimentally accessible parameters that directly depend upon $J(\omega)$, and hence on the generalized parameters of motion (i.e., $\{S^2, \tau_m, \tau_e\}$ or $\{S^2, \tau_m, \tau_1, \tau_2\}$), are provided by the longitudinal relaxation time $T_1$, the transverse relaxation time $T_2$, and the heteronuclear NOE. Each of these parameters is explicitly dependent upon $J(\omega)$ evaluated at specific frequencies.[17] For an $^{15}$N–$^1$H group in which the influence of both dipolar and CSA interactions is accounted for, the corresponding $^{15}$N relaxation parameters are expressed by

$$1/T_1 = d^2[J(\omega_H - \omega_N) + 3J(\omega_N) + 6J(\omega_H + \omega_N)] + c^2J(\omega_N) \tag{3}$$

$$1/T_2 = (^1/_2)d^2[4J(0) + J(\omega_H - \omega_N) + 3J(\omega_N) + 6J(\omega_H) + 6J(\omega_H + \omega_N)]$$
$$+ (^1/_6)c^2[4J(0) + 3J(\omega_N)] \tag{4}$$

$$\text{NOE} = 1 + (\gamma_H/\gamma_N)d^2[6J(\omega_H + \omega_N) - J(\omega_H - \omega_N)]T_1 \tag{5}$$

where the constants $d$ and $c$ denote the strength of the static dipolar and chemical shift anisotropy interactions, respectively, $\gamma_i$ is the gyromagnetic ratio for nucleus $i$, and $\omega_i$ denotes the Larmor frequency of nucleus $i$. It should be noted that the above nuclear spin relaxation rates are inherently dependent upon the internuclear NH bond distance $r$ and the magnitude of the chemical shielding anisotropy ($\sigma_\parallel - \sigma_\perp$), as described in detail in Chapter 3. Specifically, the dipolar contribution (scaled by $d^2$) depends on $r^{-6}$, while the CSA contribution (scaled by $c^2$) depends on ($\sigma_\parallel - \sigma_\perp$)$^2$. When the spectral density function expressed by Equation 1 is assumed, the value of $J(\omega)$ at each of the five specific frequencies in Equations (3–5) is determined by the values of $S^2$, $\tau_m$, and $\tau_e$. Hence, by measuring $T_1$, $T_2$, and NOE values, the spectral density function is being probed at five points, but the value of $J(\omega)$ at each of these points is determined by the three parameters of motion ($S^2$, $\tau_m$ and $\tau_e$), which determine the lineshape of the function. For a given set of $S^2$, $\tau_m$, and $\tau_e$, the theoretical $T_1$, $T_2$, and NOE values can be calculated and compared with the measured values. In this manner the experimental relaxation data are fit to yield the optimal set of parameters describing the motion of individual NH groups within the protein. Experimental approaches for accurate measurement of $^{15}$N $T_1$, $T_2$, and NOE values, and analytical approaches for extraction of the parameters of motion have been described in detail elsewhere, and will not be presented here.[12,18,19]

In order to appreciate the information content of the measured relaxation parameters, it is useful to visualize the sensitivity of $T_1$, $T_2$, and NOE values to internal protein motions. Using Equation (1) and Equations (3–5), theoretical $T_1$, $T_2$, and NOE values were calculated as functions of $S^2$ and $\tau_e$ for an overall correlation time of 9.1 ns; these values are plotted in Figure 4, with the different curves corresponding to different $S^2$ values. It should be kept in mind that all three parameters are scaled by overall tumbling $\tau_m$, and that the plots in Figure 4 represent application of the Lipari and Szabo formalism Equation (1), to a protein in the 20-kDa size range. These plots are useful because they point out the sensitivity of the different relaxation parameters to the generalized parameters describing internal motion. For example, the $T_2$ curves are relatively flat, but are well separated vertically; hence, $T_2$ is relatively insensitive to the time scale of internal motion $\tau_e$, but is very sensitive to the amplitude of motion $S^2$. Similarly, $T_1$ is more sensitive to amplitude and less sensitive to the time scale of internal motion. The NOE is sensitive to both $S^2$ and $\tau_e$ when the time scale of motion is longer than 10 ps. These sensitivities can be

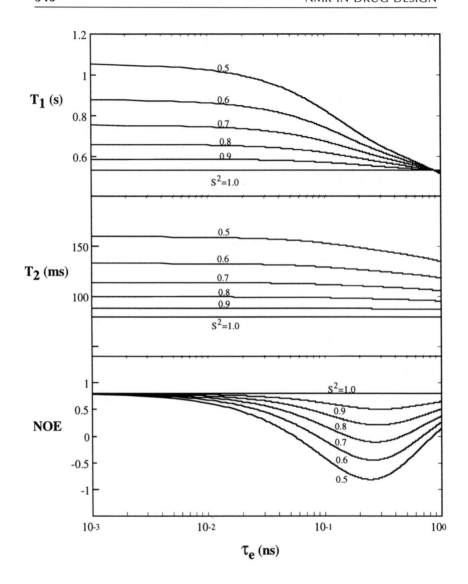

**FIGURE 4**
Theoretical plots of $T_1$, $T_2$ and NOE values as functions of $S^2$ and $\tau_e$ for a correlation time for overall tumbling of 9.1 ns. These plots were generated from Equations (3–5), assuming the spectral density function given by Equation (1). The individual curves represent different values of $S^2$, as noted. These plots illustrate the sensitivity of each of the relaxation parameters to the amplitude and time scale of internal motion for a protein in the 20-kDa size range tumbling isotropically in solution.

combined to yield an initial estimate of $S^2$ and $\tau_e$ for a given site without numerical fitting. The $T_1$ and $T_2$ relaxation times yield an approximate $S^2$

value, and the NOE value yields an approximate $\tau_e$ corresponding to this $S^2$. Hence, the plots in Figure 4 can be used to obtain an initial qualitative idea of the amplitude and time scale of motion for a given site, based on the $T_1$, $T_2$, and NOE values observed.

## 2   The Influence of Chemical-Exchange Processes

The internal motions discussed in the previous sections have been limited to rapid time scale (picosecond to nanosecond) motions, which provide relaxation pathways for all three NMR relaxation parameters measured. An additional type of motion that contributes to relaxation of transverse magnetization only $T_2$ is chemical exchange. As discussed in detail in Chapter 3, chemical exchange refers to any process that alters the chemical environment of the nucleus on a time scale that is on the order of the magnitude of change in chemical shift, typically in the milli- to microsecond time frame. Such processes may include transitions between different ionization forms, different positions of protonation, different conformations, and different complexed forms. In the simplest case, an exchange process involving two states that have equal populations in fast exchange ($\tau_{ex} < T_{CP}$), the contribution to the relaxation rate of transverse magnetization ($1/T_2$) is given by[20]

$$R_{ex} = (\Delta\omega/2)^2\tau_{ex}[1 - (2\tau_{ex}/T_{CP})]  \tag{6}$$

where $\tau_{ex} = 2/k$, with $k$ being the rate constant for the exchange process, $T_{CP}$ is the time interval between the $^{15}N$ 180° pulses in the Carr–Purcell–Meiboom–Gill (CPMG) segment of the $T_2$ pulse sequence[9] (900 µs for the experiments reported herein), and $\Delta\omega$ is the difference in $^{15}N$ chemical shifts in the two states (rad/s). Since $R_{ex}$ is dependent on $(\Delta\omega)^2$, the effect of chemical exchange on $T_2$ scales with the square of the applied static magnetic field. Hence, $T_2$ measurements at different field strengths can be used to confirm the presence of chemical exchange. However, in order to obtain a value for $\tau_{ex}$, $\Delta\omega$ must be known or assumed. Depending on the relative values of $\Delta\omega$ and $\tau_{ex}$, it is sometimes possible to determine both of these parameters from measurements of $1/T_{1\rho}$, the relaxation rate of spin-locked $^{15}N$ transverse magnetization (i.e., $T_1$ in the rotating frame). For two equally populated states, the chemical exchange contribution to $1/T_{1\rho}$ is given by[20,21]

$$R_{ex} = (\Delta\omega/2)^2\tau_{ex}/[1 + (\omega_1\tau_{ex})^2]  \tag{7}$$

where $\omega_1$ is the strength of the applied spin-lock field. Hence, provided that $\omega_1\tau_{ex} \geq 0.5$, measurements of $R_{ex}$ as a function of $\omega_1$ yield both $\tau_{ex}$ and $\Delta\omega$.

### 3  Hydrogen–Deuterium Exchange as a Probe of Structural Stability

The stability of hydrogen bonds within a protein in solution can be probed by measurement of hydrogen–deuterium exchange rates.[22] Briefly, amide proton exchange rates can be determined by lyophilizing a protein from $H_2O$ buffer, dissolving the protein in $D_2O$, and measuring the $^{15}N-^1H$ cross-peak signal intensities in a series of two-dimensional heteronuclear single quantum correlation (HSQC) spectra as a function of time. These exchange rates indicate the level of competition of solvent for structural hydrogen bonds, and can be used as a qualitative measure of structural stability. These results, together with the dynamics information extracted from $^{15}N$ NMR relaxation parameters, provide a dynamic description of hydrogen bonds that otherwise may not be apparent in structural information obtained from X-ray crystallography or NMR. It should be noted that the intrinsic exchange rates of labile amide NH protons are extremely sensitive to pH, since the propensity of an amide proton to be pulled off is directly dependent upon the concentration of base catalyst. For example, exchange rates measured at pH 6.5 will be approximately 18 times faster than at pH 5.2. Hence, when comparing exchange rates in a quantitative manner, care should be take to ensure that differences in pH are accounted for. Furthermore, inherent effects of primary structure, in the form of inductive and steric blocking effects due to neighboring side chains, can influence the rate of exchange of peptide group NH hydrogen atoms as demonstrated for unstructured oligo- and polypeptides.[22] Thus, when quantitatively comparing measured exchange rates for different residues, the influence of primary sequence should also be considered.

---

## III  APPLICATION TO THE HIV-1 PROTEASE

The HIV-1 protease provides an excellent system in which to investigate the relationships between structure, dynamics, and function. A wealth of structural and functional information is available, with more than 170 X-ray crystal structures solved[23,24] and the effects of site-directed mutagenesis of each residue on enzyme activity evaluated.[25-30] By comparing backbone motions in the protease when bound to two different inhibitors with significantly different $K_i$ values, we can ask whether entropic energy associated with backbone flexibility contributes significantly to the free energy of the bound complexes. Furthermore, by looking at the common features of backbone flexibility in the two complexes, we can consider backbone motions that may play important functional roles and, hence, may point to regions of the protein that could be vulnerable to destabilization by properly designed compounds.

## A  Targeting the HIV-1 Protease

The viral life cycle of HIV involves the use of proteins found in the host as well as proteins coded for by the virus. The virus produces most of its own proteins as part of one of two long, continuous strings of protein, coded for by the *gag* and *pol* viral genes. These long polyproteins are subsequently cleaved at the appropriate places to produce a repertoire of structural proteins and enzymes required by the virus for replication and infection. The HIV-1 protease is the cutting tool that accomplishes this vital proteolytic processing. Inhibition or specific mutation of the protease leads to the production of noninfectious viral particles;[31,32] hence, this enzyme has become a primary target for rational drug design approaches. It is a member of the aspartic acid protease family, a class of enzymes in which aspartic acid residues positioned at the active site play a key catalytic role. Normal cellular aspartic acid proteases such as pepsin differ from the viral form in a number of ways, and these differences are crucial in designing protease inhibitors that are specific for the viral rather than the cellular form of the enzyme.

To achieve specificity of inhibitors for the target enzyme, the focus has been on structural differences between the retroviral protease and related cellular proteases. The HIV-1 protease is active as a dimer composed of identical subunits (Figure 5c), while the larger cellular aspartic acid proteases are functional as monomers. Related to this global difference, the viral form has two flaps, one contributed by each subunit, that close down over the active site and participate in specific interactions with ligands, while the cellular counterparts have a single flap. In addition, in the viral form there is a conserved structural water that forms a hydrogen bonded network between the tips of the flaps and the ligand, while there is no such water molecule in the cellular form.

Rational drug design approaches applied to the HIV-1 protease have keyed in on the absence of the structural water in the cellular form. Dupont Merck Pharmaceutical Company has designed an inhibitor that displaces the structural water molecule bound at the tips of the flaps. The inhibitor DMP323 ($K_i = 0.27$ n$M$)[2] is a cyclic urea compound that employs a strategically placed carbonyl oxygen to mimic the hydrogen-bonding features of the key structural water, thereby excluding the water molecule and imparting specificity for the viral protease.[2,33] In contrast, the linear diol inhibitor P9941 ($K_i = 9$ n$M$)[34] has no such functional group, and retains the structural water at the active site.[33] The DMP323 and P9941 structures are illustrated in Figure 5, along with the backbone fold of the viral enzyme. The difference in binding constants between these two

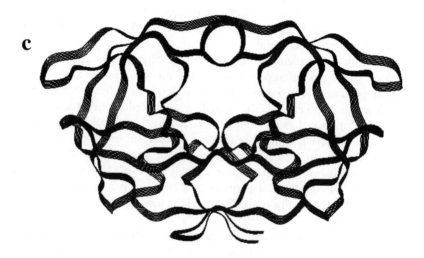

**FIGURE 5**

Structures of the inhibitors employed in dynamics studies: (a) DMP323 ($K_i$ = 0.3 n$M$); (b) P9941 ($K_i$ = 9 n$M$); (c) a ribbon diagram of the homodimeric HIV-1 protease illustrating the backbone fold of the viral enzyme.

inhibitors has been partly rationalized by the relative entropic losses of the inhibitors upon binding, since the linear P9941 has significantly greater conformational freedom in solution than the cyclic DMP323 compound. However, little is known about the entropic contribution of the protein to binding energy, particularly from the protein backbone.

B   CHARACTERIZATION OF BACKBONE FLEXIBILITY IN PROTEASE/
INHIBITOR COMPLEXES

### 1   Symmetry of the Dimer When Bound to Symmetric Inhibitors

A salient question that has arisen from the numerous X-ray crystal structures is the symmetry of the dimer, since structures of the protease bound to symmetric inhibitors have revealed various asymmetric hydrogen bonding networks involved in dimer stabilization.[23] Each complex that we have studied in the solution state is composed of two identical monomers (residues 1–99 and 1'–99') and a symmetric inhibitor. If a complex is asymmetric, resonances arising from a given residue involved in an asymmetric interaction will be different in each of the two monomers, reflecting the different electronic environments. If a complex is fully symmetric, resonances arising from a given residue will be identical in each of the two monomers, reflecting the identical electronic environments. Hence, if viewed from a static perspective, the sequence-specific assignment of the backbone should reveal asymmetries, if they exist. Assignments of protease backbone $^{15}$N and $^1$H resonances have been made for both the DMP323[35] and P9941[33] complexes. The $^{15}$N–$^1$H HSQC spectrum for $^{15}$N-labeled protease bound to DMP323 is shown in Figure 6. The solution state of each complex gives rise to a single set of backbone $^1$H–$^{15}$N cross peaks, indicating a fully symmetric dimer conformation. However, as will be described herein, this is the result of a *dynamic symmetry*, and we find evidence for a conformational exchange between asymmetric hydrogen bonded states at the tips of the flaps. As described below, it is only through dynamics measurements, specifically the measurement of transverse relaxation times $T_2$ that are inherently sensitive to slow chemical exchange processes, that this asymmetry is revealed.

### 2   Comparison of Chemical Environments

A qualitative picture of inhibitor-sensitive regions of the HIV-1 protease is provided by a comparison of chemical shift frequencies for the two complexes. As discussed in Chapter 3, the chemical shift frequency (or chemical shielding) is dependent upon the electronic environment of the nucleus; hence, a change in chemical shift frequency for a given nucleus indicates that the distribution of electrons surrounding the nucleus is influenced differently by the two inhibitors. Quantitative interpretation of chemical shift differences in terms of structure, particularly for $^{15}$N nuclei, is not currently feasible although progress toward this end has recently been reported.[36] Differences in $^{15}$N frequencies between the two complexes for each site are plotted in Figure 7a, and for $^1$H$_N$ frequencies in Figure 7b. Differences in both the $^{15}$N and $^1$H$_N$ chemical shift frequencies

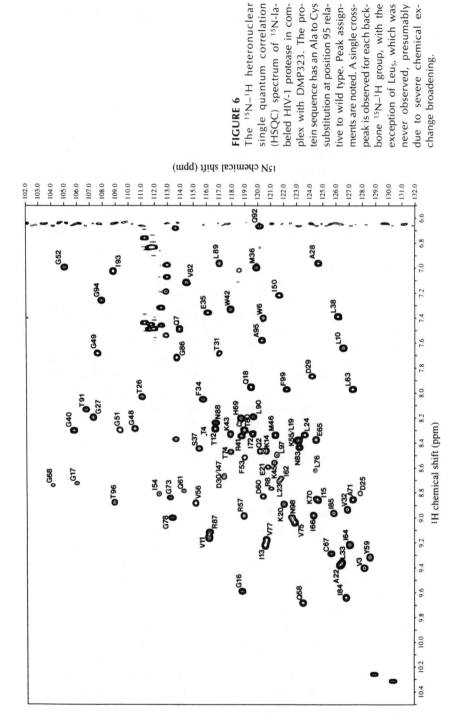

**FIGURE 6**

The $^{15}N-^{1}H$ heteronuclear single quantum correlation (HSQC) spectrum of $^{15}N$-labeled HIV-1 protease in complex with DMP323. The protein sequence has an Ala to Cys substitution at position 95 relative to wild type. Peak assignments are noted. A single cross-peak is observed for each backbone $^{15}N-^{1}H$ group, with the exception of Leu$_5$, which was never observed, presumably due to severe chemical exchange broadening.

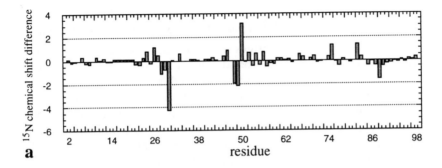

a

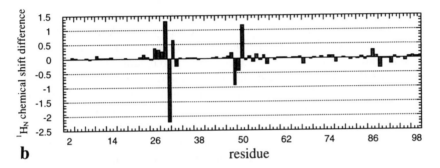

b

**FIGURE 7**

Chemical shift δ differences for backbone $^{15}N-^{1}H$ groups between the two complexes. (a) Backbone $^{15}N$ chemical shift difference for each residue, $\delta^{N}_{P9941}-\delta^{N}_{DMP323}$; (b) backbone $^{1}H_{N}$ chemical shift difference for each residue, $\delta^{H}_{P9941}-\delta^{H}_{DMP323}$.

correlate quite well, and the similar responses in residues 46–57 is striking. The alternating pattern observed in both the $^{15}N$ and $^{1}H$ chemical shift differences for residues 50–57 corresponds to a stretch of β-sheet that forms one edge of the flap. The alternation in peptide plane orientation in a β-sheet structure might contribute to such an alternating pattern in chemical shift frequency change upon a nonuniform change in chemical environment. It is interesting to note that the active site loop (residues 25–30) and the flap region (residues 45–60) exhibit substantial changes, as well as residues 75 and 82 and sites in the helix (residues 87–89), particularly $Asn_{88}$. Residues $Arg_{87}$ and $Asn_{88}$, at the beginning of the helix, are required for proteolytic activity,[26] and both of these residues participate in a hydrogen-bonding network involving the active site loop, the helix, and the N-terminal loop ($Trp_6$–$Arg_8$) of the opposing monomer.[37] As described below, this region of the protease backbone exhibits interesting motional characteristics as well. It has been shown that $Asn_{88}$ is essential for dimer formation, presumably because of its role in stabilizing this hydrogen-bonding network.[27] Thus, although qualitative in nature, differences in chemical shifts between the two complexes correlate strongly with sites that play crucial roles in the stability and function of the enzyme.

### 3 Comparison of Backbone Motions in the Two Complexes

It is possible to gain insight into the role of dynamics in protease specificity by comparing the backbone motions in the protease when bound to each of the two inhibitors, which differ substantially in binding affinity. It has been postulated that the 30-fold difference in $K_i$ between DMP323 and P9941 is largely due to the difference in the entropic price paid by each inhibitor upon binding.[2] The DMP323 inhibitor is a rigid cyclic urea ring that preorganizes its constituents into a conformation that favors binding to the protease, while the linear P9941 inhibitor has much greater conformational freedom in solution. Hence, P9941 undergoes a much greater loss in configurational entropy upon binding to the protease than does DMP323. These arguments are based upon knowledge of the structure and conformational freedom of the inhibitors in the free and bound states. What can we learn about the complementary flexibility of the protease? Does backbone flexibility play a role in determining the change in free energy upon inhibitor binding that translates into a contribution to $K_i$? At present, it is not possible to study the free protease in solution due to autolysis. However, given that the entropy of the free protease is identical in the two systems studied (i.e., is independent of inhibitor), we can compare the flexibility of the protease backbone when bound to each inhibitor to reveal differences in the change in backbone entropy upon binding each inhibitor due to NH bond motions in the nano- to picosecond time frame.

Relaxation parameters ($^{15}N$ $T_1$, $T_2$, and the heteronuclear NOE) were measured for individual $^{15}N$ nuclei in the protease backbone of both complexes using inverse-detected heteronuclear NMR experiments, as described in detail elsewhere.[19] These values are plotted in Figure 8 and are listed in Table 1. The Lipari and Szabo formalism,[14,15] Equation (1) was applied to analyze the measured relaxation parameters to yield the overall correlation time $\tau_m$ as well as the residue-specific parameters of motion for each complex $S^2$ and $\tau_e$.[19] When necessary, the extended form of the spectral density function, Equation (2), was employed, or the influence of chemical exchange was included by the addition of $R_{ex}$ to the right-hand side of Equation (4) to obtain a satisfactory fit to the data.[19] Sites requiring application of these extended models are noted in Table 1. The rate of global tumbling in solution is essentially the same for the two complexes, 9.2 ns (DMP323) and 9.3 ns (P9941), reflecting the compact shape of the protein and the comparable size of the inhibitors. These correlation times are in agreement with what is expected from overall correlation times reported for proteins having a variety of molecular weights.[12,38-40] The order parameter $S^2$ for each residue in each complex is also listed in Table 1. The average order parameter across the backbone is nearly identical for the two complexes ($<S^2>$ = 0.85, DMP323; $<S^2>$ = 0.87, P9941). In general, sites within well-defined regions of secondary structure have small-amplitude, fast internal

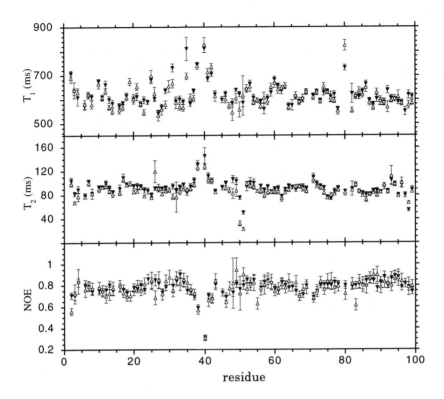

**FIGURE 8**

Experimental $^{15}$N relaxation parameters. (a) $T_1$, (b) $T_2$, and (c) NOE measured for backbone sites in the HIV-1 protease in complex with inhibitors DMP323 (▼) and P9941 (Δ). The $T_1$ and $T_2$ values were measured at 500 MHz, and the NOE values at 600 MHz. (From Nicholson, L. K., et al., *Nature Struct. Biol.,* 1995, 2, 274–280. With permission.)

motions, which occur on a typical time scale of approximately 50 ps. However, for such small-amplitude motions in the fast exchange limit, the correlation time for internal motion is not well defined.

The largest difference in backbone motion between the two complexes occurs at Gly$_{48}$. For linear inhibitors that are close analogs of P9941, X-ray crystal structures have shown that the Gly$_{48}$ NH group is hydrogen bonded to a carbonyl group in the inhibitor P3 subsite.[24] The cyclic DMP323 inhibitor does not contain a P3 site,[2] and the Gly$_{48}$ NH group does not form a hydrogen bond in the crystal structure of the protease/ DMP323 complex. The absence of a Gly$_{48}$ hydrogen bond acceptor in the DMP323 inhibitor is consistent with the significantly larger amplitude of motion (small $S^2$ value) observed for the Gly$_{48}$ site in DMP323 complex.

There are additional backbone NH groups that are potential hydrogen bond donors within the active site of the protease. These include Ile$_{50}$, Asp$_{29}$, and Asp$_{30}$. As mentioned previously, the largest $^{15}$N and $^1$H$_N$

## TABLE 1

Backbone [15]N Relaxation Parameters and Order Parameters for the HIV-1 Protease in Complex with DMP323 ($\tau_m$ = 9.2 ns) and P9941 ($\tau_m$ = 9.3 ns)

| | DMP323 | | | | P9941 | | | |
|---|---|---|---|---|---|---|---|---|
| aa | $T_1$(ms) [±13] | $T_2$(ms) [±4] | NOE [±0.04] | $S^2$ [±0.03] | $T_1$(ms) [±17] | $T_2$(ms) [±4] | NOE [±0.06] | $S^2$ [±0.03] |
| P1 | | | | | | | | |
| Q2 | 710 | 105 | 0.708 | 0.74 | 689 | 99 | 0.562 | 0.76 |
| V3 | 634 | 83 | 0.707 | ™0.82 | 640 | 68 | 0.725 | ™0.82 |
| T4 | 609 | 90 | 0.831 | 0.88 | 631 | 78 | 0.843 | 0.88 |
| L5 | | | | | | | | |
| W6 | 574 | 80 | 0.801 | 0.94 | 581 | 78 | 0.763 | 0.96 |
| Q7 | 617 | 103 | 0.797 | 0.84 | 622 | 101 | 0.798 | 0.84 |
| R8 | 612 | 83 | 0.746 | ™0.88 | 580 | 83 | 0.777 | 0.92 |
| P9 | | | | | | | | |
| L10 | 676 | 94 | 0.754 | 0.79 | 664 | 91 | 0.786 | 0.82 |
| V11 | 611 | 94 | 0.744 | 0.85 | 609 | 94 | 0.752 | 0.85 |
| T12 | 663 | 101 | 0.761 | 0.79 | 635 | 95 | 0.702 | 0.83 |
| I13 | 601 | 93 | 0.808 | 0.88 | 568 | 88 | 0.728 | 0.92 |
| K14 | 584 | 86 | 0.755 | 0.91 | 552 | 82 | 0.776 | 0.96 |
| I15 | | | | | | | | |
| G16 | 575 | 91 | 0.788 | 0.92 | 557 | 84 | 0.798 | 0.95 |
| G17 | 587 | 110 | 0.767 | †0.67 | 569 | 108 | 0.732 | †0.67 |
| Q18 | 617 | 98 | 0.736 | 0.84 | 610 | 98 | 0.699 | 0.84 |
| L19 | | | | | 675 | 100 | 0.706 | 0.78 |
| K20 | 602 | 96 | 0.783 | 0.87 | 603 | 86 | 0.765 | 0.90 |
| E21 | 613 | 96 | 0.772 | 0.85 | 654 | 87 | 0.803 | 0.84 |
| A22 | 582 | 95 | 0.809 | 0.90 | 583 | 92 | 0.759 | 0.89 |
| L23 | 599 | 89 | 0.767 | 0.88 | 547 | 79 | 0.816 | 0.99 |
| L24 | 590 | 88 | 0.864 | 0.91 | | | | |
| D25 | 682 | 81 | 0.827 | ™0.78 | 699 | 76 | 0.848 | ™0.77 |
| T26 | 606 | 92 | 0.854 | 0.88 | 625 | 120 | 0.689 | 0.83 |
| G27 | 543 | 91 | 0.824 | 0.95 | 535 | 92 | 0.854 | 0.97 |
| A28 | 571 | 92 | 0.739 | 0.91 | 560 | 83 | 0.721 | 0.94 |
| D29 | 637 | 93 | 0.791 | 0.83 | 580 | 87 | 0.844 | 0.92 |
| D30 | | | | | 656 | 89 | 0.879 | 0.85 |
| T31 | 732 | 95 | 0.800 | ™0.73 | 667 | 78 | 0.756 | ™0.80 |
| V32 | 592 | 88 | 0.842 | 0.90 | 587 | 77 | 0.872 | 0.93 |
| L33 | 601 | 94 | 0.907 | 0.89 | 569 | 87 | 0.817 | 0.94 |
| E34 | 590 | 98 | 0.827 | 0.88 | 566 | 90 | 0.856 | 0.91 |
| E35 | 811 | 85 | 0.755 | ™0.65 | 697 | 90 | 0.828 | ™0.77 |
| M36 | 583 | 95 | 0.741 | 0.89 | 608 | 91 | 0.765 | 0.87 |
| S37 | 636 | 105 | 0.700 | 0.81 | 604 | 98 | 0.727 | 0.86 |
| L38 | 746 | 132 | 0.592 | †0.58 | 740 | 126 | 0.569 | †0.60 |
| P39 | | | | | | | | |
| G40 | 812 | 146 | 0.310 | 0.59 | 827 | 128 | 0.313 | 0.59 |
| R41 | 686 | 112 | 0.705 | 0.75 | 713 | 105 | 0.664 | 0.73 |
| W42 | 706 | 104 | 0.673 | 0.74 | 736 | 105 | 0.679 | 0.72 |
| K43 | 622 | 87 | 0.810 | 0.87 | 614 | 85 | 0.843 | 0.91 |
| P44 | | | | | | | | |
| K45 | 600 | 93 | 0.734 | 0.87 | | | | |

**TABLE 1 (continued)**

Backbone $^{15}N$ Relaxation Parameters and Order Parameters for the HIV-1 Protease in Complex with DMP323 ($\tau_m$ = 9.2 ns) and P9941 ($\tau_m$ = 9.3 ns)

| | DMP323 | | | | P9941 | | | |
|---|---|---|---|---|---|---|---|---|
| aa | $T_1$(ms) [±13] | $T_2$(ms) [±4] | NOE [±0.04] | $S^2$ [±0.03] | $T_1$(ms) [±17] | $T_2$(ms) [±4] | NOE [±0.06] | $S^2$ [±0.03] |
| M46 | 623 | 100 | 0.695 | 0.83 | 600 | 92 | 0.646 | 0.86 |
| I47 | | | | | 574 | 88 | 0.772 | 0.92 |
| G48 | 585 | 107 | 0.734 | †0.70 | 546 | 83 | 0.821 | 0.97 |
| G49 | 640 | 104 | 0.814 | 0.83 | 604 | 88 | 0.947 | 0.89 |
| I50 | 622 | 76 | 0.767 | ™0.85 | 558 | 32 | 0.726 | ™0.95 |
| G51 | 587 | 51 | 0.800 | ™0.93 | 616 | 23 | 0.905 | ™0.87 |
| G52 | 639 | 95 | 0.857 | 0.84 | 646 | 99 | 0.769 | 0.81 |
| F53 | 664 | 101 | 0.815 | 0.80 | 653 | 95 | 0.811 | 0.82 |
| I54 | 607 | 101 | 0.852 | 0.87 | 587 | 94 | 0.826 | 0.90 |
| K55 | | | | | 596 | 87 | 0.630 | 0.88 |
| V56 | 592 | 95 | 0.780 | 0.88 | 572 | 87 | 0.774 | 0.93 |
| R57 | 561 | 89 | 0.833 | 0.92 | 606 | 80 | 0.808 | 0.92 |
| Q58 | 605 | 94 | 0.846 | 0.88 | 592 | 85 | 0.844 | 0.92 |
| Y59 | 628 | 87 | 0.819 | 0.87 | 652 | 86 | 0.830 | 0.85 |
| D60 | 684 | 91 | 0.771 | ™0.77 | 667 | 86 | 0.746 | ™0.80 |
| Q61 | 659 | 92 | 0.749 | 0.81 | 640 | 86 | 0.772 | 0.85 |
| I62 | 635 | 78 | 0.833 | ™0.84 | 647 | 75 | 0.811 | ™0.83 |
| L63 | 651 | 90 | 0.804 | ™0.82 | 657 | 84 | 0.780 | ™0.81 |
| I64 | 574 | 95 | 0.780 | 0.90 | 566 | 89 | 0.845 | 0.94 |
| E65 | 575 | 93 | 0.786 | 0.88 | | | | |
| I66 | 609 | 89 | 0.746 | 0.87 | 616 | 95 | 0.825 | 0.85 |
| C67 | 590 | 94 | 0.688 | 0.87 | 592 | 95 | 0.699 | 0.86 |
| G68 | 598 | 93 | 0.715 | 0.87 | 606 | 92 | 0.766 | 0.88 |
| H69 | 631 | 91 | 0.798 | 0.85 | 632 | 87 | 0.784 | 0.85 |
| K70 | | | | | | | | |
| A71 | 614 | 111 | 0.691 | †0.68 | 611 | 105 | 0.684 | †0.72 |
| I72 | 628 | 100 | 0.746 | 0.83 | 631 | 94 | 0.747 | 0.84 |
| G73 | 594 | 95 | 0.802 | 0.89 | 593 | 93 | 0.839 | 0.90 |
| T74 | 628 | 92 | 0.806 | 0.85 | 655 | 84 | 0.763 | ™0.81 |
| V75 | 632 | 78 | 0.802 | ™0.84 | 632 | 76 | 0.839 | ™0.94 |
| L76 | 610 | 74 | 0.800 | ™0.87 | 605 | 80 | 0.839 | 0.92 |
| V77 | 621 | 87 | 0.829 | 0.87 | 595 | 82 | 0.782 | 0.92 |
| G78 | 561 | 92 | 0.812 | 0.94 | 551 | 89 | 0.791 | 0.94 |
| P79 | | | | | | | | |
| T80 | 733 | 86 | 0.802 | ™0.72 | 824 | 84 | 0.723 | ™0.64 |
| P81 | | | | | | | | |
| V82 | 624 | 91 | 0.787 | 0.85 | 554 | 88 | 0.818 | 0.94 |
| N83 | 609 | 96 | 0.798 | 0.86 | 616 | 98 | 0.615 | 0.83 |
| I84 | 610 | 85 | 0.812 | 0.89 | 634 | 87 | 0.833 | 0.87 |
| I85 | 633 | 84 | 0.802 | ™0.84 | 621 | 79 | 0.805 | ™0.86 |
| G86 | 663 | 81 | 0.845 | ™0.81 | 650 | 73 | 0.798 | ™0.82 |
| R87 | 596 | 81 | 0.853 | ™0.90 | 588 | 82 | 0.868 | 0.94 |
| N88 | 582 | 87 | 0.851 | 0.92 | 567 | 84 | 0.899 | 0.94 |
| L89 | 602 | 87 | 0.777 | 0.88 | 629 | 80 | 0.902 | 0.88 |
| L90 | 589 | 85 | 0.826 | 0.91 | 594 | 85 | 0.786 | 0.91 |

**TABLE 1 (continued)**

Backbone $^{15}N$ Relaxation Parameters and Order Parameters for the HIV-1 Protease in Complex with DMP323 ($\tau_m$ = 9.2 ns) and P9941 ($\tau_m$ = 9.3 ns)

| | DMP323 | | | | P9941 | | | |
|---|---|---|---|---|---|---|---|---|
| aa | $T_1$(ms) [±13] | $T_2$(ms) [±4] | NOE [±0.04] | $S^2$ [±0.03] | $T_1$(ms) [±17] | $T_2$(ms) [±4] | NOE [±0.06] | $S^2$ [±0.03] |
| T91 | 588 | 94 | 0.879 | 0.91 | 588 | 97 | 0.833 | 0.88 |
| Q92 | 638 | 86 | 0.798 | 0.85 | 568 | 86 | 0.821 | 0.93 |
| I93 | 605 | 105 | 0.870 | 0.88 | 596 | 112 | 0.801 | 0.90 |
| G94 | 599 | 98 | 0.890 | 0.89 | 603 | 99 | 0.876 | 0.87 |
| A95 | 590 | 81 | 0.878 | 0.90 | 611 | 78 | 0.868 | 0.90 |
| A96 | 585 | 97 | 0.787 | 0.89 | 585 | 101 | 0.841 | 0.91 |
| L97 | 550 | 80 | 0.817 | 0.97 | | | | |
| N98 | 619 | 55 | 0.787 | ™0.86 | 576 | 67 | 0.786 | ™0.93 |
| F99 | 611 | 89 | 0.744 | 0.86 | 585 | 86 | 0.796 | 0.91 |

*Note:* Standard errors for each parameter were determined via conjugate gradient minimization of the fit to the experimental data in combination with a Monte Carlo approach as described in detail elsewhere.[19] The average standard error in each parameter is noted in square brackets in each column heading.

†   Required extended model for motion on intermediate time scale.

™   Required inclusion of chemical exchange term.

chemical shift differences between the two complexes occur at $Asp_{30}$. Unfortunately, the $Asp_{30}$ resonance overlaps the $Ile_{47}$ peak for the DMP323 complex, and its volume could not be quantitatively analyzed for measurement of relaxation parameters. Hence, the motion of this site could not be compared for the two complexes. For the remaining two potential hydrogen bond donor NH groups ($Ile_{50}$ and $Asp_{29}$), similar $S^2$ values (>0.8) were observed in each complex, consistent with restricted, well-ordered structure (Table 1). Solution NMR experiments have demonstrated that the $Ile_{50}$ NH bond is hydrogen bonded to the structural water in the P9941 complex,[33] and the X-ray crystal structure of the DMP323 complex shows that $Ile_{50}$ is hydrogen bonded to the cyclic urea oxygen in DMP323. The $Asp_{29}$ NH group exhibited rapid hydrogen–deuterium amide proton exchange in both complexes, indicating that in both structures it is exposed to solvent. This site is an example of a case where, in the absence of a structural hydrogen bond, the NH group is still relatively restricted in space in the bound complex, and an inhibitor with a hydrogen bond acceptor positioned to interact with the $Asp_{29}$ NH group would gain a favorable enthalpic reduction in free energy without paying a high entropic price for restriction of the backbone. However, the net gain will also depend on the energy required for desolvation of this site as well as of the corresponding acceptor group on the inhibitor.

In general, the flexibility in the protease backbone is essentially the same for the two complexes with the exception of $Gly_{48}$. Excluding $Gly_{48}$, the difference between $S^2$ values for individual residues between the two complexes has an rms value of 0.042. This value, which expresses the average difference in backbone mobility between the two complexes, is in accord with the average standard errors in $S^2$ (0.031) for each complex. This illustrates that, although the DMP323 inhibitor has a $K_i$ that is 30-fold lower than that of P9941, the flexibility of the protease backbone is not significantly different in the two complexes with the exception of the $Gly_{48}$ NH bond vector, which is attributed to a loss of a hydrogen bond. It is interesting to note that the difference in entropy at $Gly_{48}$ between the two complexes, calculated by the method of Akke et al.,[41] is equivalent to approximately one hydrogen bond. Thus, the change in free energy of the protease backbone between the two complexes, due to loss of the $Gly_{48}$ hydrogen bond for the DMP323 complex, appears to be at least partly compensated for by an increase in entropy due to larger-amplitude motions of the $Gly_{48}$ NH bond vector on the nanosecond to picosecond time frame. In terms of rational drug design, this result illustrates that a consideration of which potential hydrogen bond donors and acceptors should be targeted might be aided by knowledge of the intrinsic flexibility of the individual donor and acceptor sites. In general, a drug design target possesses a set of potential hydrogen bond donors and acceptors for interaction with an inhibitor (the HIV-1 protease has 18 such potential interactions[23]). Typically, maximizing the fulfillment of potential hydrogen bond interactions does not result in the highest-affinity inhibitor, and it is found that inhibitors with very few hydrogen bond interactions with the protease are quite potent.[23] The priority of fulfilling a potential hydrogen bond could be weighted by the potential flexibility of the donor or acceptor on the protein, which raises the question: is the favorable enthalpic energy associated with forming a hydrogen bond going to be compensated for by an unfavorable entropic energy associated with spatially restricting the potential donor or acceptor?

The hydrogen–deuterium exchange rates were measured for the backbone amide protons in both complexes, and a comparison of peak intensities at comparable time points is shown in Figure 9. The exchange rates were measured at pD = 6.5 and 5.2 for the DMP323 and P9941 complexes, respectively. Hence, the time points at 5 and 64 min (DMP323 complex) and at 2 and 24 hr (P9941 complex) are compared. The patterns of protection from exchange can essentially be superimposed for the two complexes, although this is a qualitative comparison due to the difference in pD. Those residues found to undergo large-amplitude motions are not protected, with the exception of $Ala_{71}$ and $Thr_{80}$ in both complexes, and $Thr_{31}$ and $Glu_{35}$ in the DMP323 complex. Primary structure effects on

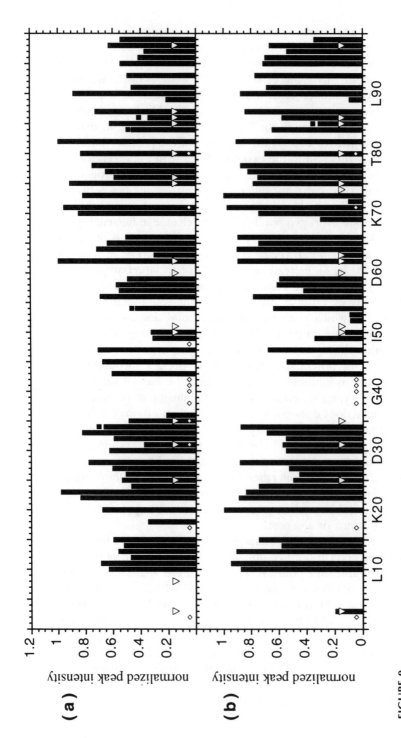

**FIGURE 9**

Comparison of hydrogen–deuterium exchange in the two protease/inhibitor complexes: (a) DMP323 (measured at pD = 6.5); (b) P9941 (measured at pD = 5.2). Bar heights represent peak intensities (normalized to the strongest peak in the spectrum) observed at comparable initial time points in each complex (5 min, DMP323; 2 h, P9941), and denote normalized peak intensities observed at comparable long time points (64 min, DMP323; 24 h, P9941). Residues undergoing large-amplitude, fast motions (◇) and those affected by chemical exchange (▽) are noted.

amide NH hydrogen exchange rates may play a role in the protection from exchange observed at these sites,[22] particularly for $Thr_{80}$, which is preceded by a Pro (see Table II in Reference 22). It is interesting to note that the residues that comprise the interleaved four-stranded β-sheet formed by the N- and C-termini of the two monomers follow the hydrogen bonding pattern expected from the X-ray crystal structures. The N-terminus contributes the outer edges of the sheet, and only the NH group of $Val_3$ participates in a hydrogen bond. The inner two strands are formed by the C-termini of each monomer, with the NH groups of $Ala_{96}$, $Leu_{97}$, $Asn_{98}$, and $Phe_{99}$ all participating in hydrogen bonds. Due to the difference in pD, the minor differences between complexes, such as when an initial time point is observed in one complex and not the other, should not be interpreted quantitatively. Hence, there are no major differences between the two complexes, which is in general agreement with the comparison of $S^2$ values. It should be noted that the $Gly_{48}$ cross peak was observed in the P9941 complex at 5-, 15, and 25 min, but had disappeared at 45 min. Hence, this NH group is relatively protected from exchange with $D_2O$ in the P9941 complex, in agreement with the presence of a hydrogen bond. No cross peak was observed for this NH group at the initial exchange time point for the DMP323 complex.

### 4  Characteristics of Backbone Flexibility in Both Complexes

It is possible to gain insight into the role of dynamics in protease function by considering the dynamic variations across the backbone that are common to both complexes, and by correlating these observations with structural information from X-ray crystal studies and with functional information from site-directed mutagenesis studies. There are several regions of the protease backbone in both complexes where small-amplitude, fast internal motions do not fit the relaxation data, revealing parts of the protein where other dynamic processes are taking place. These regions include loops and points of contact between monomers. Several residues undergo large-amplitude, fast internal motions, while some exhibit the effects of slow chemical exchange processes.

#### a  Residues Undergoing Large-Amplitude, Fast Internal Motions

While most residues in both complexes have relatively small-amplitude motions ($S^2 > 0.8$, Figure 10a), indicative of well-ordered secondary structure, 11 residues in the DMP323 complex (Figure 11a and Table 1) and eight residues in the P9941 complex (Table 1) have $S^2$ values in the range 0.5 to 0.76. If a simple model of motion such as wobble in a cone[14,15] is applied, this range of order parameters corresponds to NH bond vector amplitudes of ±24° to ±38°. As illustrated in Figure 11a, most residues undergoing large-amplitude internal motions are in loops of the

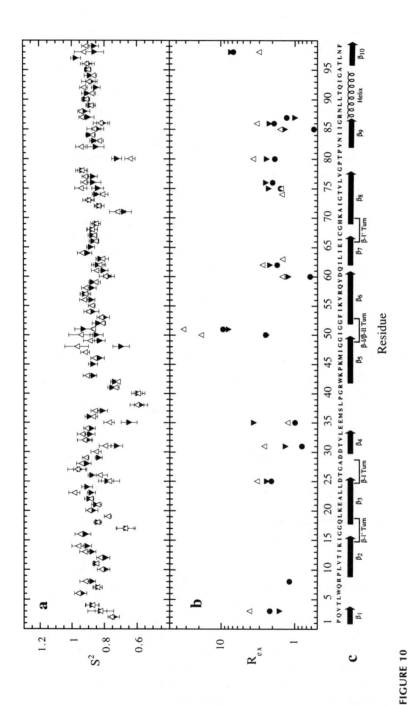

**FIGURE 10**

(a) Generalized order parameters $S^2$, (b) the chemical exchange contribution to $1/T_2$ ($R_{ex}$), and (c) the NMR-derived secondary structure for the HIV-1 protease, plotted as a function of residue number for the two complexes (▼) DMP323 using three relaxation parameters, $T_1$, $T_2$ at 500 MHz, and NOE at 600 MHz; (●) DMP323 using four relaxation parameters, $T_1$, $T_2$ at 500 MHz and $T_2$, NOE at 600 MHz; and (△) P9941 using three relaxation parameters, $T_1$, $T_2$ at 500 MHz, and NOE at 600 MHz. (From Nicholson, L. K., et al., *Nature Struct. Biol.*, 1995, 2, 274–280. With permission.)

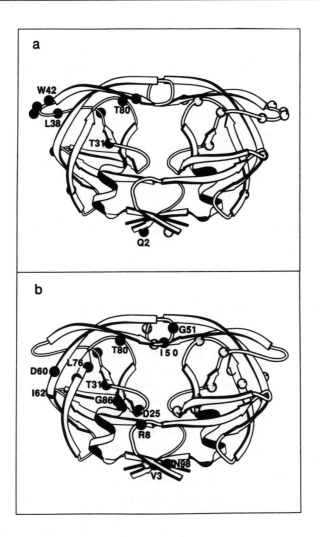

**FIGURE 11**

Protease amide sites in the DMP323 complex (a) undergoing rapid large-amplitude motions ($S^2 < 0.76$, three standard deviations less than the average value of $S^2$), and (b) affected by chemical exchange. Black and stippled spheres identify and distinguish equivalent sites in the two monomer units. The NH bonds of the residues depicted in (a) reorient internally on the time scale of approximately 1–100 ps. In the P9941 complex, all sites identified in (a), with the exception of residues 31, 35, and 48, have $S^2 < 0.76$. The amide sites depicted in (b) are affected by chemical exchange processes on the time scale of milli- to microseconds. These residues, and essentially the same residues in the P9941 complex, required the inclusion of an exchange term $R_{ex}$ to fit the relaxation data. Residues were mapped onto the crystal structure of the protease/DMP323 complex[2] using *Molscript*[44] software. (From Nicholson, L. K., et al., *Nature Struct. Biol.*, 1995, _2_, 274–280. With permission.)

protease backbone. The largest cluster of these flexible residues is formed by $Leu_{38}$, $Gly_{40}$, $Arg_{41}$, and $Trp_{42}$ ($Pro_{39}$ is not observed due to the lack of an amide proton). These residues are in a loop preceding one of the flap-forming β-strands, and comprise an "elbow" for the flap. These sites exhibit high $T_1$ and $T_2$ values and low NOE values in both complexes, consistent with large-amplitude internal motions. These residues also have elevated B-factor values in the X-ray crystal structure of the protease/DMP323 complex. In mammalian aspartic proteases, this region forms a well-structured helix. However, in both the solution and crystalline states of the HIV-1 protease, residues 36–42 form a broad, solvent-exposed loop, which would be expected to undergo large segmental motions. Protease activity is negatively affected by nonconservative amino acid substitutions at $Leu_{38}$ and $Gly_{40}$, indicating that specific characteristics of this loop are indeed important for function or folding.[25] Crystallographic studies have indicated that flexibility of the flaps is required to allow access of substrates and inhibitors to the active site of the protease.[24] It is possible that flexibility of this elbow is necessary for the flaps in the apoenzyme to open sufficiently to accommodate entrance of the substrate and to facilitate product release from the bound complex. In light of drug design, this loop region could be a potential target; it is not difficult to imagine a small bridging compound that, with the proper specificity, could interact with the loop region in such a way that its flexibility was hindered, possibly impairing substrate binding and product release.

The remaining residues that undergo large-amplitude motions, $Gln_2$, $Gly_{17}$, and $Thr_{31}$ (DMP323 only), $Glu_{35}$ (DMP323 only), $Ala_{71}$ and $Thr_{80}$, are distributed across the backbone and represent isolated sites of high mobility. The $Gln_2$ NH group resides in the first peptide plane of the protease (preceded by the amide $NH_2^+$ of $Pro_1$), which is on the outside edge of the interleaved four-stranded β-sheet. In X-ray crystal structures, the carbonyl group in this peptide plane is hydrogen bonded to the NH group of $Phe_{99}$, while the $Gln_2$ NH group is solvent exposed. Hence, the rapid amide proton exchange rate is expected, and the large-amplitude of motion most likely reflects the "looseness" of the first peptide plane of the protease. Similarly, the rapid amide proton exchange rate and the large-amplitude motion of the $Gly_{17}$ NH group is not surprising, since it is in the β–I' turn separating the $\beta_2$ and $\beta_3$ strands (Figure 10c), and is solvent exposed (Figure 9). In X-ray crystal structures, the $Thr_{31}$ NH group participates in a hydrogen bond with the side-chain oxygen of $Asn_{88}$[37]; in solution we observe a slow proton–deuterium exchange rate, which concurs with the crystallograhic results, but also an apparent large-amplitude of motion in the DMP323 complex. This may possibly be explained by correlated large-amplitude motions of the $Asn_{88}$ side chain and the $Thr_{31}$ NH group, which allows the hydrogen bond between these groups to be maintained. The $Glu_{35}$ NH group, which is located just upstream of the flexible loop discussed above (residues 38–42) also displays large-amplitude motions in the DMP323 complex in spite of a significant level of protection from amide exchange, implying correlated motions of hydrogen bond partners. A similar case is found for the $Ala_{71}$ NH group, located in the $\beta_4$-strand, which undergoes large-amplitude motions in both complexes, yet exhibits very slow hydrogen–deuterium exchange rates. $Thr_{80}$ is sandwiched between two proline residues, the dynamics of which can not be evaluated with the $^1H$–$^{15}N$-filtered experiments employed for these studies due to the lack of an amide proton. The $Pro_{79}$–$Thr_{80}$–$Pro_{81}$ triad forms a partially solvent-exposed loop that is also involved in inhibitor binding; the slow amide proton exchange rate observed at this site in both complexes indicates that the $Thr_{80}$ NH group is possibly involved in a stable hydrogen bond in spite of its apparently large orientational excursions. It is possible that for the residues exhibiting both large-amplitude motions and significant protection from amide NH hydrogen exchange, local structural features may be responsible for the observed effects. Deviations in NH bond length and/or in the magnitude of chemical shielding anisotropy from the values assumed in the analysis (1.02 Å and 160 ppm for all sites, respectively) could significantly influence the measured relaxation parameters in a way that is not accounted for in the fitting, leading to an artificially large-amplitude for the best fit of the data. Alternatively, as previously mentioned, the primary sequence effects on the amide NH proton exchange rate may lead to a significant protection of this site from exchange, independent of formation of a stable hydrogen bond. In summary, although residues in loops, in turns, and at the N-terminus of the protease exhibit predictable large-amplitude motions that are accompanied by rapid amide proton–deuterium exchange, four residues scattered across the backbone display somewhat anomolous behavior in that large-amplitude motions apparently take place in spite of protection of these NH groups from amide NH hydrogen exchange with the solvent. These results could indicate the presence of coordinated motions of hydrogen bond partners, or could possibly be explained by deviations from the typical local structural features assumed in the analysis.

### b    Residues Affected by Chemical Exchange

Our analysis of the measured relaxation parameters revealed that 15 residues in the protease/DMP323 complex are affected by chemical exchange on the milli- to microsecond time scale, and virtually the same residues are affected in the protease/P9941 complex (Figure 10b). Many of these residues either are involved in intermonomer contacts (residues $Val_3$, $Gly_{51}$, $Ala_{96}$, and $Asn_{98}$) or interact with the inhibitor (residues $Asp_{25}$, and $Ile_{50}$). Sequential correlations are immediately apparent in Figure 10b (residues 50–51, 60–63, 74–76, and 85–87); when viewed in light of the three-dimensional structure, spatial groupings of these residues emerge

(Figure 11b). One cluster extends across the $\beta$-sheet core (residues $Asp_{60}$, $Ile_{62}$, $Leu_{63}$, $Thr_{74}$, $Val_{75}$, and $Leu_{76}$); another cluster is formed by residues in the beginning of the helix (residues $Ile_{85}$, $Gly_{86}$, and $Arg_{87}$), near the active site loop ($Thr_{31}$), and in a loop near the N-terminus ($Arg_8$); and a third cluster involves residues in the four-stranded $\beta$-sheet formed by the N- and C-termini of the protease ($Val_3$ and $Asn_{98}$). It is interesting to note that three of the four residues displaying anomolous behaviour, as discussed in the previous section (large-amplitude motion accompanied by slow proton–deuterium exchange), also require the inclusion of a chemical exchange term in order to satisfactorily fit the data (residues $Thr_{31}$, $Glu_{35}$, and $Thr_{80}$). While it is possible to correlate some of these residues to conformational dynamic equilibria, as discussed below, the nature of the chemical exchange processes affecting some of the sites is unclear. However, observance of the effects of chemical exchange at a given site indicates that a slow dynamic process is occurring in the vicinity of this site, involving movement of the site itself or of neighboring groups.

The chemical exchange observed at $Asp_{25}$ appears to be associated with fluctuations in an intermolecular hydrogen bond network between the protease and inhibitor. Based on both NMR and X-ray data, it was previously proposed that the catalytic $Asp_{25}/Asp_{25'}$ side chains can form two possible hydrogen bond networks with the diol groups of the DMP323 inhibitor, and that the two networks are in dynamic equilibrium.[42] Transitions between these two possible networks may be responsible for the observation of exchange broadening for the NH group of $Asp_{25}$ and could also contribute to the exchange broadening observed for neighboring residues $Arg_8$, $Ile_{85}$, $Gly_{86}$, and $Arg_{87}$.

Residues at the tips of the flaps, $Ile_{50}$ and $Gly_{51}$, are strongly affected by chemical exchange. In nearly all protease crystal structures, asymmetric $\beta I/\beta II$ turn conformations are observed, with a single hydrogen bond formed between the same peptide plane on each monomer (the peptide plane containing the $Gly_{51}$ NH group and the Ile50 carbonyl group). Hence, formation of this hydrogen bond imparts asymmetry to the dimer, with the $Gly_{51}$ NH group of one monomer interacting with the $Ile_{50'}$ carbonyl group of the opposing monomer, and the remaining $Ile_{50}$ carbonyl and $Gly_{51'}$ NH not hydrogen bonded. This asymmetric hydrogen bond places the $Gly_{51}$ NH groups on each monomer in very different chemical environments that would be expected to have different $^1H$ and $^{15}N$ chemical shifts. However, we observe a single cross peak for this residue that is severely exchange broadened, indicating that the NH group is in dynamic equilibrium between different chemical environments. Analysis of the three-dimensional $^{15}N$-separated NOESY spectrum of the protease/DMP323 complex shows that, in solution, the conformation at the tips of the flaps is a mixture of $\beta I$ and $\beta II$ turns. Hence, the structural data from both X-ray crystallographic and solution NMR studies, taken together with the dynamics results, suggests a dynamic equilibrium in which the single peptide plane at the tip of the flap of each monomer undergoes conformational exchange between asymmetric hydrogen bonded orientations. However, since the X-ray crystal structure of the protease/DMP323 complex shows a symmetric $\beta II/\beta II$ conformation at the tips of the flaps, which does not allow formation of the hydrogen bond, we cannot rule out the occurrence of this conformation in solution as well. Hence, the dynamic model depicted in Figure 12 is proposed, in which the three flap conformations (two asymmetric hydrogen bonded and one symmetric nonhydrogen bonded) undergo exchange.

It should be noted that the conformational exchange depicted in Figure 12 is highly localized, and involves a flip of the $Ile_{50}/Gly_{51}$ peptide plane by approximately 180°. This results in a large reorientation of the $Gly_{51}$ NH group, which resides in this plane, and explains the large value of $R_{ex}$ that is observed for this site. However, the orientation of the $Ile_{50}$ NH group, which resides in the preceding peptide plane, is not affected by the proposed conformational exchange. This is consistent with both NMR and X-ray data, which show that the $I_{50}$ NH group participates in a hydrogen bond to an internal water molecule in the P9941 complex[33] and to the cyclic urea oxygen in the DMP323 complex.[2] Hydrogen–deuterium exchange experiments[19] show protection factors[22] of at least 100-fold for the $Ile_{50}$ NH group in both complexes, confirming the hydrogen bonding of this site in solution. Hence, we conclude that the observed chemical exchange for the $Ile_{50}$ NH site is not due to its own flexibility, but rather to the fluctuations in its electronic environment caused by motions of neighboring atoms of the $Ile_{50}/Gly_{51}$ peptide plane that participate in the conformational exchange at the tips of the flaps.

Residues $Ile_{50}$ and $Gly_{51}$ are highly conserved in retroviral protease primary sequences, and nonconservative substitutions of these residues strongly diminish protease activity,[26] indicating that the structure and dynamics at the tips of the flaps are related to function. We suggest that the conformational exchange at the tips of the flaps generates a low-energy dynamic symmetry that stabilizes the structure of the protease/substrate complex, yet has the flexibility to facilitate product release following catalysis.

Additional residues at the dimer interface that participate directly in intermonomer interactions and that are affected by chemical exchange include $Val_3$ and $Asn_{98}$. All available crystal structures show that the NH groups of $Val_3$ and $Asn_{98}$ are hydrogen bonded within the highly ordered $\beta$-sheet that interlocks the N- and C-termini of the two monomers. All NMR data, including [15]N- and [13]C-separated NOESY spectra and hydrogen–deuterium exchange data, confirm that these structural features are also present in solution. Hence, it is very unlikely that the backbone NH groups of $Val_3$ and $Asn_{98}$ are flexible. Crystal structures also show an asymmetric hydrogen bond network involving the side chains of $Gln_2$ and $Asn_{98}$ of each monomer that spans across the solvent-exposed face of the

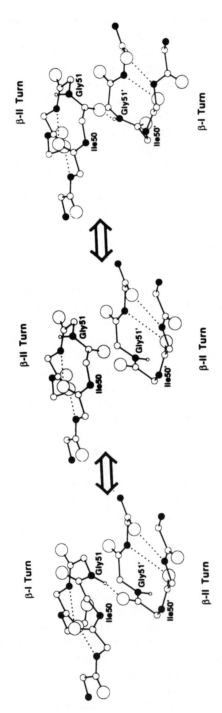

**FIGURE 12**

Proposed model of internal motion at the tips of the protease flaps: a conformational switch involving residues $Ile_{(50,50')}$ and $Gly_{(51,51')}$. In order to form the hydrogen bond between the $Ile_{50}$ carbonyl and the $Gly_{51'}$ NH group observed in most crystal structures of protease/inhibitor complexes[23,24], the $Ile_{50}/Gly_{51}$ peptide plane in one monomer (containing the $Ile_{50}$ carbonyl and the $Gly_{51}$ NH group) must be oriented in opposite directions from the $Ile_{50'}/Gly_{51'}$ plane in the other monomer. Hence, only the asymmetric conformations will result in the formation of the $Ile_{50}/Gly_{51'}$ and $Ile_{50'}/Gly_{51}$ hydrogen bonds. Even though the hydrogen-bonded protease conformations are asymmetric, they are isoenergetic, and their rapid exchange results in a symmetric NMR spectrum reflecting the dynamic averaging of the homodimer bound to a symmetric inhibitor. The chemical exchange reduces the $T_2$ values of the $Ile_{50}$ and $Gly_{51}$ [15]N nuclei, necessitating the inclusion of a chemical exchange term in the data analysis. (From Nicholson, L. K., et al., *Nature Struct. Biol.*, 1995, 2, 274–280. With permission.)

interleaved β-sheet.[37] If this side-chain lattice were similarly structured in solution, it is likely that two resonances would be observed for individual nuclei in this region, reflecting the asymmetric chemical environments of the two monomers. A dynamic symmetry involving a 180° flip of each side chain in this hydrogen bond network would average these resonance frequencies and would be able to account for the exchange broadening observed for the nearby NH groups of $Val_3$ and $Asn_{98}$. However, we have seen no evidence for exchange broadening or for multiple conformations in the $^1H$, $^{13}C$, or $^{15}N$ signals of the $Gln_2$ or $Asn_{98}$ side chains. Hence, it is very unlikely that the solvent-exposed side chains of these residues are restricted in a hydrogen-bonded network. Therefore, the chemical exchange experienced by $Val_3$ and $Asn_{98}$ is ascribed to the backbone flexibility of nearby residues $Thr_4$ and $Leu_5$, which are in a solvent-exposed loop but do not exhibit large-amplitude, fast internal motions. This hypothesis is supported by the observations that (a) the backbone amide signal of $Thr_4$ is very weak due to a large proton line width, and (b) the backbone amide signal of $Leu_5$ has not been observed, presumably because it is severely exchange broadened.[35] It is noteworthy that the primary autolysis site in the HIV-1 protease is the $Leu_5$–$Trp_6$ peptide bond, and it has been suggested that the rate of cleavage of this bond may regulate the activity of the protease *in vivo*.[43] If this is the case, the conformational dynamics of these residues could significantly affect the viral life cycle.

The slow motion of the $Thr_4$–$Leu_5$ loop region may also account for the exchange broadening observed for residues $Ala_{85}$, $Gly_{86}$, $Arg_{87}$, $Thr_{31}$, and $Arg_8$. As mentioned above, these residues form a cluster involving regions near the beginning of the helix ($Ala_{85}$–$Arg_{87}$), at the end of the active site loop ($Thr_{31}$), and in the N-terminal loop ($Arg_8$). It is interesting to note that residues $Gly_{86}$, $Arg_{87}$, and $Asn_{88}$ form a highly conserved region that is present in all retroviral aspartic proteases, but is absent in the cellular counterparts. Conservative site-directed mutation of $Arg_{87}$ to Lys (maintaining the positive side-chain charge) and a major mutation of this residue to Glu (shortening the side chain and reversing its charge) both abolished proteolytic activity, illustrating the sensitivity of $Arg_{87}$ to even minor disruptions.[26] Similarly, site-directed mutagenesis of $Asn_{88}$ indicated that the domain surrounding this residue affects the potential of the protease to form stable and active dimers, and it was suggested that this domain might be a promising target for antiviral compounds.[27] This region is at the transition point between the β9 strand and N-terminal end of the helix, and participates in both inter- and intramonomer hydrogen bonds. In X-ray crystal structures, this region forms hydrogen bonds with residues in the active site loop (residues 29–31) and with residues in the loop near the N-terminus (residues 5–8).[37] The NH bonds of $Arg_{87}$, $Asn_{88}$, and $Thr_{31}$ are involved in this hydrogen bond network, and both $Arg_{87}$ and $Thr_{31}$ exhibit chemical exchange, as does $Arg_8$.

It is interesting that in both P9941 and DMP323 complexes, the hydrogen–deuterium exchange rate for the amide proton of $Asn_{88}$ is fast, indicating that the hydrogen bond between this NH group and the carbonyl group of $Asp_{29}$ observed in X-ray crystal structures[37] is not stable. However, the order parameter for this NH group indicates that motion of this bond vector is highly restricted. Similarly, the NH groups of residues $Thr_4$, $Trp_6$, $Gln_7$, and $Arg_8$ in the N-terminal loop and residue $Asp_{29}$ in the active site loop display rapid hydrogen–deuterium exchange rates, while remaining highly restricted in space on the pico- to nanosecond time frame. In contrast, the hydrogen–deuterium exchange rate for amide protons of residues $Ala_{95}$, $Gly_{86}$, $Arg_{87}$, and $Thr_{31}$ is slow, indicative of stable hydrogen bonding of these NH groups.

The apparent structural stability of the $Thr_4$–$Arg_8$ loop on the pico- to nanosecond time scale is quite interesting, considering that none of the NH groups appears to be involved in stable hydrogen bonds (all exhibit rapid hydrogen–deuterium exchange rates). The factors that stabilize this region in X-ray crystal structures include hydrogen bonds between the side-chain guanidinium group of $Arg_{87}$ and the backbone carbonyls of $Leu_5$ and $Arg_8$ from the opposing monomer.[37] The side chains of the $Thr_4$–$Arg_8$ loop also contribute to stabilization through hydrogen bonding (between the $Arg_8$ guanidinium group and a side-chain carbonyl group of $Asp_{29}$ on the opposing monomer[37]) and through hydrophobic interactions between the $Thr_4$, $Leu_5$, and $Trp_6$ side chains and their local environments. These stabilization forces restrict this loop to small-amplitude motions on the pico- to nanosecond time frame, but allow a slow conformational exchange in this region that appears to centrally involve the $Thr_4$ and $Leu_5$ residues.

Taken together, these data indicate that this crucial structural region formed by residues in and near the beginning of the helix, near the active site loop, and in the $Thr_4$–$Arg_8$ loop of the opposing monomer may present a potential target for inhibition of protease function, with NH groups in each of these three clustered subdomains available to solvent yet relatively restricted in space. A compound with a complementary constellation of hydrogen bond acceptors may succeed in disrupting the forces that stabilize this highly conserved structural domain, and the slow conformational fluctuation of the loop containing $Thr_4$ and $Leu_5$ could possibly provide a favorable situation for induced fit of the protease to an inhibitor designed to interact with this region.

# IV   CONCLUSIONS AND PERSPECTIVE

There have been two major obstacles to designing successful drugs that inhibit the HIV-1 protease *in vivo*. Since therapy based on HIV protease inhibition is likely to be long term, oral administration is a top priority in design of protease inhibitors. Although hundreds of compounds have been developed that are highly effective inhibitors of this enzyme *in vitro*, only a handful have progressed into full-scale clinical trials. The main stumbling block has been low bioavailability. *Bioavailability* refers to the concentration of drug in the blood following administration. Since the targeted protease-binding region is quite large and has a strong hydrophobic character, most protease inhibitors have been on the high end of the molecular weight distribution of all marketed oral and systemic drugs,[3] and they suffer relatively low aqueous solubility. Hence, these compounds typically have not been efficiently absorbed into the bloodstream when orally administered, and have tended to be rapidly cleared by the liver. For compounds that have been clinically tested, significant reductions in antiviral effectiveness have been observed over time, a consequence of the ability of HIV to rapidly mutate and, hence, to develop drug resistance.

Based on experience gained thus far, two points have emerged as being crucial for the design of successful anti-HIV protease agents. The frustrations of low bioavailability have led to the conclusion that "small is good," and that the probability of a compound reaching plasma concentrations high enough to be effective is much higher for compounds in the 200- to 500-Da molecular weight range.[3] Fortunately, relatively small (600-700 Da) inhibitors can be quite potent, even though they form relatively few hydrogen bonds with the protease.[3,23] Hence, it is essential that key interactions between protease and inhibitor be identified and targeted in order to minimize molecular weight. A second point concerns mutationally induced drug resistance. It is apparent that the problems encountered with the development of HIV drug resistance are not unique for RT inhibitors such as AZT, and that the mutational ability of HIV must also be addressed in HIV protease inhibition. By only targeting potential interactions that are required for enzyme function, such as hydrogen bonds to the active site Asps, the chance of mutationally induced drug resistance to an inhibitor will be minimized. Furthermore, it has been suggested that a combination of several antiviral drugs is likely to be the most effective therapeutic strategy, since the probability that HIV will develop resistance to all the drugs at once is greatly reduced. Therefore, the chances of blocking HIV over the long term through inhibition of the HIV protease will increase with the number of different angles of attack on this enzyme.

In the context of the work presented here, it has been found that flexibility of the HIV-1 protease backbone correlates strongly with highly conserved and mutationally sensitive regions, implying important functional roles of backbone flexibility. Three regions have been identified where, if motional characteristics were either disrupted or exploited, protease function might be significantly affected. Disruption of the large-amplitude, fast internal motions of the "elbow" of the flap (the loop formed by residues $Leu_{38}$–$Trp_{42}$) by a small bridging compound could possibly impair the ability of the protease to bind substrate and release products. The proposed conformational exchange at the tips of the flaps, involving a single peptide plane containing the $Ile_{50}$ carbonyl and the $Gly_{51}$ NH, implies that a crucial hydrogen bond stabilizing the flaps is transient. Hence, both the $Ile_{50}$ carbonyl and $Gly_{51}$ NH groups, along with every other NH and carbonyl group in the $Gly_{43}$–$Ile_{50}$, and $Gly_{43'}$–$Ile_{50'}$ stretches of solvent-exposed β-strands, would be vulnerable to competition from an inhibitor that might attack the protease from outside the active site. A compound with recognition sites on both flaps and centered at the flap tips might lock the flaps together upon binding, blocking access of substrate to and release of products from the active site. The slow motion observed for the $Thr_4$ and $Leu_5$ residues in the solvent-exposed $Thr_4$–$Arg_8$ loop brings attention to a structural domain involving regions from both monomers, that has previously been highlighted as a potentially promising drug target.[26,27,37] This domain is formed by residues near the beginning of the helix ($Ala_{85}$–$Arg_{87}$), near the end of the active site loop ($Asp_{29}$–$Thr_{31}$), and in the $Thr_4$–$Arg_8$ loop of the opposing monomer.[37] It is found that several NH groups in these three clustered subdomains are accessible to solvent yet remain relatively restricted in space, on the pico- to nanosecond time frame. Hence, a compound with a complementary arrangement of hydrogen bond acceptors may, through specific interactions with this region, disrupt the forces that stabilize the dimer and promote the formation of monomeric, inactive protease.

In addition, it is suggested that knowledge of the inherent flexibility of the potential hydrogen bond donors and acceptors in the targeted region of the protease could be useful in establishing criteria for deciding which hydrogen bonds an inhibitor should attempt to form with the protein target. Inhibitor binding is stabilized by a reduction in free energy of the system (composed of the enzyme, inhibitor, and solvent) upon formation of the enzyme/inhibitor complex. The total change in free energy of the system is determined by changes in entropy ($\Delta S$) and changes in enthalpy ($\Delta H$) of all system components. Currently, changes in the conformational freedom of the inhibitor ($\Delta S_I$), changes in entropic energy associated with the hydrophobic effect, and changes in entropic and enthalpic energies associated with desolvation of and pairwise interactions between polar, ionic, and hydrogen bond donor and acceptor groups on both enzyme and inhibitor are typically considered in the rational drug design process. It is suggested that changes in entropy of the backbone might be a useful criterion in deciding which potential hydrogen bond donors and acceptors on a protein that an inhibitor should target. The one major difference in backbone flexibility found between the two inhibitor complexes studied is the mobility of the $Gly_{48}$ NH group, and this difference is attributed to the formation of a hydrogen bond between this site and the inhibitor in one complex and not in the other. Due to the inherent flexibility of this site, the favorable enthalpic contribution to free energy due to hydrogen bond formation in one complex is at least partly compensated for in the non-hydrogen-bonded complex by favorable entropic contributions due to large-amplitude motion of this site. It is suggested that other potential hydrogen bond donors and acceptors that are inherently more rigid might offer greater reductions in free energy upon hydrogen bond formation, and the $Asp_{29}$ NH group is presented as an example.

It is hoped that the information presented herein may provide insight into possible new avenues of attack for the HIV-1 protease. We are in the beginning stages of understanding the importance of protein flexibility in enzyme function and ligand binding, and additional dynamics studies of systems in which structural and functional information is available will further our understanding of the fundamental relationships between structure, dynamics, and function.

# ACKNOWLEDGMENTS

The authors wish to thank Dennis Torchia of NIH/NIDR for his expert guidance in the performance of the studies presented here, and for many helpful discussions during preparation of this manuscript. This work was made possible through collaboration with DuPont Merck Pharmaceutical Company, which generously provided the DMP323 and P9941 inhibitors, the protein expression system and purification scheme, and the X-ray crystal coordinates of the protease/DMP323 complex. In particular, the authors wish to thank Peter Domaille, Patrick Lam, Prabhakar Jadhav, and Sharon Campbell Burk for their invaluable contributions toward making this collaborative project possible. The authors also wish to thank Stephen Stahl, Joshua Kaufman, and Paul Wingfield of the Protein Expression Lab at NIH for providing purified protease/inhibitor complexes, Stephan Grzesiek and Ad Bax of the Laboratory of Chemical Physics at NIH for measurement of the heteronuclear NOE values for both complexes and $T_2$ measurements at 600 MHz for the DMP323 complex, Toshimasa Yamazaki of NIDR/NIH for assistance in backbone resonance assignments, Frank Delaglio and Dan Garrett of the Laboratory of Chemical Physics at NIH for their invaluable software tools, and Rolf Tschudin of the Laboratory of Chemical Physics at NIH for expert technical support. This work was supported by the AIDS-targeted Anti-Viral Program of the Office of the Director of the National Institutes of Health.

# REFERENCES

1. Clare, M. *Perspect. Drug Discovery Design* 1993, 1, 49-68.
2. Lam, P. Y.-S.; Jadhav, P. K.; Eyermann, C. J.; Hodge, C. N.; Ru, Y.; Bacheler, L. T.; Meek, J. L.; Otto, M. J.; Rayner, M. M.; Wong, Y. N.; Chang, C.-H.; Weber, P. C.; Jackson, D. A.; Sharpe, T. R.; Erickson-Viitanen, S. *Science* 1993, 263, 380-384.
3. Kim, E. E.; Baker, C. T.; Dwyer, M. D.; Murcko, M. A., Rao, B. G., Tung, R. D.; Navia, M. A. *J. Am. Chem. Soc.* 1995, 117, 1181-1182.
4. Harte, W. E.; Swaminathan. S.; Mansuri, M. M.; Martin, J. C.; Rosenberg, I. E.;. Beveridge, D. L. *Proc. Natl. Acad. Sci.* 1990, 87, 8864-8868.
5. Venable, R. M.; Brooks, B. R.; Carson, F. W. *Proteins: Struct. Function, Genet.* 1993, 15, 374-384.
6. York, D. M.; Darden, T. A.; Pedersen, L. G.; Anderson, M. W. *Biochemistry* 1993, 32, 1443-1453.
7. Bax, A; Grzesiek, S., in *NMR of Proteins* Clore, G. M.; Gronenborn, A. M., Eds.; Macmillan Press: London, 1993; chap. 2.
8. Clore, G. M.; Gronenborn, A. M., in *NMR of Proteins* Clore, G. M.; Gronenborn, A. M., Eds.; Macmillan Press: London, 1993; chap. 1.
9. Kay, L. E.; Nicholson, L. K.; Delaglio, F.; Bax, A.; Torchia, D. A. *J. Magn. Reson.* 1992, 97, 359-375.
10. Kay, L. E.; Bull, T. E.; Nicholson, L. K.; Griesinger, C.; Schwalbe, H; Bax, A.; Torchia, D. A. *J. Magn. Reson.* 1992, 100, 538-558.
11. Grzesiek, S.; and Bax, A. *J. Am. Chem. Soc.* 1993, 115, 12593-12594.
12. Farrow, N. A.; Muhandiram, R.; Singer, A. U.; Pascal, S. M.; Kay, C. M.; Gish, G.; Shoelson, S. E.; Pawson, T.; Forman-Kay, J. D.; and Kay, L. E. *Biochemistry* 1994, 33, 5984-6003.
13. Yamazaki, T.; Muhandiram, R.; Kay, L. E. *J. Am. Chem. Soc.* 1994, 116, 8266-8278.
14. Lipari, G.; Szabo, A. *J. Am. Chem. Soc.* 1982, 104, 4546-4559.
15. Lipari, G.; Szabo, A. *J. Am. Chem. Soc.* 1982, 104, 4559-4570.
16. Clore, G. M.; Szabo, A.; Bax, A.; Kay, L. E.; Driscoll, P. C.; Gronenborn, A. *J. Am. Chem. Soc.* 1990, 112, 4989-4991.
17. Abragam, A. *The Principles of Nuclear Magnetism* Oxford University Press: Oxford, 1961.
18. Nicholson, L. K.; Kay, L. E.; and Torchia, D. A., in *NMR Spectroscopy and its Application to Biological Research* Sarkar, S., Ed.; Elsevier Science: New York, in press.
19. Nicholson, L. K.; Yamazaki, T.; Torchia, D. A.; Grzesiek, S.; Bax, A.; Stahl, S. J.; Kaufman, J. D.; Wingfield, P. T.; Lam, P. Y.-S.; Jadhav, P. K.; Hodge, C. N.; Domaille, P. J.; Chang, C.-H. *Nature Structural Biology* 1995, 2, 274–280.
20. Farrar, T. C.; Becker, E. D. *Pulse and Fourier Transform NMR* Academic Press: New York, 1971; pp. 1-115.
21. Szypersky, T; Luginbuhl, P.; Otting, G.; Guntert, P.; Wüthrich, K. *J. Biomol. NMR* 1993, 3, 151.
22. Bai, Y.; Milne, J. S.; Mayne, L.; Englander, S. W. *Proteins, Struct. Function Genet.* 1993, 17, 75.
23. Appelt, K. *Perspect. Drug Discovery Design* 1993, 1, 23-48.
24. Wlodawer, A.; Erickson, J. W. *Annu. Rev. Biochem.* 1993, 62, 543-585.
25. Loeb, D. D.; Swanstrom, R.; Everitt, L.; Manchester, M.; Stamper, S. E.; Hutchison, C. A., III, *Nature* 1989, 340, 397-400.

26. Louis, J. M.; Dale Smith, C. A.; Wondrak, E. M.; Mora, P. T.; Oroszlan, S. *Biochem. Biophy. Res. Commun.* 1989, 164, 30-38.
27. Guenet, C.; Leppik, R. A.; Pelton, J. T.; Moelling, K.; Lovenberg, W.; Harris, B. A. *Eur. J. Pharmacol. Mol. Pharmacol. Sect.* 1989, 172, 443-451.
28. Cheng, Y.-S. E.; Yin, F. H.; Foundling, S.; Blomstrom, D.; Kettner, C. A. *Proc. Natl. Acad. Sci. USA* 1990, 87, 9660-9664.
29. Le Grice, S. F. J.; Mills, J.; Mous, J. *EMBO J.* 1988, 7, 2547-2553.
30. Sardana, V. V.; Schlabach, A. J.; Graham, P.; Bush, B. L.; Condra, J. H.; Culberson, J. C.; Gotlib, L.; Graham, D. J.; Kohl, N. E.; La Femina, R. L.; Schneider, C. L.; Wolanski, B. S.; Wolfgang, J. A.; Emina, E. A. *Biochemistry* 1994, 33, 2004-2010.
31. Seelmeier, S.; Schmidt, H.; Turk, V.; van der Helm, K. *Proc. Natl. Acad. Sci. USA* 1988, 85, 6612-6616.
32. Kohl, N. E.; Emini, E. A.; Schleif, W. A.; Davis, L. J.; Heimbach, J. C.; Dickson, R. A. F.; Scolnik, E. M.; Sigal, I. S. *Proc. Natl. Acad. Sci. USA* 1988, 85, 4686-4690.
33. Grzesiek, S.; Bax, A.; Nicholson, L. K.; Yamazaki, T.; Wingfield, P. T.; Stahl, S. J.; Eyermann, C. J.; Torchia, D. A.; Hodge, C. N.; Lam, P. Y. S.; Jadhav, P. K.; Chang, C.-H. *J. Am. Chem. Soc.* 1994, 116, 1581-1582.
34. Jadhav, P. K.; Woemer, F. J. *Bioorg. Med. Chem. Lett.* 1992, 2, 353.
35. Yamakaki, T.; Nicholson, L. K.; Torchia, D. A.; Stahl, S. J.; Kaufman, J. D.; Wingfield, P. T.; Domaille, P. J.; and Campbell-Burk, S. *Eur. J. Biochem.* 1994, 219, 707-712.
36. Le, H.; Oldfield, E. *J. Biomol. NMR* 1994, 4, 341-348.
37. Weber, I. T. *J. Biol. Chem.* 1990, 265, 10492-10496.
38. Torchia, D. A.; Nicholson, L. K.; Cole, H. B. R. ; Kay, L. E., in *NMR of Proteins* Gore, G. M.; Gronenborn, A. M., Eds.; Macmillan Press: London, 1993; pp. 190-219.
39. Kordel, J.; Skelton, N. J.; Akke, M.; Palmer, A. G.; Chazin, W. J. *Biochemistry* 1992, 31, 4856-4859.
40. Clore, G. M.; Driscoll, P. C.; Wingfield, P. T.; Gronenborn, A. *Biochemistry* 1990, 29, 7387-7401.
41. Akke, M.; Bruschweiler, R.; Palmer , A. G., III, *J. Am. Chem. Soc.* 1993, 115, 9832-9833.
42. Yamazaki, T.; Nicholson, L. K.; Wingfield, P. T.; Stahl, S. J.; Kaufman, J. D.; Domaille, P. J.; Torchia, D.A. *J. Am. Chem. Soc.* 1994, 116, 10791-10792.
43. Rose, J. R.; Salto, R.; Craik, C. S. *J. Biol. Chem.* 1993, 268, 11939-11945.
44. Kraulis, P. *J. Appl. Crystallogr.* 1991, 24, 946-950.

# CHAPTER 11

# DNA AS A TARGET FOR DRUG ACTION: COMPLEXES OF INTERCALATING ANTIBIOTICS

*Mark S. Searle*

## CONTENTS

I    DNA as a Target for Drug Action ................................................. 378

II   Anthracycline Antibiotics ................................................. 381
     A   Nogalamycin–DNA Interactions ......................................... 381
         1   $^1$H Resonance Assignment Methodologies:
             The Nogalamycin–$d$(GACGTC)$_2$ Complexes .................... 382
         2   Nogalamycin Binding to the 5′-CpG Site of
             $d$(GACGTC)$_2$ ................................................. 389
             a   Ligand-Induced Changes in DNA
                 Conformation ................................................. 389
             b   Intermolecular Hydrogen Bonding ............................ 392
             c   Hydrophobic Interactions .................................... 393
         3   Nogalamycin Specificity for CpA vs. CpG
             Binding Sites ................................................. 393
         4   Deoxyribose Conformation and Dynamics in the
             Nogalamycin Complex with $d$(GCATGC)$_2$ ..................... 394
         5   Drug–DNA Interactions Probed by $^{31}$P NMR ................. 395
             a   $^{31}$P Chemical Shift Assignments and $^1$H–$^{31}$P
                 Coupling Constants ....................................... 396
             b   $^1$H and $^{31}$P NMR Relaxation Studies of the
                 Nogalamycin Complex with $d$(GCATGC)$_2$ ................ 398

0-8493-7824-9/96/$0.00+$.50
© 1996 by CRC Press, Inc.

B   Arugomycin–DNA Interactions ............................................. 399
    1   Structure of the (Arugomycin)$_2$–$d$(GCATGC)$_2$
        Complex ................................................................................ 401
    2   The Role of the Sugar Residues of Arugomycin
        in Binding ......................................................................... 403

III Quinomycin Antibiotics and Luzopeptin .................................... 404
    A   Quinomycin Antibiotics ............................................. 404
    B   Interaction of UK-65,662 (QN) with $d$(ACGT)$_2$
        and $d$(GACGTC)$_2$ ......................................................... 407
        1   Hoogsteen vs. Watson–Crick Base Pairing ...................... 407
        2   Intermolecular Interactions Between QN and the
            DNA Minor Groove ........................................................ 408
        3   Drug-Induced Helix Unwinding ..................................... 413
    C   Luzopeptin–DNA Interactions ............................................. 414
    D   Hydrogen Exchange Studies of Luzopeptin and
        Echinomycin Complexes ......................................................... 417

IV  Summary and Conclusions ............................................................ 418

References ................................................................................ 420

# I  DNA AS A TARGET FOR DRUG ACTION

Intracellular DNA represents the primary target for a wide variety of clinically important antibiotics and synthetic compounds that exhibit antitumour activities. A substantial body of research has been directed toward understanding the molecular basis for DNA sequence specificity by identifying the preferred binding sequences of many key drugs with "natural" DNA. Patterns of endonuclease protection (so-called "footprinting" data) have proven invaluable in designing short, synthetic DNA fragments suitable for structural analysis in complexes with drug molecules in solution[1] and in the crystal.[2] The results have had considerable impact in advancing our understanding of the microscopic structural heterogeneity of DNA[2-4] and the molecular basis for ligand–DNA recognition,[1,2,5,6] providing principles upon which medicinal chemists can base design strategies for new chemotherapeutic agents.

A structurally diverse set of drug molecules and their DNA complexes have now been investigated, characterised, and modelled on the basis of high-resolution solution NMR data.[1] Undoubtedly, progress in the chemistry of nucleic acid synthesis, which has enabled milligram quantities of defined-sequence oligonucleotides to be generated routinely, has helped to expand the interest in drug–DNA recognition.[1] The synthesis of relatively short fragments of DNA (4 to 12 bp have been employed) enables a single high-affinity binding site (or several) to be isolated for study while maintaining spectral complexity at a tractable level. The assumption that such small DNA fragments are, to at least some degree, representative of larger segments of "real" DNA seems reasonably well founded.[3,4] Invariably, the length of sequence chosen represents a compromise between what can be considered as representative of real DNA and what will enable features of the molecular-recognition complex to be characterised. Many naturally occurring antibiotics have high sequence specificities and their DNA complexes long lifetimes, making them particularly suitable for high-resolution NMR studies in solution.

The great architectural diversity found amongst the natural antibiotics reflects not only the effects of evolution on the producing organism's strategy for survival in repelling other organisms, but perhaps also the *flexibility* of DNA as a *receptor*. Although the DNA major groove has greater recognition potential and is the site of binding for many gene regulatory proteins,[7] the majority of small molecule ligands are minor-groove specific. This, in large part, appears to be a consequence of better complementarity between the ligand structure and the closely spaced walls of the minor groove of the B-DNA helix. Van der Waals and hydrophobic interactions appear to play a key part in complex stabilisation.[6]

A number of recent studies highlight the induced-fit nature of the drug–DNA interaction; in particular, the minor groove has been shown to expand to accommodate bulky dimers of chromomycin[8,9] and distamycin[10,11] (Figure 1A), as is further described in Chapter 12. Alternatively, structural distortions of the sugar-phosphate backbone are necessary to allow intercalators to thread chains of sugar residues between the DNA base pairs. These observations lead to the conclusion that *intrinsic* conformational properties of the B-DNA double helix, such as the width of the

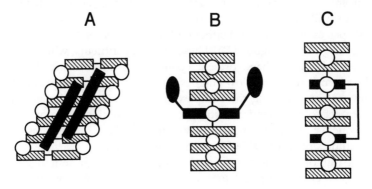

**FIGURE 1**
Schematic representation of drug–DNA complexes: (A) minor groove binding dimer (B) monointercalator, (C) bisintercalator. Hatched planks represent base pairs, circles are connecting phosphate groups, and DNA is presented as a ladder structure.

minor groove, may be less important in determining ligand-binding specificity than perhaps previously concluded. In this regard, the studies with chromomycin and distamycin dimers have introduced the concept of *binding stoichiometry* as an additional parameter in the design of DNA-specific ligands. The notion of *induced-fit*, but involving significant conformational changes in the drug, has been illustrated for the antibiotic luzopeptin.[12] *Trans* to *cis* isomerisation of several drug peptide bonds, which transforms intramolecular hydrogen bonds (stabilising a β-sheet like depsipeptide structure) into intermolecular interactions in the minor groove and which simultaneously optimises the interchromophore separation suitable for a bisintercalative mode of binding, has been identified. Approaches to ligand design aimed at altering the recognition properties of A–T specific ligands (such as distamycin, netropsin, and Hoechst 33258) to those capable of recognising mixed sequences of A·T and G·C base pairs, but which simultaneously reject rather than tolerate purely A–T sequences, have proven successful.[13-15] These approaches hold the potential for new insight into DNA recognition, ligand design, and targeting of new drugs to cognate sequences of DNA.

In this chapter, the results of solution NMR studies are highlighted for a number of DNA intercalators within the anthracycline and quinomycin families of antibiotics, including luzopeptin. The intercalative mode of binding is characterised by the insertion of a polyaromatic ring system between the unstacked base pairs of a partially unwound DNA helix. Subsequent stacking interactions between the DNA bases and the aromatic rings of the intercalating molecule make a major contribution to complex stabilisation. The anthracycline antibiotics typify the monofunctional binding mode. The planar aromatic ring system intercalates "head on" between the DNA base pairs positioning the long axis of the chromophore at right angles to the long axis of the adjacent base pairs. In the case illustrated for nogalamycin, this mode of binding simultaneously places drug sugars on either end of the chromophore in the major and minor grooves (Figure 1B). These bulky substituents, which give the molecule a dumbbell shape, present a considerable mechanistic obstacle to binding, which results in slow kinetics for both the association and dissociation processes, placing the complex in the very-slow-exchange regime with respect to the chemical-shift time scale. Slow kinetics, coupled with high sequence selectivity, make this system a paradigm for high-resolution NMR studies of drug–DNA interactions in solution.

The quinomycin antibiotics and luzopeptin are representative of the bifunctional class of intercalators; two aromatic ring systems attached at opposite ends of a relatively rigid cyclic depsipeptide structure allow the drug to intercalate in a staple-like manner, bracketing two base pairs (Figure 1C). The depsipeptide rings form additional structure-stabilising interactions in the minor groove by hydrogen bonding through peptide NHs to the edges of the base pairs. As is also the case for the anthracyclines, the sugar or peptide domains that reside in the minor groove have a striking complementarity for the right-handed twist that allows them to match the groove's natural curvature and contours.

## II  ANTHRACYCLINE ANTIBIOTICS

### A  NOGALAMYCIN–DNA INTERACTIONS

The antibiotic nogalamycin (Figure 2) is an active antitumour agent and a member of the anthracycline family of widely used chemotherapeutic agents that bind to DNA through the process of intercalation.[16-19] Nogalamycin represents a step up in structural complexity compared with the simpler, and better known, daunomycin-like anthracyclines (Figure 2), in that the aglycon chromophore is substituted at both ends with bulky sugar residues. The positive charge on nogalamycin (a protonated $N,N$-dimethylamino group) resides on the fused bicycloaminoglucose sugar, which daunomycin lacks altogether. An uncharged hydrophobic nogalose sugar is located at the 7 position where daunomycin has the positively charged daunosamine sugar. These structural differences, particularly the location of the positive charge, led to some uncertainty regarding the binding orientation and disposition of the antibiotic sugar residues with respect to the DNA major and minor groove.[6] DNA-binding studies have clearly established that nogalamycin forms a stable intercalation complex; however, the formidable mechanistic obstacle to binding presented by its bulky structure is reflected in slow rates of association and dissociation.[20] The kinetic observations have been interpreted in terms of a transient disruption (or melting) of the DNA structure as the rate-limiting step to

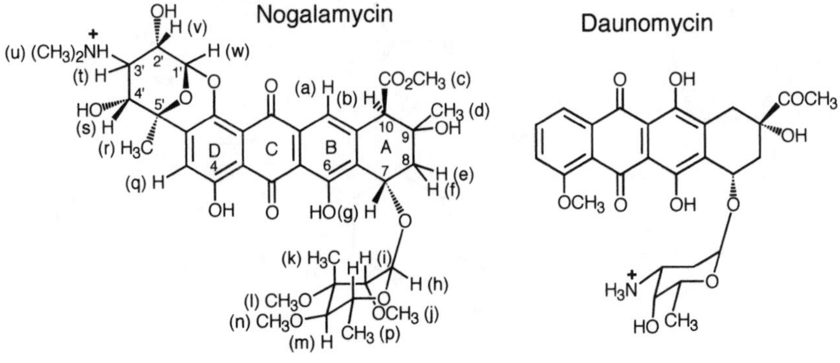

**FIGURE 2**
Structure of nogalamycin with proton-labelling scheme and carbon atom numbering. Structure of daunomycin is shown for comparison.

binding (or complex dissociation),[20] which then allows the aglycon chromophore to thread through the distorted DNA helix and locate sugar residues in both grooves.

## 1  *¹H Resonance Assignment Methodologies: The Nogalamycin–d(GACGTC)₂ Complexes*

The ¹H assignment methodologies outlined for oligonucleotides in solution[3,4,21] are potentially complicated by disruption of the pattern of sequential NOE connectivities as a consequence of structural distortions associated with ligand intercalation. The assignment procedure is outlined, with examples, for the complex of nogalamycin with the hexamer duplex d(GACGTC)₂.[22] The asymmetric antibiotic intercalates at the central 5'-CpG step, lifting the dyad symmetry of the self-complementary duplex, leading to a nonequivalence of the two nucleotide strands. The 12 distinguishable deoxyribose spin systems are labelled according to the scheme

$$5'\text{--G1 A2 C3 G4 T5 C6}$$

$$\text{C12 T11 G10 C9 A8 G7--}5'$$

and are partially assigned on the basis of scalar coupling interactions identified in DQF-COSY and HOHAHA spectra. The numbering scheme for sugar and base protons is shown below:

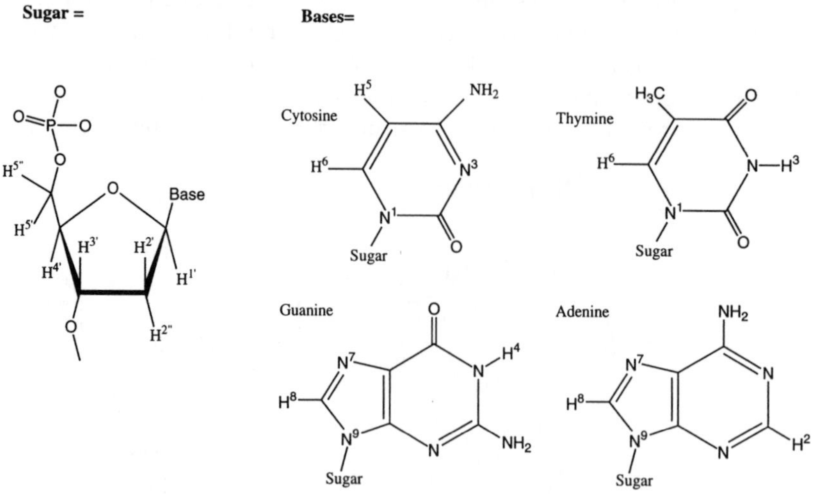

While couplings between H1' (5.0–6.5 ppm) and H2'/H2" (1.8–3.0 ppm) are readily identified in phase-sensitive DQF-COSY spectra (Figure 3A),[1] extensive overlap of the H3' (4.5–5.2 ppm) and H4', H5'/H5"

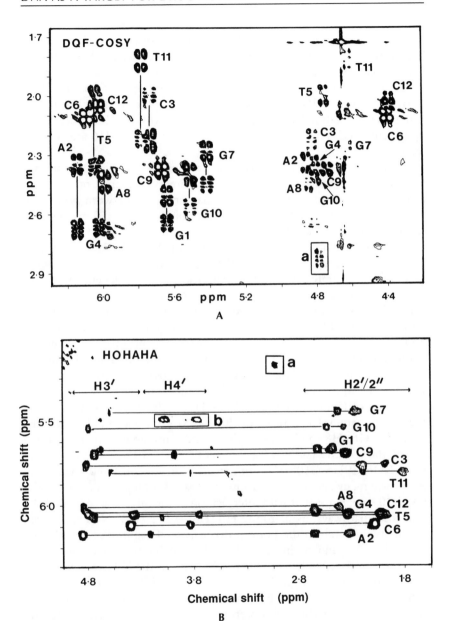

**FIGURE 3**
(A) Phase-sensitive double-quantum filtered COSY spectrum of the nogalamycin–
d(GACGTC)$_2$ complex identifying H1'-H2'/H1'-H2" and H2'-H3'/H2"-H3' correlations
within the 12 nonequivalent deoxyribose spin systems. H1' (5.2–6.2 ppm), H2'/H2" (1.7–
2.9 ppm), and H3' (4.4–5.0 ppm). Cross-peak (a) corresponds to H$_g$-H$_e$ of the bound
antibiotic. (B) Expanded portion of the HOHAHA spectrum (100-ms mixing time) of the
nogalamycin–d(GACGTC)$_2$ complex correlating deoxyribose H1' resonances (5.2–6.2
ppm) with H2'/H2"/H3', and in several cases, H4' resonances. (Data from Searle, M.S.,
and Bicknell, W., *Eur. J. Biochem.*, 205, 45–58, 1992.)

(3.5–4.5 ppm) resonances precludes a complete assignment of all deoxyribose protons using COSY. The relatively well-resolved H1′ resonances permit spin-system assignments to be extended to all H3′ and a number of H4′ resonances from an analysis of coherence transfer through H1′ in isotropic mixing (HOHAHA) experiments, as illustrated in Figure 3B. Additional three-bond couplings arising from cytosine H5-H6 (5.5–7.5 ppm), and weak four-bond couplings for thymine $CH_3$-H6 are also detected.

The assignment of individual base protons and deoxyribose spin systems to specific nucleotides within the primary sequence relies on an analysis of the pattern of nuclear Overhauser effects between protons in nearest-neighbour residues. The contour plot of the 250-ms NOESY spectrum of the nogalamycin–$d$(GACGTC)$_2$ complex is illustrated in Figure 4, together with the equivalent region of the HOHAHA spectrum. The highlighted regions of the NOESY spectrum are expanded in Figure 5, and they illustrate NOE connectivities within the independent assignment pathways involving the correlations H6/H8 → H1′ and H6/H8 → H2′/2″, respectively. With the exception of the base proton of the 5′-terminal nucleotide in each strand, which exhibits only intranucleotide NOEs, the right-handed twist of the B-DNA conformation places the pyrimidine H6 and purine H8 of residue $i$ in close proximity to the H1′ of residue $i$, and H1′ of the 5′-linked deoxyribose ($i - 1$) (both < 4 Å in B-DNA[21]), but *not* the H1′ of the 3′-linked deoxyribose ($i + 1$). In the top two panels of Figure 5, the H6/H8 → H1′, assignment pathways within the two nonequivalent strands of the complex are traced independently. While the H6/H8 → H1′ connectivities are contiguous along the G1–C6 strand, the G7–C12 pathway is broken at the C9–G10 step; the internucleotide NOE C9H6-G10H1′ is not detected (proton–proton distance >5.0 Å), providing evidence for a disruption of base-stacking interactions at the C9–G10 step, consistent with intercalation at this site. The second of the sequential pathways, highlighting H6/H8 → H2′/H2″ NOEs, is traced for the two strands in the bottom two panels of Figure 5. Similarly, the pyrimidine H6 and purine H8 of residue $i$ exhibits interactions to the H2′/H2″ of the 5′-linked residue ($i - 1$), but not the 3′-linked nucleotide ($i + 1$). In the bottom right-hand panel of Figure 5, NOEs between purine H8 and pyrimidine $H5/CH_3$, characteristic of 5′-pur-pyr steps with a right-handed twist (but *not* observed for the 5′-pyr-pur step), are also highlighted and are a valuable additional assignment check; NOEs corresponding to the two 5′-GpT steps in the sequence (G4H8 → $T5CH_3$ and G10H8 → $T11CH_3$) are illustrated.

The only nonexchangeable protons to demonstrate interstrand NOEs are the base H2 of adenine, which is often correlated with the deoxyribose H1′ of the base-paired thymine residue (on the opposite strand) and also with the H1′ of the 5′-flanking residue of the base-paired thymine.

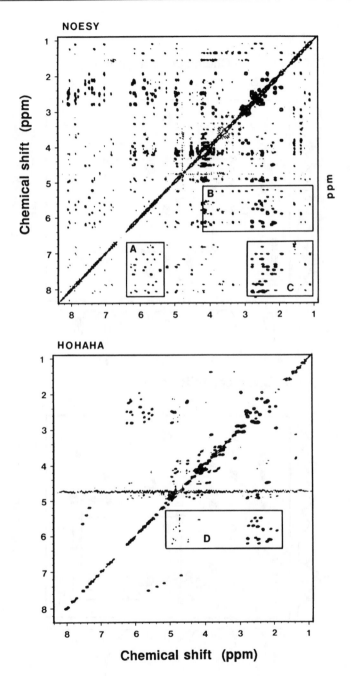

**FIGURE 4**
The 400-MHz pure-absorption phase-sensitive NOESY (250 ms) and HOHAHA (33 ms) spectra of the nogalamycin–$d$(GACGTC)$_2$ complex (20°C in D$_2$O). Boxed regions appear in expanded form in subsequent figures. (Data from Searle, M.S., and Bicknell, W., *Eur. J. Biochem.*, 205, 45–58, 1992.)

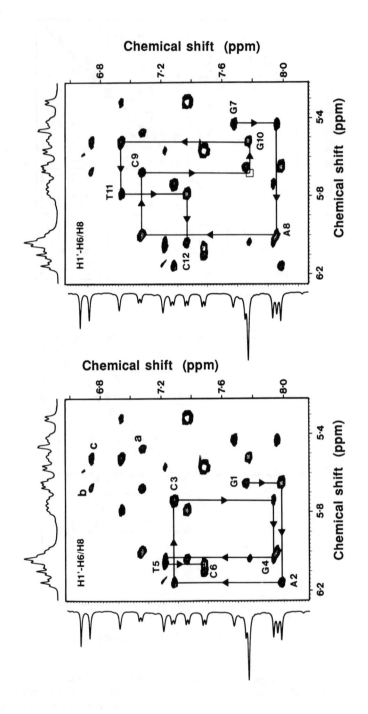

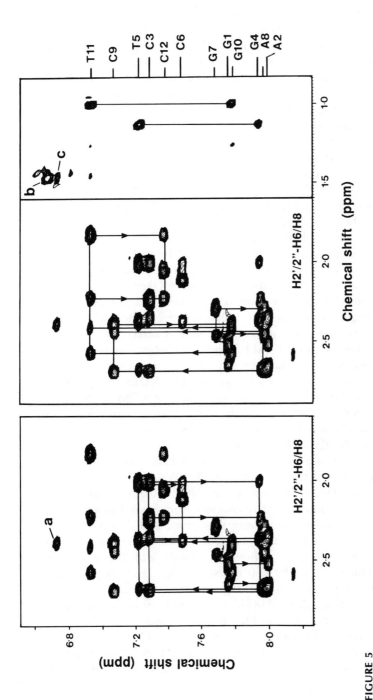

**FIGURE 5**

Expanded portions of the NOESY spectrum of Figure 4 highlighting intranucleotide and sequential correlations involving base H6/H8 and deoxyribose H1' resonances (top), and base H6/H8 and deoxyribose H2'/H2'' resonances (bottom). The assignment pathways for the two nonequivalent strands in both cases are traced in separate panels; intranucleotide NOEs are labelled according to sequence position. In the bottom right-hand panel NOEs are also highlighted from the thymine methyl groups of T5 and T11 to their respective T H6 and the H8 of the adjacent guanine base. Several additional NOEs are highlighted: in the top panel — (a) C9H6 → H$_a$, (b) C9H1' → H$_a$, (c) G10H1' → H$_a$; in the bottom panels — (a) C9H2'' → H$_a$, (b) H$_q$ → Me$_r$, (c) H$_q$ → Me$_d$. (Data from Searle, M.S., and Bicknell, W., *Eur. J. Biochem.*, 205, 45–58, 1992.)

Observations of these cross-peaks, though generally weak, prove useful in confirming adenine H2 assignments in complex spectra.

The exchangeable protons of A·T and G·C base pairs provide particularly important monitors of hydrogen bonding interactions and dynamic processes in drug–DNA complexes. Gueron et al.[23] have recently reviewed solvent-suppression schemes for detecting exchangeable proton resonances. The amino protons (cytidine N4, guanosine N2, and adenosine N6) generally exhibit broad signals, although their involvement in intermolecular hydrogen bonds in ligand complexes can appreciably modify their rate of exchange with solvent. The thymine (N3) and guanine (N1) imino proton resonances in the $H_2O$ spectrum of the nogalamycin–$d$(GACGTC)$_2$ complex (Figure 6) are identified between 12 and 14 ppm; the lowest field resonances at ca. 13.6 ppm corresponding to thymine H3 of T5 and T11. The amino protons generally overlap with the nonexchangeable base proton resonances between 6.0 and 8.5 ppm. Two resonances are identified between 11.0 and 11.5 ppm (Figure 6) that correspond to the slowly exchanging 4-OH and 6-OH of the bound antibiotic. Many NOE cross-peaks from 4-OH and 6-OH unambiguously locate the antibiotic between the G4·C9 and G10·C3 base pairs.[22] A consequence of ligand intercalation between the G·C base pairs is that sequential NOEs are lost (e.g., no NOE is detected between the imino protons G4H1 and G10H1). If, however, nogalamycin is considered a surrogate base pair, then the sequential assignment pathway, via exchangeable proton resonances, is completed by NOEs from 6-OH to both G4H1 and G10H1 (Figure 6). With the exception of the imino proton resonances of the terminal base pairs, which are appreciably broadened, the following sequence of NOEs is observed: T11H3 → G10H1 → Nog 6-OH → G4H1 → T5H3.

The assignment of a large number of resonances due to the bound antibiotic is paramount to securing a detailed description of the drug–DNA interaction through intermolecular NOEs. Correlations used in the assignment of a number of resonances from bound nogalamycin, corresponding to protons on the nogalose sugar and ring A, are illustrated in Figure 7 from an analysis of through-bond interactions identified in HOHAHA spectra (above diagonal) and through-space connectivities identified in the 250-ms NOESY spectrum (below diagonal). The nogalamycin proton labelling scheme is indicated in Figure 2. For example, in Figure 7, HOHAHA correlations (above diagonal) are readily identified for $H_m \rightarrow H_o \rightarrow Me_p$ (nogalose sugar), and between the geminal protons $H_e \rightarrow H_f$ (ring A). The orientation of the nogalose sugar relative to ring A is defined by the occurrence and relative intensities of the NOEs $H_o \rightarrow H_e$, $H_o \rightarrow H_f$, $Me_k \rightarrow Me_d$ and $H_g \rightarrow H_h$ (below diagonal).

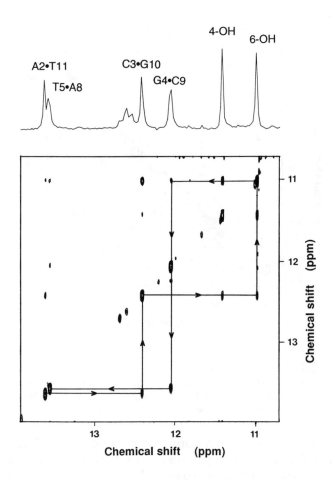

**FIGURE 6**

The 500-MHz 2D NOESY spectrum (300-ms mixing time) of the nogalamycin–*d*(GACGTC)₂ complex recorded at 5°C in 90% H₂O solution. Sequential NOEs are highlighted between imino protons, with the 6-OH of the intervening antibiotic completing the pathway by mediating between the two central C·G base pairs.

## 2   Nogalamycin Binding to the 5′-CpG Site of d(GACGTC)₂

### a   Ligand-Induced Changes in DNA Conformation

The interaction of nogalamycin with the single unique 5′-CpG binding site at the centre of the sequence *d*(GACGTC)₂ has been modelled using energy minimisation and restrained molecular dynamics calculations guided by the NMR data already described.[22] The antibiotic threads between the G·C base pairs, its long axis approximately perpendicular to the long axis of the base pairs, locating the positively charged bicycloamino

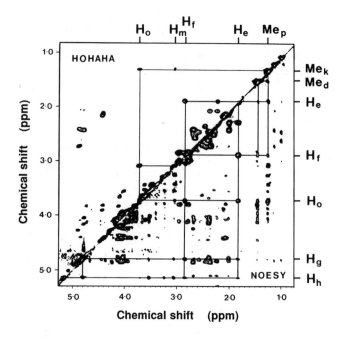

**FIGURE 7**
Combined portions of NOESY (*bottom half*) and HOHAHA spectra (*top half*) of the
nogalamycin–*d*(GACGTC)$_2$ complex (1.0–5.0 ppm) illustrating key correlations in the
assignment of a number of resonances of the nogalose and ring A sugars of the bound
antibiotic. (Data from Searle, M.S. and Bicknell, W., *Eur. J. Biochem.*, 205, 45–58, 1992.)

sugar in the major groove. A feature of the structure that is particularly
evident, and one that is emerging as a general characteristic of anthracycline
intercalation complexes, is the considerable buckling of base pairs at the
intercalation site. The base pairs wrap around the drug chromophore so as
to maximise the surface area in van der Waals contact while minimising the
occurrence of cavities in the structure. In the 'CpG' complex of
nogalamycin,[22] the pattern of H6/H8 → H1′ internucleotide NOEs is
consistent with this base-pair-buckled structure. While the internucleotide
NOEs [H6/H8 ($i$) → H1′ ($i-1$)] along the G1–C6 strand are contiguous
(even at the C3pG4 site of intercalation), the complementary G7–C12
sequence *is* interrupted at the C9pG10 step where the G10H8 → C9H1′
NOE is not observed (Figure 5, top right-hand panel). These observations
are readily rationalised by reference to the structure of the complex
presented in Figure 8 (top). The C9 and G10 bases, on either side of the
intercalation site, retain a parallel alignment and are widely separated by
the intervening antibiotic chromophore, which stacks preferentially on
these bases; Figure 8 (top). The result is a large separation (>5 Å) of
C9H1′ and G10H8 that is expected to significantly reduce the intensity of
the internucleotide NOE, as observed. In contrast, C3 and G4 adopt a

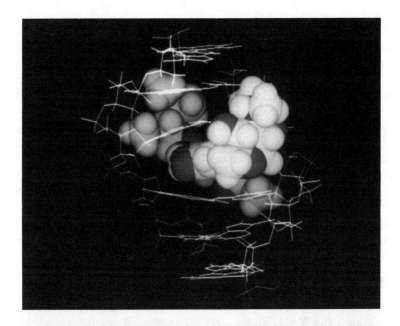

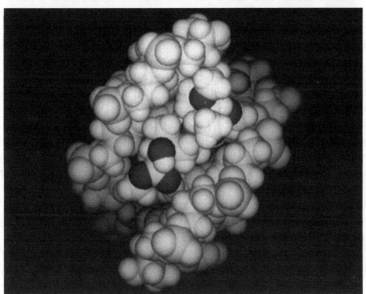

**FIGURE 8**

Energy-minimised structures of the nogalamycin–$d$(GACGTC)$_2$ complex. (*Top*) View of the complex from the major groove highlighting buckling of the G·C base pairs at the intercalation site; the base pair at the top of the figure corresponds to G1·C12. (*Bottom*) View into the minor groove illustrating the remarkable complementarity between the conformation of the nogalose and ring A sugars of the antibiotic and the walls of the minor groove. (Data from Searle, M.S. and Bicknell, W., *Eur. J. Biochem.*, 205, 45–58, 1992.)

wedge-shaped alignment that separates the bases to a sufficient extent to allow intercalation but retains C3H1' and G4H8 in close proximity, as confirmed by the observation of the corresponding internucleotide NOE (Figure 5). Measurements from the energy-minimised structures indicate that the base pairs C3·G10 and G4·C9 buckle by approximately 22 and −9°, respectively, to produce the observed binding-site geometry. The antibiotic also unwinds the duplex by 16°; the intercalation site appears to be overwound by 4°, with the net effect close to the value of 18° previously determined in solution.[16] Two high-resolution crystal structures have reported details of the interaction of nogalamycin with modified 5'-CpG sites at the terminal positions of the hexamer duplex $d$($^{m5}$CGTA$^{m5}$CG)$_2$ (where $^{m5}$C represents cytosine methylated at the 5 position on the pyrimidine ring),[24,25] and here substantial buckling of the base pairs (up to 26°) again emerges as a key feature of intercalation site geometry.

### b  Intermolecular Hydrogen Bonding

The conformationally constrained bicyclo sugar of nogalamycin preorganises the 2'-OH and 4'-OH groups[26] in orientations suitable for involvement in direct hydrogen bonding interactions with the major–groove edge of the conserved G·C base pair at the intercalation site. These hydroxyl groups are utilised as both hydrogen bond donors and acceptors. The 2'-OH donates a hydrogen bond to the guanine N7 of G10, while the 4'-OH, visible in Figure 8 (top), accepts a weaker hydrogen bond from the 4-amino group of C3. The positively charged $N,N$-dimethyamino group is located in the minor groove in a region of high electrostatic potential[27] close to O6/N7 of the same guanine base (G10), where electrostatic interactions and water-mediated hydrogen bonds are likely to impart some degree of complex stabilisation. It seems probable that these interactions in combination may account for some part of the specificity for a G·C base pair at this position. The only apparent feature of the antibiotic capable of contributing any degree of sequence specificity for the minor groove is the carbonyl group of the methyl ester on ring A that forms a direct hydrogen bond to the 2-amino group of G4.

The bulky sugar moieties at either end of the aglycon chromophore occlude both grooves of the double helix over several base pairs (see Figure 8), accounting for the marked reduction in the rate of imino proton exchange in base pairs close to the drug intercalation site. Variable-temperature studies[22] indicate that imino proton resonances attributed to the C3·G10 and G4·C9 base pairs, but also the flanking A2·T11 base pair (T5·A8 remains relatively unaffected), are slowly exchanging up to about 50°C, while resonances in the spectrum of the ligand-free duplex are broadened to baseline above about 25°C.

### c   Hydrophobic Interactions

The nogalose sugar and ring A form a continuous hydrophobic domain that interacts closely with the floor and walls of the minor groove over a span of 4 bp, as underlined $d$(GACGTC). Van der Waals contacts between antibiotic protons and, principally, deoxyribose H1′ in the minor groove are evident from NOEs observed in 40-ms NOESY spectra of the complex (data not shown, but correspond to NOEs observed in portion B of the NOESY spectrum of Figure 4). In particular, the NOEs Me$_d$ → G$_{10}$H1′, OMe$_j$ → C$_3$H1′, Me$_k$ → T$_{11}$H1′, and OMe$_l$ → C$_{12}$H1′ have high intensities that equate with interproton distances <3.0 Å and illustrate the hand-in-glove complementarity between the drug sugar domain and the right-handed twist of the DNA minor groove, as clearly illustrated in Figure 8.

## 3   Nogalamycin Specificity for CpA vs. CpG Binding Sites

Footprinting data indicate that nogalamycin binds best to alternating sequences of DNA with preferences for 5′-Y-R-3′ binding sites (Y–pyrimidine, R–purine) within several sequences of natural DNA;[28,29] both CpA (TpG) and CpG (but not TpA) binding sites are highly protected from endonuclease cleavage. Studies with the hexamer duplex $d$(GCATGC)$_2$,[30] together with the related octamer duplex $d$(AGCATGCT)$_2$,[31] confirm that nogalamycin binds with high affinity and specificity to the 5′-CpA and equivalent TpG sites in these mixed sequences of DNA. In each of these complexes, one drug molecule is bound at each of the two symmetry-related sites per duplex, giving a complex with twofold symmetry. The structural details that have emerged from studies of the interaction of nogalamycin with the key recognition sites 5′-CpA (5′-TpG) and 5′-CpG, both in solution and in the crystal,[22,24,25,30-32] permit some comparison of structure-stabilising features and some discussion of the molecular basis for DNA sequence specificity. Direct interactions between antibiotic and DNA in the major groove (principally hydrogen bonding and electrostatics) are dominated by the region of highly negative electrostatic potential associated with the N7 and O6 of guanine, as described above. These features are retained in both complexes. However, substituting a G·C with an A·T base pair in the second position (5′-CpG → 5′-CpA), eliminates the guanine 2-amino group in the minor groove and precludes the formation of a direct hydrogen bond to the carbonyl oxygen of the methyl ester on sugar ring A of the antibiotic (see Figure 8). The effect on specificity of the loss of a hydrogen bond in the minor groove of the CpA complex appears to be compensated by thymine-specific interactions in the major groove, namely, with the thymine methyl group. Hydrophobic interactions between the bridgehead atoms (H$_w$-O-Me$_r$) of the bicycloamino-glucose sugar (Figure 2) and the thymine methyl (identified through NOEs between $TCH_3$ and $H_w/Me_r$)[30,31] appear to establish the latter's importance for intercalation site specificity in the CpA complex. The majority of the hydrophobic interactions between the nogalose/ring A sugars and the minor groove deoxyribose sugars are common to both CpA and CpG complexes. Although these interactions do not appear to impart any degree of sequence specificity, their contribution to binding is undoubtedly thermodynamically significant.

## 4 Deoxyribose Conformation and Dynamics in the Nogalamycin Complex with d(GCATGC)₂

An investigation of the effects of nogalamycin binding on the conformation and dynamics of the deoxyribose rings of the hexamer duplex $d(GCATGC)_2$[33] reveals shifts in the position of the dynamic equilibrium between the C2'-endo and C3'-endo low-energy configurations. These changes reflect ligand-induced unwinding of the hexamer duplex, particularly the A–T base pairs sandwiched between the two intercalation sites. Deoxyribose conformational analysis from $^1H$–$^1H$ vicinal coupling constants and sums of coupling constants[34] (primarily $J_{1'-2'}$, $J_{1'-2''}$, $\Sigma_{1'} = J_{1'-2'} + J_{1'-2''}$, $\Sigma_{2'} = J_{1'-2'} + J_{2'-2''} + J_{2'-3'}$ and $\Sigma_{2''} = J_{1'-2''} + J_{2'-2''} + J_{2''-3'}$ measured from 1D and phase-sensitive 2D COSY and DQF-COSY experiments; see Table 1), assuming a rapid dynamic equilibrium between N and S states, reveals quite different predominant conformations for the deoxyribose rings of the 2C·5G and 3A·4T base pairs that form the drug-intercalation site. While the deoxyribose rings of the 2C·5G base pairs are best described in terms of an equilibrium heavily weighted in favour of the S conformer (>95%, with the pseudorotation phase angle $P$, lying in the range 170–175°; see Table 1), the analysis shows a higher proportion of the N conformer for the sugars of the 3A·4T base pairs. The data show that the C2'-endo (S) and C3'-endo (N) conformers are equally populated for 3A, as indicated by a particularly small value for $\Sigma 1'$, and a larger than average value for $\Sigma 2''$ (see Table 1). A more limited data set for the deoxyribose of 4T restricts the equilibrium to ca. 65–75% C2'-endo. The relationship between the magnitude of the active coupling and the relative intensity of cross-peaks in both DQF-COSY and isotropic mixing experiments (HOHAHA), enables a semiquantitative estimate to be made of the value of $J_{3'-4'}$. A high proportion of the C3'-endo conformer is anticipated to produce a large average value for $J_{3'-4'}$, reflecting a value of $J_{3'-4'}$ close to zero for the pure C2'-endo conformer, but a substantially larger value (ca. 9 Hz) for the C3'-endo conformer. The deoxyribose of 3A and 4T (and also that of the terminal 6C) give much more intense H3'–H4' cross-peaks than 2C and 5G, consistent with a higher proportional of the C3'-endo conformer. Further, in HOHAHA spectra, coherence transfer is observed from H1' through to H4' only for those nucleotides (3A, 4T, and 6C) that

## TABLE 1

$^1$H–$^1$H Coupling Constants (Hz), Sums of Coupling Constants (Hz), and Conformation (Phase Angle P, Pucker Amplitude $\Phi$) of the Deoxyribose Rings of the (Nogalamycin)$_2$–$d$(GCATGC)$_2$ Complex at 25°C

| Base | $J_{1'-2'}$ | $J_{1'-2''}$ | $\Sigma 1'$ | $\Sigma 2'$ | $\Sigma 2''$ | $J_{3'-4'}$ | %S | $P_s$ | $\Phi$ | RMS |
|------|-------------|--------------|-------------|-------------|--------------|-------------|-----|-------|--------|-----|
| 1G | 8.2 | 5.8 | 14.0 | 28.3 | 22.1 | w | 80 | 180 | 40 | 0.11 |
|    | (8.2) | (5.8) | (14.0) | (27.3) | (23.1) | | | | | |
| 2C | 9.8 | 5.6 | 15.4 | 28.9 | 20.6 | w | >95 | 171 | 35 | 0.02 |
|    | (9.8) | (5.7) | (15.5) | (29.4) | (21.0) | | | | | |
| 3A | 5.7 | 6.7 | 12.4 | 26.9 | 26.0 | s | 50 | 162 | 35 | 0.06 |
|    | (5.8) | (6.7) | (12.5) | (26.5) | (26.2) | | | | | |
| 4T | — | — | 14.2 | — | — | s | 65–75 | 128–189 | 35 | — |
| 5G | 10.0 | 5.2 | 15.2 | 29.2 | 20.8 | w | >95 | 175 | 40 | 0.11 |
|    | (10.1) | (5.2) | (15.3) | (28.8) | (20.8) | | | | | |
| 6C | 7.9 | 6.3 | 14.2 | 28.9 | 23.4 | s | 70 | 126 | 35 | 0.28 |
|    | (7.9) | (6.4) | (14.2) | (29.4) | (23.9) | | | | | |

*Note:* Coupling constants from 1D spectra are ±0.2 Hz; sums of coupling constants from 2D spectra are ±0.8 Hz. $J_{3'-4'}$ is assigned a value of weak (w) or strong (s) on the basis of cross-peak intensities in TOCSY and DQF-COSY spectra. Values in parentheses are coupling constants calculated using the two-state model and the data on the limiting structures described by Rinkel and Altona[34]. The two-state model describes the percentage of C2'-endo (%S), with phase angle $P$, and pucker amplitude $\Phi$, in dynamic equilibrium with the C3'-endo conformer described by $P = 9°$ and $\Phi = 40°$; RMS is the root-mean-square difference between the experimental and calculated coupling constants. The limited amount of data for 4T reflects the virtually coincident chemical-shift values of the H2' and H2" of this residue.

Data from Searle, M.S. and Wakelin, L.P.G., *Biochem. J.*, 269, 341–346, 1990. With permission.

have a substantial proportion of the C3'-endo conformer (i.e., where coherence transfer is mediated by a significant value of $J_{3'-4'}$).[33]

The preference of the A and T nucleotides for a higher proportion of the C3'-endo conformer than typically found for non-terminal nucleotides in the B-DNA conformation appears to reflect the extent to which the helix is unwound within the A–T sequence of $d$(GC**AT**GC)$_2$ (underlined) by two drug molecules intercalated in such close proximity at the 5'-CpA and 5'-TpG steps. Theoretical energy-minimisation studies addressed the relationship between local helical twist angle and backbone conformation in DNA and concluded that in unwound helices there is a tendency for sugars to repucker to the O4'-endo or C3'-endo configurations.[35]

## 5 *Drug–DNA Interactions Probed by* $^{31}P$ *NMR*

The negatively charged phosphodiester groups lie on the outside of the DNA double helix and are thought to play an important role in protein–DNA recognition.[36,37] [31]P NMR has long been recognised as a useful probe for monitoring changes in phosphodiester torsion angles that accompany ligand binding to DNA duplexes. Intercalation phenomena, in particular, are frequently characterised by large downfield shifts (up to 2 ppm) of the [31]P resonances corresponding to the phosphate groups at the intercalation sites.[30,38] Such large chemical-shift perturbations are not exclusively the domain of intercalators; ligands that bind covalently to DNA in the minor groove, such as anthramycin, have been shown to produce comparable effects.[1,39] Theoretical studies[40-42] indicate that changes in conformation involving $\alpha$ and $\zeta$ torsion angles appear to be the most important in determining [31]P chemical-shift values. These studies suggest that deshielding effects of up to 2 ppm are possible for a conformational transition from a *gauche, gauche* (B-DNA) to a *gauche, trans* configuration, in agreement with the magnitude of effects observed for a number of intercalation complexes.

### a  [31]P Chemical Shift Assignments and [1]H–[31]P Coupling Constants

The [31]P assignment procedure is based on the observation of [31]P–[1]H scalar coupling interactions with H3′, H4′ and H5′/H5″, with [1]H resonances first assigned using the combination of methods described above. While H3′ and H4′ are generally unambiguously identified in the spectra of relatively short oligonucleotides, those for H5′/H5″ are frequently ill resolved; the [31]P–H5′/H5″ correlations provide confirmation of the latter [1]H assignments. Correlations in the [31]P-detected HETCOR spectrum of the 2:1 complex of nogalamycin with the hexamer duplex $d(GCATGC)_2$ are illustrated in Figure 9.[43] Drug molecules are bound at each of the symmetry-related 5′-CpA and 5′-TpG steps with full retention of the twofold symmetry of the duplex. The five phosphate resonances in the 1D [31]P spectrum of the complex are well dispersed as a consequence of ligand-induced downfield shifts of up to 1.5 ppm. Each phosphate group shows [31]P–[1]H scalar coupling interactions to the H4′ and H5′/H5″ resonances of the 3′-flanking deoxyribose, and to the H3′ of the 5′-flanking sugar, which permits the two downfield-shifted resonances to be assigned to the phosphate groups at the C2pA3 and T4pG5 steps that form the intercalation sites.

The [1]H–decoupled [31]P spectrum of the 2:1 complex of nogalamycin with $d(GCATGC)_2$ shows little variation in [31]P linewidths, indicative of comparable spin–spin relaxation times. In contrast, the fully [1]H-coupled spectrum (Figure 9B) shows significant variation (contrast two lowest-field resonances in Figure 9B), reflecting variations in the magnitude of one or more [1]H–[31]P spin-coupling constants indicative of differences in backbone torsion angles. In phase–sensitive coupled [1]H–[31]P shift correlation experiments (data not shown), C2pA and G1pC phosphates show large antiphase

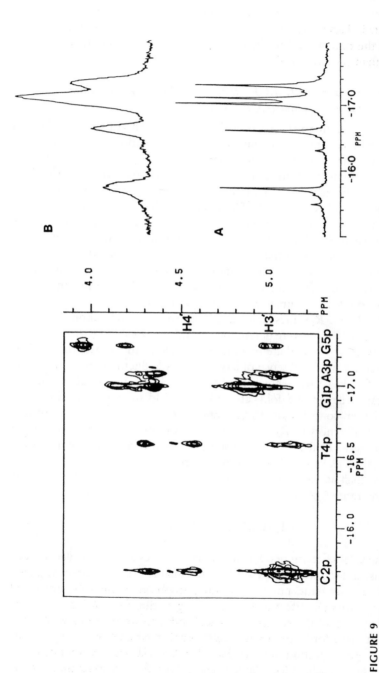

**FIGURE 9**

[31]P NMR spectra of the (nogalamycin)$_2$–d(GCATGC)$_2$ complex. (*Left panel*) 2D heteronuclear shift correlation spectrum recorded at 298 K, highlighting cross-peaks to H3'/H4' and H5'/H5" between 3.8 and 5.4 ppm. (A) [1]H-decoupled and (B) [1]H-coupled 1D [31]P NMR spectra. (Data from Searle, M.S. and Lane, A.N., *FEBS Lett.*, 297, 292–296, 1992. With permission.)

splittings of 6–8 Hz for coupling to H3′, whereas all other H3′–$^{31}$P couplings are <3 Hz. Roongta et al.[44] have related the H3′–$^{31}$P coupling constant to the backbone torsion angle ε through a Karplus relationship. The data indicate that the ε torsion angle for the C2pA step (together with that of the terminal G1pC linker) is closer to the $B_{II}$ conformation (ε = - 105°) than the other residues.

### b   $^1$H and $^{31}$P NMR Relaxation Studies of the Nogalamycin Complex with d(GCATGC)₂

A lower limit to the rotational correlation time of the complex has been estimated from measurement of the reorientational correlation time of the cytosine H5–H6 vectors of the d(GCATGC)₂ duplex.[43] The $^1$H–$^1$H time-dependent NOE measurements (irradiating the cytosine H6 of C2 and C6) indicate a cross-relaxation rate constant of –0.56 s$^{-1}$ for both cytosines at 298 K and 9.4 T. This equates with a correlation time of 2.3 ± 0.3 ns (assuming the H5–H6 distance to be 2.46 Å). This value is approximately 30% higher than that of an equivalent hexamer duplex with no bound ligand. Given that each nogalamycin molecule extends the helix by the equivalent of 1 bp, a correlation time for the 2:1 complex equivalent to that of an octamer duplex is anticipated (i.e., 33% greater than for a hexamer duplex), in agreement with experiment.

The $R_1$ and $R_2$ values (spin–lattice and spin–spin relaxation constants) for each phosphorus were determined at 4.7 and 9.4 T, together with $^1$H– $^{31}$P NOE at 4.7 T, and are presented in Table 2. In all cases the NOE is small, indicating the absence of large-amplitude fluctuations in the orientation of P–H vectors, which might affect relaxation. The $R_2$ values are significantly larger (2.5-fold) at the higher field strength, indicative of a much larger contribution to relaxation from chemical-shift anisotropy (CSA). Differences in $R_2$ values are also more pronounced at the higher field strength; $R_2$ for C2pA is substantially smaller than the average while $R_2$ for A3pT is larger (Table 2). As the contribution from dipolar relaxation is small at 9.4 T, the effective correlation time τ, can be obtained from the ratio $R_2/R_1$.[43]

$$\tau = 1/(\omega_p)^2 \; [3/2 \; (R_2/R_1 - 7/6)]^{1/2} \qquad (1)$$

The values determined for the five phosphates are very similar, τ = 3.2 ± 0.1 ns, and slightly larger than for the cytosine H5–H6 vector, suggesting that any substantial mobility of the phosphates on the subnanosecond time scale does not affect relaxation. Using a value for τ of 3.2 ns permits the calculation of the effective chemical shift anisotropy χ (Table 2). It is apparent that χ for C2pA is significantly smaller, while A3pT is larger, than the average, reflecting nonstandard DNA backbone conformations at these positions, which for C2pA, is also reflected in the magnitude of the

**TABLE 2**

$^{31}$P NMR Chemical Shifts and Relaxation Parameters at 298K[a]

| Parameter | G1p | C2p | A3p | T4p | G5p |
|---|---|---|---|---|---|
| $\delta$(ppm)[b] | −17.0 | −15.7 | −17.1 | −16.6 | −17.3 |
| *4.7 T* | | | | | |
| $R_1$ (s$^{-1}$) | 0.81 | 0.79 | 0.84 | 0.79 | 0.81 |
| $R_2$ (s$^{-1}$) | 2.89 | 2.66 | 3.13 | 2.97 | 2.95 |
| $\Delta R$ (s$^{-1}$) | 2.49 | 2.27 | 2.71 | 2.58 | 2.55 |
| $R_2/R_1$ | 3.6 | 3.4 | 3.7 | 3.8 | 3.6 |
| NOE | 1.08 | 1.05 | 1.07 | 1.05 | 1.06 |
| *9.4 T* | | | | | |
| $R_1$ (s$^{-1}$) | 0.84 | 0.80 | 0.95 | 0.86 | 0.92 |
| $R_2$ (s$^{-1}$) | 7.2 | 6.2 | 8.3 | 7.1 | 7.4 |
| $\Delta R$ (s$^{-1}$) | 6.8 | 5.8 | 7.8 | 6.7 | 7.0 |
| $R_2/R_1$ | 8.6 | 7.8 | 8.7 | 8.3 | 8.0 |
| $\tau$ (ns) | 3.3 | 3.1 | 3.3 | 3.2 | 3.1 |
| $\chi$ (ppm)[c] | 142 | 130 | 154 | 141 | 144 |

[a] Errors in $R_1$, $R_2$, and NOE ±10%; $\chi$ ±5% and $\tau$ ±10%.
[b] Chemical shifts with respect to methylene diphosphate.
[c] Chemical shift anisotropy $\chi$ is defined by $\chi^2 = \Delta\sigma^2 (1 + \eta^{2/3})$ where $\Delta\sigma$ and $\eta$ are the anisotropy and asymmetry of the shielding tensor, respectively.

Data from Searle, M.S. and Lane, A.N., *FEBS Lett.*, 297, 292–296, 1992. With permission.

H3′–$^{31}$P spin-coupling constant (see above). The considerable binding-site asymmetry in calculated solution structures alluded to above, and also found in crystal structures, is also reflected in $^{31}$P chemical-shift and relaxation measurements. The correlation times calculated from Equation (1) must represent lower limits, as the effects of internal motions have not been considered. However, it is interesting that the phosphates, which are usually regarded as the most mobile portion of the DNA structure, give correlation times larger than the cytosine bases, generally regarded to be a rigid part of the molecule.[45,46]

## B    ARUGOMYCIN–DNA INTERACTIONS

Arugomycin (Figure 10) has the most complex molecular architecture of all the anthracyclines so far isolated and, remarkably, also binds to the DNA double helix through intercalation.[47,48] Parallel footprinting studies with nogalamycin indicate that both drugs have similar sequence specificities with "natural" DNA.[48] A combination of NMR data and molecular

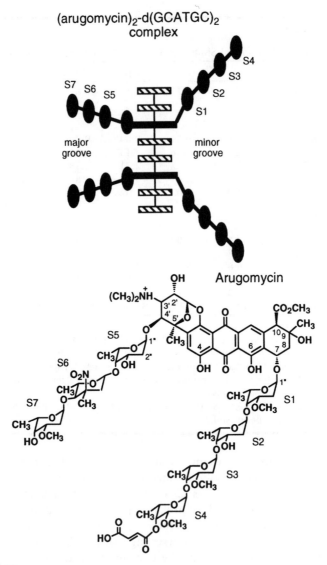

**FIGURE 10**

Structure of arugomycin (bottom) and a schematic representation (top) of the 2:1 complex with $d$(GCATGC)$_2$.

modelling (energy minimisation and molecular dynamics calculations) has been used to investigate the interaction of arugomycin with the hexamer duplex $d$(GCATGC)$_2$, permitting comparison of structural features with earlier studies of the same hexamer with nogalamycin (see above).[47] Surprisingly, the hexamer duplex is able to accommodate two drug molecules in close proximity at the symmetry-related 5′-CpA and 5′-TpG binding sites in the manner described for nogalamycin,[30,31] and as represented schematically in Figure 10. Ligand-induced complexation shifts observed for the nucleotide resonances H1/H3, H1′, H6/H8, and H2/H5/CH$_3$ are plotted against sequence position in Figure 11 for both nogalamycin (Nog) and arugomycin (Aru) binding to $d$(GCATGC)$_2$. The sequence-dependent pattern of chemical-shift perturbations suggests many common features between the binding interactions of the two antibiotics. The aromatic rings of the drug appear to stack in a similar fashion with the DNA bases in each complex, inducing large perturbations to the chemical shifts of protons within the 5′-CpA (5′-TpG) step (notably, ca. 0.8 ppm for both 4TH3 and 3AH2 in each complex).

## 1   Structure of the (Arugomycin)$_2$–d(GCATGC)$_2$ Complex

Molecular-modelling studies, guided by 24 intermolecular NOE constraints, point to many structure-stabilising interactions that are common to both arugomycin and nogalamycin. The orientation of the 2′-hydroxyl of arugomycin is defined similarly by the constrained bicyclo sugar in such a way as to form a direct hydrogen bond (1.8 Å) to the N7 of the guanine base at the 5′-TpG step (Figure 12A),[47] while the charged $N,N$-dimethylamino group is also located in the major groove close to the guanine O6/N7 at the (C·G)·(A·T) intercalation site, as discussed for nogalamycin. The intermolecular hydrogen bond found for the 4′-hydroxyl substituent of nogalamycin is absent in the case of arugomycin. Modification at the C4′ position on the bicyclo sugar of arugomycin, together with a change of stereochemistry (see Figure 10), provides the point of attachment for one of the extended sugar chains. The proposed interaction of the 2′-hydroxyl with guanine N7 in the major groove is conserved and emerges as a likely contributor to DNA sequence recognition

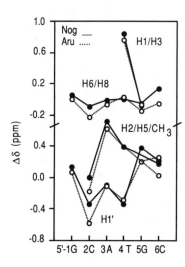

**FIGURE 11**

Perturbations to the ¹H chemical shifts of $d$(GCATGC)$_2$ induced by nogalamycin (Nog) and arugomycin (Aru). (Data from Searle, M.S., et al., *Nucleic Acids Res.*, 19, 2897–2906, 1991. With permission of Oxford University Press.)

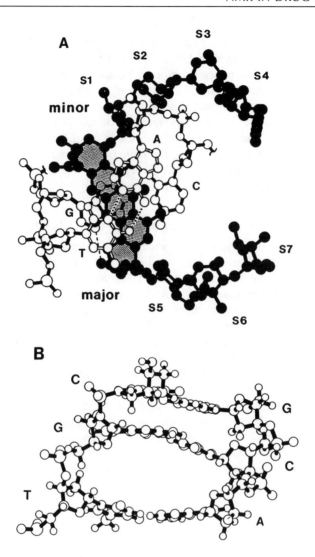

**FIGURE 12**

(A) Portion of the energy-minimised structure of the (arugomycin)$_2$–$d$(GCATGC)$_2$ complex (viewed down the helix axis) illustrating the stacking geometry at one of the $d$(5'-CA)·$d$(5'-TG) intercalation sites. Antibiotic sugar chains are located in both the major and the minor groove. (B) Base-pair buckling at one of the $d$(5'-GCA)·$d$(5'-TGC) intercalation sites of arugomycin in the energy-minimised structure of the complex. Drug removed for clarity. (Figures from Searle, M.S., et al., *Nucleic Acids Res.*, 19, 2897–2906, 1991. With permission of Oxford University Press.)

within this group of anthracyclines. Potential differences in binding contributions between the two antibiotics are evident in the extent and complementarity of their interactions with the minor groove. The nogalose sugar has five methyl/methoxy substituents and fits snugly into the minor groove with excellent van der Waals complementarity (Figure 8); in contrast, arugomycin appears to be significantly less hydrophobic than nogalamycin, having only two methyl groups on the equivalent sugar residue (S1; Figure 10); this structural difference is reflected in many fewer intermolecular NOEs between arugomycin sugar S1 and nucleotide protons located in the minor groove.

Semiquantitative interpretation of the NOE data, together with the results of modelling studies on the 2:1 complex of arugomycin with $d(GCATGC)_2$, again indicates a buckled, wedge-shaped intercalation site. The structure of the trinucleotide binding site $d(GCA) \cdot d(TGC)$, illustrating the base-pair geometry (drug removed for clarity), is highlighted in Figure 12B.[47] While the internucleotide separation 4TH1'-5GH8 is significantly increased (>5 Å) compared with the standard B-DNA geometry, with the subsequent loss of the corresponding NOE (data not shown), the distance between 2CH1' and 3AH8 on the opposing strand is only slightly increased, and the corresponding NOE remains within the detectable limit (<5 Å), consistent with this binding-site geometry. Although these features appear to be common to both arugomycin and nogalamycin complexes with $d(GCATGC)_2$, arugomycin produces far less dramatic downfield shifts in the $^{31}P$ NMR spectrum of the hexamer (0.5 vs. 1.5 ppm for nogalamycin), which suggests, at least qualitatively, that arugomycin may unwind the helix less markedly at the intercalation site than nogalamycin. High-resolution crystal structures will undoubtedly be required to resolve these subtle conformational differences.

## 2   The Role of the Sugar Residues of Arugomycin in Binding

The hexamer duplex chosen for the above study is too short to be able to fully accommodate the sugar chains of the antibiotic within the grooves; consequently, only a limited opportunity is available to examine the role of the sugar chains of arugomycin in the binding interaction with DNA *in vivo*. However, intramolecular NOE data, together with the modelling studies, do shed some light on the involvement of these sugars in the DNA-recognition process. The orientation of S5, attached at the C4' position on the bicyclo sugar, is defined by intramolecular NOEs to protons on the adjacent bicyclo sugar, and aglycon ring D. Coupled with the apparent absence of NOEs between protons of S5 and any DNA protons, the data indicate that S5 plays little part in the binding interaction and extends away from the major groove into solution (see Figure 12A). In the minor groove, intra- and intermolecular NOEs position the S1 sugar in a conformation similar to that found for the nogalose sugar (as described above). In the complex with $d(GCATGC)_2$, the 3"-OMe (OMe$_j$) of both nogalamycin and arugomycin gives a strong NOE to the deoxyribose H1' of the terminal nucleotide 6C, which confirms that the two sugars appear to adopt the same orientation and occupy the same region of conformational space within the minor groove.[47] The arugomycin sugar rings S2, S3, and S4 extend beyond the ends of this short duplex, and it remains to be established whether this extended, apparently flexible chain would interact with the minor groove in a longer sequence of DNA. It is noteworthy that none of the sugar units involved has particularly suitable hydrogen bond donors or acceptors, nor offers significant hydrophobic surface areas for burial (contrast the nogalose sugar). Further, the likely repulsive interaction of the carboxylate group of S5 with the DNA phosphates would seem to preclude binding of the S2-S3-S4 chain within the minor groove of DNA *in vivo*. In the complex of arugomycin with $d(GCATGC)_2$, interactions that are likely to account for some degree of sequence recognition appear to be largely confined to structural features that are also common to nogalamycin. These conclusions seem to correlate well with the results of "footprinting" experiments with "natural" DNA, which identify a binding-site size for arugomycin that is identical to that for nogalamycin, and would appear to preclude any significant role for arugomycin sugars, at least in protecting against DNAse I cleavage.[48]

---

# III  QUINOMYCIN ANTIBIOTICS AND LUZOPEPTIN

## A  QUINOMYCIN ANTIBIOTICS

The quinomycin antitumour antibiotics are a family of cyclic depsipeptides, of which echinomycin is probably the best known. Their biological properties are associated with their ability to bind to the DNA of susceptible cells[49] through the process of bisintercalation.[50] The two quinoxaline-2-carboxyl chromophores of echinomycin give the molecule the necessary staplelike configuration for bracketing its preferred 5'-CpG binding site. Molecular details of the structure of the drug–DNA complex were first elucidated by X-ray crystallographic analysis and revealed a remarkable drug-induced feature.[51] The A·T base pairs flanking the intercalation sites in the 2:1 complex with the hexamer duplex $d(CGTACG)_2$ adopt the Hoogsteen base-pairing scheme (Figure 13), in which the adenine base is flipped into a *syn* orientation about the glycosidic bond. The consequence of such a radical drug-induced change in conformation is to make the minor groove narrower by bringing the C1' deoxyribose atoms on opposite strands approximately 2 Å closer together. The proposed benefit of such a conformational change is the opportunity for better van der Waals complementarity between the peptide antibiotic and the walls of the minor groove. A number of solution NMR studies[5,38,52-56] have focused attention on detecting such a radical drug-induced structural change in solution, with some interesting results.

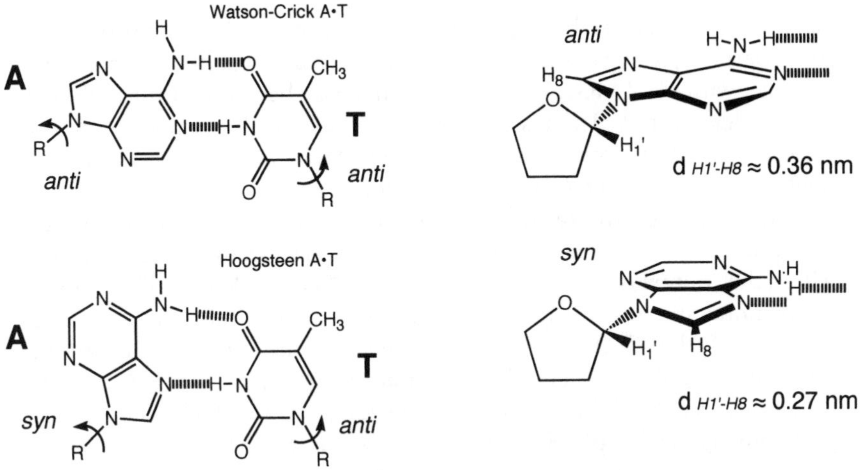

**FIGURE 13**

Hydrogen-bonding scheme in Hoogsteen and Watson–Crick A·T base pairs. Effects of purine *syn* and *anti* glycosidic torsion angles on intranucleotide H1'–H8 interproton distances (C2'-endo deoxyribose conformation).

The purine glycosidic bond angle associated with Watson–Crick (*anti*) and Hoogsteen (*syn*) base-pairing schemes (Figure 13) produces significant differences in the intensity of H8 → H1' intranucleotide NOEs such as to provide a convenient method of discriminating between the two hydrogen-bonding schemes. In the *syn* orientation the H8 → H1' NOE (proton–proton separation 2.5–2.7 Å) is of intensity comparable to that for the cytosine H5 → H6 (reference distance 2.5 Å); in contrast, in the *anti* orientation the H8 → H1' NOE is considerably weaker (corresponding distance 3.5–3.7 Å).

NMR studies have identified Hoogsteen A·T and G·C[+] base-pair formation at terminal sites in short DNA duplexes.[5,38] Initial focus on 5'-pur–C–G–pyr and 5'-pyr–C–G–pur tetranucleotides, containing a central CpG drug-binding site, established important sequence-dependent differences in conformation. For example, in complexes of echinomycin with $d(ACGT)_2$,[38] the terminal A·T base pairs were shown to adopt the Hoogsteen conformation (Figure 13), while with $d(TCGA)_2$ the preferred configuration involves Watson–Crick base pairing throughout. In analogous studies with the duplexes $d(GCGC)_2$ and $d(CCGG)_2$,[5] a pH-dependent structural transition is detected for the echinomycin–$d(GCGC)_2$ complex; downfield shifts of the phosphate resonances of G1-p-C2 and G3-p-C4 occur with a transition p$K_a$ of 5.1. A quantitative examination of the intensity of H8 → H1' intranucleotide NOEs readily attributes this transition to a change from a G1 *anti* to a G1 *syn* glycosidic conformation at low pH. The observation is consistent with the formation of a protonated cytosine, which permits the formation of a G1·C4[+] Hoogsteen base pair at low pH, and establishes a pH-dependent switch from Watson–Crick to Hoogsteen pairing under acidic conditions. In contrast, the echinomycin complex with $d(CCGG)_2$ remains Watson–Crick base paired throughout, independent of pH. The results from the studies with tetramer duplexes indicate that Hoogsteen pairing is more stable in 5′-pur-C-G-pyr sequences than in 5′-pyr–C–G–pur sequences.

Feigon and co-workers have described the bisintercalation complexes of echinomycin with the same -ACGT- and -TCGA- binding sites but within the context of the duplexes $d(ACGTACGT)_2$ and $d(TCGATCGA)_2$, each containing two drug-binding sites,[52,54] and within the sequence $d(ACGTATACGT)_2$,[55] where the binding sites are separated by several intervening A·T base pairs. The magnitude of adenosine H8 → H1′ intramolecular NOEs indicates that at low temperature (1°C) the A·T base pairs flanking the 5′-CpG binding sites in the complex with $d(ACGTACGT)_2$ adopt the Hoogsteen conformation. However, as the temperature is raised, the interior Hoogsteen base pairs are destabilised, with the possibility of exchange between Hoogsteen and a Watson–Crick paired state, or an open state.[52] The terminal A·T base pairs, which are not constrained by the helix in the same way as the internal base pairs, are stably Hoogsteen base paired up to ca. 45°C. In the complex with $d(TCGATCGA)_2$, no A·T Hoogsteen base pairing is detected;[54] moreover, the internal Watson–Crick A·T base pairs even appear to be stabilised by drug binding, with little structural change over a wide temperature range (0 to 45°C).

The effects of echinomycin binding on the conformation of an extended sequence of A·T base pairs has been investigated within the duplex $d(ACGTATACGT)_2$.[55] As previously concluded, the terminal A·T base pairs are stably Hoogsteen paired; however, none of the four internal A·T base pairs are either stable or Hoogsteen-paired, but all appear to be destabilised relative to those in the ligand-free DNA. Drug binding is reported to lead to significant helix unwinding that is propagated from the two bisintercalation sites into the intervening region of A·T base pairs. Long-range conformational changes induced by echinomycin binding have been examined with the sequence $d(AAACGTTT)_2$.[5] By analogy with studies of $d(ACGT)_2$, it was anticipated that the complex would contain a Hoogsteen alignment of A·T base pairs flanking the ligand-binding site, and the possibility of a similar configuration for the remaining A·T base pairs. Quantitative NOE measurements reveal that the intensities of all H6/H8 → H1′ NOEs are weak with respect to the cytosine H5 → H6 internal reference, demonstrating *anti* glycosidic torsion angles and Watson–Crick A·T base pairing throughout. Additional support for this scheme is the observation of NOEs from thymine imino proton (H3) to base-paired adenine H2 that characterise the Watson–Crick hydrogen-bonding scheme, but that are expected to be absent in the Hoogsteen arrangement (see Figure 13).

The structural data so far reported from solution NMR studies of DNA complexes with the quinomycin antibiotics emphasise the importance of DNA helical constraints, particularly base pair–base pair stacking interactions, on the stability of Hoogsteen base pairs adjacent to drug-binding sites. In studies with 5′-pur-C-G-pyr binding sites, the NMR results have identified a destabilisation of A·T base pairs in the flanking positions when these base pairs occupy nonterminal sites in DNA duplexes. Binding to such sites also appears to be associated with considerable drug-induced helix unwinding. In the light of these data, helix unwinding and base-pair destabilisation present a more plausible alternative explanation for the increased sensitivity to "footprinting" reagents observed for A – T rich regions flanking echinomycin-binding sites,[57] rather than a model invoking Hoogsteen base pairing.[58] Recent results suggest that structural changes induced by echinomycin are not confined to regions immediately adjacent to the drug-binding site but are able to be cooperatively propagated over several turns of the DNA helix.[59] Together these data cast considerable doubt on the biological relevance of ligand-induced Hoogsteen base pairing in DNA complexes *in vivo*.

## B    Interaction of UK-65,662 (QN) with D(ACGT)$_2$ and D(GACGTC)$_2$

### 1    Hoogsteen vs. Watson–Crick Base Pairing

Many of the structural features of the drug–DNA interaction are now illustrated for complexes of d(ACGT)$_2$ and d(GACGTC)$_2$ with UK-65,662 (B), a closely related member of the quinomycin family of antibiotics (Figure 14).[53,56] UK-65,662 (B), henceforth denoted QN, contains several novel residues, including 3-hydroxy-quinaldic acid chromophores as replacements for the quinoxaline rings of echinomycin, and methyl-cyclopropyl groups replacing the valine residues. The binding of the antibiotic to d(ACGT)$_2$ is characterised by similar ligand-induced features to those reported for echinomycin,[38] namely, stable Hoogsteen A·T base pairs. In the portion of the 100-ms NOESY spectrum of the QN-d(ACGT)$_2$ complex illustrated in Figure 15, the A1H8 → H1′ NOE is of comparable intensity to the C2 H5 → H6 reference peak, while all remaining H6/H8 → H1′ interactions are weak by comparison, indicative of a predominantly *syn* conformation for A1, but *anti* conformations for C2, G3, and T4. In contrast, all base pairs in the QN-d(GACGTC)$_2$ complex, including the A·T base pairs within the same ACGT binding site, exhibit very weak AH8 → H1′ NOE cross-peaks (Figure 15), indicative of glycosidic torsion angles that are predominantly *anti* and that equate with Watson–Crick hydrogen bonding throughout.

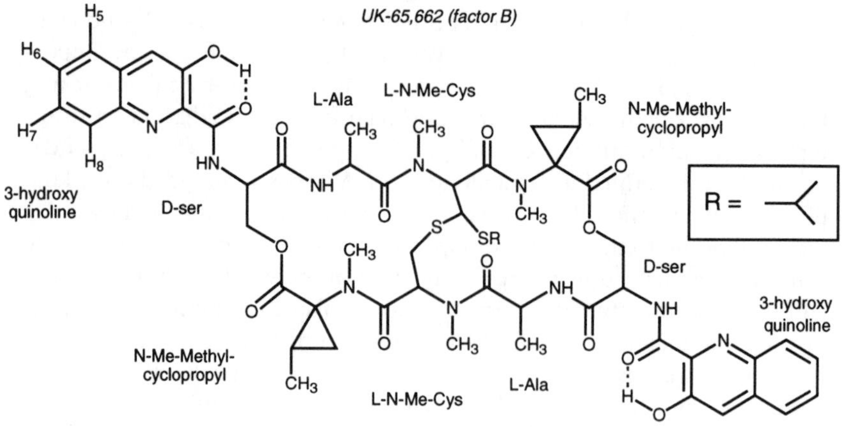

**FIGURE 14**

Structure of UK-65,662 (QN). In the structure of echinomycin, L-N-methylvaline residues replace the methylcyclopropyl units, while the quinoxaline ring system replaces the hydroxy-quinoline substituents shown.

An analysis of the preferred deoxyribose conformations from $^1$H–$^1$H coupling constant data (see above), and relative intensities of intranucleotide NOEs (H6/H8 → H3' vs. H6/H8 → H2'), indicates that the cytosine deoxyribose at the intercalation site in both $d(A\underline{C}GT)_2$ and $d(GA\underline{C}GTC)_2$ complexes (base underlined) adopts a predominantly $N$-type (C3'-endo) conformation, as also found in crystal structures of quinomycin and triostin complexes.[51] Coupling constants for C2 in the $d(ACGT)_2$ complex ($J_{1'-2'}$ = 3.2 Hz and $J_{1'-2''}$ = 8.8 Hz) can be described in terms of a single conformer with pseudorotation phase angle ($P$) in the range 34–36°, with a pucker amplitude of 35°[34]. A consequence of a predominantly $N$-type conformation is the considerable shortening of the H6 → H3' distance ($\approx$2.7 Å[21]) compared with that found for the standard (C2'-endo) B-DNA geometry where the H6 → H3' NOE appears as a relatively weak interaction ($\approx$3.6 Å[21]); such differences in average proton–proton distances are readily discerned in the 50-ms NOESY spectrum of the complex, where the C2H6 → C2H3' NOE is of comparable intensity to the cytosine H5 → H6 reference distance ($\approx$2.5 Å). All other deoxyribose conformations in both $d(ACGT)_2$ and $d(GACGTC)_2$ complexes are described by predominantly (70–90%) C2'-endo conformations.[56]

## 2   Intermolecular Interactions Between QN and the DNA Minor Groove

Many strong intermolecular NOEs are detected in both complexes between the bound antibiotic and the DNA minor groove that point to very similar binding interactions with the 5'-CpG step at the centre of each

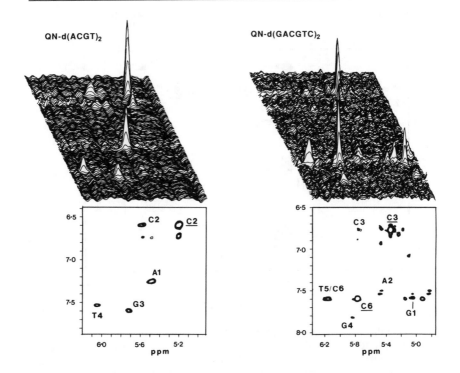

**FIGURE 15**

Stack plots and contour plots of the 100-ms NOESY spectra of complexes of UK-65,662 (QN) with the duplexes $d$(ACGT)$_2$ and $d$(GACGTC)$_2$ recorded at 20°C. The portions of the spectra highlight relative intensities of H1'-H6/H8 inter- and intranucleotide NOEs. Intranucleotide cross-peaks are labelled, together with cytosine H5–H6 reference peaks (underlined). The antibiotic lacks a twofold symmetry axis and partially removes the twofold symmetry of the two duplexes under study. This is clearly visible only for the A2H8 resonances in the QN–$d$(GACGTC)$_2$ complex. (Data from Searle, M.S. and Wickham, G., *FEBS Lett.*, 272, 171–174, 1990. With permission.)

duplex, despite the fact that the flanking A·T base pairs on either side of this site have quite different conformations. Some of these interactions are now highlighted for the QN complex with $d$(GACGTC)$_2$ (Figure 16).[56] The C$_\beta$H$_3$ of the Ala residues are pushed into van der Waals contact with the deoxyribose rings of both C3 and G4, with NOEs readily detected in 50-ms NOESY spectra. Similarly short-range interactions are observed between the methyl group of the cyclopropyl residues and the deoxyribose of A2 (in particular A2H1'). The orientation of the quinoline chromophores with respect to the depsipeptide are defined by NOEs between quinoline H8 and C$_\alpha$H/C$_\beta$H$_3$ of the methylcyclopropyl residues; the long axis of the chromophores are aligned parallel with the minor axis of the depsipeptide, giving the antibiotic the staplelike geometry necessary for bisintercalation. Strong interactions are evident between the quinoline H7 of the antibiotic and A2H1' and A2H2'/2", while the adjacent C$\alpha$Hs of

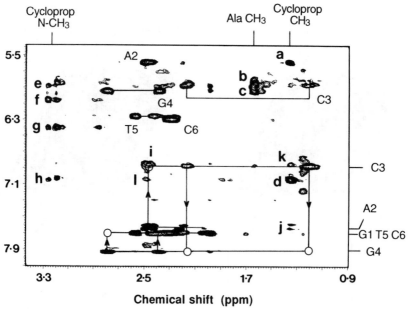

**FIGURE 16**

Portion of the 400-MHz NOESY spectrum (250-ms mixing time) of the complex of QN with d(GACGTC)₂ in D₂O solution at 20°C. The sequential-assignment pathway is traced via base H6/H8 and deoxyribose H2'/H2" resonances. Small circles represent the positions of NOEs that are normally diagnostic of a standard B-DNA conformation but which are not observed in this spectrum. Labels on the right-hand axis indicate specific base H6 or H8 assignments (e.g., G1 = G1H8). In the upper part of the figure, cross-peaks are labelled pairwise corresponding to deoxyribose H1'–H2' and H1'–H2" of each nucleotide. The positions of several antibiotic methyl groups are identified along the top of the figure. The following NOEs are highlighted: (a) cycloprop CH₃ → A2H1', (b) Ala CH₃ → C3H1', (c) Ala CH₃ → G4H1', (d) cycloprop CH₃ → QN H8, (e) cycloprop N-CH₃ → C3H1', (f) cycloprop N-CH₃ → Cyst CαH (2), (g) cycloprop N-CH₃ → Cyst CαH (1), (h) cycloprop N-CH₃ → QN H8, (i) QN H7 → A2H2'/H2", (j) cycloprop CH₃ → A2H2, (k) cycloprop CH₃ → QN H7, (l) QN H8 → A2H2'/H2". (Data from Searle, M.S. *Biochem. J.* 1994, <u>304</u>, 967–979. With permission.)

the Ser residues are in close proximity to T5H1'. The structure of the QN-d(GACGTC)₂ complex is shown in stereo in Figure 17. NOE data collected in H₂O solutions (Figure 18) reveal many inter- and intramolecular interactions that provide additional conformational constraints. The slowly exchanging (nonequivalent) 3-OH groups give an array of intermolecular NOEs to the deoxyribose H1', H2', and H2" of G4, suggesting that the quinoline chromophores stack on the G4 base with the 3-OH in van der Waals contact with the deoxyribose ring; an NOE from the T5 methyl group to 3-OH positions the thymine bases on top of the quinoline rings. The NOEs from C3 and G4 deoxyribose protons, but also the G4 imino proton (Figure 18), locate the alanine methyl groups and N-Me of the cyclopropyl residues in close contact with the minor groove. NOEs from Ala NH to G4H1, G4H1', and G4H2' locate the NH close to the edge

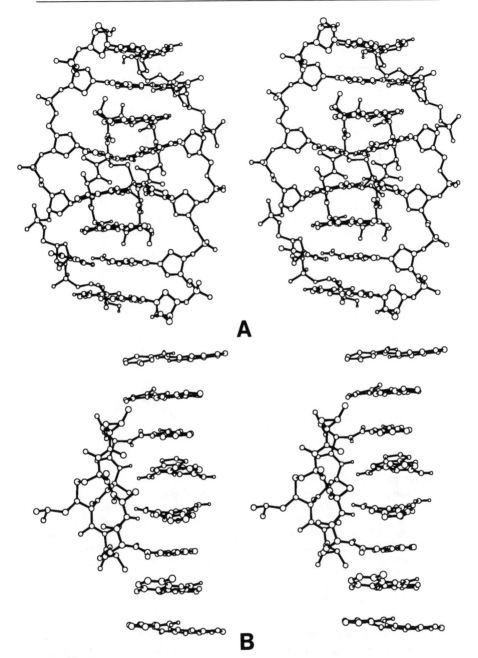

**FIGURE 17**

Stereoview of the QN-$d$(GACGTC)$_2$ complex determined from NOE-restrained molecular dynamics calculations. In A, the complex is viewed directly into the major groove with the drug intercalated around the central two base pairs. Significant unwinding of the DNA duplex is apparent. In B, the complex has been rotated by 90 degrees and the sugar-phosphate backbone removed to show the intercalation geometry more clearly. (Data from Searle, M.S. *Biochem. J.* 1994, <u>304</u>, 967–979. With permission.)

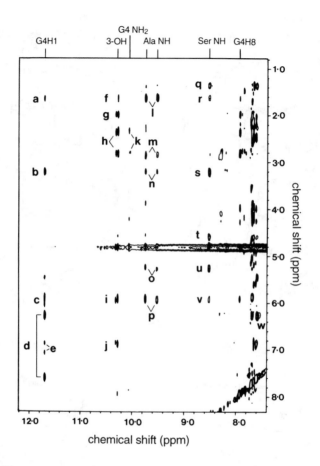

**FIGURE 18**

Downfield portion (8–12 ppm) of the 500-MHz NOESY spectrum (300-ms mixing time) of the complex of QN with $d(GACGTC)_2$ in 90% $H_2O$/10% $D_2O$ solution at 20°C. The following NOEs (a)–(w) are highlighted: [NOEs from G4H1; (a)–(e)] (a) Ala $CH_3$; (b) cycloprop N-$CH_3$; (c) G4H1'; (d) C3N$H_2$; (e) QN H7/H8; [NOEs from 3'-OH; (f)–(j)] (f) Ala $CH_3$; (g) T5$CH_3$; (h) G4H2'/H2"; (i) G4H1'; (j) QN H7; (k) G4N$H_2$ → G4H2'/H2"; [NOEs from Ala NH; (l)–(p)] (l) Ala $CH_3$; (m) G4H2'; (n) cycloprop N-$CH_3$; (o) Ser CαH; (p) G4H1'; [NOEs from Ser NH; (q)–(v)] (q) cycloprop $CH_3$; (r) Ala $CH_3$; (s) cycloprop N-$CH_3$; (t) Ser CβH$_2$; (u) Ser CαH; (v) G4H1'; and (w) G4H1 → C3N$H_2$. (From Searle, M.S. *Biochem. J.* 1994, <u>304</u>, 967–979. With permission.)

of the guanine base consistent with their involvement in hydrogen-bonding interactions with guanine N3, as identified in echinomycin and triostin crystal structures.[51] Large downfield shifts of the Ala NH resonances of ca. 3.0 ppm add further support to the persistence of these interactions in solution complexes of QN. The intermolecular NOE data for the $d(GACGTC)_2$ complex is summarised in Table 3.

**TABLE 3**

Intermolecular NOE Data for the QN–$d$(GACGTC)$_2$ Complex at 20°C

| Drug Proton | DNA Proton |
|---|---|
| c-prop-N-Me | C3H1′ (m), G3H1 (m) |
| Me | A2H1′ (s), A2H2/A2H8 (w), A2H4′ (m), C3H1′ (w), C3H4′ (m), C3H2′/H2″ (w) |
| CβH | C3H2′/H2″H1′ (w), C3H4′ (w), C3H6 (w) |
| Ala CβH$_3$ | C3H1′ (s), C3H2′/H2″ (s), C3H4′ (m), G4H1′ (s), G4H2′/H2″ (s), G4H4′ (s), G4H1 (w) |
| CαH | G4H4′ (m) |
| NH | G4H1 (s), G4H1 (m), G4H2′ (w) |
| Quin H7/H8 | A2H2′/H2″ (s), A2H3′ (w), A2H1′ (s), A1H8/H2 (w), C3H1′ (w), C2H5 (H7) (m), C3H6 (H8) (m/s), G4H1 (w) |
| 3-OH | G4H1 (m), G4H2′/H2″ (m), T5CH$_3$ (m) |
| Ser CαH | T5H1′ (s), T5H4′ (m), T5H5′/H5″ (m) |
| CβH$_2$ | A2H2 (w), T5H1′ (w) |
| NH | G4H1′ (w), G4H1 (m) |

*Note:* NOEs are designated strong (s), medium (m), or weak (w). NOEs designated strong are detected at mixing times between 50 and 100 ms.

Data from Searle, M.S. *Biochem. J.* 1994, <u>304</u>, 967–979. With permission.

## 3   *Drug-Induced Helix Unwinding*

The effects of drug binding on DNA conformation are highlighted in the expanded portion of the 250-ms NOESY spectrum of the QN–$d$(GACGTC)$_2$ complex (Figure 16) by illustrating the intensity of the internucleotide NOEs H6/H8 ($i$) → H2′/H2″ ($i$ – 1). While the intranucleotide NOEs [H6/H8 ($i$) → H2′/H2″ ($i$)] are generally readily detected (reflecting standard B-DNA glycosidic torsion angles), the internucleotide interactions [H6/H8 ($i$) → H2′/H2″ ($i$ – 1)], by comparison, are generally very weak, indicative of nonstandard helical twist. While such perturbations to NOE intensities are expected at the sites of intercalation, drug binding also produces significant unwinding at the C3pG4 step. The G4H8 → C3H2″ correlation, which corresponds to a short-range interaction in B-DNA (guanine H8 → pyrimidine H2″ ≈ 2.5 Å[21]), is undetected in the 250-ms NOESY spectrum of the QN–$d$(GACGTC)$_2$ complex (Figure 16). The very low intensity of this interaction is indicative of a dramatically increased proton–proton separation (>5 Å). Coupled with the fact that the C3 deoxyribose sugar of $d$(GA<u>C</u>GTC)$_2$ repuckers to a predominantly C3′-endo conformation (see above), the data lend support for a pronounced drug-induced unwinding of the duplex in solution as is evident for the structure shown in Figure 17. These effects are also apparent for the complex of QN with $d$(ACGT)$_2$, and have been noted in earlier studies with echinomycin complexes in solution (see above).

## C   LUZOPEPTIN–DNA INTERACTIONS

Luzopeptin is a cyclic depsipeptide antibiotic that exhibits activity against a variety of experimental animal tumours and bears structural resemblance to the quinomycin antibiotics. The structure of luzopeptin is illustrated in Figure 19 and incorporates several unusual amino acid residues such as L-β-hydroxy-N-methylvaline and *trans* (3S,4S)-4-acetoxy-2,3,4,5-tetrahydropyridazine-3-carboxylic acid, together with two 3-hydroxy-6-methoxyquinaldic acid chromophores per molecule. X-ray crystallography[60] and $^1$H NMR spectroscopy in CDCl$_3$[61] have shown that luzopeptin possesses twofold symmetry in both the crystalline and solution environments. The depsipeptide ring of luzopeptin adopts a right-handed, twisted rectangular β-sheetlike conformation stabilised by two *trans*-annular hydrogen bonds (Figure 19).[60] Luzopeptin can adopt the necessary "staplelike" conformation suitable for a bisintercalative mode of binding to DNA, reminiscent of its quinomycin and triostin relatives. An estimated interchromophore separation of between 12 and 14.5 Å (based upon the antibiotic crystal structure) suggested that luzopeptin has the capacity to span up to 3 base pairs when bound to DNA. The $^1$H NMR studies of the interaction of luzopeptin with the hexamer duplex $d$(GCATGC)$_2$[62] established that binding occurs with full retention of the dyad symmetry of the duplex. Intermolecular NOE data, together with chemical-shift perturbations to base and imino proton resonances are consistent with the quinoline chromophores in the complex bracketing the two A·T base pairs by intercalating at the 5′-CpA and 5′-TpG steps with the depsipeptide ring lying in the minor groove. No sequential NOEs are detected between the

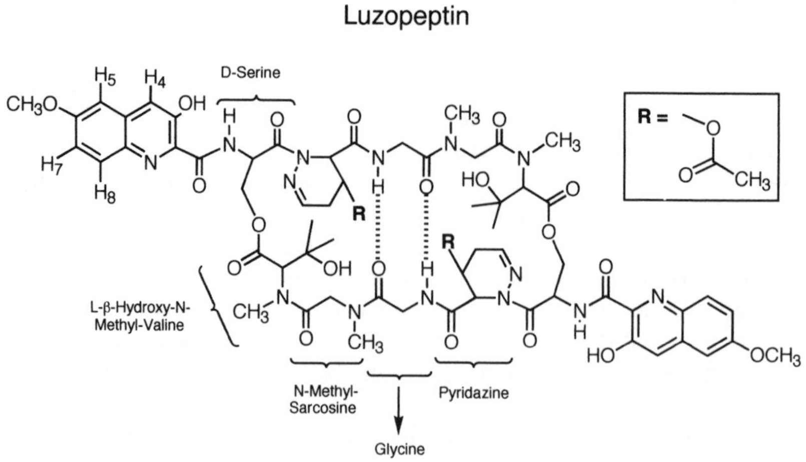

### Luzopeptin

**FIGURE 19**
Structure of luzopeptin.

imino protons of 4T and 5G, confirming that G·C on A·T base-pair stacking interactions in the complex are disrupted by intercalation of the drug chromophores. The quinoline H5, H7, and methoxy protons give NOEs to 2CH5/H6 and 3AH8, indicating that the chromophores are intercalated with their substituted edge lying in the major groove, the chromophores stacking principally on the adenine base. There is no evidence for drug-induced Hoogsteen base pairing in the complex, as observed with some echinomycin complexes; all glycosidic bond angles in the luzopeptin–$d$(GCATGC)$_2$ complex are typical of B-DNA. A model of the complex was proposed in which the *trans*-annular hydrogen bonds (Figure 19) between facing glycine residues across the depsipeptide ring are broken, followed by rotation of the amide groups by 90° toward the DNA minor groove, enabling the glycine NHs to hydrogen bond to the thymine O2s at the A–T binding site.[62] NMR studies by Zhang and Patel on a luzopeptin complex with the tetramer $d$(CATG)$_2$ have produced a high-resolution structure of the complex utilising a large body of both intra- and intermolecular NOE data as restraints for molecular dynamics calculations.[12]

The data provide a detailed description of significant conformational changes in the antibiotic on binding that accounts for the 2-base pairs-sandwich-binding model, and the subsequent alignment of the glycine residues to form intermolecular hydrogen bonds to the thymine O2s in the minor groove. These hydrogen-bonding interactions appear to be achieved by a conformational change on binding from a *trans*-peptide configuration at the pyridazine–glycine and glycine–sarcosine linkages (as found in the crystal structure of luzopeptin[60]) to *cis*-peptide bonds in the $d$(CATG)$_2$ complex in solution.[12] Intense NOE cross-peaks in the 75-ms NOESY spectrum from the Gly C$_\alpha$H$_2$ protons to the Sar C$_\alpha$H$_2$ characterise the formation of a *cis*-peptide conformation. The consequence of *cis*-peptide bonds in these positions is to increase the separation of the long sides of the rectangular β-sheetlike structure with subsequent reorientation of the glycine amide protons to form direct hydrogen bonds with thymine O2 on the floor of the minor groove. The structural transition from free ligand to bound conformation is illustrated in Figure 20.[12] The bound conformation is readily accommodated within the minor groove of a Watson–Crick base-paired duplex. Additional intermolecular hydrogen-bonding potential is identified in these structures between the peptide carbonyl groups at the serine-valine steps (located on the short sides of the rectangular depsipeptide of the antibiotic) and the exposed 2-amino protons of the two G4 bases. Intermolecular contacts (van der Waals/hydrophobic interactions) between the cyclic depsipeptide extend over much of the two interacting surfaces, illustrating the excellent complementarity between the "induced-fit" conformation of luzopeptin and the minor groove. Features of the interaction are well illustrated by the structure of the complex viewed from the minor groove (Figure 21).

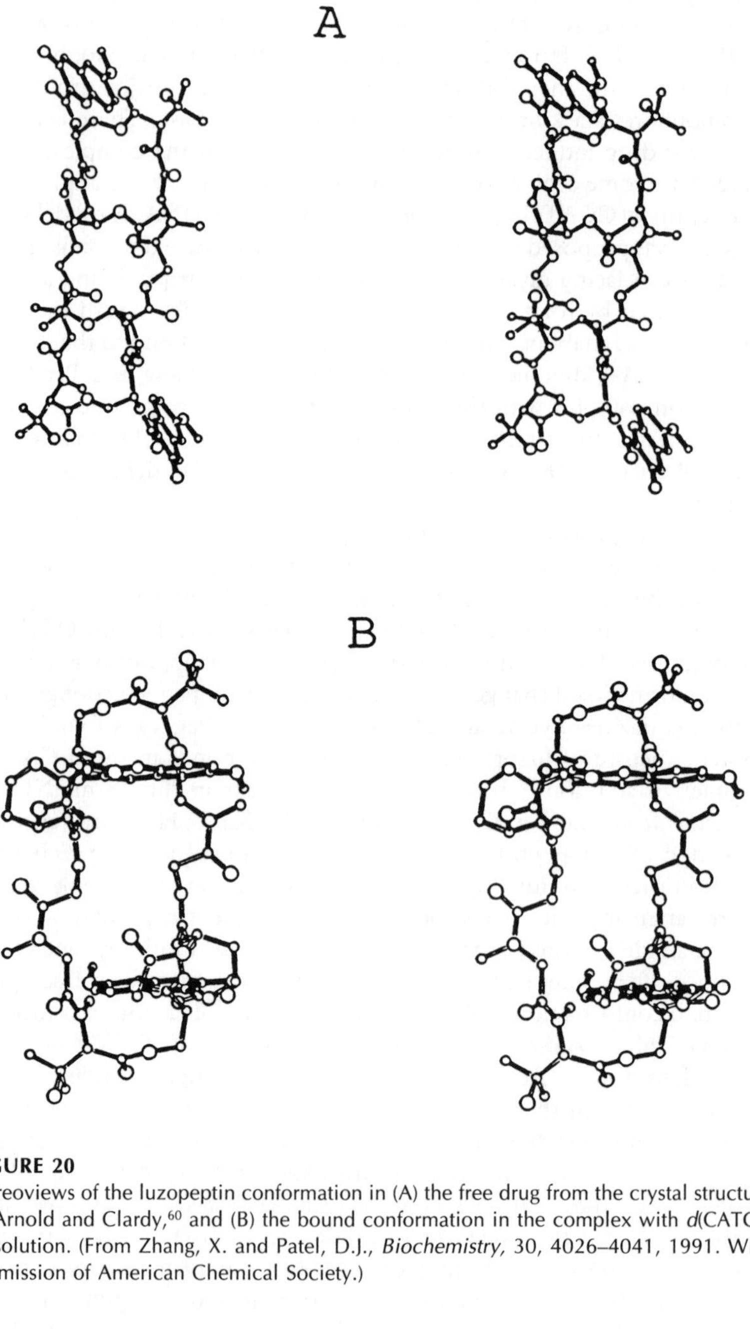

**FIGURE 20**
Stereoviews of the luzopeptin conformation in (A) the free drug from the crystal structure of Arnold and Clardy,[60] and (B) the bound conformation in the complex with $d(CATG)_2$ in solution. (From Zhang, X. and Patel, D.J., *Biochemistry*, 30, 4026–4041, 1991. With permission of American Chemical Society.)

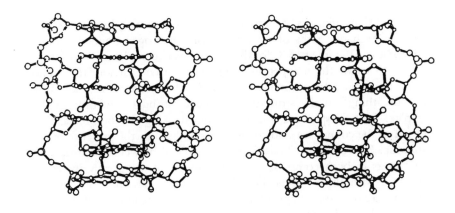

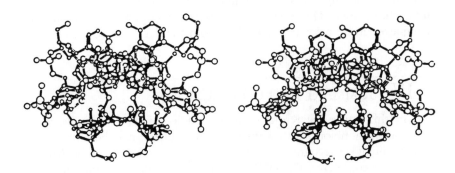

**FIGURE 21**
Stereoviews of the luzopeptin–*d*(CATG)₂ complex. (TOP) View into the minor groove. (BOTTOM) View down the helix axis emphasising the positioning of the cyclic depsipeptide in the minor groove. (From Zhang, X. and Patel, D.J., *Biochemistry*, 30, 4026–4041, 1991. With permission of American Chemical Society.)

### D   HYDROGEN EXCHANGE STUDIES OF LUZOPEPTIN AND ECHINOMYCIN COMPLEXES

Investigations of proton exchange rates in a number of DNA complexes of sequence-specific antibiotics have been reported by Leroy and co-workers.[63,64] These studies have provided new insights into the ability of drug molecules to perturb DNA stability and dynamics. Studies of complexes of luzopeptin bound to the central ApT sites of the duplexes *d*(CCCATGGG)₂ and *d*(AGCATGCT)₂, and echinomycin bound to the CpG sites of *d*(AAACGTTT)₂ and *d*(CCAAACGTTTGG)₂ have been described.[64] The lifetimes of these complexes are extremely long, estimated from the exchange rates of intermolecularly hydrogen-bonded peptide NHs to be ca. 20 min at 15°C for the echinomycin complexes, and ca. four days at 45°C for the luzopeptin complexes. By comparison, the imino proton exchange rates are much faster under these conditions, indicating that "breathing" of the structure can occur during the lifetime of the complex. Broadly speaking, the base pairs flanking the bisintercalation sites, in all the complexes studied, are not stabilised by the presence of the antibiotic. However, the 2 base pairs sandwiched between the drug aromatic rings in both complexes have lifetimes that are greatly increased compared with those of the ligand-free duplex. Base-pair dissociation constants are correspondingly reduced, but overall the lifetime of the open state is unchanged compared with the ligand-free duplexes, perhaps indicating a common base-pair opening pathway toward the major groove.[64] The action of both luzopeptin and echinomycin appears to be to "clamp" the inner base pairs tightly together, although the kinetic effects observed seem likely to be a consequence of a cooperative effect involving all the complex-stabilising interactions simultaneously, rather than from stacking interactions alone. The kinetic data for both luzopeptin and echinomycin complexes are summarised in Table 4 from the data of Leroy et al.[64]

---

# IV SUMMARY AND CONCLUSIONS

In this article the results of NMR studies of several complexes of intercalating antibiotics with synthetic DNA fragments have been presented that highlight key recognition features in solution and aspects of the dynamics of these complexes. The DNA intercalators produce dramatic effects on DNA conformation; drug molecules bind by inserting aromatic ring systems between unstacked DNA base pairs and produce substantial local unwinding of the DNA duplex. The anthracycline antibiotics intercalate "head-on" between the DNA base pairs positioning the drug aromatic rings at right angles to the long axis of the adjacent base pairs. This orientation, coupled with the unique structure of nogalamycin and arugomycin, results in bulky sugar substituents (at either end of the aromatic ring system) binding to both the major groove and the minor groove. In contrast, the quinomycin antibiotics, which are representative of the bifunctional class of intercalators, interact principally with the minor groove. Two quinoxaline rings, attached at opposite ends of a relatively rigid cyclic depsipeptide structure, stack in a parallel alignment with the DNA base pairs bracketing the preferred 5'-CpG binding site. Substantial helix unwinding appears to be a characteristic feature of the interaction. Structure-stabilising interactions in the minor groove are provided through van der Waals contacts and hydrogen bonding between the depsipeptide of the antibiotic and the edges of the base pairs,

**TABLE 4**

Base-Pair Lifetime $\tau_0$, Apparent Dissociation Constant $\alpha K_d$, and
Apparent Open State Lifetime $\alpha\tau_{open}$ of Base Pairs at, or Flanking
Bisintercalator Binding Sites in Complexes of Luzopeptin and
Echinomycin

| Complex (ns) | AT/GC | $\tau_0$(ms) | $\alpha K_d \times 10^{-6}$ | $\alpha\tau_{open}$ |
|---|---|---|---|---|
| d(CCCATGGG)$_2$ | AT[a] | 517 (0.7) | 0.09 (19) | 46 (13) |
| + Luzopeptin | GC[b] | 23 (4.0) | 1.70 (8.3) | 39 (33) |
| d(AGCATGCT)$_2$ | AT[a] | 610 (1.0) | 0.04 (18) | 24 (18) |
| + Luzopeptin | GC[b] | 15 (5.0) | 0.17 (4.7) | 2.5 (23) |
| d(AAACGTTT)$_2$ | GC[c] | 220 (3.0) | 0.12 (27) | 26 (81) |
| + Echinomycin | | | | |
| d(CCAAACGTTTGG)$_2$ | GC[d] | 78 | 0.15 | 12 |
| + Echinomycin | | | | |

*Note:* Values in parentheses are for ligand-free duplex.
[a] Complex at 35°C; free duplex at 15°C.
[b] All data at 15°C.
[c] All data at 25°C.
[d] All data at 38°C.
Data from Leroy, J.L. et al., *Biochemistry* 1992, 31, 1407–1415. With permission.

coupled with aromatic stacking interactions. Cooperatively these interactions produce significantly increased base-pair lifetimes for the G·C base pairs clamped between the drug aromatic rings. While the anthracyclines and quinomycins have essentially preorganised conformations for binding to DNA, the antibiotic luzopeptin introduces the notion of induced fit. Significant conformational changes, involving *trans* to *cis* isomerisation of several drug peptide bonds, have been shown to optimise both intermolecular interactions (hydrogen bonds) in the minor groove and the separation between quinoline moieties suitable for bisintercalative binding. A particularly striking feature of all of the complexes described here, and as illustrated by many of the figures, is the highly evolved complementarity of the interaction with the minor groove; the sugar domains (in the case of the anthracyclines) and peptide domains (in the case of the quinomycins and luzopeptin) have the necessary right-handed twist that allows them to match the groove's natural curvature and contours.

The problems associated with DNA as a target for drug action have been discussed recently.[65,66] The design strategy must take on-board sequence specificity in targeting the desired cognate sequence of DNA, and also the type of DNA modification required to produce the desired biological response. Mediation of the effects of drug binding by DNA binding proteins such as topoisomerases and transcription factors[67-69] suggests that examining drug–DNA complexes in isolation is likely to reveal only part of the impact of drug–DNA recognition on the mechanism of drug action. A detailed thermodynamic and structural description of existing sequence-specific drugs and their complexes provides an important first step toward an understanding of the recognition process.

# REFERENCES

1. Searle, M.S. *Prog. NMR Spect.* 1993, 25, 403-480.
2. Kennard, O.; Hunter, W.N. *Q. Rev. Biophys.* 1989, 22, 327-379.
3. Patel, D.J.; Shapiro, L.; Hare, D. *Q. Rev. Biophys* 1987, 20, 35-112.
4. Reid, B.R. *Q. Rev. Biophys.* 1987, 20, 1-34.
5. Gao, X.; Patel, D.J. *Q. Rev. Biophys.* 1989, 22, 93-138.
6. Neidle, S.; Pearl, L.H.; Skelly, J.V. *Biochem. J.* 1987, 243, 1-13.
7. Freemont, P.S.; Lane, A.N.; Sanderson, M.R. *Biochem. J.* 1991, 278, 1-23.
8. Gao, X.; Mirau, P.; Patel, D.J. *J. Mol. Biol.* 1992, 223, 259-279.
9. Gao, X.; Patel, D.J. *Biochemistry* 1989, 28, 751-762.
10. Pelton, J.G.; Wemmer, D.E. *Proc. Natl. Acad. Sci. USA* 1989, 86, 5723-5727.
11. Pelton, J.G.; Wemmer, D.E. *J. Am. Chem. Soc. USA* 1990, 112, 1393-1399.
12. Zhang, X.; Patel, D.J. *Biochemistry* 1991, 30, 4026-4041.
13. Kumar, S.; Joseph, T.; Singh, M.P.; Yadagiri, B.; Lown, J.W. *J. Biomol. Struct. Dyn.* 1992, 9, 853-880.
14. Dwyer, T.J.; Geierstanger, B.H.; Bathini, Y.; Lown, J.W.; Wemmer, D.E. *J. Am. Chem. Soc.* 1992, 114, 5911-5919.
15. Mrksich, M.; Wade, W.S.; Dwyer, T.J.; Geierstanger, B.H.; Wemmer, D.E.; Dervan, P.B. *Proc. Nat. Acad. Sci. USA* 1992, 89, 7586-7590.
16. Gale, E.F.; Cundliffe, E.; Reynolds, P.E.; Richmond, M.H.; Waring, M.J. *The Molecular Basis of Antibiotic Action*, 2nd ed.; John Wiley & Sons: New York, 1981; pp 258-401.
17. Bhuyan, B.K.; Deitz, A. *Antimicrob. Agents Chemother.* 1965, 836-844.
18. Bhuyan, B.K.; Reusser, F. *Cancer Res.* 1970, 30, 984-989.
19. Li, L.H.; Kuentzel, S.L.; Murch, L.I.; Pschigoda, L.M.; Kreuger, W.C. *Cancer Res.* 1979, 39, 4816-4818.
20. Fox, K.R.; Waring, M.J. *Biochim. Biophys. Acta* 1984, 802, 162-168.
21. Wüthrich, K. *NMR of Proteins and Nucleic Acids;* Wiley-Interscience: New York, 1986.
22. Searle, M.S.; Bicknell, W. *Eur. J. Biochem.* 1992, 205, 45-58.
23. Gueron, M.; Plateau, P.; Decorps, M. *Prog. NMR Spect.* 1991, 23, 135-210.
24. Liaw, Y.-C.; Robinson, H.; van der Marel, G.; van Boom. J.H.; Wang, A.H.-J. *Biochemistry* 1989, 28, 9913-9918.
25. Williams, L.D.; Egli, M.; Gao, Q.; Bash, P.; van der Marel, G.; van Boom, J.H.; Rich, A.; Frederick, G. *Proc. Natl. Acad. Sci. USA* 1990, 87, 2225-2229.
26. Arora, S.K. *J. Am. Chem. Soc.* 1983, 105, 1328-1332.
27. Hunter, C.A. *J. Mol. Biol.* 1993, 230, 1025-1054.
28. Fox, K.R. *Anti-Cancer Drug Design* 1988, 3, 157-168.
29. Fox, K.R.; Waring M.J. *Biochemistry* 1990, 29, 9451-9466.
30. Searle, M.S.; Hall, J.G.; Denny, W.A.; Wakelin, L.P.G. *Biochemistry* 1988, 27, 4340-4349.
31. Zhang, X.; Patel, D.J. *Biochemistry* 1990, 29, 9451-9466.
32. Robinson, H.; Liaw, Y.-C.; van der Marel, G.; van Boom, J.H.; Wang, A.H-J. *Nucleic Acids Res.* 1990, 18, 4851-4858.

33. Searle, M.S.; Wakelin, L.P.G. *Biochem. J.* 1990, 269, 341-346.
34. Rinkel, L.J.; Altona, C. *J. Biomol. Struct. Dyn.* 1987, 4, 621-649.
35. Kollman, P.; Keepers, J.W.; Weiner, P. *Biopolymers* 1982, 21, 2345-2376.
36. Lane, A.N.; Lefevre, J.-F.; Jardetzky, O. *Biochem. Biophys. Acta.* 1987, 876, 45-56.
37. Otwinowski, Z.; Schevitz, R.W.; Zhang, R.G.; Lawson, C.L.; Joachimiak, A.; Marmorstein, R.Q.; Luisi, B.F.; Sigler, P.B. *Nature* 1988, 335, 321-329.
38. Gao, X.; Patel, D.J. *Biochemistry* 1988, 27, 1744-1751.
39. Boyd, F.L.; Cheatham, S.F.; Remers, W.; Hill, G.C.; Hurley, L.H. *J. Am. Chem. Soc.* 1990, 112, 3279-3289.
40. Gorenstein, D.G.; Schroeder, S.A.; Fu, J.M.; Metz, J.T.; Roongta, V.; Jones, C.R. *Biochemistry* 1988, 27, 7223-7237.
41. Gorenstein, D.G.; Lai, K. *Biochemistry* 1989, 28, 2804-2812.
42. Schroeder, S.A.; Roongta, V.; Fu, J.M.; Jones, C.R.; Gorenstein, D.G. *Biochemistry* 1989, 28, 8292-8303.
43. Searle, M.S.; Lane, A.N. *FEBS Lett.* 1992, 297, 292-296.
44. Roongta, V.A.; Jones, C.R.; Gorenstein, D.G. *Biochemistry* 1990, 29, 5245-5258.
45. McCammon, J.A.; Harvey, S.C; *Dynamics of Proteins and Nucleic Acids;* Cambridge University Press: Cambridge, 1987.
46. Swaminathan, S.; Ravishanker, G.; Beveridge, D.L. *J. Am. Chem. Soc.* 1991, 113, 5027-5040.
47. Searle, M.S.; Bicknell, W.; Wakelin, L.P.G.; Denny, W.A. *Nucleic Acids Res.* 1991, 19, 2897-2906.
48. Fox, K.R. *Anti-Cancer Drug Des.* 1988, 3, 147-168.
49. Ward, D.; Reich, E.; Goldberg, I.H. *Science* 1965, 149, 1259-1263.
50. Waring, M.J.; Wakelin, L.P.G. *Nature* 1974, 252, 653-657.
51. Wang, A.H.; Ughetto, G.; Quigley, G.J.; Hakoshima, T.; van der Marel, G.A.; van Boom; J. H.; Rich, A. *Science* 1984, 225, 1115-1121.
52. Gilbert, D.E.; van der Marel, G.A.; van Boom, J.H.; Feigon, J. *Proc. Natl. Acad. Sci. USA* 1989, 86, 3006-3010.
53. Searle, M.S.; Wickham, G. *FEBS Lett.* 1990, 272, 171-174.
54. Gilbert, D. E.; Feigon, J. *Biochemistry* 1991, 30, 2483-2494.
55. Gilbert, D.E.; Feigon, J. *Nucleic Acids Res.* 1992, 20, 2411-2420.
56. Searle, M.S. *Biochem. J.* 1994, 304, 967–979.
57. McLean, M.J.; Waring, M.J. *J. Mol. Recogn.* 1988, 1, 138-151.
58. Mendel, D.; Dervan, P.B. *Proc. Natl. Acad. Sci. USA* 1987, 84, 910-914.
59. Fox, K.R.; Kentebe, E. *Nucleic Acids Res.* 1990, 18, 1957-1963.
60. Arnold, E.; Clardy, J. *J. Am. Chem. Soc.* 1981, 103, 1243-1244.
61. Searle, M.S.; Hall, J.G.; Wakelin, L.P.G. *Biochem. J.* 1988, 256, 271-278.
62. Searle, M.S.; Hall, J.G.; Denny, W.A.; Wakelin, L.P.G. *Biochem. J.* 1989, 259, 433-441.
63. Leroy, J.L.; Gao, X.; Gueron, M.; Patel, D.J. *Biochemistry* 1991, 30, 5653-5661.
64. Leroy, J.L.; Gao, X.; Misra, V.; Gueron, M.; Patel, M. *Biochemistry* 1992, 31, 1407-1415.
65. Hurley, L.H.; Boyd, F.L. *Trends Pharmacol. Sci.* 1988, 9, 402-407.
66. Hurley, L.H. *J. Med Chem.* 1989, 32, 2027-2033.
67. Nelson, E.M.; Tewey, K.M.; Liu, L.F. *Proc. Natl. Acad. Sci. USA* 1984, 81, 1361.
68. Ross, W.E.; Glaubiger, D.L.; Kohn, K.W. *Biochem. Biophys. Acta* 1978, 519, 23.
69. Tewey, K.M.; Rowe, T.C.; Yang, L.; Halligan, B.D.; Lui, L.F. *Science* 1984, 22, 466-468.

# CHAPTER 12

# DRUG BINDING TO THE MINOR GROOVE OF DNA

*David J. Craik, Spiro Pavlopoulos, and Geoffrey Wickham*

## CONTENTS

I  Introduction ................................................................ 424

II  Hoechst 33258 ............................................................ 427
  A  Stoichiometry and Kinetics ..................................... 428
  B  Resonance Assignments in DNA Complexes ........................ 430
  C  Binding Site ..................................................... 435
  D  Hydrogen Bonding ................................................ 437
  E  Dynamic Processes ............................................... 439
  F  Summary of Solution Studies ..................................... 440
  G  Comparison of NMR and X-Ray Structures .......................... 440

III  Other Minor Groove Binders ........................................... 442
  A  CC-1065 .......................................................... 443
  B  Netropsin and Distamycin ........................................ 443
  C  SN-6999 .......................................................... 445
  D  Terephthalamides ................................................ 446
    1  Titration Experiments ......................................... 447
    2  Evidence for Minor Groove Binding ............................. 451
    3  Location of Binding Site ...................................... 453
    4  Ligand Design ................................................. 454
    5  Comparison with Other Minor Groove Binders .................... 457

0-8493-7824-9/96/$0.00+$.50
© 1996 by CRC Press, Inc.

**IV**  Drug Design ............................................................................. 458

Acknowledgments  ................................................................... 462

**References**  ............................................................................. 463

# I    INTRODUCTION

In the preceding chapter a description of the role of DNA as a potential drug target was given and we saw examples of compounds that bind via intercalation between DNA base pairs. In this chapter the focus is on compounds that target the minor groove of DNA (Figure 1). Examples of this class include antiviral antibiotics such as netropsin and distamycin, bisquaternary ammonium heterocycles, bisamidines such as berenil, and terephthalamides. The common classification of these compounds was initially based on the observation that while they bound to DNA, as indicated by changes to UV and CD spectra, hydrodynamic changes in DNA, and ethidium displacement assays,[1,2] they did not cause unwinding of closed circular DNA as occurs with intercalating agents. These studies implicated the minor groove as the binding site for these compounds, and subsequent studies have demonstrated that many of them bind preferentially to AT-rich regions of DNA. The basis for this sequence selectivity has been examined using X-ray crystallography and NMR spectroscopy for a number of compounds including netropsin,[3,4] distamycin,[5-8] SN-6999,[9,10] DAPI,[11] CC-1065,[12] and Hoechst 33258.[13-21] These structural studies confirmed that compounds of this type bind specifically and sequence selectively in the minor groove of B-form duplex DNA.

Members of this class contain a number of common structural features that have been shown from the X-ray and NMR studies to contribute most significantly to their binding mode. Figure 2 shows some examples of minor groove–binding compounds and illustrates their structural similarities. The essentially planar nature of the ligands allows them to fit edgewise between the walls of the minor groove formed by the sugar phosphate backbone of the DNA strands, and to make van der Waals contacts between their aromatic $\pi$-systems and the deoxyribose sugar rings of the DNA. Furthermore, the aromatic rings of the ligands can rotate with respect to each other and are therefore able to stay parallel with the groove walls despite the helical twist of the duplex. The minor groove has been shown to be deeper and narrower in poly($d$A-$d$T) sequences than in poly($d$G-$d$C) sequences because of the projection of guanine 2-amino groups into the minor groove, and because of the ease with which AT base pairs may be propeller twisted.[22-24] Thus, van der Waals contacts between

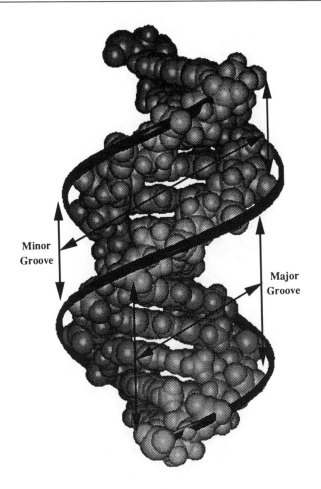

**FIGURE 1**
Structure of DNA showing the relative sizes of the major and minor grooves.

the ligand and the minor-groove walls are maximised in poly($d$A-$d$T) sequences.

Minor groove binders adopt a curved conformation that allows the concave edge of the ligand to be presented to the convex floor of the minor groove formed by the edges of the helically twisted nucleotide bases. The complementary shape of the ligand and the floor of the groove provides scope for further van der Waals interactions. As close contact with the floor of the groove is hindered by projecting guanine 2-amino groups, interaction between these two surfaces is again favoured in poly($d$A-$d$T) sequences.

Electrostatic forces also contribute significantly to binding. Most of the known minor groove binders contain at least one charge-bearing

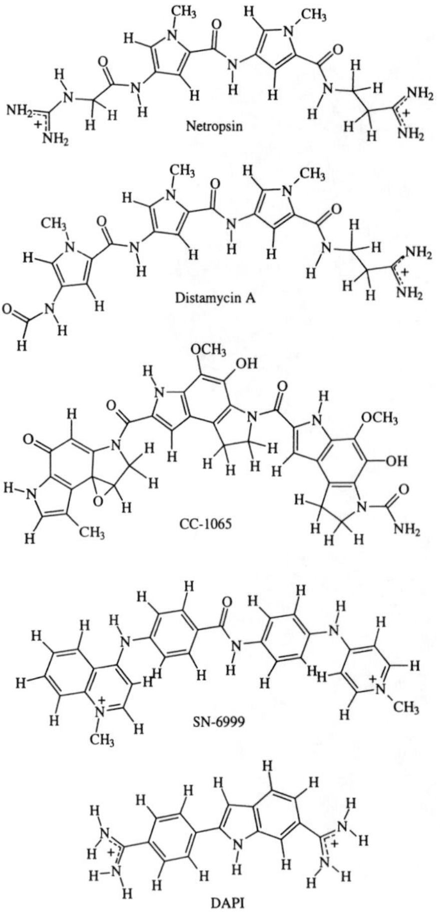

**FIGURE 2**

Structures of some well-characterized minor groove binders.

group, the majority of them possessing a positive charge at both ends of the molecule. X-ray studies have shown that, when complexed to DNA, the positive charges of the ligands lie close to the floor of the minor groove. The greatest negative potential within the minor groove of DNA occurs in AT base-pair tracts, which thus offer the greatest stabilisation to cationic ligands.[25] Minor groove-binding compounds such as netropsin, distamycin, DAPI, and Hoechst 33258, which have NH groups on their concave face, have been shown to form bridging (bifurcated) hydrogen bonds to the thymine O2 and adenine N3 positions on the floor of the groove at AT base pairs.[26]

To illustrate the NMR approaches that may be used to examine the interactions of minor groove–binding ligands with DNA, some recent studies on the bisbenzimidazole-based compound Hoechst 33258 will be described. As noted in the previous chapter, synthetic oligonucleotide sequences provide useful models for DNA in such studies. The information derived from these studies, as well as from NMR studies of the interactions of other minor groove binders with DNA, is useful for the design of ligands with altered specificity or increased binding affinity, with the overall goal being the development of novel drugs.

# II  HOECHST 33258

Hoechst 33258 is a synthetic compound consisting of two linked benzimidazole rings with phenol and N-methylpiperizine moieties attached at either end of the structure (Figure 3). It has been used widely as a fluorescent cytological DNA stain and is also active as an anthelmintic agent. It also has activity against intraperitoneally implanted L1210 and P388 leukemias in mice. Footprinting studies[27] have shown that sequences of four AT base pairs are a prerequisite for strong binding to DNA, consistent with similar observations for other structurally related molecules such as distamycin and netropsin.[3-8]

The first structural studies of Hoechst 33258 complexed to short sequences of synthetic oligonucleotides were done using X-ray crystallographic methods.[13-15] NMR and further X-ray studies followed.[16-21] Three of the X-ray studies[13,14,16] used the EcoR1 sequence $d$(CGCGAATTCGCG)$_2$, and another[15] used the oligonucleotide sequence $d$(CGCGATATCGCG)$_2$. Both sequences fulfil the requirement of at least four consecutive AT base pairs, and the resulting complexes showed similar modes of binding. In all the X-ray studies, the Hoechst ligand was found to bind to the minor groove. This interaction was found to involve (1) van der Waals contacts between the planar aromatic rings and the walls and floor of the minor groove, (2) hydrogen bonding between the NH groups of the benzimidazole residues and electronegative atoms on the floor of the groove such as N3 of adenine and O2 of thymine, and (3) electrostatic interactions between the negative potential of the groove and the positively charged piperizine ring.

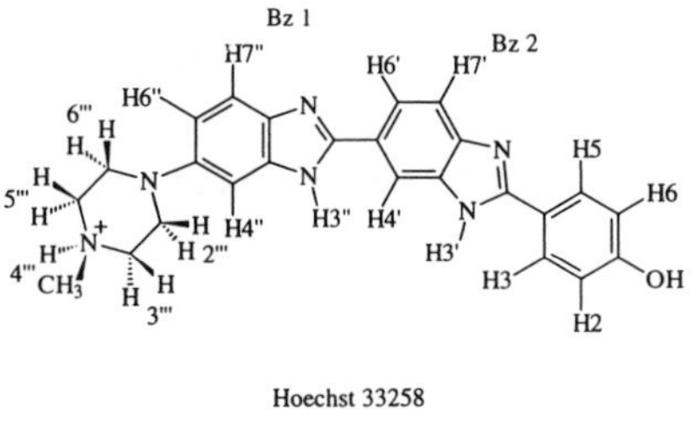

Hoechst 33258

**FIGURE 3**
Structure of Hoechst 33258 and proton-labelling scheme. The two benzimidazole rings are labelled Bz-1 and Bz-2.

Differences were observed with respect to the positioning of the ligand within the AT tract and its orientation with respect to the binding site. In the structures reported by Teng et al.[14] and Quintana et al.,[16] the ligand interacts with the four central AT base pairs. However, Pjura et al.[13] and Carrondo et al.[15] reported that the position of the ligand in their structures was displaced by 1 bp so that in each case the charged piperizine ring extended into the GC region flanking the AT tract. It was postulated that the minor groove at this position would be wider than in the AT tract and better able to accommodate this bulkier portion of the ligand. The Hoechst molecule was found to have opposite orientations in these two structures. Pjura et al.[13] found the piperizine ring to be located toward the 3′ end of the AT tract so that the binding site encompassed 5′-ATTC-3′. In contrast, Carrondo et al.[15] proposed that the piperizine portion of the molecule was located toward the 5′ end of the AT tract, so that in their structure the binding site encompassed 5′-GATA-3′.

A number of NMR studies of complexes between Hoechst 33258 and oligonucleotide sequences have been conducted to determine the nature of the interaction in solution and for comparison with the crystal structure data.[17-21] As the binding is reversible, the NMR data offer the opportunity to derive information about the kinetics of the interaction. As with the crystallographic studies, the oligonucleotide sequences were designed to contain runs of AT base pairs. Some NMR studies were performed with dodecanucleotide sequences used in crystallographic studies, including $d(CGCGAATTCGCG)_2$,[19] which allowed a direct comparison with the crystallographic data. Experiments were also performed with sequences specifically designed to investigate different aspects of the interaction. The sequence $d(CTTTTGCAAAAG)_2$ was designed to offer two binding sites, and it was shown that two Hoechst molecules interacted with the DNA duplex in symmetry-related orientations at the 5′-TTTT-3′ and 5′-AAAA-3′ sites.[17]

The oligonucleotide sequence $d(GGTAATTACC)_2$ was used to probe the reported displacement of the ligand toward the flanking GC base pair.[18] It had previously been shown to possess a very narrow minor groove[28] and subsequently was shown to form a 1:1 complex with Hoechst 33258.[18] This sequence contains five possible binding sites, two of which contain one GC base pair at the periphery. The related sequence, $d(GTGGAATTCCAC)_2$, which also contains a central AATT tract, has also been studied by NMR.[20,21] The results of these various studies are summarized below.

## A　STOICHIOMETRY AND KINETICS

The starting point in studies of ligand–DNA complexes is usually a titration experiment to establish the nature and stoichiometry of the complex. Complexes between the ligand and DNA duplex are obtained by adding small aliquots of ligand solution to a sample of the DNA duplex with one-dimensional $^1$H NMR spectra acquired after each addition. The effects observed on the NMR spectrum after each addition reveal whether an interaction is taking place and allow the interaction to be characterized as fast or slow exchange on the NMR time scale. The stoichiometry of the interaction can also be determined from the titration.

In general, the addition of Hoechst 33258 to the oligonucleotide duplexes noted above causes a decrease in the intensity of free DNA resonances and a concomitant increase in the intensity of new resonances, which appear in previously unoccupied spectral regions. This is consistent with the free and bound forms of the DNA duplex being in slow exchange with each other. For example, when Hoechst 33258 is added to $d(\text{GGTAATTACC})_2$, the free DNA signals completely disappear at a DNA to drug ratio of 1:1, and the number of new resonances is twice the number of previously observed free DNA resonances[18] (Figure 4). This is a common feature of complexes with 1:1 stoichiometry and reflects a loss of the dyad symmetry of the duplex due to ligand binding.

Upon addition of Hoechst 33258 to $d(\text{CTTTTCGAAAAG})_2$, the free DNA signals completely disappeared at a ratio of 2:1 drug to DNA, and

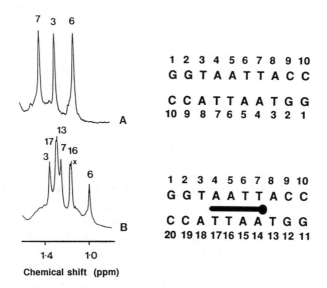

**FIGURE 4**

The 1D $^1$H NMR spectra (recorded at 20°C) illustrating the thymine methyl region (A) for the symmetrical ligand-free duplex and (B) for the 1:1 Hoechst–$d(\text{GGTAATTACC})_2$ complex, which is no longer symmetrical due to the ligand binding; x corresponds to a small impurity peak. The DNA strands are numbered to the right of the spectra and the approximate location of the ligand is indicated by a black bar. (Adapted from Embrey, K.J., et al., *Eur. J. Biochem.*, 211, 437–447, 1993.)

there was no doubling of the number of DNA resonances in the spectrum.[17] From this, it could be concluded that two molecules were bound per duplex in a manner that retained the dyad symmetry of the DNA duplex. The binding was also determined to be cooperative, as no intermediate 1:1 complex was detected.[17] The formation of a 1:1 complex would have resulted in a very complicated spectrum at intermediate ligand to DNA ratios, as resonances arising from the free DNA, the 1:1 complex and the 2:1 complex would have produced four times as many observable peaks relative to the free DNA species. At intermediate ligand concentration, however, only two sets of peaks arising from DNA molecules were detected, as illustrated in Figure 5 for the methyl region of the spectrum. In the 2:1 complex only four thymine methyl resonances were detected (1.0–1.5 ppm), as expected for a symmetrical DNA duplex. These are all overlapped in the free DNA spectrum (upper trace). In the 1:1 mixture, only signals from free DNA and from the 2:1 complex were detected.

The reversible nature of the Hoechst to DNA interaction is illustrated by the observation of chemical exchange cross-peaks in NOESY spectra of mixtures of free and complexed oligonucleotides.[17,19] This may be seen in the NOESY spectrum of a mixture of free and complexed $d$(CTTTTCGAAAAG)$_2$ shown in Figure 6, in which many chemical-exchange cross-peaks are observed between resonances arising from the free and bound oligonucleotide. In a NOESY spectrum acquired at lower temperature, the intensity of these chemical exchange cross-peaks is significantly reduced, indicating that the exchange is slowed at lower temperatures. The exchange rate was estimated to be <10 s$^{-1}$ at 10°C.[17] The ability to observe dynamic phenomena is one of the strengths of NMR relative to X-ray crystallography, and several examples of these phenomena will be described later in the chapter.

## B  RESONANCE ASSIGNMENTS IN DNA COMPLEXES

The $^1$H NMR resonances of oligonucleotide duplexes can be assigned using well-established techniques,[29-31] which were mentioned briefly in the previous chapter. The deoxyribose spin systems as well as cytosine H5–H6 and thymine CH$_3$–H6 correlations are identified through $J$-coupling interactions observed in COSY spectra. Cross peaks observed in NOESY spectra, including H6/H8($i$) → H1'($i$) → H6/H8 ($i$ + 1) and H6/H8($i$) → H2'/2'' ($i$) → H6/H8($i$ + 1), allow the sequence-specific assignment of the base and deoxyribose spin systems. Figure 7 summarizes some of the useful connectivities derived from COSY and NOESY spectra.

Methods for the assignment of DNA resonances of oligonucleotide–ligand complexes are similar to those for the free oligonucleotide duplexes. However, in favourable circumstances chemical exchange cross peaks (such as those illustrated in Figure 6) in NOESY spectra of mixtures of free and complexed DNA can be used to confirm assignments. This approach has

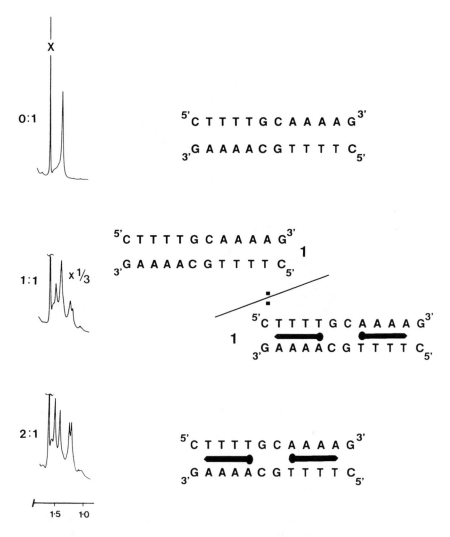

**FIGURE 5**
Portions of the 1D $^1$H NMR spectra of $d$(CTTTTGCAAAAG)$_2$ recorded at 10°C at the various ratios of Hoechst to DNA indicated. The upper trace corresponds to uncomplexed DNA, and x marks the position of an impurity peak due to sodium acetate. The nature of species present in solution at the various mole ratios is schematically illustrated to the right of the spectra. No evidence for an intermediate 1:1 complex is detected. (Adapted from Searle, M.S. and Embrey, K.J., *Nucleic Acids Res.*, 18, 3753–3762, 1990. With permission of Oxford University Press.)

been used for both 1:1 and 2:1 complexes and is similar to the examples described in Chapter 8, where chemical exchange was used to assign bound ligand signals based on the known assignment of free ligands. In the case of the 2:1 complex of Hoechst 33258 with $d$(CTTTTCGAAAAG)$_2$,

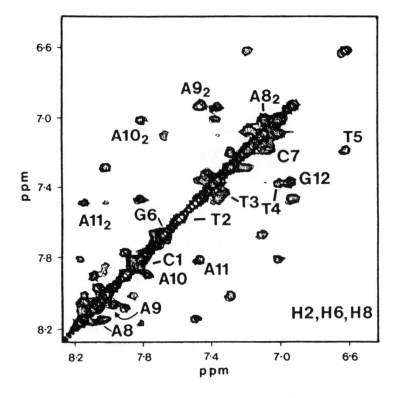

**FIGURE 6**

Aromatic region of NOESY spectrum of a 1:1 mixture of Hoechst vs. $d$(CTTTTCGAAAAG)$_2$ recorded with a 200-ms mixing time. Chemical-exchange cross-peaks between protons of the free DNA and the 2:1 Hoechst–DNA complex are labelled with their identifying base pair. Below the diagonal the H6 and H8 cross-peaks are shown, while those of the adenine H2 resonances are highlighted in the upper portion of the figure and labelled with a subscript 2. (From Searle, M.S. and Embrey, K.J., *Nucleic Acids, Res.,* 18, 3753–3762, 1990. With permission of Oxford University Press.)

only one connectivity pathway is observed due to the symmetry of the DNA duplex.[17] However, in complexes where there is a 1:1 stoichiometry and the duplex is no longer symmetrical, connectivity pathways can be traced for each oligonucleotide strand of the duplex[18] (Figure 8).

Imino proton resonance assignments can be obtained from spectra recorded in 90% $H_2O$/10% $D_2O$ solution. Exchange between solvent and these protons is generally slow, allowing NOEs to be detected. Two assignment pathways are available for the determination of imino resonances. The first involves interresidue NOEs between imino protons of sequentially neighbouring base pairs;[20] for example, in the case of the 2:1 complex $NH(i) \rightarrow NH(i+1)$, sequential NOEs were observed for all steps along the AT tract.[17] The second pathway involves the observation of interstrand NOEs; for example, the assignment of thymine H3 resonances

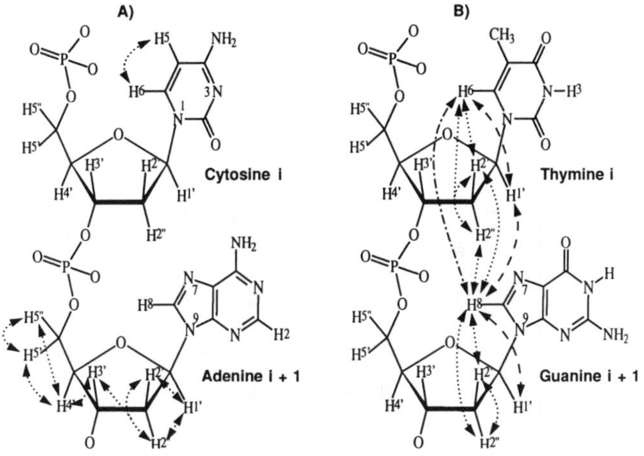

**FIGURE 7**
Strategies of sequential resonance assignments for B-DNA. Double-pointed arrows indicate observable COSY and NOESY correlations that can be used in sequential assignments. (A) Intranucleotide COSY correlations; (B) intranucleotide and internucleotide NOEs that make up three different connectivity pathways. These are indicated by dashed, dotted, and broken arrowed lines.

in the 2:1 complex was based on the observation of NOEs to the H2 of the base-paired adenine. This also confirmed the AH2 assignments made from chemical-exchange data.

Amino proton resonances of cytosine and adenine residues can be assigned based on interstrand NOEs to the imino protons of the base-paired guanine and thymine residues.[17,18] Cytosine amino protons also show strong NOEs to the base H5 proton, which assists in assignment.[20]

Assignment of ligand resonances in complexes may be accomplished using well-established methods, as described below for Hoechst 33258. Hoechst 33258 contains three aromatic spin systems, which were assigned from a combination of TOCSY, COSY, and NOESY spectra.[17,18] Scalar-coupling interactions of the oligonucleotide in the aromatic region of the spectrum are limited to cytosine H5–H6 interactions, resulting in an uncluttered aromatic region of DQF-COSY and TOCSY spectra, and enabling easy identification of aromatic signals from the bound ligand. DQF-COSY spectra of the 1:1 and 2:1 complexes described above contain three cross-peaks (in addition to the cytosine H5–H6 cross-peaks), which are readily assigned and originate from the ortho-coupled protons H2/6–H3/5, H6′–H7′ and H6″–H7″ of the bound Hoechst molecule.[17,18] TOCSY spectra have also proved to be useful in the assignment of the benzimidazole protons in Hoechst 33258.[20] NOESY spectra have been used to distinguish between the two benzimidazole spin systems,[17,20] as one of them displays NOEs to two upfield resonances belonging to the

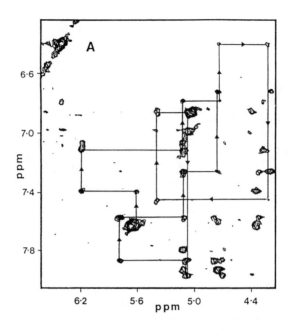

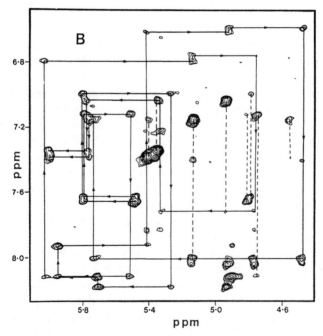

**FIGURE 8**

Fingerprint regions of NOESY spectra for (A) 2:1 complex of Hoechst–d(CTTTTCGAAAAG)₂, and (B) 1:1 complex of Hoechst vs d(GGTAATTACC)₂. (Adapted from Searle, M.S. and Embrey, K.J., *Nucleic Acids Res.*, 18, 3753–3763, 1990, and Embrey, K.J., *Eur. J. Biochem.*, 211, 437–447, 1993.)

piperizine moiety. These two resonances, assigned as H2‴/6‴ and H3‴/5‴, also show NOEs to each other as well as to the easily distinguishable N-methyl resonance. Acquiring NOESY spectra in 90% $H_2O$/10% $D_2O$ allows the assignment of the exchangeable ligand resonances. The benzimidazole NH protons appear well downfield of the nonexchangeable resonances (11-12 ppm). The NH of Bz-2 (Figure 3) can be distinguished from that of Bz-1 on the basis of NOEs to the phenolic H3/5 and H2/6 resonances. NOEs are also observed between NH protons and neighbouring H4′ and H4″ protons.

## C  BINDING SITE

A combination of chemical-shift and NOE information can be used to locate and characterize binding sites. Chemical-shift differences between resonances arising from free and bound forms of DNA are indicative of the nature of the interaction. In all studies of the Hoechst complexes described above,[17-21] significant changes to the chemical shifts of thymine H1′ protons and adenine H2 protons were observed, in contrast to the generally small perturbations observed for the base H8/H6 and $CH_3$ resonances located in the major groove. Perturbations of this nature are consistent with binding to the minor groove. In some instances, significant perturbations were observed to major groove protons located well within the binding site, reflecting changes in the conformation of the DNA duplex (e.g., base roll, propeller twisting).[17,20]

Further evidence of minor groove binding is provided by the fact that resonances arising from protons on the floor of the groove, such as the adenine H2 and imino resonances, are shifted downfield, whereas resonances from protons on the minor groove walls, such as the H1′ protons, are shifted upfield. This is a consequence of the ligand being inserted edge-on into the minor groove. The deoxyribose protons that form the walls of the minor groove are positioned above the π-plane of the aromatic rings and consequently receive upfield perturbations to their chemical shifts. Protons positioned on the floor of the groove, however, generally lie in the plane of the aromatic rings and experience downfield perturbations to their chemical shifts, as illustrated in Figure 9.

The magnitude of chemical-shift changes is a strong indicator of the location of the binding site. In the case of the 2:1 complex with $d$(CTTTTCGAAAAG)$_2$ the largest chemical-shift changes occur over the 5′-TTTT-3′ and 5′-AAAA-3′ regions of the duplex.[17] In the case of 1:1 complexes, where the DNA duplex contains an AT base-pair segment located at the centre of the sequence, greater chemical-shift perturbations are observed for resonances in that region,[18-20] consistent with the binding site being located there. It is interesting to note, particularly with the sequence $d$(GGTAATTACC)$_2$,[18] that significant chemical-shift changes

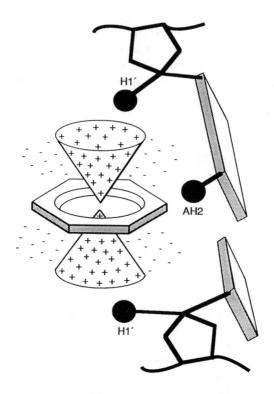

**FIGURE 9**
Schematic representation of ligand-induced ring-current effects on nucleotide protons that form the walls (deoxyribose H1′) and floor (adenine H2) of the minor groove. (+) shielding effects, (–) deshielding effects. (Adapted from Embrey, K.J., et al., *Eur. J. Biochem.*, 211, 437–447, 1993.)

did not occur for resonances of GC base pairs on the periphery of the AT regions.

Assignment of the bound ligand and DNA resonances enables the identification of intermolecular NOEs, which are required for a precise determination of the binding site. The interaction of Hoechst 33258 with the oligonucleotides produced a large number of intermolecular NOEs (~25–30), placing considerable constraints on the structure of the complex and enabling the orientation of the ligand within the binding site to be determined. The NOE contacts observed for different complexes have a few features in common. The contacts generally involve DNA protons associated with the minor groove, such as ribose H1′ and adenine H2, clearly locating Hoechst in the minor groove. Protons of all four spin systems of the ligand show NOEs to protons of the DNA, demonstrating that the interaction occurs along the entire length of the drug. Typically, protons along one edge of the ligand, for example, NH and H4′/H4″, exhibit close contacts to protons on the floor of the minor groove, showing that the bound drug is crescent shaped and isohelical with the DNA.[17-20]

Some interesting interstrand NOEs were observed by Searle and Embrey[17] in the 2:1 complex of Hoechst 33258 with $d(\text{CTTTTCGAAAAG})_2$. In particular, NOEs were observed between adenine H2 protons and the H1′ protons of complementary thymine nucleotides which are located well onto the backbone of the opposite strand. Such interactions are indicative of a high degree of propeller twisting and a particularly narrow minor groove.

Models of the interaction of Hoechst 33258 with the oligonucleotides studied were generated based on the intermolecular NOEs. The models of the 1:1 complexes indicated that the ligand interacted with the four AT base pairs located at the centre of the sequence. Interestingly, there was no evidence for interactions with GC base pairs on the periphery of the binding sites. In the 2:1 complex reported by Searle and Embrey[17] the array of contacts observed located the ligand in the minor groove at the centre of the 5′-TTTT-3′ and 5′-AAAA-3′ sites as illustrated in Figure 10.

As well as defining the location of the binding site, intermolecular NOEs can be used to determine the orientation of the ligand at that site. In the case of the 2:1 complex, the $N$-methylpiperizine moieties were found to point towards the centre of the duplex, as indicated by NOEs between the protons from the piperizine ring and the 5′-terminus of the adenine tract (Figure 10). Corresponding NOEs were also observed between the drug phenolic protons and the 5′-terminus of the thymine tract, as well as the 3′-terminus of the adenine tract of the complementary strand. This model did not indicate any interaction with the central GC base pairs.[17]

The orientation of the ligand was similarly determined in the 1:1 complexes based on intermolecular NOEs between protons located at the extremities of the Hoechst molecule and protons of the binding site. For example, in the interaction with $d(\text{GTGGAATTCCAC})_2$, Fede et al.[20] reported NOEs between protons from the piperizine moiety and the H2 and H1′ protons of the dinucleotide fragment $d(\text{A}_5\text{T}_5)\cdot d(\text{A}_6\text{T}_6)$.

## D  HYDROGEN BONDING

In the studies of Hoechst–DNA complexes described so far, the intermolecular hydrogen bonds were not detected directly by two-dimensional NMR methods, but were deduced from molecular models based on the NOE data. (It has been established, however, that the $^{15}$N chemical shifts of thymine N3 resonances are sensitive to the formation of hydrogen bonds to the adjacent thymine O2 atom, making $^{15}$N resonances a sensitive marker for hydrogen bonding.[25,32]) The general conclusion drawn from the solution studies is that there is a system of bifurcated hydrogen bonds

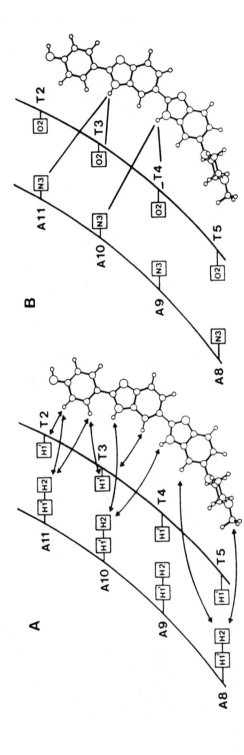

**FIGURE 10**

Schematic representation of Hoechst 33258 bound to the minor groove of the 5'-TTTT sequence. (A) Highlights of some of the NOEs that determine the position and orientation of the Hoechst molecule within the minor groove. (B) Intermolecular hydrogen-bonding scheme. Molecular-modelling studies with an idealized B-DNA helical structure indicate that the benzimidazole H3' is capable of forming bifurcated interactions with A11N3 and T302, while the benzimidazole H3" hydrogen bonds in a similar manner, but with A10N3 and T402. In the proposed model of the complex, these distances fall within 3.5 Å and are thus within acceptable hydrogen-bonding limits. (From Searle, M.S. and Embrey, K.J. *Nucleic Acids Res.* 1990, 18, 3753–3762. With permission of Oxford University Press.)

that involves the NH groups of the benzimidazole rings and the adenine N3 and thymine O2 atoms. (Figure 10). This is consistent with the slow-exchange rates and the small temperature dependence of the chemical shifts observed for the exchangeable benzimidazole protons. Fede et al.[21] interpreted their data for the binding of Hoechst 33258 to $d$(GTGGAATTCCAC)$_2$ in terms of two coexisting bound conformations that had hydrogen-bonding patterns slightly different from each other.

## E  DYNAMIC PROCESSES

The binding of the Hoechst molecule to the self-complementary oligonucleotide duplexes in a 1:1 ratio lifts the dyad symmetry of the duplexes so that two sets of DNA resonances are observed. This indicates that the drug is in slow exchange between the free and the bound forms. Close examination of the 2D NOE data, however, reveals the presence of chemical-exchange cross-peaks between symmetry-related protons on opposite sides of the dyad axis of the DNA duplex. The mechanism by which this occurs has been described as dissociation of the Hoechst molecule from the duplex, followed by a 180° reorientation and rebinding.[18,20] The self-complementary nature of the sequences ensures that the same complex is formed for either ligand orientation but with the net effect of interchanging the two strands with respect to the orientation of the Hoechst molecule. The rate at which this process occurs was estimated using Equation (1), where $k_{ex}$ is the exchange rate, $R$ is the ratio of exchange cross-peak intensity to diagonal cross-peak intensity, and $\tau_m$ is the mixing time used in the NOESY experiment.[20]

$$k_{ex} = \ln\left[(1 + R)/(1 - R)\right]/2\tau_m \tag{1}$$

When interacting with $d$(GGTAATTACC)$_2$ and $d$(GTGGAAT TCCAC)$_2$, the lifetime of the complex in each state $(1/k_{ex})$ was reported to be approximately 0.8 and 0.45 s, respectively.[18,20] These values indicate a small but significant difference in the affinity of Hoechst for TAATTA and GAATTC sites.

Intramolecular dynamic processes that are fast on the NMR time scale are also observable in the $^1$H NMR spectrum of the bound Hoechst molecule. Resonance averaging is observed for the H2/H6 and H3/H5 protons of the phenol group, which is consistent with the environments on either side of the ring being averaged by rapid ring-flipping motions about the C4–C2′ axis. This occurs despite the apparent tight fit between the phenyl ring and the walls of the minor groove, which in a static model of the complex, must present a large barrier for rotation. It was estimated[18] that the rate for this process is as high as 1000 s$^{-1}$. This is much higher than the rate of interconversion between free and bound forms of the duplex;

thus dissociation of the drug from the complex cannot be the rate-limiting factor for phenol ring flipping. Dynamic fluctuations of the DNA conformation are more likely to provide the rate-limiting step.

The piperizine ring has been reported to exist in at least two conformations, as suggested by the appearance of two resonances arising from the bound N-methyl of the piperizine ring in the complex with d(CTTTTCGAAAAG)$_2$. Interestingly, only protons from one of these two resonances showed NOE contacts to an adenine H2 proton located on the floor of the minor groove.[20] Two signals were not observed for other solution structures; however, Embrey et al. reported that the N-methyl resonance of their 1:1 complex was appreciably broadened, indicative of an intermediate rate of exchange between two nonequivalent sites.[18] They also observed dynamic effects for the resonances H2'''/H6'''(axial), H2'''/6''' (equatorial), and H3'''/H5'''(equatorial) of the N-methylpiperizine, and in this case ring flipping or free rotation also appears to be fast in the bound form of Hoechst, as observed for the free ligand.

## F  Summary of Solution Studies

The data obtained from these NMR studies are consistent with the bound ligand fitting tightly within the minor groove of AT tetramers, with the aromatic rings of the ligand being roughly coplanar. The AT tract provides the key recognition features required for binding, including the narrowness of the minor groove. The importance of van der Waals interactions is evident, given the large number of NOE contacts between the ligand and the walls and floor of the groove. Hydrogen bonding also plays a significant role in stabilizing the interaction, as do electrostatic interactions between the positively charged piperizine ring and the minor groove. Electrostatic interactions are also likely to play a significant role in orienting the ligand within the binding site, as shown in the 2:1 complex, where the piperazine rings point towards the centre of the duplex, where the positive charge is best stabilized.[17] Hydrogen bonds do not play a role in orientation of the ligands, as they can be formed in either of the two possible orientations.

## G  Comparison of NMR and X-Ray Structures

The results from the X-ray and NMR analyses of the Hoechst 33258–oligonucleotide complexes indicate a similar mode of binding of the ligand to the DNA duplex. The structure of the DNA duplex is similar in the solution and the X-ray structures. The overall B-DNA conformation of the helix is retained upon binding of the ligand; however, significant local variations do occur at the binding site. The X-ray studies in particular showed that base pairs buckle away from the binding site toward each end of the helix and that the helix axis becomes bent.[16] This is consistent with the chemical-shift changes observed for major groove protons such as thymine H6 and $CH_3$.

The crystal structures reported by Pjura et al.[13] and Carrondo et al.[15] differed in the orientation of the piperizine moiety in the different sequences. Pjura et al. had the piperizine moiety displaced toward the lower end of the helix (i.e., C12·G13), whereas Carrondo et al. had the ligand rotated 180° and the piperizine moiety extended to the flanking GC base pair toward the upper part of the helix (i.e., G1·C24). It is important to note that, with the self-complementary oligonucleotide sequences used in these studies, the distinction between the two ends of the helix only occurs in the crystal as a result of a slight bend in the upper part of the helix, which is not seen in the lower region.[33] In solution the distinction between upper and lower ends of the helix is lost, and the binding modes reported by Pjura et al. and Carrondo et al. would be identical. The NMR solution structures do show that the ligand effectively undergoes a 180° flipping process at the binding site. This flipping process may explain the different orientations observed in the two crystal structures.

The selectivity for GC base pairs on the periphery of the AT runs, which was observed by Pjura et al.[13] and Carrondo et al.[15] in the crystal structures, was not observed in the solution structures. Some of the crystal data also support a model of the ligand located centrally within an AT tract. It has been suggested[16] that the GC selectivity may arise from the fact that for Hoechst, only the phenol and the two benzimidazole moieties are involved in sequence-recognition reactions with the DNA (i.e., hydrogen bonding and van der Waals interactions with protons on the floor of the groove). This would require the molecule to bridge either the first three central AT base pairs or the last three, depending on the orientation of the piperizine. The piperizine ring could then occupy the remaining part of the AT centre or could extend into the adjacent GC zone. It may be possible that this latter mode of binding does occur in solution if the ligand is able to slide along the AT tract. However, as there is no evidence of such a binding mode from the NOESY data, it must be very transitory in nature if present.

The conformation of the Hoechst molecule in the complex is governed by two main factors. Resonance delocalization between the aromatic rings makes it favourable for adjacent rings to be coplanar; however, it is also energetically favourable to follow the curvature of the walls of the minor groove, so that a twist is introduced at each connecting bond. The degree of twist is not great, however, and it has generally been found that the aromatic portions of the ligand, in particular the two benzimidazole rings are close to coplanar (Table 1). The solution studies confirm this finding. In the study by Fede et al.[21] the NMR data were interpreted in terms of two conformations for the bound ligand, but the range of angles between the two benzimidazole rings was small in both conformers. By

**TABLE 1**

Angles Between Aromatic Groups in
Hoechst 33258 as a Function of
Temperature

| Temperature (°C) | α1 (deg) | α2 (deg) | α3 (deg) | Ref. |
|---|---|---|---|---|
| Room | 0 | 36 | 60 | 13 |
| 15 | 18 | 13 | 21 | 15 |
| 15 | 8 | 32 | 14 | 14 |
| 0 | 8 | 15 | 3 | 16 |
| −25 | 10 | 12 | 8 | 16 |
| −100 | 30 | 2 | 6 | 16 |

Note: α1 is the angle between the phenol ring
and its adjacent benzimidazole (Bz-2,
see Figure 3); α2 is the angle between Bz-
1 and Bz-2, and α3 is the angle between
the piperazine ring and Bz-3.

contrast, the solution studies indicate that the phenol and piperizine rings at each end of the molecule are conformationally flexible.[21]

# III OTHER MINOR GROOVE BINDERS

A number of other minor groove binders, including netropsin, distamycin SN-6999, CC-1065, and DAPI, have been studied extensively and have been shown to bind sequence selectively to AT-rich regions of DNA. This sequence selectivity is based on varying combinations of the interactions described above for the binding of Hoechst 33258 to the minor groove of DNA duplexes. In some cases, these interactions lead to a regional specificity so that the ligand shows a preference for regions that contain mostly AT base pairs and, in other cases, lead to local specificity so that a specific base pair is required at a specific site.[16]

Important factors that lead to regional specificity include the high degree of propeller twisting in AT regions, which leads to a narrower minor groove, the absence of amino groups that cause the minor groove of GC-rich regions to be shallower, and the lower electrostatic potential of AT regions compared to GC regions. Factors that lead to local specificity include close van der Waals contacts (evidence for which is seen in NOEs between drug protons and adenine H2 protons) as well as hydrogen-bonding interactions.

The study of different minor groove binders highlights different aspects of the overall binding and allows an assessment of the relative importance of individual interactions. A comparison of the findings from binding studies on different ligands therefore contributes to the development of general models for small molecule–DNA recognition in the minor groove.

## A   CC-1065

The importance of the complementarity between the crescent shape of ligands and the minor groove of DNA duplexes, and the resulting van der Waals interactions when the two are bound, is illustrated by the antibiotic CC-1065 (Figure 2). This ligand does not bear any charge, and has exhibited two types of binding to AT-rich regions: one reversible and noncovalent in nature and the other irreversible and covalent.[34] The ligand is capable of covalently binding to the N3 of adenine via the cyclopropyl group.[12] The complex of CC-1065 with the DNA duplex $d$(CGATTAGC)·$d$(CGATTAGC) showed that the ligand was indeed located in the minor groove at the 5′-ATTA-3′ site, and computer modelling indicated a snug fit to the floor of the minor groove. The interaction of this ligand involves insertion into the minor groove in a reversible fashion, as seen for other minor groove binders, followed by alkylation of the adenine N3, which is also located in the minor groove. The absence of any charge-bearing groups on the ligand implies that the complementarity between the minor groove and the ligand and the resulting van der Waals interactions alone can induce AT selectivity.

## B   Netropsin and Distamycin

Netropsin[3,4] and distamycin[5-8] are crescent shaped di- and tripeptides containing aromatic $N$-methylpyrrole rings linked together by amide groups. They are probably the most extensively studied of the minor groove binders, and their binding is generally similar to that described earlier for Hoechst 33258. The pyrrole rings fit snugly in the narrow minor groove, with many van der Waals contacts to the walls and floor of the groove. The amide protons form bifurcated hydrogen bonds to the acceptor atoms on the floor of the minor groove (N3 of adenine and O2 of thymine). The preference for AT regions arises from clashes that would occur between the $NH_2$ group of guanine in GC regions and the aromatic hydrogens of the pyrrole rings.

An interesting observation regarding these compounds is that they bind more tightly to consecutive runs of A or T than to stretches of alternating A and T residues.[35] A study of the interaction of netropsin with $d$(CGCGATATCGCG)$_2$ revealed that the basis for this was the fact that the high degree of propeller twisting prevalent in contiguous runs of A and T is not present in alternating AT segments.[4] A continuous high-propeller twist is unlikely to occur in alternating AT stretches because of the repulsion of the N6 atoms of consecutive adenines from opposite strands in the major groove.[4] This phenomenon was also observed in the interaction of Hoechst 33258 with the same oligonucleotide.[15]

Given that a narrow minor groove was observed in the complex of netropsin with this DNA duplex, the question arises as to what causes the narrowness of the groove in this case. There is evidence to suggest that the netropsin molecule is more than a passive ligand attracted to the binding site and is capable of helping to collapse a "normal" minor groove into a narrow minor groove. The ligand has a structural effect on the DNA duplex, analogous to the unwinding of DNA caused by intercalators.[4]

Distamycin shows the typical mode of binding to the minor groove.[5] However, it also displays a unique property in being able to bind to the DNA duplex $d$(CGCAAATTGGC)·$d$(GCCAATTTGCG) in a 2:1 ratio[7] so that two drug molecules bind simultaneously in the minor groove and are in close contact with the DNA and each other, as illustrated schematically in Figure 11. This binding can be envisaged as the typical mode of binding in which the distamycin undergoes exchange between two symmetry-related binding sites via a flip-flop mechanism, except that both binding sites are occupied by a distamycin molecule at the same time. The presence of two distamycin molecules in the minor groove causes the minor groove to expand in width to accommodate them. The complex is stabilised, however, by stacking interactions between the two ligand molecules and the walls of the minor groove in addition to electrostatic forces and hydrogen-bond formation.[8]

This mode of binding was explored further with the oligonucleotide duplex $d$(CGCAAATTTGCG)$_2$.[8] The addition of a sixth AT base pair effectively creates two adjacent binding sites, 5'-AATT-3' and 5'-ATTT-3', on each strand of the helix. This leads to a total of three different binding

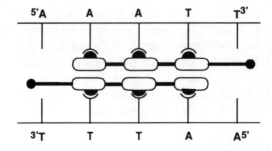

**FIGURE 11**
The 2:1 binding mode of distamycin to the binding site of the oligonucleotide duplex $d$(CGCAAATTGGC)·$d$(GCCAATTTGCG). Hydrogen bond acceptors on the floor of the groove are represented schematically by semicircles.

modes. The two stacked ligands can both occupy the 5'-AATT-3' site of each strand, the 5' ATTT-3' site of each strand, or one ligand molecule can occupy the 5'-AATT-3' site of its adjacent strand while the second ligand molecule occupies the 5' ATTT-3' site of its adjacent strand. As only one set of drug and DNA resonances was observed, it is assumed that the drug molecules slide past each other between the two sites at a rate approaching the fast-exchange limit. No evidence is observed for drug binding in the opposite orientation with the two positively charged propylamidinium groups in close contact.

The findings from the NMR data differ from those of an X-ray study of the same ligand and oligomer, where a 1:1 binding mode was observed.[22] NMR spectra of the complex in phosphate buffer, as well as in the buffer used in the X-ray study, revealed that the 2:1 complex was the primary species present. Thus, the observation of a 1:1 complex in the crystalline state appears to be due to selection by crystal-packing forces rather than it being the dominant form in solution.

## C  SN-6999

Dynamic aspects of ligand binding are conveniently illustrated using the bisquaternary ammonium heterocycle SN-6999, the structure of which is shown in Figure 2. This ligand binds specifically to AT regions of oligonucleotide sequences;[1] however, its affinity is not as high as other minor groove binders. When it was complexed with the oligonucleotide $d$(CGTAATTACG)$_2$, the kinetics of binding were found to be intermediate to fast on the NMR time scale, and a rapid exchange between equivalent binding sites was observed.[10] This was best illustrated by the behaviour of a DNA methyl resonance, which was a single, relatively narrow line at 305 K but split into two lines of equal intensity at temperatures below 289 K. The retention of the twofold symmetry of the duplex at higher temperatures is due to exchange of the drug between two symmetry-related binding sites that is fast enough on the NMR time scale to cause signal averaging. The rate at which this occurs was estimated to be $\geq 96$ s$^{-1}$ at 289 K and of the order of 200 s$^{-1}$ at 300 K. Exchange between binding sites could be achieved by the ligand sliding along the minor groove, but sliding motions do not account for the NMR equivalence of the two DNA strands at high temperatures. The data were more consistent with a model whereby the ligand was flipped by 180° to the symmetry-related binding site. It was proposed that this may involve transient dissociation of the complex, possibly with exchange of ligands between different DNA duplexes, or it may be intramolecular in nature. Tentative evidence cited[10] for the latter mechanism was that the ligand inhibits solvent accessibility of imino protons.

This flip-flop exchange process was confirmed when SN-6999 was bound to the oligonucleotide duplex $d$(GGTTAATGCGGT)·$d$(ACCGCATTAACC).[9] This sequence was designed to provide a nonpalindromic DNA duplex that would simplify interpretation of the spectra as well as containing an optimum binding site of five AT base pairs and thereby limit any potential sliding of the ligand in the binding site. The AT site is flanked by GC base pairs so that the guanine amino groups protruding into the minor groove provide a structural restriction on sliding. Inspection of the intermolecular NOEs revealed that the ligand bound to the minor groove of the AT region in two orientations relative to the helix axis. The linewidths of a number of resonances showed a strong temperature dependence and, in the case of one adenine H2 resonance, two sets of signals were observed in a NOESY spectrum acquired at 276 K. It was not possible to freeze out two sets of signals for thymine methyl resonances as in the previous complex. This indicates that the ligand exchanges rapidly between the two binding sites and the rate at which this occurs was estimated to be >300 s[-1] at 315 K. The similarities in the exchange rates, estimated activation energies for the exchange, and the effects observed in NMR spectra suggest that the exchange processes in the two complexes are due to the same physical phenomenon, that is, flipping of the molecule by 180° relative to the DNA duplex.[9] Evidence for such a mechanism has also been observed for Hoechst 33258, as discussed above, as well as for netropsin, distamycin, and lexitropsins. This flip-flop process would therefore seem to represent a property inherent in complexes between minor groove binders and duplex DNA.

## D   TEREPHTHALAMIDES

The terephthalamides (or terephthalanilides) comprise a class of synthetic compounds for which high levels of activity against leukaemias and lymphomas in mice have been observed.[1,36] Representative members of this series are triaryl bisamides derived from terephthalic acid and substituted anilines, with the aniline substituent being an amidine or guanidine functional group (e.g., NSC 57153 in Figure 12). The basic terminal groups in these symmetrically substituted compounds are protonated at physiological pH, so that each end of the molecule is positively charged. The terephthalamides can adopt a curved, coplanar conformation where the two amide hydrogens form part of the concave edge, suitably placed for forming hydrogen bonds to acceptor groups (e.g., adenine N3 and thymine O2) in the floor of the minor groove.

In the first structural study of molecules of this type, Gago et al.[37] used molecular mechanics methods to model the interaction between NSC 57153 and the minor groove of short segments of DNA. In their model of the complex with 5'-ATAT-3', the ligand covered the 4 bp, with one

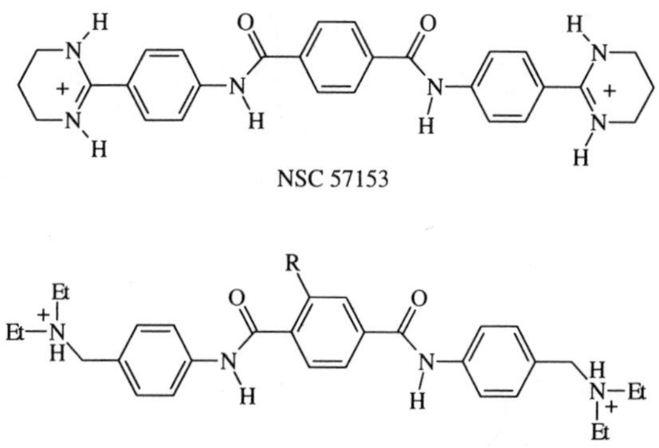

NSC 57153

| Compound | R |
|----------|---|
| L(NO₂) | NO₂ |
| L(NH₂) | NH₂ |
| L(Gly) | NHCOCH₂NH₂ |

**FIGURE 12**
Structures of NSC 57153 and the terephthalamide derivatives $L(NH_2)$, $L(NO_2)$, and $L(Gly)$.

amide NH forming a bifurcated hydrogen bond to two adjacent thymine O2 atoms and the other amide NH forming a single hydrogen bond to an adenine N3 atom. While this model predicts similarities in binding between terephthalamides and established minor groove-binding ligands (e.g., netropsin and distamycin), it was of interest to confirm the binding mode of terephthalamides using experimental methods.

This was done in a study aimed at the development of DNA-binding antitumour agents, in which a series of terephthalamides having different substituents on the central benzene ring and tertiary amines as the terminal charge-bearing groups in place of amidine or guanidine groups, was prepared.[38] The ligands, referred to as $L(NO_2)$, $L(NH_2)$, and $L(Gly)$, are shown in Figure 12. To establish whether these terephthalamides bound in the minor groove of AT-rich DNA, a series of NMR titration experiments was undertaken. During the course of these studies it became clear that the ligands bind more weakly to DNA than the other classes of compounds described earlier and that the spectra exhibit fast-exchange characteristics. Nevertheless, considerable information on their binding mode was derived, and this is described below to illustrate approaches that can be used for weakly binding ligands.

## 1  Titration Experiments

Figure 13 shows an expansion of the aliphatic region of a series of $^1$H NMR spectra of 0.5-m$M$ $d$(GGTAATTACC)$_2$, to which increasing amounts

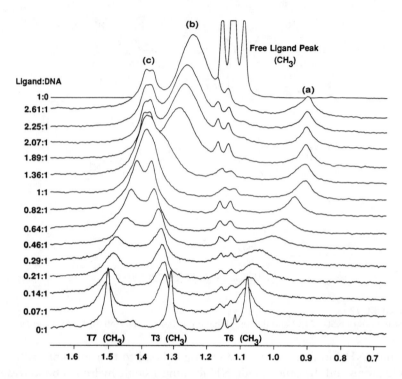

**FIGURE 13**

Expanded regions from 300-MHz $^1$H NMR spectra for complexes between $L(NH_2)$ and $d(GGTAATTACC)_2$ recorded at 10°C. The two small peaks at 1.12 and 1.14 ppm arise from an impurity. Increasing ligand concentration causes an upfield shift of the T6 methyl resonance (a), and causes the T7 and T3 resonances to become overlapped at later stages of the titration (c). Peak (b) is an averaged resonance from the ligand methyl groups intermediate in shift between the bound and free forms of the ligand.

of $L(NH_2)$ have been added.[38] The spectra cover mole ratios of ligand to DNA duplex ranging from 0:1 to 2.6:1. While the spectra are complicated by overlap in some regions, it is clear that addition of the ligand causes significant changes to the DNA resonances. A typical example is seen for the T6 methyl resonance, where addition of ligand causes both an upfield shift and broadening of the resonance at certain stages of the titration. The chemical shift moves monotonically with ligand concentration up to a mole ratio of 1:1 and then reaches a plateau, remaining constant as larger amounts of ligand are added. Broadening of the resonance reaches a maximum at a ligand to DNA mole ratio of approximately 0.3. Both observations are consistent with there being moderately fast exchange on the chemical-shift time scale between the free and ligand-bound forms of the DNA in solution.[39-41] In this case, the observed spectral peaks reflect neither the free nor the bound form of DNA, but are averaged resonances.

Ligand resonances are also in fast exchange, as seen with the $L(NH_2)$ methyl resonance, which first appears at a ligand to DNA ratio of 1.36:1 as a shoulder on the overlapped T3 and T7 methyl resonances at approximately 1.27 ppm. This resonance is not initially visible in spectra at low ligand to DNA mole ratios because of the small population of bound species and the overlapping DNA peaks. It moves upfield with increasing ligand concentration and, again, represents an averaged resonance intermediate in chemical shift between free and bound forms, reflecting fast-exchange kinetics. Eventually, the chemical shift of this signal approaches that of the free ligand of 1.1 ppm (measured in a separate experiment with a solution of ligand alone).

In the fast-exchange cases such as this, it is possible to obtain an estimate of the dissociation constant for the complex $K_d$ and the bound chemical shift $v_b$ of DNA resonances by fitting the observed chemical shift changes as a function of ligand concentration to Equation (2).[39]

$$v_{obs} - v_f = \frac{[ML]}{M_T}(v_b - v_f) \tag{2}$$

Here, $v_{obs}$, $v_f$, and $v_b$ are the observed chemical shift, the free chemical shift and the bound chemical shift, respectively. The total concentration of the macromolecule $M_T$ in this case is equal to the initial DNA concentration, and $[ML]$ is the concentration of the macromolecule–ligand complex. Values for $[ML]$ at any point in the titration are readily obtained by solving the quadratic equation Equation (3) pertaining to the binding equilibrium, Equation (4) between the ligand and DNA.[39] In Equation (3), $L_T$ is the total ligand concentration.

$$[ML] = \frac{1}{2}\left\{(M_T + L_T + K_d) - \left[(M_T + L_T + K_d)^2 - 4M_T L_T\right]^{1/2}\right\} \tag{3}$$

$$M + L \underset{k_{off}}{\overset{k_{on}}{\rightleftarrows}} ML \tag{4}$$

The observed shift data were fitted to Equation (2) by iteratively adjusting values of $K_d$ and $(v_b - v_f)$ until the error between the calculated and observed values of $(v_{obs} - v_f)$ was minimized. The parameters that best fitted the experimental data for the T6 methyl resonance were $K_d = 1.2 \times 10^{-6}$ $M$ and $(v_b - v_f) = 46$ Hz, as shown in Figure 14. Limitations on the accuracy of $K_d$ values derived in this way have been described previously.[39]

To further define the thermodynamic constants associated with binding, the linewidth data were also quantitatively examined using Equation (5).

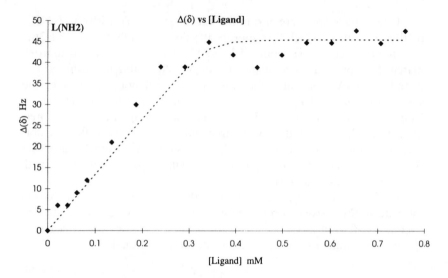

**FIGURE 14**

Experimental and theoretical plots of changes in chemical shift vs. ligand concentration for the T6 methyl of $d(GGTAATTACC)_2$ interacting with $L(NH_2)$. Experimentally determined chemical shifts are shown as filled diamonds. The dashed line is the theoretical fit to Equation 2 with $\Delta(\delta) = \nu_{obs} - \nu_f$, $K_d = 1.2 \times 10^{-6}$ M, and $\nu_b - \nu_f = 46$ Hz.[38]

$$LW_{obs} = LW_f\left(1 - \frac{[ML]}{M_T}\right) + LW_b\,\frac{[ML]}{M_T} + \frac{\dfrac{[ML]}{M_T}\left(1 - \dfrac{[ML]}{M_T}\right)^2 4\pi\left(\nu_b - \nu_f\right)^2}{k_{off}} \tag{5}$$

In this equation, $LW_{obs}$, $LW_f$, and $LW_b$ are the observed, the free, and the bound linewidths, respectively. The last term is referred to as the exchange contribution to linewidth. In the case of moderately fast exchange, a maximum linewidth is predicted at a ligand to DNA mole ratio of 0.33,[39,40] as observed in the current case.

The experimental results were iteratively fitted to Equation (5) by adjusting parameters $K_d$, $k_{off}$, $(\nu_b - \nu_f)$, and $LW_b$. Figure 15 shows calculated and experimental linewidths vs. ligand concentration. The best fit was achieved with $K_d \leq 1.0 \times 10^{-6}$ M, $k_{off} \approx 250$ s$^{-1}$, $(\nu_b - \nu_f) = 49$ Hz, and $LW_b = 12$ Hz. These values are consistent with those derived from Equation (3).

The overall effect on the DNA spectrum caused by $L(NO_2)$ binding is similar to the effects caused by $L(NH_2)$. An example of this is shown in Figure 16, where the upfield methyl resonances of the duplex are seen to shift in a similar fashion upon binding of these two terephthalamide derivatives. This figure also demonstrates the perturbation plateau achieved at a 1:1 ligand to DNA ratio, confirming the 1:1 stoichiometry. Broadening of the peaks is also observed, with the maximum linewidth occurring at a ratio of ~0.3. Equation (2) was used to derive values of $K_d$ and ($v_b$ – $v_f$) using the observed shift changes for several clearly resolved resonances in the DNA spectrum, including the T6 $CH_3$ resonance.[38] These are summarized in Table 2, and are similar to the results obtained from $L(NH_2)$.

## 2   Evidence for Minor Groove Binding

Figure 17 summarizes the chemical-shift perturbations for various DNA protons along the sequence and confirms the expected minor groove binding of the terephthalamide ligands $L(NH_2)$ and $L(NO_2)$. Residues A4, A5, and A8 are the only ones that contain easily detectable minor groove protons (H2). These resonances, which originate from the floor of the minor groove, are shifted downfield with ligand binding, whereas other resonances are shifted upfield. This observation is consistent with the ligands binding in the minor groove, as noted earlier, and has been reported for other minor groove binders such as Hoechst 33258,[8] and SN-6999,[9,10] where adenine H2 protons on the floor of the groove experience deshielding ring-current effects.

Significant chemical-shift changes were also observed for some major groove protons. The largest effects observed were for A5 and T6. Large perturbations in the major groove have also been observed for other

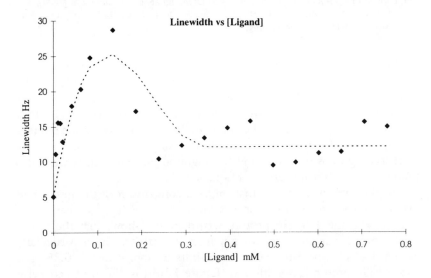

**FIGURE 15**
Experimental and theoretical plots of linewidth of the T6 methyl resonance of $d$(GGTAATTACC)$_2$ vs. concentration of $L(NH_2)$.[38]

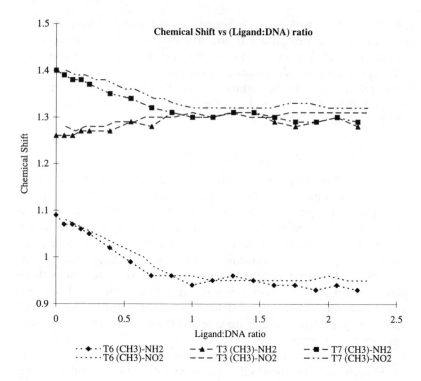

**FIGURE 16**
Comparison of chemical-shift perturbations to DNA signals upon binding of $L(NH_2)$ and $L(NO_2)$. (From Pavlopoulos, S. et al., *Anti-Cancer Drug Design* 1995, in press. With permission of Oxford University Press.)

established minor groove binders such as distamycin,[5] netropsin,[3] and Hoechst 33258.[17] Not all these perturbations could be explained by ring-current effects. Based on NOE and crystallographic data, it was concluded that the effects were caused by distortions of the B-DNA duplex, including changes in the "base roll" of residues within the binding site, upon complexation. Electronic effects arising from the close proximity of charged groups on the ligand to neighbouring nucleotides were also found to perturb major groove resonances.

In the case of the terephthalamides a comparison of the minor and major groove perturbations for a particular residue (i.e., comparison of adenine H2 and H8/H6 proton perturbations) shows that the minor groove protons are affected to a much greater extent. This is particularly evident for A8, where the H2 proton shifts by approximately 0.25 ppm and the H8 proton is not affected (Figure 17). It is difficult to conceive of a binding mode in the major groove that would account for such a large effect on the minor groove A8 H2 resonance without a simultaneous effect

**TABLE 2**

Calculated Values of $K_d$ and $(\nu_b - \nu_f)$ for Several Perturbed Resonances from the Titration of $d$(GGTAATTACC)$_2$ with $L$(NO$_2$) and $L$(NH$_2$)

| Resonance | $K_d \times 10^6$ M | | $(\nu_b - \nu_f)$ Hz | |
|---|---|---|---|---|
| | $L$(NH$_2$) | $L$(NO$_2$) | $L$(NH$_2$) | $L$(NO$_2$) |
| T6 CH$_3$ | ≤1.23 | ≤1.0 | 45 | 42 |
| T7 CH$_3$ | ≤2.66 | ≤1.0 | 32 | 24 |
| A5 H8 | ≤1.21 | ≤1.0 | 45 | 58 |
| T6 H6 | ≤0.62 | ≤1.0 | 87 | 76 |

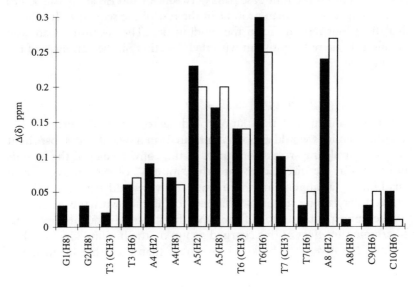

**FIGURE 17**

Chemical-shift perturbations of DNA protons upon ligand binding. The lighter and darker columns represent shifts due to $L$(NO$_2$) and $L$(NH$_2$) derivatives, respectively. (From Pavlopoulos, S. et al., *Anti-Cancer Drug Design* 1995, in press. With permission of Oxford University Press.)

on the major groove protons of T7 and A8. The observed 1:1 stoichiometry of the complex excludes the possibility that the ligand binds to the major and minor groove at the same time. It is more likely, therefore, that binding in the minor groove causes distortion of the DNA structure so that perturbations are observed for the major groove protons of A5 and T6, but not neighbouring nucleotides.

## 3    Location of Binding Site

Molecular mechanics modelling of NSC 57153[37] predicted that terephthalamides would interact predominantly with four base pairs. This suggests the possibility of up to three different binding sites (Figure 18) along the oligonucleotide AT tract used in the NMR study.[38] The terephthalamide derivatives studied are similar in size to established minor groove binders such as distamycin-A[5,8] and Hoechst,[18,21] which interact with a four-base pair binding site. Binding of these ligands causes much larger chemical-shift perturbations to the nucleotides that make up the binding site than to the rest of the oligonucleotide sequence. This has also been observed for other minor groove binders and was thus expected to apply for the terephthalamides.[3,10]

Figure 17 shows that, upon binding of the terephthalamides, the DNA protons on the four base pairs between A5 and A8 are perturbed to a much larger degree than protons in the rest of the sequence. It is likely that these four residues form the binding site. The A4 protons are also significantly altered, consistent with their location on the periphery of the binding site.

## 4   Ligand Design

It was anticipated that, upon binding to the minor groove, the terephthalamides would adopt a conformation in which the substituent on the central ring would form part of the convex edge of the ligands and therefore be directed toward the "mouth" of the groove. Given this binding arrangement, the ligand $L$(Gly) would have a positively charged alkylamine group positioned to interact with the negatively charged phosphate groups of the DNA backbone. It was of interest to determine the effect of this charged group on the binding kinetics. The $L$(Gly) derivative has a bulkier substituent than the other ligands, and

a) GG**TA A T**TACC

b) GGT**A A T T**ACC

c) GGTA**A T T A**CC

**FIGURE 18**
DNA sequence used in the terephthalamide-binding study, highlighting possible ligand binding sites: (a) TAAT, (b) AATT, (c) ATTA.

this was also expected to lead to some differences in its binding. In a titration of the oligonucleotide with $L(\text{Gly})$,[38] significant perturbations were observed to those resonances most affected by binding of $L(\text{NH}_2)$ and $L(\text{NO}_2)$. In the methyl region of the titration spectra shown in Figure 19, the T7 $CH_3$ signal moves upfield and the T3 $CH_3$ signal moves slightly downfield, as seen previously, with increasing ligand concentration. However, in contrast to the case for the other ligands, the characteristic broadening of resonances at intermediate ratios is non-Lorentzian, suggesting kinetics in the intermediate-exchange regime. The T6 $CH_3$ resonance does not shift in the characteristic fast-exchange manner but, instead, a new broad resonance appears close to the expected position of the bound T6 $CH_3$ chemical shift on the first addition of ligand and increases in intensity with increasing ligand concentration. This observation is consistent with the ligand being in slow to intermediate exchange between the free and bound forms, with $k_{\text{off}} \approx (v_b - v_f)$. Based on the magnitude of $v_b - v_f$ for this resonance, $k_{\text{off}}$ for $L(\text{Gly})$ is estimated to be 50 s$^{-1}$, which is significantly slower than for $L(\text{NO}_2)$ and $L(\text{NH}_2)$.

At a ligand to DNA ratio of approximately 1:1, the ratio of the integrals of the T6 methyl resonance and the overlapped T3 and T7 methyl resonances is ~1:6. The expected value is 1:2, which indicates that the bound ligand methyl resonance ($4 \times CH_3$) is overlapped with the T7 and T3 methyl resonances, as observed with $L(\text{NH}_2)$ and $L(\text{NO}_2)$. When the ligand-to-DNA ratio is increased beyond 1:1, a new peak appears at ~1.15 ppm and increases in intensity as the ligand concentration is increased. This new peak corresponds to the methyl resonance of the free ligand, and its appearance in this manner is consistent with slow exchange on the chemical-shift time scale. To confirm this, spectra of a 2:1 mixture of $L(\text{Gly})$ and $d(\text{GGTAATTACC})_2$ were acquired at different temperatures[38] (Figure 20). This mixture contains equimolar amounts of free and bound $L(\text{Gly})$.

At low temperatures, signals at 1.15 and 1.30 ppm (overlapped with the T7 $CH_3$ and T3 $CH_3$ resonances) attributable to the methyl groups from the free and bound ligand, respectively, are distinguishable. As the temperature is increased, a broad peak appears between these two resonances (at ~1.22 ppm). At the lower temperatures $k_{\text{off}} \leq (v_b - v_f)$, so that methyl resonances of the ligand have complex characteristics reflecting slow–intermediate exchange. At higher temperatures, $k_{\text{off}} \geq (v_b - v_f)$, so the resonance appears as a fast-exchanged average between the free and bound resonances. From a qualitative analysis of the spectra, $k_{\text{off}}$ for $L(\text{Gly})$ was estimated to be 50–60 s$^{-1}$ at 283 K.

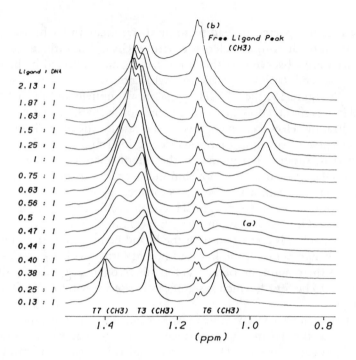

**FIGURE 19**

Expansions from the 600-MHz $^1$H NMR spectra for complexes formed between $L$(Gly) and $d$(GGTAATTACC)$_2$ showing the methyl resonances. The two small peaks at 1.12 and 1.14 ppm are due to an impurity. The complex nature of the T6 methyl resonance at ligand to DNA ratios less than 1:1 (a), and the manner in which signal intensity increases at ~1.15 ppm at DNA to ligand ratios greater than 1:1 (b), are indicative of intermediate exchange. (From Pavlopoulos, S. et al., *Anti-Cancer Drug Design* 1995, in press. With permission of Oxford University Press.)

The fact that some resonances (e.g., the oligonucleotide T7 and T3 methyl signals) exhibit fast exchange, while others in the same spectrum of the same complex exhibit slow–intermediate character-istics is a reflection of the different $(v_b - v_f)$ values for different resonances. This emphasizes the point made in Chapter 3 that "ex-change regime" is a relative expression and depends not only on the rate of exchange, but also on the size of the chemical-shift differences involved.

Changes were also observed for several resonances in the aromatic region of the spectrum as a function of ligand to DNA ratio and temperature, and the findings support the results above. In sum-mary, the observations suggest that $k_{off}$ for binding of $L$(Gly) to the oligonucleotide duplex is much slower than for the other two derivatives. This provides an illustration of the value of NMR as a quick method for

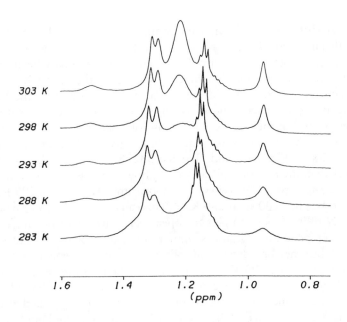

**FIGURE 20**
Expansions of ¹H NMR spectra of a 2:1 mixture of L(Gly) and d(GGTAATTACC)₂ acquired
at different temperatures. (From Pavlopoulos, S. et al., *Anti-Cancer Drug Design* 1995, in
press. With permission of Oxford University Press.)

comparing the binding of different ligands, and for confirming ligand-
binding hypotheses, as was discussed in Chapters 7 and 8.

## 5 Comparison with Other Minor Groove Binders

The observed binding kinetics for the terephthalamide derivatives
studied indicate moderate affinity for DNA. The $L(NH_2)$ and $L(NO_2)$
were calculated to have $K_d \approx 1.0 \times 10^{-6}$ M at 283 K with $k_{off} \approx 250$ s⁻¹. The
$L(Gly)$ displayed a fivefold slower off rate, and thus a fivefold-higher
affinity for DNA, than $L(NH_2)$ or $L(NO_2)$. These are comparable to
affinities of other minor groove binders. Netropsin and distamycin-A have
$K_d \approx 10^{-7}$ M, and the rate constant for dissociation $k_{off}$ is less than 5 s⁻¹ at
300 K.[3,5,8] Hoechst 33258 also shows similar binding kinetics at 293 K,
and as a result, the titration spectra for these compounds displayed no
averaging between free and bound DNA resonances. SN-6999 exhibits
weaker binding, with $K_d \approx 2 \times 10^{-6}$ M at 298 K and does exhibit signal
averaging when a 1:1 complex is formed with the oligonucleotide
$d(GCATTAATGC)_2$.[10] In this case, the DNA spectrum and the observed

chemical-shift perturbations are similar to the results from the terephthalamide study.

As noted earlier, a number of minor groove binders have been shown to exchange between equivalent binding sites across the dyad axis of a self-complementary oligonucleotide sequence in such a way that the ligand reverses its position from head to tail to become associated with the opposite strand of the duplex. In the case of distamycin-A, the exchange rate between the two sites was found to be approximately half the $k_{off}$ value, that is, $\approx 2$ s$^{-1}$.[5] Netropsin and Hoechst 33258 showed similar exchange rates between the two sites.[3,18] SN-6999, however, was shown to have an exchange rate between the two sites of approximately 200 s$^{-1}$ at 299 K, and this decreases to ~100 s$^{-1}$ at 289 K.[9,10] This caused some DNA resonances of the SN-6999–DNA complex to appear as relatively narrow, single lines at high temperatures because symmetry-related resonances were being averaged, but they broadened and split into two lines of equal intensity at temperatures below 290 K.[10] At no stage in the titrations with $L(NH_2)$, $L(NO_2)$, and $L(Gly)$ was there an increase in the number of bound DNA resonances with increasing ligand concentration. This suggests that there is a dynamic equivalence of the two ATTA symmetry-related binding sites and that the flip-flop exchange common to the other minor groove-binding ligands also occurs for the terephthalamides.

---

# IV DRUG DESIGN

A detailed analysis of the interaction of small molecules with the minor groove has highlighted the factors that are important in sequence recognition. This information has been used to design analogues of these compounds with altered sequence specificities and affinities. These studies serve the dual purpose of confirming binding hypotheses deduced from structural studies and further improving our understanding of drug–DNA interactions, as well as testing the notion of inducing a desired property in a compound by a process of rational design. The importance of such studies to therapeutic applications is illustrated by the recent publication of a book devoted to nucleic acid targeted drug design.[42]

The terephthalamide derivatives described above provide one example of this approach. It was shown[38] that $L(NH_2)$, $L(NO_2)$, and $L(Gly)$ bind to the minor groove of DNA and that the binding site on the oligonucleotide duplex $d(GGTAATTACC)_2$ spans the four bases A5–A8. Molecular mechanics studies predict terephthalamides will have a decreased affinity for the minor groove of AT-rich regions compared to other minor groove binders such as netropsin and distamycin.[37] This was found to be the case for $L(NH_2)$ and $L(NO_2)$. However, the tethering of a charged group to the central benzene ring of a terephthalamide in place of an aromatic $-NO_2$ or $-NH_2$ led to an increase in binding affinity.

Efforts to increase the binding affinity of distamycin have also been made, although a different approach was utilized. Molecules were designed with an increased number of $N$-methyl pyrrolcarboxamides, which had the effect of increasing the size of the binding site and improving the sequence specificity for longer tracts of AT-rich regions. These studies led to the general rule that $n$-amide NHs afford binding-site sizes of $n + 1$ base pairs.[43-46]

A range of other approaches have been applied to netropsin[47-50] and distamycin.[51-53] Structural studies of these molecules with DNA indicated that a major component of the binding to AT-rich regions was the close van der Waals contacts of the aromatic protons of the pyrrole groups with the floor of the minor groove. The steric clash that would occur between the 2-amino group of the guanine and these aromatic protons prevents the molecules from binding to GC regions. Any attempt to induce GC selectivity would require the removal of these aromatic hydrogens, which led to the suggestion that one or more of the pyrrole groups be replaced by imidazole.[47,48] This modification not only improves the compatibility with GC regions but also provides a hydrogen bond acceptor on the concave surface of the ligand, which then has the potential to form H bonds with the $NH_2$ of guanine (Figure 21). This approach was partially successful, with analogues showing decreased AT specificity and a corresponding increase in GC specificity.[47] However, it became clear that factors other than H bonding and van der Waals interactions were important. The requirement of locating the charged end groups in the high negative potential of AT regions imposes a substantial opposing influence on the structural modifications.[47,49]

This led to the idea of reducing the AT bias of the ligands by reducing the cationic charge of the molecule in addition to introducing guanine reading groups. To achieve this, the cationic guanidino and amidino groups were removed. This approach proved successful when an analogue that had the guanidinium moiety replaced by an $N$-formyl group showed greatly enhanced binding to GC-containing sites.[48]

A similar concept was used in an attempt to induce GC specificity in Hoechst 33258 by replacing the benzimidazole moieties with pyridoimidazole and benzoxazole moieties.[54,55] The concave face of the ligand would then contain hydrogen bond acceptors with the potential to form H bonds with the $NH_2$ groups present in the minor groove of GC-rich regions (Figure 21). This strategy was again partially successful, and studies of the interaction with the oligonucleotide duplex $d$(CATGGCCATG)$_2$ showed that the preferred binding site was $d$(CCAT)·$d$(GGTA).[55] The orientation of the ligand was such that the piperizine moiety was located in the GC region where the minor groove

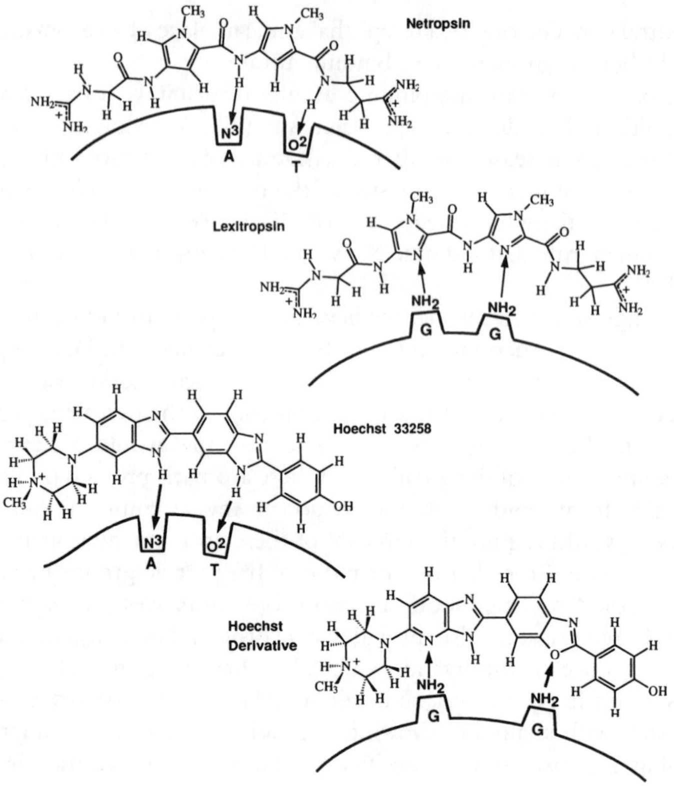

**FIGURE 21**

The design rationale for lexitropsins and Hoechst derivatives. Replacement of pyrole groups of netropsin with imidazoles provides better complementarity with the floor of the minor groove of GC regions and also provides an H-bond acceptor as opposed to a donor. Replacement of the benzimidazole moieties of Hoechst 33258 with pyridoimidazole and benzoxazole moieties employs the same strategy for GC recognition.

is wider, and the phenol moiety extended toward the AT region. Calculations showed that the analogue could easily adopt the shape required for isohelical binding to DNA and that the distance between the hydrogen-bonding elements was optimal for hydrogen-bonding to consecutive base pairs. The pyridoimidazole moiety clearly showed a selectivity toward GC base pairs. Hydrogen bonding was observed to the $NH_2$ of the guanine in the binding domain and the N proton was placed so that it showed H bonds to the O2 of T3 and the O2 of C7 on the opposite strand, thus providing a clear basis for the observed GC selectivity.

In the structure of the complex of modified Hoechst 33258 with $d(CATGGCCATG)_2$ the benzoxazole moiety is located in the AT region, indicating that the presence of a hydrogen bond acceptor oxygen, as proposed in the design hypothesis in Figure 21, is alone not enough to achieve GC selectivity.[55] In the actual complex, van der Waals interactions occur between the adenine H2 protons and the aromatic proton that is adjacent to the oxygen atom of the benzoxazole moiety. This suggests a potential steric clash between this aromatic proton and the $NH_2$ of guanines, thus inhibiting interaction with GC base pairs. In contrast to the prediction in Figure 21, the benzoxazole oxygen in the complex did not exhibit any H bonding to the minor groove floor, but the NH of the neighbouring pyridoimidazole does show the familiar, strong H bonding to donors on the floor of the groove. The results of this study indicate that if the interfering aromatic hydrogen of the benzoxazole were removed, GC recognition would be achieved. The successful binding of the pyridoimidazole moiety suggests that GC recognition would best be achieved by a derivative consisting of two pyridine oxazole moieties.[55]

This idea was also applied in the modification of distamycin to achieve GC selectivity. The replacement of the terminal N-methyl-pyrrolecarboxamide of distamycin with pyridine-2-carboxamide was expected to bind to one GC base pair followed by three AT base pairs. It was anticipated that the amide hydrogens would form bifurcated H bonds with adenine N3 and thymine O2 atoms, while the pyridine nitrogen would participate in a key hydrogen bond with the $NH_2$ group of a GC base pair.[52] Pyridine-3-carboxamide and pyridine-4-carboxamide were also synthesised to test whether the placement of the ring nitrogen would have any effect on specificity. It was found that the pyridine 2-carboxamide analogue bound to three AT rich sites, 5′-TTTTT-3′, 5′-AATAA-3′, and 5′-CTTTT-3′, as well as 5′-TGTCA-3′, which was not predicted. The pyrrole-3 and 4-carboxamide analogues bound only to AT regions, showing that the 2 position is important as it locates the nitrogen on the concave face of the ligand.

The binding to the CTTTT sequence was consistent with the design rationale; however, it was clear that this was not the highest-affinity binding site. The recognition of two GC base pairs separated by one AT base pair was difficult to explain with a 1:1 binding model. However, given that distamycin has also displayed a 2:1 binding mode, it is possible to explain the observed specificity[52] (Figure 22).

With two molecules of this analogue bound in a side-by-side motif within the minor groove, each of the two guanine amino groups in the binding site can hydrogen-bond to the pyridine ring nitrogens of the ligands. To further explore the binding to the 5′-TGTCA-3′ sequence, the pyridine ring was replaced with N-methylimidazole (i.e., a six-membered nitrogen-containing ring was replaced with a five-membered ring). This derivative bound to 5′-TGTCA-3′ with a higher sequence specificity. Two-dimensional NMR studies confirmed that this analogue bound with 2:1 stoichiometry, in a side-by-side motif, and also showed that the two ligands bind with positive cooperativity.[52]

In a separate study, a distamycin analogue containing a central imidazole was shown to interact with 5′-AAGTT-3′ as a side-by-side antiparallel

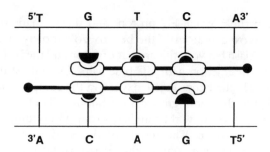

**FIGURE 22**
Recognition of GC base pairs separated by one AT base pair due to the 2:1 binding mode of distamyacin.

dimer.[51] Furthermore, the modification was successful not only in recognising mixed GC and AT sequences, but also in actively rejecting AT sequences. These models established that the minor groove expands to accommodate both molecules and that each ligand participates in hydrogen bonds only with bases on a single strand, as opposed to the bifurcated H bonds to both strands that are prevalent in the 1:1 binding modes of netropsin and distamycin.

These studies indicated that if one of the $N$-methyl imidazole analogues in the 2:1 complex with 5′-TGTCA-3′ was replaced by a distamycin A molecule the absence of the imidazole nitrogen should favour the selection of an AT base pair relative to a GC base pair, so that the sequence $(A,T)G(A,T)_3$ would be favoured. Footprinting experiments have indicated that distamycin A and its $N$-methylimidazole analogue bind as an antiparallel side-by-side heterodimer in the minor groove of 5′-TGTAA-3′.[53] This design rationale differed in that each ligand of the dimer is targeted to a single strand of the binding site in the minor groove of DNA, independent of the other ligand–strand interactions. So far this approach has been the most successful in attempts to specifically target mixed sequences.

In conclusion, further advances in the technology described in this chapter should lead to the development of improved sequence-specific DNA-binding agents, ideally to target any predetermined sequence. Such agents will be invaluable for the study of gene expression and control, and should have many applications in molecular biology, diagnosis, and therapy.[55] NMR promises to play a vital role in the design of such agents.

## ACKNOWLEDGMENTS

We are grateful to our colleagues Kevin Embrey and Mark Searle for their valuable collaborations cited in this chapter. We thank John Gehrmann,

Justine Hill, and Robyn Craik for their helpful comments on the manuscript. Some of the studies described in the chapter were funded in part by a grant from the NH & MRC (Australia).

# REFERENCES

1. Baguley, B.C. *Mol. Cell. Biochem.* 1982, 43, 167-181.
2. Braithwaite, A.W.; Baguley, B.C. *Biochemistry* 1980, 19, 1101-1106.
3. Patel, D.J.; Shapiro, L. *J. Biol. Chem.* 1986, 261, 1230-1240.
4. Coll, M.; Aymami, J.; van der Marel, G.A.; van Boom, J.H.; Rich, A.; Wang, A.H.-J. *Biochemistry* 1989, 28, 310-320.
5. Klevit, R.E.; Wemmer, D.E.; Reid, B.R. *Biochemistry* 1986, 25, 3296-3303.
6. Pelton, J.G., Wemmer, D.E. *Biochemistry* 1988, 27, 8088-8096.
7. Pelton, J.G.; Wemmer, D.E. *Proc. Natl. Acad. Sci. USA* 1989, 86, 5723-5727.
8. Pelton, J.G.; Wemmer, D.E. *J. Am. Chem. Soc.* 1990, 112, 1393-1399.
9. Chen, S.; Leupin, W.; Rance, M.; Chazin, W.J. *Biochemistry* 1992, 31, 4406-4413.
10. Leupin, W.; Chazin, W.J.; Hyberts, S.; Denny, W.A.; Wüthrich, K. *Biochemistry* 1986, 25, 5902-5910.
11. Trotta, E.; D'Ambrosio, E.; Del Grosso, N.; Ravagnan, G.; Cirilli, M.; Paci, M. *J. Biol. Chem.* 1993, 268, 3944-3951.
12. Scahill, T.A.; Jensen, R.M.; Swenson, D.H.; Hatzenbuhler, N.T.; Petzold, G.; Wierenga, W.; Brahme, N.D. *Biochemistry* 1990, 29, 2852-2860.
13. Pjura, E.P.; Grzeskowiak, K.; Dickerson, R.E. *J. Mol. Biol.* 1987, 197, 257-271.
14. Teng, M.K.; Usman, N.; Frederick, C.K.; Wang, H.J. *Nucleic Acids Res.* 1988, 16, 2671-2690.
15. Carrondo, M.A.A.F. de C.T.; Coll, M.; Aaymami, J.; Wang, A.H-J.; van der Marel, G.A.; van Boom, J.H.; Rich, A. *Biochemistry* 1989, 28, 7849-7859.
16. Quintana, J.R.; Lipanov, A.A.; Dickerson, R.E. *Biochemistry* 1991, 30, 10294-10306.
17. Searle, M.S.; Embrey, K.J. *Nucleic Acids Res.* 1990, 18, 3753-3762.
18. Embrey, K.J.; Searle, M.S.; Craik, D.J. *Eur. J. Biochem.* 1993, 211, 437-447.
19. Parkinson, J.A.; Barber, J.; Douglas, K.T.; Rosamond, J.; Sharples, D. *Biochemistry* 1990, 29, 10181-10190.
20. Fede, A.; Labhardt, A.; Bannwarth, W.; Leupin, W. *Biochemistry* 1991, 30, 11377-11388.
21. Fede, A.; Billeter, M.; Leupin, W.; Wüthrich, K. *Structure* 1993, 1, 177-186.
22. Coll, M.; Frederick, C.A.; Wang, A.H.; Rich, A. *Proc. Natl. Acad. Sci. USA* 1987, 84, 8385-8389.
23. Nelson, H.C.M.; Finch, J.T.; Luisi, B.F.; Klug, A. *Nature* 1987, 330, 221-226.
24. Searle, M.S.; Wakelin, L.P.G. *Biochim. Biophys. Acta* 1990, 1049, 69-77.
25. Pulman, B. *Advances in Drug Research* 1989, 18, 1-113.
26. Searle, M.S. *Prog. Nucl. Magn. Reson. Spectrosc.* 1993, 25, 403-480.
27. Harshman, K.D.; Dervan, P. *Nucleic Acids Res.* 1985, 13, 4825-4835.
28. Embrey, K.J.; Searle, M.S.; Craik, D.J. *Biochem Int.* 1991, 24, 567-576.
29. Gronenborn, A.M.; Clore, G.M. *Proc. Nucl. Magn. Reson. Spectrosc.* 1985, 17, 1-32.
30. Hosur, R.V.; Govil, G.; Miles, H.T. *Magn. Reson. Chem.* 1988, 26, 927-944.
31. Wüthrich, K. *NMR of Proteins and Nucleic Acids*; Wiley-Interscience: New York, 1986.

32. Ashcroft, J.; Live, D.H.; Patel, D.J.; Cowburn, D. *Biopolymers* 1991, 31, 45-46.
33. Drew, H.R.; Wing, R.M.; Takano, T.; Broka, C.; Tanaka, S.; Itakura, K.; Dickerson, R.E. *Proc. Natl. Acad. Sci. USA* 1981, 78, 2119-2183.
34. Swenson, D.H.; Li, L.H.; Hurley, L.H.; Rokem, J.S.; Petzolo, G.L.; Dayton, B.D.; Wallace, T.L.; Lin, A.H.; Krueger, W.C. *Cancer Res.* 1982, 42.
35. Zimmer, C.; Wähnert, U. *Prog. Biophys. Molec. Biol.* 1986, 47, 31-112.
36. Bennet, L.L., Jr. *Prog. Exp. Tumor Res.* 1965, 7, 259-325.
37. Gago, F.; Reynolds, C.A.; Richards, W.G. *Mol. Pharmacol.* 1989, 35, 232-241.
38. Pavlopoulos, S.; Rose, M.; Wickham, G.; Craik, D.J. *Anti-Cancer Drug Design*, 1995, in press.
39. Feeney, J.; Batchelor, J.G.; Albrand, J.P.; Roberts, G.C.K. *J. Magn. Reson.* 1979, 33, 519-529.
40. Lian, L-Y; Roberts, G.C.K., Effects of Chemical Exchange on NMR spectra, in *NMR of Macro-molecules: A Practical Approach*; Roberts, G.C.K., Ed.; Oxford University Press: Oxford, U.K., 1993.
41. Craik, D.J.; Higgins, K.A., in *Annual Reports on NMR Spectroscopy, Vol. 22*; Webb, G.A., Ed.; Academic Press: London, 1990.
42. Propst, C.L.; Perun, T.J., Eds.; *Nucleic Acid Targeted Drug Design*; Marcel Dekker: New York, 1992.
43. Schultz, P.G.; Dervan, P.B. *J. Am. Chem. Soc.* 1983, 105, 7748-7750.
44. Youngquist, R.S.; Dervan, P.B. *J. Am. Chem. Soc.* 1985, 107, 5528-5529.
45. Youngquist, R.S.; Dervan, P.B. *J. Am. Chem. Soc.* 1987, 109, 7564-7566.
46. Griffin, J.H.; Dervan, P.B. *J. Am. Chem. Soc.* 1986, 108, 5008-5009.
47. Lown, J.W.; Krowicki, K.; Bhat, U.G. *Biochemistry* 1986 25, 7408-7416.
48. Kissinger, K.; Krowicki, K.; Dabrowiak, J.C.; Lown, J.W. *Biochemistry* 1987, 26, 5590-5595.
49. Lee, M.; Pon, R.T.; Korwicki, K.; Lown, J.W. *J. Biomol. Struct. Dyn.* 1988, 5, 939-949.
50. Kumar, S.; Bathini, Y.; Joseph, T.; Pon, R.T.; Lown, J.W. *J. Biomol. Struct. Dyn.* 1991, 9, 1-21.
51. Dwyer, T.J.; Geierstanger, B.H.; Bathini, Y.; Lown, J.W.; Wemmer, D.E. *J. Am. Chem. Soc.* 1992, 114, 5914-5919.
52. Wade, W.S.; Mrksich, M.; Dervan, P.B. *J. Am. Chem. Soc.* 1992, 114, 8783-8794.
53. Mrkisch, M.; Dervan, P.B. *J. Am. Chem. Soc.* 1993, 115, 2572-2576.
54. Kumar, S.; Joseph, T.; Singh, M.P.; Bathini, Y.; Lown, J.W. *J. Biomol. Struct. Dyn.* 1991, 9, 853-880.
55. Kumar, S.; Bathini, Y.; Zimmermann, J.; Pon, R.T.; Lown, J.W. *J. Biomol. Struct. Dyn.* 1990, 8, 331-357.

# Index

## A

ACE inhibitors, 8
Acetazolamide, 5
Actinomycin D, 88–89
Adenosine triphosphate, see ATP
Aggregation of proteins, 116, 118, 119
AIDS, 338
Alanine racemase, 27
Allosteric effector, 250
Amide exchange, 69, 129, 348, 363
p-Aminobenzoic acid, 4, 6
γ-Aminobutyric acid, 203
Aminotetralins, 203
Anaesthetics, 206
Analgesics, 205
Angiotensin-converting enzyme, see ACE inhibitors
Angular order parameter, 187
Anipamil, 23–24
Antamanide, 235
Anthracycline antibiotics, 380–381
  nogalamycin, see Nogalamycin
  arugomycin, see Arugomycin
Antibacterial compounds, 3, 276
Antibodies, 250
Anticoagulant compounds, 91
Antidepressants, 204
Antidiuretics, 5
Antihypertensive drugs, 3, 92
Anti-inflammatory compounds, 89, 207
Antimalarial compounds, 276
Antineoplastic compounds, 276

Antiprotozoal drugs, 318
Antipsychotic drugs, 203
Antitumour antibiotics, 92, 380
Antiulcer drugs, 7
Antiviral antibiotics, 424
(R)-Apomorphine, 203
Arginine kinase, 256
Arginine vasopressin, 72–74
Arugomycin, 399–401
  binding to d(GCATGC)$_2$, 401–404
  sugar residues, 403–404
Ascomycin, 27, 95, 231
Aspirin, 5
Assignments in peptides and proteins
  bound ligands, 285–288
  diastereotopic protons, 222
  in DHFR, 281–285
  heteronuclear strategies
    coherence transfer via couplings, 132–135, 222
    heteronuclear-edited homonuclear experiments, 135–140, 222–223
    triple resonance experiments, 140–148
  homonuclear strategies
    minor conformers, 224
    proteins, size limitations, 125–127
    spin system identification, 127–129, 222–224
    sequential assignments, 129–130
    three-dimensional methods, 130–132

two-dimensional methods, 122–125, 222

sequential, see Sequential assignments

strategy overview, 148–152, 222–224

ATP (Adenosine triphosphate), 22, 250, 256

*Atropa belladonna*, 3

Atropine, 2

Auxotrophic strains, 116

Azide, 118

AZT, 338, 371


**B**

*Bacillus subtilis*, 106–109

Backbone dynamics, 339

Bacteriorhodopsin, 233

Barbiturates, 205

Benzodiazepines, 205

Bicarbonate ion, 5

Binding modes

multiple bound conformers, 26, 40, 294–306

prediction from computer graphics, 27

Binding sites of drugs, 33, 35, 55–56

Binding stoichiometry, 380

Bioavailability, 238, 371

Biochemical energetics, 19

Biomolecular structure, 37–39, 170–186

Bisbenzimidazole derivatives, 427

Bisintercalators, 379

Boltzmann's law, 45, 78

Bound conformations of ligands, 26, 40, 231–233, 248–255, 258, 285

Bounds smoothing, 171

Bradykinin antagonist, 233

Brodimoprim, 292–293

Brookhaven Protein Data Bank, see PDB

Burimamide, 7

(+)-Butaclamol, 203–205


**C**

Calcium binding, 316, 319–320

Calcium channel blockers, 207

Calicheamicin, 92–94

Calmidazolium, 318, 321–331

Calmodulin, 316–334

Cannabinoids, 206

Captopril, 8–9

Carbon-13

chemical shifts, 221, 227, 259, 261, 305

labelling, 95, 261, 269, 283–287

relaxation times, 230, 261, 306–307

spectra, 295, 302

Carbonic anhydrase, 37

Carboxypeptidase A, 8

Cardiac metabolism, 22

Catalytic antibody, 251

CAVEAT, 237

cDNA libraries, 105

Central nervous system drugs, see CNS drugs

Chelex, 118

Chemical diversity, 10

Chemical exchange, 55–66

cross-peaks, 224, 229, 299, 430

fast, see Fast exchange

intermediate exchange, 60, 455–456

lineshape effects, 55–64, 307, 365–370

multi-site exchange, 63–64, 294–306

relaxation effects, 64–65, 306–307, 365

scalar coupling, 66

slow, see Slow exchange

Chemical shielding, see Chemical shifts

Chemical shift anisotropy, 62, 65, 340, 345

Chemical shift indices, 170

Chemical shifts

assignments, 43

factors which determine, 41–43

ranges for various nuclei, 40
ring–current effects, 42, 298,
    452
secondary structure correlations,
    137, 170
Chemotherapy, 3–4
Chloramphenicol, 118
Chloramphenicol acetyltransferase,
    263
Chorismate, 251, 252
Chromomycin, 379, 380
Cimetidine, 7
*Cis* peptide bonds, 223, 265–269
*Cis-trans* isomerases, 93
*Cis-trans* isomerization, 73, 224,
    229, 380
Clinical observations, 4
Cloning, see Recombinant proteins
CNS drugs, 205
Coalescence rate, 57
Coherence, 46
Combinatorial chemistry, 10
Computer-based drug design, 8, 26,
    253–254, 291–294
Computer graphics, 26, 28, 292
Conformation
    of bound ligands, see Bound
        conformations of ligands
    of drugs in solution, 202–209,
        246
Conformational isomerization, 224,
    230
Conformational parameters, 202,
    221, 224–228
Convulsant activity, 205
Cooperative binding, 277
Correlation time
    definition, 50, 125, 341
    internal motion, 341–344
    linewidth effects, 62
    molecular weight relationship,
        50
    nulling of NOE cross-peaks, 80,
        85
    relaxation equations, 50–51, 54,
        80
    temperature effects, 62

COSY (correlated spectroscopy), 91,
    122, 266, 269, 283; see also
    DQFCOSY
Coupling constants
    decoupling, 44
    in DNA complexes, 395
    E.COSY, 168
    HMQC-*J* experiment, 166–167
    *J*-modulated HMQC, 165–166
    magnitude of, 44
    P.E.COSY. 168
    in peptides, 221
    use in structure determination, 41,
        132–133, 165, 279
CPMG pulse sequence, 347
Cr(III)ATP, 256
Crystal-packing forces, 445
Cyclophilin, 27, 94, 231, 264–269
Cyclosporin A, 27, 231–232, 235,
    246, 264–269


D

DAPI, 424
ddC, 338
ddI, 338
Debye-Stokes-Einstein equation,
    49–50, 126
Decoupling, 44, 66, 168
Deoxyribose conformation, see DNA
Deuteration, 113–115, 190,
    283–284, 317, 326–328
DG, see Distance geometry
DG-II, 171
DGEOM, 171
DHFR (Dihydrofolate reductase),
    75, 250, 261, 276–308
    assignment of resonances
        enzyme, 281–285
        ligands, 285–288
    fluorinated ligands, 75, 261
    inhibitor design, 291–294
    ionization states, 288–291
    ligand binding, 261,
        inhibitors, 288–294
        substrates, 301–306
    mechanism of action, 276–281

multiple binding modes,
    294–306
resistance to antibacterials, 250
1,3-Diacetyl-chloroamphenicol,
    263
DIANA, 174, 176
Diastereotopic assignments, 220
Dielectric relaxation, 50
3′,5′-Difluoromethotrexate, 76,
    307
Digitalis, 2
Dihedral angles, 38, 44, 95, 165;
    see also Coupling constants
7,8-Dihydrofolate, 276, 278, 279
Dihydrofolate reductase, see DHFR
Diltiazem, 207
Dipole-dipole interactions, 33
Disaccharide-antibody complex,
    249
Disaccharides, 249, 251
DISGEO, 171
DISMAN, 174, 176
Dissociation rates, 66–77
Distamycin, 379, 380, 443–444
Distance geometry
    metric-matrix DG algorithms,
        171–174
    in peptide calculations, 221
    torsion-space DG algorithms,
        174–176
Distances between protons, see
    Interproton distances
Dithiothreitol, 118
DMP323, 339, 349–373
DNA
    arugomycin complex, see
        Arugomycin
    calicheamicin complex, 94
    deoxyribose conformation,
        394–395,
    ligand-induced conformational
        changes, 389–392
    luzopeptin complex, see
        Luzopeptin
    major groove, 379
    minor groove binders, see Minor
        groove binding

QN complex, see
    QN-oligonucleotide complex
target for drug action, 378–381,
    419–420
Dopamine receptors, 203
Dopaminergic compounds, 205
DQFCOSY (double quantum
    filtered COSY), 122–128
    of calmidazolium, 325
    in DHFR complexes, 283–284
    in oligonucleotide complexes with
        Hoechst 33258, 433
    of nogalamycin complex,
        382–383
    pulse sequence, 123
Drug abuse, 205
Drug discovery, 2–13, 15, 34–37,
    103, 216, 269–270
Drug metabolism, 17, 19
DSPACE, 171
d4T, 338
Dyes, 3
Dynamic light scattering, see
    Molecular weight estimation
Dynamic lineshape analysis, 75–76
Dynamic processes, 40, 96, 103,
    277, 306–308


E

Echinomycin, 404
Ecochemical drug discovery, 10
E.COSY, 168
EDTA, 118
Elastase, 250
Entropy, 235, 354, 372
Enzymatic catalysis, 259
Enzymatic degradation, 235
Enzyme inhibitors, 33
Ergot alkaloids, 206
Escherichia coli, 95, 252, 306
E-selectin, 251
ESR (electron spin resonance),
    50
Ethnobotany, 2–3
Exchange spectroscopy, 71–75
Experamicins, 92

Expression systems, see Recombinant
    proteins

F

Fast exchange, 56, 229, 445–446,
    448–449
Field inhomogeneity, 47
FK-506, 27, 231–232, 267–269
FK-506-binding protein, 94–95,
    231, 267–269
Flexibility of structures, 40
Fluorescence, 50
Fluorine-19 NMR, 75–76, 89, 90,
    249, 261–262, 283, 287
Folate, 276, 278, 280, 301–306
Food and Drug Administration, 338
Force-fields for solvents, 221
Formaldehyde, 27
Four-dimensional NMR, 137–139
    heteronuclear-edited experiments,
        138
    HMQC-NOESY-HSQC, 137
    triple resonance experiments,
        140–148; see also
        Three-dimensional NMR

G

β-Galactosidase, 38
Gastrointestinal infections, 6
Glutamic acid analogues, 203
Glycosylation, 107
G proteins, 255
Gradient methods, see PFG

H

Half filters, 263, 266
Hansch relationships, 6
H2-antagonists, 7
HCCH experiments, 138–139
HCP, see Heteronuclear cross
    polarisation
HEHOHEHAHA, 158
Herpes simplex virus, 252
HETCOR, 396–397

Heteronuclear cross polarisation,
    157–158
Heteronuclear editing, 135–139,
    229
Heteronuclear multiple quantum
    coherence spectroscopy, see
    HMQC
HETLOC, 227
Hinge peptide of Gl
    immunoglobulin, 223
Hirudin, 253, 255
Histamine, 7
Histaminergic compounds, 205,
    206
History of NMR, 16
HIV (Human immunodeficiency
    virus), 338
HIV protease, 338, 348–350
    amide exchange, 359–361,
        365–370
    backbone flexibility, 351–373
    bound water molecules, 270, 349
    chemical shifts, 351–353
    dynamic symmetry, 351
    hydrogen bonding, 365–370
    inhibitors, 262, 349, 351–361
    relaxation parameters, 354–358
    target in drug design, 37, 103,
        349–350
    β-turns, 366–367
    X-ray studies, 351
HMQC, 133, 257
HMBC, 222, 227
HMQC-COSY, 222
HMQC-NOESY, 224–225, 264,
    286, 303
HMQC-TOCSY, 222–223
HOE140, 233–234
Hoechst 33258-DNA complexes
    binding site, 435–437
    comparison of NMR and X-ray
        structures, 440–447
    dynamic processes, 439–440
    hydrogen bonding, 437–439
    resonance assignments, 430–435
    selectivity, 380
    stoichiometry and kinetics, 428–430

HOHAHA, see TOCSY
Hoogsteen base pairing, 404–407
Hormones, 250
HSA (human serum albumin), 90,
    91
HSQC, 133–135, 351–352
HSQC-NOESY, 269
HSQC-TOCSY, 269
Human immunodeficiency virus,
    see HIV
Human serum albumin, see HSA
4-Hydroxy-2,2,6,6-
    tetramethylpiperidinyl-oxy,
    53
Hypertension, 34
Hypotensive drugs, 5
HyTEMPO, 266, 269


I

Imino protons, 432
Imipramine, 205
Immunosuppressant-immunophilin
    complexes, 93–95, 264–269
Immunosuppressive drugs, 27,
    264–269
Induced-fit, 379, 380
INEPT, 133
Influenza, 8, 37, 103
Integrin inhibitors, 237
Intercalation, 379–380
Interleukins, 35
Interproton distances
    calibration of, 161–164
    in peptides, 220
Inversion transfer, 70
Ion-dipole interactions, 33
Ionisation states, 286, 288–291
Ischaemia, 23–24
Isolated spin pair approximation,
    see ISPA
Isotope filters, 262–269, 365
Isotope labelling, 38, 132
    costs, 113
    fractional deuteration, 113–115;
        see also Deuteration
    selective, 115, 259–261

uniform ($^{13}C/^{15}N$), 112–113
ISPA (Isolated spin pair
    approximation), 163, 208


J

$J$ coupling, see Coupling constants
Jun transcription factors
    c-Jun, 106
    sJunLZ, 128


K

Karplus equation, 165–167, 227,
    228
Kedarcidins, 92


L

Labelling, see Isotope labelling
Lactate dehydrogenase, 250
Lactobacillus casei, 278
Langendorff perfusion, 22
Lectin, 250
Leucine zipper domain, 111
Leukotrienes, 207
Linear prediction, 160
Lineshape analysis, 75–76
Linewidths, 55–64, 114,
    450–451
Lipari and Szabo analysis, 230,
    307, 342, 345, 354
Lovastatin, 10
Luzopeptin, 414–418


M

Major histocompatability complex,
    see MHC
Maximum entropy method (MEM),
    159–160
MCD (main-chain directed)
    assignment method, 130
Medicinal chemistry, 28, 246
Membrane mimics, 218, 233
Membrane proteins, 35
Methotrexate, 75, 261, 276

*N*-Methyl-D-aspartate, 203
MHC (Major histocompatability complex), 264
Micelles, 218, 221, 233
Microbial contamination, 118
Mimetics, see Peptides
Minor groove binding,
  calicheamicin, 93
  CC-1065, 443
  characteristics, 424–427
  distamycin, 443–444
  Hoechst 33258, see Hoechst 33258
  netropsin, 443–444
  QN, see QN-oligonucleotide complexes
  SN-6999, 445–446
  structures, 426
  terephthalamides, see Terephthalamide-oligonucleotide complexes
Minoxodil, 34
MLCK (Myosin light chain kinase), 316
Molecular dynamics, 221; see also RMD
Molecular mechanics, 203
Molecular modelling, 37, 292; see also Computer-based drug design; Computer graphics
Molecular optimisation, 5
Molecular pharmacology, 6
Molecular weight estimation
  correlation time, 50
  dynamic light scattering, 117
  PFGSE (pulsed-field-gradient spin echo), 117
  sedimentation equilibrium, 116–117
Monointercalators, 339
Morphine, 205–206
Multidimensional NMR, 122; see also Two-, Three-, and Four-dimensional experiments
Muscarine, 203

Muscarinic agonists/antagonists, 203
Myosin light chain kinase, see MLCK

**N**

NADP, 276–281, 290
NADPH, 276–281, 285, 290
Natural products, 11
Neocarzinostatins, 92
Netropsin, 380, 443–444
Neuraminidase, 103; see also Sialidase
Neuroactive drugs, 203–206
Neuroleptic agents, 203
Neurophysin, 251
Neutron diffraction, 37
Nicotine, 203
Nicotinic agonists/antagonists, 203
3-Nitro-4-fluoropyrimethamine, 297–301
Nitrogen-15
  labelling, 95, 261, 285–286
  chemical shifts, 290
Nitroxide radicals, 53
NMR assignments, see Assignments
NMR spectrometers
  overview, 18–20
  probes, 19–20
  sensitivity, 19
NMR timescale, 58, 229–230, 247, 306–308, 448
NOE (Nuclear Overhauser Enhancement), 77–80
  buildup, 82, 250
  definition, 48
  distance dependence, 162–164
  distances in peptides, 219
  heteronuclear, 344–347
  motion dependence, 345–346
  rotating-frame, 85
  steady-state, 81
  transferred, see Transferred NOE
  transient, 83

two-dimensional, 83–85; see also
    NOESY
NOESY (nuclear Overhauser
    enhancement spectroscopy),
    122–123, 257
  in calmodulin complexes, 326–328
  in DHFR complexes, 299
  in oligonucleotide complexes,
    432–434
  peptide assignments, 224
  pulse sequence, 123
Nogalamycin, 381
  binding to d(GACGTC)$_2$,
    389–399
  DQFCOSY spectra, 382–384
  HOHAHA spectra, 384–385
  hydrogen bonding, 392
  NOESY spectra, 384–387
  $^{31}$P NMR studies, 395–399
  resonance assignments in
    oligonucleotide complexes,
    382–389
  sequence specificity, 393–394
Nonlinear sampling, 159
NSC-57153, 453
Nuclear Overhauser Enhancement,
    see NOE
Nucleotide binding, 250


O

Oligosaccharides, 251
Opiate agonists, 205
Opiate receptor, 206
Order parameter, 341, 354–358
Oxazines, 27
Oxytocin, 72, 251


P

P9941, 339, 350–373
Paramagnetic species, 52, 118, 247,
    255–257, 266
PCR (polymerase chain reaction),
    105
PDB (Protein Data Bank), 35, 103,
    189, 331

P.E.COSY, 168, 227
Penicillin, 34
Pepsin, 231, 261, 263
Pepstatin analogues, 261
Peptides, 12, 26
  aggregation, 219
  bioavailability, 12, 238
  backbone conformations, 219
  complexes with receptors, 231
  cyclic, 219, 221, 235–237
  libraries, 10, 216, 238
  metal complexes, 233–235
  mimetics, 216
  receptor-bound conformation,
    231
  retro-inverso analogues, 237
  structural studies
    conformational parameters,
      222–227
    limitations, 216–218
    solvent effects, 228
    strategies for, 221–222
    surface-to-core ratio, 219
Peptidomimetics, 12, 216, 237
Peptoids, 216
Perfused heart, 23
PFG, (Pulsed field gradients),
    153–157
PFGSE (Pulsed field gradient spin
    echo), see Molecular weight
    estimation
pH
  amide exchange effects, 118–119
  intracellular, 22
  NMR titrations, 289
  sample preparation, 39, 118–119
Phage libraries, 216
Pharmacokinetics, 262, 317
Phosphatidylcholine, 252
Phosphatidylethanolamine, 252
Phosphocreatine, 22–24
3-Phosphoglycerate, 256
Phosphoglycero kinase, 256
Phospholipase A$_2$ inhibitors, 252,
    254, 257, 260
Phosphorus-31 NMR, 286, 290,
    295, 395–399

Piperazine ring, 440
pKa, 6, 288–291
Platelet aggregation, 5, 91
Polymerase chain reaction, see PCR
Post-translational modifications,
    107
Prephenate, 252
PROCHECK, 189
Proline-containing peptides, 229
Prontosil, 4, 5
Propeller twisting in DNA, 442
Prostoglandins, 207
Protein Data Bank, see PDB
Protein dynamics, 103
    function, effects on, 370–373
    relaxation analysis, see Relaxation
    theoretical description,
        340–344
Protein-protein interactions, 250
Protein structure determination by
    NMR, 103
    amount of sample required, 104
    data acquisition, see Assignments
    sample preparation, 116–121
        aggregation, 116–117, 118,
            119
        microbial contaminants, 118
        paramagnetic contaminants,
            118
        pH, see pH
        temperature, 120–121
    size limitations, 26
    structural constraints, see
        Structural constraints
    structure calculations,
        see Structure calculations
Pulsed field gradients, see PFG
Pulsed field gradient spin echo
    methods, see PFGSE
Pyrimethamine, 261, 276,
    296–301

**Q**

QN-oligonucleotide complex, 407
    base pairing, 407–408
    helix unwinding, 413

minor groove interactions,
    408–413
Quantitative-structure-activity-
    relationships, see QSAR
Quaternary carbons, 222
Quinine, 3
Quinomycin antibiotics, 404–407
QSAR, 6; see also Structure-activity
    relationships

**R**

Radial distribution functions, 228
Ramachandran plots, 219
Random screening in drug discovery,
    8–10, 34
Ranitidine, 7
Rapamycin, 231–232
Rational drug design, 2, 20–21,
    35–37, 103, 216–217,
    291–294
*Rauwolfia serpentina*, 3
Receptors, see also Binding sites
    charge distribution, 33
    location, 32
Recombinant proteins, 104–105
    cloning vectors, 109–112
    DNA for cloning, 105–106
    expression systems
        *Bacillus subtilis*, 106, 107, 109
        baculovirus, 108, 109
        yeast (*Saccharomyces cerevisiae*),
            107, 109
    isotope labelling, see Isotope
        labelling
Relaxation
    chemical exchange effects, 347
    chemical shift anisotropy, 54
    dipole-dipole, 49
    distance dependence, 51–52
    in drug DNA complexes, 398–399
    molecular dynamics applications,
        339–344
    parameters, 344–347
    rates, 41
    spin-lattice, see Spin-lattice
        relaxation

transverse, see Transverse
  relaxation
Reperfusion injury, 316
Replication termination protein,
  133–134
Resonance assignments, see
  Assignments
Restrained molecular dynamics, see
  RMD
Reverse transcriptase, 338
R factor, 187–189
Ribonucleotide reductase, 252
Ricin B-chain, 249, 251
RGD sequence, 236–237
Rhodopsin, 255
Ring current effects, see Chemical
  shifts
Ring flipping, 297, 307, 440
RMD (Restrained molecular
  dynamics), 176–179
RMSD (root mean square deviation),
  187; see also Structure
  calculations
ROE, 48
  advantages, 85, 229
  buildup rates, 207–208
  2-dimensional, see ROESY
ROESY (rotating Overhauser
  enhancement spectroscopy),
  85, 224–227, 229, 253
Rogaine, see Minoxodil
Rotating frame experiments, see
  ROE, ROESY
Rotational correlation time, see
  Correlation time
Rotamer populations, 203


S

Saturation transfer, 67–69, 286,
  304
Scalar coupling, see Coupling
  constants
Screening, 2, 8, 262
SCUBA, 127
SDS, 233
Secondary metabolites, 10

Sedimentation equilibrium analysis,
  see Molecular weight
  estimation
Segmental motions, 306
Selective labelling, see Isotope
  labelling
Selective toxicity, 3–4
Septicaemia, 4
Sequential assignments
  in peptides and proteins, 125,
  129
  in nucleic acids, 433
Serendipity in drug discovery, 34
Sialidase, 8, 37; see also
  Neuraminidase
Side effects, 35
Site-directed mutagenesis, 279,
  361
Sleeping sickness, 318
Slow exchange, 56, 58
  calmodulin-calmidazolium
  complexes, 319
  conformers of butaclamol, 204
  limit for free and complexed
  molecules, 247
  in peptides, 229
Snake venom, 10
Soil microorganisms, 10
Solid-phase peptide synthesis, 104
Solid-state NMR, 269
Solomon equations, 79–80
Somatostatin, 236
Spectral assignments, see
  Assignments
Spectral density function, 342–345
Spectrometers, see NMR
  spectrometers
Spin coupling, see Coupling
  constants
Spin diffusion, 225, 228, 249
Spin echo experiments, 76–77
Spin labels, 52
Spin-lattice relaxation
  definition, 45–46
  equation for, 50
  in HIV protease, 356–358
  rotating frame, 77

Spin-spin coupling, see Coupling constants
Spin system identification, 127–129
Staphylococcal nuclease, 256, 258
STEREOSEARCH, 169
Stereospecific assignment, 169, 283
Stoichiometry of complexes, 39, 447–448, 453, 461–462
Stokes-Einstein equation, 117; see also Debye-Stokes-Einstein equation
Streptococcal infections, 33
Structural constraints
 amide protein exchange, 169–170
 chemical shifts, 170
 coupling constants, 165–169; see also Coupling constants
 NOEs, 161–164
Structural water, 358
Structure-activity relationships, 238, 246; see also QSAR
Structure calculations, 170–189
 direct refinement, 182–185
 distance geometry, 171–176, 228
 dynamical simulated annealing, 179–180
 energy minimisation, 176–179
 optimal filtering, 185–186
 precision, 164
 quality of calculated structures, 187–189
 restrained molecular dynamics, 176–179, 228
 solvent inclusion, 228
 time-averaged constraints, 180–182, 228, 230
Substrates, 250
Sugars, 250
Sulfanilamide, 4
Sulfonamide drugs, 6
Sulfonamide group, 5
Sulindac, 89, 90
Sulindac sulfide, 89
Surface coils, 19
Surface patch analogues, 12

**T**

$T_1$, see Spin-lattice relaxation
$T_2$, see Transverse relaxation
Target function, 174, 176
Tautomeric states, 304
Taxol, 207–208
Temperature
 dependence of NH protons, 227
 optimum for peptide studies, 221
Terephthalamide-oligonucleotide complexes, 446–447
 binding site, 453–454
 drug design applications 454–457, 458–462
 minor groove binding, 451–453
 titration experiments, 447–451
Tetrahedral intermediates, 259
5,6,7,8-Tetrahydrofolate, 4, 276–279
TFE, 221
Thioamides, 237
Three-dimensional NMR, 130–132
 HCCH-COSY, 138, 281
 HCCH-TOCSY, 138, 281–282
 HMQC-NOESY, 266
 HMQC-NOESY-HMQC, 281
 HNCA, 281
 HOHAHA-NOESY, 132
 NOESY-HMQC, 135–137, 257, 281, 329–330
 NOESY-HOHAHA, 130
 NOESY-HSQC, 135–137
 NOESY-NOESY, 132
 ROESY-HMQC, 280
 TOCSY-HMQC, 136, 281, 329
 TOCSY-HSQC, 135–136
Thrombin, 92, 103, 249, 253, 255
Thymidine, 3′,5′-diphosphate, 257
Thymidylate synthase, 103
Time-dependent restraints, 230
Time-shared chemical-shift evolution, 159
TOCSY (total correlation spectroscopy), 125
 in DHFR complexes, 281–282

in peptides, 222–224
in oligonucleotide complexes,
    385–386, 433
pulse sequence, 123
spin system identification,
    127–128
TOCSY-REVINEPT, 266
Tolbutamide, 5
Total correlation spectroscopy, see
    TOCSY
Toxicity, 35
Toxicology, 317
Traditional medicine, 2
Transducin, 255
Transferred NOE, 86–88, 231–232,
    248–255, 257
Transverse relaxation
    chemical exchange contribution,
        450
    definition, 46–47
    equation for, 51
    in HIV protease, 356–358
    structure determination, limiting
        effects in, 190
    linewidth effects, 47, 113, 231
    in multi-step pulse sequences, 137
Tricyclic antidepressants, 205
Trifluoroethanol, see TFE
Trimethoprim, 250, 261, 276, 286,
    295
Triple resonance experiments, 135,
    140–148
    CBCA(CO)NH, 145, 150
    CBCANH, 145, 148
    HBHA(CBCACO)NH, 146
    HCACO, 146, 152
    HCA(CO)N, 146
    H(CCO)NH-TOCSY, 146, 151
    H(C)NH-TOCSY, 146, 151
    HNCA, 141, 149, 152
    HNCACB, 145,
    HN(CA)CO, 140, 152
    HN(CA)HA, 141–145, 150
    HNCO, 140, 149, 150, 152
    HN(CO)CA, 141–145, 149
    HN(CO)CAHA, 141, 145, 149
    HN(COCA)HA, 145
    pulse sequences, 142–143

Tritium NMR, 285
*Trypanosoma bruceirhodesiense*, 318
Trypanosomes, 318
Trypsin-BPTI complex, 253
β-Turns in peptides, 224, 226, 236
γ-Turns in peptides, 236–237
Two-dimensional NMR, see also
        DQFCOSY, NOESY, TOCSY
    exchange spectroscopy, 71–74
    HMBC, 222
    HMQC, 133
    HMQC-COSY, 222
    HMQC-NOESY, 224–225
    HMQC-TOCSY, 222–223
    NOESY-HMQC, 136–137
    processing, 124
    pulse sequences, 123;
    TOCSY-HMQC, 136–137
Typhoid fever, 5
Tyrosine hydroxylase, 256

U

Ubiquitin, 144
Urinary tract infections, 6

V

Valium, 70–71
van der Waals interactions, 33, 424,
    427, 441, 443
Verapamil, 207
Vesicles, 218
Viscosity, 50, 62, 126

W

Water molecules in protein
        structures, 280, 358
Water suppression
    gradient methods, 156
    pre-saturation, 127
Watson-Crick base pairing, 405–407

X

X-ray crystallography, 25, 28, 35, 39,
    103, 217–218, 257, 270, 277